Pediatric Dentistry

Antonella Polimeni

Full Professor of Odontostomatological Diseases,
Department of Oral and Maxillo-facial Sciences, Sapienza Università di Roma
Director of Pediatric Dentistry Specialty School, Sapienza Università di Roma
Director of Pediatric Dentistry Unit,
Azienda Ospedaliero Universitaria Policlinico Umberto I, Roma

Pediatric Dentistry

SECOND EDITION

edra

Original title
Antonella Polimeni – Odontoiatria pediatrica seconda edizione
©2019 EDRA s.p.A. – All rights reserved
ISBN: 978-88-214-5036-5

Book Publishing Manager: Costanza Smeraldi
Paper, Printing and Binding Manager: Michele Ribatti

Translation and editing: Enago
Cover: Paolo Ballerini

ISBN: 978-88-214-5153-9
eISBN: 978-88-214-5154-6

Edra S.p.A.
Via G. Spadolini 7, 20141 Milano (Italy)
Tel. 02 881841
www.edizioniedra.it

Printed in Italy by "Printer Trento" S.r.l., June 2020

(*) Edra S.p.A. is part of LSWR GROUP

Autors

Susanna Annibali
Former Associate Professor
Sapienza University of Rome

Tiziano Baccetti†
Researcher
University of Florence

Ersilia Barbato
Full Professor
Sapienza University of Rome

Elena Bardellini
Associate Professor
University of Brescia

Maurizio Bossù
Associate Professor
Sapienza University of Rome

Lorenzo Breschi
Full Professor
University of Bologna

Mauro Celli
Hospital Medical Director
University Hospital
Policlinico Umberto I, Rome

Claudio Chimenti
Full Professor
University of L'Aquila

Massimo Cordaro
Full Professor
Catholic University of the Sacred Heart, Milan

Denise Corridore
Orthodontic specialist
Sapienza University of Rome

Paola Cozza
Full Professor
Tor Vergata University of Rome

Natale D'Alessandro
Former Full Professor
University of Palermo

Ferdinando D'Ambrosio
Full Professor
Sapienza University of Rome

Efisio Defraia
Associate Professor
University of Florence

Elettra De Stefano Dorigo
Former Full Professor
University of Trieste

Gianni Di Giorgio
Ph.D. Researcher
Sapienza University of Rome

Carlo Di Paolo
Associate Professor
Sapienza University of Rome

Giampietro Farronato
Full Professor
University of Milan

Roberto Favaro
Former Associate Professor
Sapienza University of Rome

Marco Ferrari
Full Professor
University of Siena

Lorenzo Franchi
Associate Professor
University of Florence

Gabriella Galluccio
Associate Professor
Sapienza University of Rome

Giovanna Giuliana
Full Professor
University of Palermo

Gaetano Ierardo
Researcher
Sapienza University of Rome

Roly Kornblit
Private Practitioner, Rome

Giuseppina Laganà
Orthodontic Specialist
Tor Vergata University of Rome

Valeria Luzzi
Researcher
Sapienza University of Rome

Alessandra Majorana
Full Professor
University of Brescia

Ambrosina Michelotti
Full Professor
University Federico II, Naples

Livia Ottolenghi
Full Professor
Sapienza University of Rome

Gabriela Piana
Associate Professor
University of Bologna

Silvia Pizzi
Full Professor
University of Parma

Gianfranco Prada
Dentist
Vice-President, ANDI

Umberto Romeo
Associate Professor
Sapienza University of Rome

Gian Luca Sfasciotti
Associate Professor
Sapienza University of Rome

Enrico Spinas
Researcher
University of Cagliari

Andrea Spota
Researcher
Sapienza University of Rome

Laura Strohmenger
Former Full Professor
University of Milan

Claudio Voglino
Architect, Rome

The following people also contributed to the project

Francesco Antonucci
Rossano Botto
Elisabetta Cretella Lombardo
Alexandros Galanakis
Alberto Libero
Saveria Loberto
Luca Mazzucchelli
Gianpaolo Migliardi
Giuseppina Pieragostini
Paolo Tordiglione

Preface

This second edition is being published seven years after the first one at a time at which pediatric dentistry is consolidating its prestige as an autonomous clinical discipline in the academic field with the founding of a dedicated post-graduate school that finally connects the aforementioned specialized training with a focus on the *core* education in essential areas of dental practice.

As in the first edition, the intention here too has been to present a didactic text in which all the topics are comprehensively covered using language that is easy to understand and a rich graphic design that highlights the didactic and clinical experience of the authors.

The contents of the book are organized in the same way as in the first edition, although it has been updated with a revision of the chapter on endodontics and the introduction of some new chapters: one dedicated to the prevention and treatment of snoring and obstructive sleep apnea syndrome during the developmental age—which incorporates the national guidelines issued by the Italian Ministry of Health in 2016; one on the therapeutic procedures to be followed in patients affected by systemic pathologies and syndromes; one on myofunctional therapy; and one on pharmacological treatment.

The second edition continues to offer a sound base for studying the topics of pediatric dentistry, thereby proving to be a valid tool for consultation and for diagnostic and therapeutic guidance. I am sure that it will still be a valid resource for training and refresher courses, not just for graduates and postgraduates but also for all specialists dealing with dental pathologies affecting patients in the developmental age.

Antonella Polimeni

Table of contents

Chapter 1

Communication and approach in pediatric dentistry

V. Luzzi, A. Polimeni

Let us consider the following quote: "*we increase shared knowledge, in other words, common sense, the fundamental precondition for the existence of any community*" (Rosengren, 2001); the fluid communication with other individuals and with work settings activates cognitive and emotional aspects that may turn a profession into a place of growth, creativity, and gratification.
By analyzing both the environmental and specific conditions of a therapy, it is evident that relational aspects comprise a large part of the time and commitment of the participants involved. Furthermore, the level of work-related discomfort and fatigue are often caused by the difficulties and burdens associated with the management of relational issues, which may work either as an ally or, in contrast, as a reason for the discontinuation of therapy.
In this context, for simplicity, communication will be first considered from the perspective of its pragmatic aspects within the health procedures and second as a by-product of more complex emotional processes.
Communication is defined as three interrelated processes essentially based on "making it common," "being in touch," and "conveying." Therefore, communication is an articulated process by which information is transmitted from one system to another using special signals. It is achieved through real information flow as follows:

- Motivation or will, which gives added value to communication
- Knowledge, intended as the capacity to receive and interpret information
- Ability to formulate messages
- Competence, intended as the ability to behave in an appropriate manner so as to benefit health.

Goals of communication

The communication goals of pediatric dentistry coincide with those of generic dentistry and are based on five essential points that define the dentist–patient relationship.
In communication, the dentist should clearly understand the patients' *expectations and requests* using "active listening" techniques and by empathizing with them, thereby showing a great capacity of understanding and decoding their moods.
Communication occurs via verbal messages that express the "what" and nonverbal and paraverbal messages that express the "how." Nonverbal messages are susceptible of a lower level of conscious control and involve most of the communication. When

it comes to talking to children, verbal communication involves the use of simple language, which is clear and appropriate for their age: communicating with technical terms should be avoided, and technical terms should always be explained to children. The amount of information shared must therefore be adequate for the attention and processing abilities of the children, which are often reduced in the dental setting because of anxiety and physical discomfort. In fact, it is necessary to consider those factors that affect the feedback of the child's verbal communication. Among these are the quality of information, anxiety control, and, last but not least, the surrounding settings, which includes the visual, acoustic, smell, taste, and tactile perception. The next step is to provide *information* to obtain the parent's consent for performing therapeutic procedures. This is followed by the so-called "*behavioral management*," which defines the important distinction between adult and child. While for adults the approach is based on the *problem-solving* principle, which requires proposing and discussing several therapeutic possibilities with the patient, for children, there are several behavioral management strategies that will be described below.

Another communication goal is persuasion, something that requires the collaboration of the child by using specific methods since the first check-up, which will be described below as deviation, curiosity, and introduction targeted to treatment.

The communication cycle ends with the last phase, which is represented by the *gain of the patient's trust*, in other words, the establishment of a trustworthy relationship between the patient and dentist.

Communication interface

The uniqueness of communication in pediatric dentistry is the existence of three entities that communicate with each other: the *child*, *parent*, and *pediatric dentist*. Among these entities, the child undoubtedly plays the role of the main character. The dialog between the pediatric dentist and the child should, in any case, take into consideration the parents and their influence on the child's dental attitude. As a guideline, in the authors' clinical practice, it is possible to identify several types of parents that generally correspond to specific behavioral profiles of children. If parents appear reasonable, calm, available, and collaborative toward the proposed therapies, the child will be collaborative and serene; on the contrary, if parents appear anxious, uncertain, and doubtful about the practitioner's skills and the therapeutic procedures, the child will be anxious and will show little inclination to cooperate. In situations in which the parents feel guilty, i.e. when they feel responsible for the dental pathology affecting the child, such as in the clinical cases of early childhood caries, the child will cooperate only to solve situations that need urgent intervention, for instance, the presence of painful symptomatology. With a proud, aggressive, and uncooperative parent, the child will be fearful and uncooperative.

Regardless of the several types of parents identified in the clinical practice, it is always indispensable to have a preliminary interview with the adult in charge in order to solve

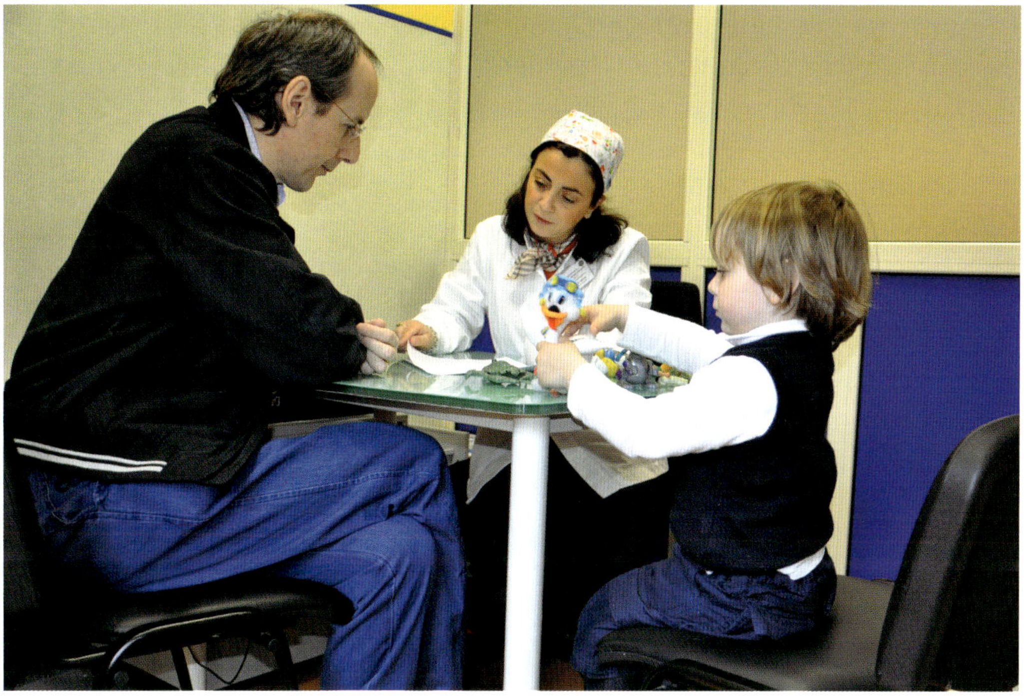

Figure 1.1 Preliminary interview with the pediatric dentist: the parent is informed about the therapeutic approach.

possible doubts and resistances to the treatment (Fig. 1.1). Only then is it possible to reassure the parents about the appropriateness of the therapeutic approach used, with the further advantage of making them an important ally to guide the child toward exhibiting a suitable behavior.

Dental fear and anxiety

Psychological aspects

Slight fear and anxiety represent an expected and significant experience in normal child psychological development. These become a serious concern and potentially require a specific treatment when are disproportionate compared with the real problem and when they hinder the implementation of normal activities. One of the most commonly accepted statements about anxiety is that it represents a multidimensional construct that comprises somatic, cognitive, and emotional elements (Kendall, 2006). *Dental fear* or *anxiety* (DFA) is a normal emotional reaction to one or more specific stimuli perceived as threatening in the dental setting. It represents a state of apprehension originating from the fear that something catastrophic is about to take place with regard to the dental treatment, and it is associated with a sense of loss of control.

Dental phobia (DP) is the most serious type of dental anxiety and is characterized by a marked and persistent anxiety in association to either clearly identifiable objects such as a turbine or a syringe needle or the dental setting in general.
In accordance with the Diagnostic and Statistical Manual of Mental Disorders (DSM-5; 2013) published by the American Psychiatric Association, the diagnostic criteria for DP are as follows:

- Marked, persistent, and excessive fear of unreasonable nature
- Exposure to phobic stimuli that almost invariably provoke an immediate anxious response
- The patient's realization that the excessive and unreasonable fear is not a requirement
- Phobic situation avoided or, alternatively, supported with intense anxiety.

In the presence of a diagnosis of DP, dental fear and anxiety can lead to complete avoidance of necessary dental treatment or endurance of the treatment with fear.
In the dental literature, the words dental fear, dental anxiety, and DP are commonly used interchangeably. In general, whether the diagnosis criteria for DP are satisfied or not, the words dental fear and dental anxiety are used when referring to strong negative feelings associated with dental treatment in children and adolescents.
Dental fear and anxiety are frequently associated with the child's difficulties in cooperating with dental treatment. Such cases refer to the behavioral management problems of the child, known as dental behavior management problems (DBMPs).
In 1982, Winer published a review regarding the anxious behavior of children in the dental setting in *Child Development*. The author reviewed the measurement of dental anxiety and uncooperative child behaviors, as well as their incidence and association with age. As revealed in the review, cooperative behavior increases with age, notably between 3 and 6 years of age. Winer suggested that anxiety in the dental setting represents a more general and basic type of anxiety and that certain personality aspects of a child emerge, such as impulse control and cognitive function organization, which can lead to a reduction of fear in the most advanced preschool age (5–6 years). This review showed the results of several correlations between dental and nondental anxieties, which support the hypothesis that dental anxiety is not highly specific but might be correlated with general anxiety.

DFA and DBMP measurement techniques

The measurement of DFA is performed through anxiety self-evaluation by children (if they belong to the teenage group) or by parents (if children are aged less than 13 years). The most psychometric self-evaluation scale used is the Children's Fear Survey Schedule-Dental Subscale (CFSS-DS) (Scherer and Nakamura, 1968). This scale has optimal psychometric properties: it measures dental fear more precisely, covers several aspects of dentistry, has a high test-retest reliability, and shows good correlations with other behavioral factors. The CFSS-DS scale evaluates children's fear reactions on a

scale of 1 (not scared) to 5 (very scared) in relation to 15 individuals or circumstances linked to the medical–dental setting.
DBMPs are directly defined by observation by the pediatric dentist during the treatment using the so-called *behavioral assessment*, for which there are numerous scales: the most commonly used is Frankl's behavior rating scale (Frankl et al, 1962).

Prevalence and relationship between DFA and DBPM

Klingberg et al (2007) summarized several studies in the review and reported that Western countries have a prevalence of DFA and DBMP of 9%–21%. Both DFA and DBMP are more frequently observed in girls and are correlated to general fear and behavioral problems, even though these correlations have not been completely understood yet. It is important to note that DFA and DBMP do not always show an association: a substantial percentage of uncooperative children show no signs of dental fear; on the other hand, the presence of dental fear does not automatically imply noncooperation from the child (Klingberg et al, 1995).

Factors that determine behavior

It has been previously observed that parents' behavior toward pediatric dentists can influence children's reactions and their behavior during the treatment (Milgrom et al, 1995).
Over the years, researchers have focused their attention on the systematic identification of the factors that influence this behavior or that allow its prediction (Kyritsi et al, 2009; Holst et al, 1993).
These studies show that the previous dental experiences of children have a strong influence on their behavior: children that have shown dental anxiety and fear during previous dental check-ups generally tend to be less cooperative. In contrast, when they have had previous positive dental experiences, they show a cooperative behavior.
Furthermore, it was noted that the evaluation of children's dental fear and their reactions to the therapy performed by the parents is realistic in most cases; therefore, the opinion of parents about children's cooperation is highly correlated to the behavior they exhibit during treatment.
In addition, it was observed that children acquire emotional reactions to the dental treatment from their parents and that they imitate their oral health behaviors: many fearful and less cooperative children have parents that are equally fearful.
Finally, it was found that in general, the reduction in DFA and DBMP with age reflects the normal psychological development of children.

Clinical management pathway

If children do not cooperate, professionals must ask themselves why and, in particular, what to do to lead children to the treatment in a targeted manner. This is because DBMPs are not an intrinsic quality of children but an expression of the dentist–child relationship. The presence of DBMPs is the main cause (37% of cases) of referral to pediatric dentistry specialists (Klingberg et al, 2006).

It is important that all dentists acknowledge that uncooperative children are not "difficult children." Instead, they have their own personalities and *special needs* that require advanced cognitive knowledge, therapies, and abilities from pediatric dentists. The knowledge of developmental age psychology is therefore a fundamental component to make dental sessions a positive experience for children.

Child–dentist relationship among various age groups

The "dentist–child" relationship should take into consideration age-related differences. From this perspective, it is possible to distinguish three age groups: 0–2 years, 3–5 years, and 6–12 years.

In the 0–2-years age group, it is impossible to establish a mutual dialog as the child's communication ability has not yet developed. The main interlocutors are the parents, and the interventions are limited to emergency procedures. When it is necessary to visit infants, who offer no adequate cooperation, their positioning on the armchair requires a procedure that involves the parent's cooperation: this is called the "*knee-to-knee*" position. The practitioner and the parent sit facing each other with their knees in contact; the baby, in the arms of the parents, is placed with the head on the practitioner's legs; the parent holds the baby's arms. Subsequently, the practitioner proceeds with the examination or with the therapeutic procedure (Fig. 1.2). In this case, communication is predominantly nonverbal and is essentially based on the variations in the baby's voice tone and the contact modalities with him/her. Furthermore, it is not based on a direct motivational approach with the baby but rather with the parent, who will be directed at prevention through oral hygiene and nutrition education, as well as avoidance of bad habits.

In the 3–5-years age group, children have not yet developed control capacities and are unable to manage emotions as well as manage themselves. Therefore, a firm behavioral guide is needed on the dentist's part in a situation in which the main interlocutors are both the parent and the child. To get positive behavioral *imprinting*, the pediatric dentist should adopt simple verbal communication using short sentences and replacement words. For example, it is preferable to indicate the anesthesia needle using the phrase "little tube from which chamomile drops come out" or to indicate the saliva ejector using the term "vacuum cleaner" or the turbine with "spinning top." In this age group, the professional figure of the *dental assistant* plays a very important

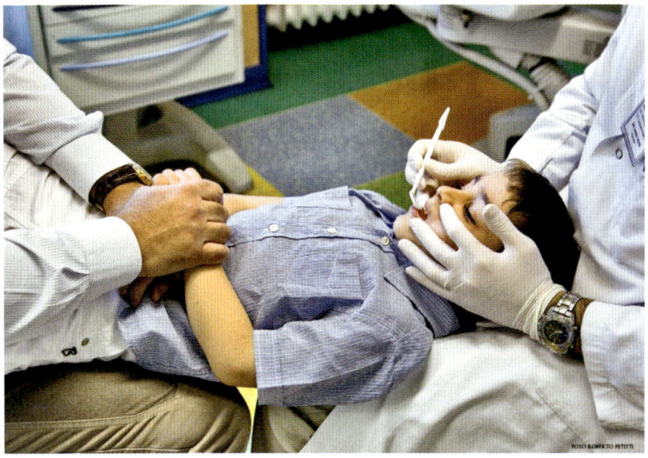

Figure 1.2 "*Knee-to-knee*" position. The practitioner and parent sit facing each other with their knees in contact; the child in the parent's arms is positioned with the head on the operator's legs and the arms held by the parent; in this position, the practitioner can proceed with the evaluation and therapeutic maneuvers.

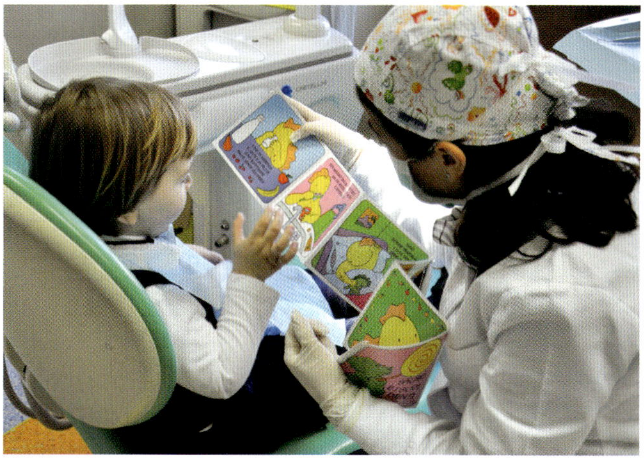

Figure 1.3 Motivational approach in a 3-year-old child. An educational booklet is shown, with figures that stimulate the simulation of correct behaviors of oral health.

role. This figure should adopt a behavior consistent with that of the pediatric dentist by favoring the cooperation with the child. Furthermore, using an adequate presentation of the *tray*, this figure should make sure to hide needles, syringes, and any other tool that may cause anxiety in children.

Additionally, a motivational approach can be directed at both the parent and child. While parents should always be given tools to obtain the appropriate dental health motivation and education for their children, it is possible to show figures to the children that stimulate the imitation of correct oral health-related behaviors (Fig. 1.3). For instance, in the educational booklet developed by a collaboration of the Chair of Pediatric Dentistry, the Chair of Preventive Dentistry, and the Department of Linguistics of the Sapienza University of Rome with the Municipality of Rome (Fig. 1.4), two characters, Dino and Sauro, who embody two opposing types of behavior toward oral and food hygiene in children, are pitted against each other.

In the 6–12-years age group, children develop their own personality and understand the reasons behind the treatment. Their thought process is linked to concrete situations, and abstraction capacity is limited. Therefore, for effective communication, the situations should be shown and simulated in a concrete manner using an adequate communication with precise and correct terms. In this age group, it is necessary to establish a direct relationship with the patient, and the main interlocutor is the child.

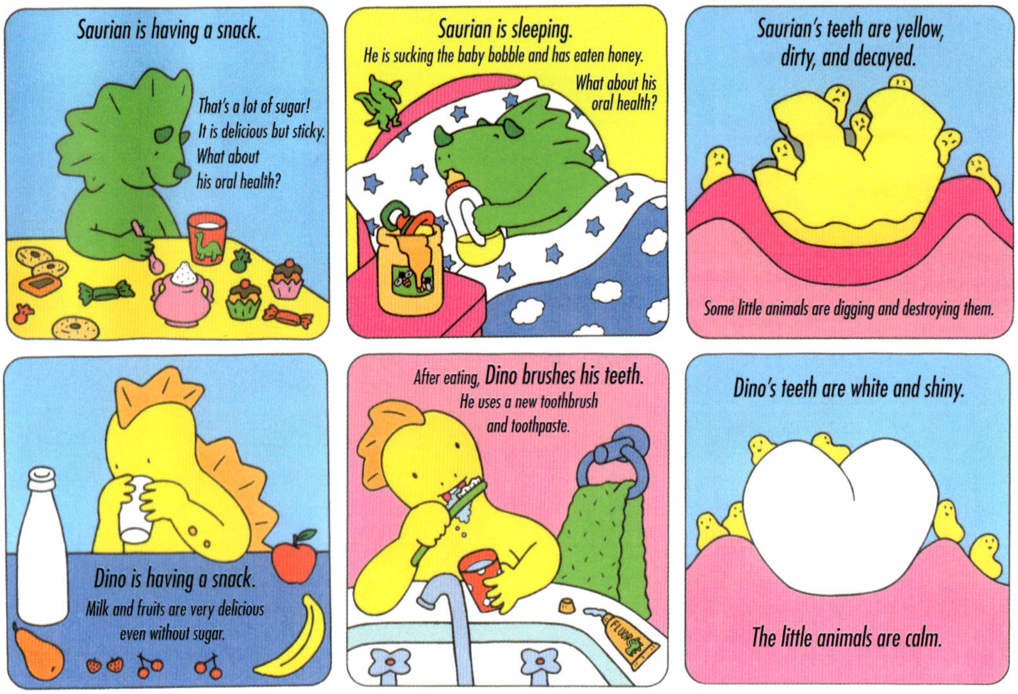
Saurian is having a snack.
That's a lot of sugar! It is delicious but sticky. What about his oral health?
Saurian is sleeping.
He is sucking the baby bobble and has eaten honey.
What about his oral health?
Saurian's teeth are yellow, dirty, and decayed.
Some little animals are digging and destroying them.
Dino is having a snack.
Milk and fruits are very delicious even without sugar.
After eating, Dino brushes his teeth.
He uses a new toothbrush and toothpaste.
Dino's teeth are white and shiny.
The little animals are calm.

Figure 1.4 Educational booklet in which two characters, Dino and Sauro, confront each other; they embody two opposite types of behavior toward oral and food hygiene measures for children.

First examination

The critical aspects regarding the relationship with the child specifically express the dynamics contained in each care relation and make the establishment of trust particularly crucial from the beginning. Upon arrival of the children and their parents, the emotional aspects involved in the therapeutic request should always be taken into consideration because this can help establish a cooperative and mutually trustworthy relationship and can allow appropriate formulation of the therapeutic solution in order to avoid a clash with ideal expectations that frequently occur with every request and to face the inevitable resulting disappointments.

In this regard, the five steps recommended by the *evidence-based* model introduced by Robert Smith (University of Michigan) at the American College of Physicians (Smith, 2005) is useful because it seems to meet both the medical needs and the need to establish a cooperative relationship. The five steps are listed below:

- welcome and introduction of the practitioner and search for an adequate setting, where the patient's privacy and comfort can be guaranteed
- determination of the time available for the search and determination of the patient's needs
- medical history collection starting from the long-term questions, as well as evaluation of the patients' behavior, their physical characteristics, and nonverbal communication
- specific investigation aimed at evaluating the physical, personal, and emotional history, giving a name to emotions, and understanding, respecting, and supporting them
- summary of the clinical report for the evaluation of data focused on providing care

The behaviors that should be adopted by medical professionals during the doctor-centered interview are precisely conceptualized in these five steps, as well as places and times for drafting the therapeutic project. From the relational perspective, the attention to the patient's emotional needs through both the welcome and interview is pivotal.

Since the initial entry into the operating room, the child can be faced by a sense of insecurity and fear that should be considered as expected experiences and normal reactions when confronted by new situations and stimuli (Fig. 1.5).

The following methods are suggested during the approach before the *first examination*:

- deviation
- curiosity
- induction targeted at the treatment

At the initial examination, the child's attention should be deviated from the dental issue and directed at topics related to school, sports, and personal hobbies, thereby inducing a mental relaxation state. Subsequently, the practitioner stimulates the children by asking questions that assess the knowledge they have about their own body and questions related to the number of eyes, hands, and feet up to those related to the number of teeth inside the mouth. During the first session, it is also important to perform diagnostic and therapeutic maneuvers that generate no unpleasant sensation in order to comply with what can be defined as an induction targeted at the treatment. Therefore, radiological investigations and temporary dressings that do not involve the use of rotating tools and digging procedures on cavities of necrotic elements should be performed.

The subsequent phase includes the implementation of the treatment by the practitioner to treat the dental problems. This phase requires the knowledge of specific techniques to manage the child's behavior that will be different from those usually adopted in the case of adult patients.

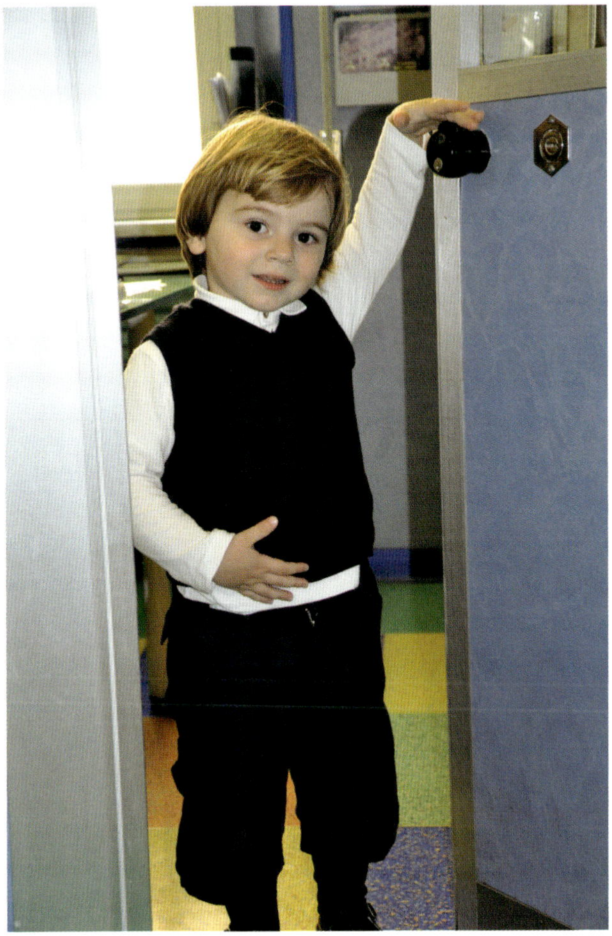

Figure 1.5 First entry of the child in the operating room. Confronted by new situations and stimuli, the child can show insecurity and fear, which are to be considered expected experiences and normal reactions.

Behavior management techniques

It is necessary to distinguish the basic behavior management techniques from the behavior management techniques in the strict sense.
The term "*basic techniques*" refers to a set of general techniques that should be performed with all children, including those who are very cooperative. The *behavior management techniques in the strict sense* should be applied in cases of noncooperation in order to reduce anxiety and help the patient undergo treatment in a more relaxed manner.

Basic techniques

The basic techniques include the *tell-show-do* approach, which is also called suggestion or explanation technique, and the *technique of reinforcement*.
The *tell-show-do* technique (Fig. 1.6) is based on a preliminary explanation given to children about the operation of a tool and the sensations they might feel, followed by a practical–clinical simulation and presentation. The *tell-show-do* technique has its theoretical basis on the children's rejection of surprise and deception and on their suggestibility, which requires a correct framing for the sensations felt.
In contrast, the technique of reinforcement takes advantage of the capability of a given behavior to cause a psychological reaction. In general, reinforcements can be positive or negative, depending on whether the practitioner wants to stimulate or inhibit the repetition of a given behavior.
Furthermore, there can be innate, social, material, and activity reinforcements.
The innate reinforcements used in pediatric dentistry can only be positive, and their purpose is to express approval toward the child's behaviors showed during the operating sessions.
Social reinforcements are the basis of communication with children. They are distinguished between verbal and facial expression reinforcements, as well as reinforcements of contact, proximity, and separation. In this case, it is pivotal not to use positive social reinforcements when the child has shown an uncooperative behavior on the chair, showing little attitude to cooperation.
Material reinforcements correspond to final prizes that are linked to the child's cooperation. The examples include toys, balloons, oral hygiene kits, etc. (Fig. 1.7)
Finally, activity reinforcements take advantage of the natural competitive tendency of an individual who, while in a group, is stimulated to surpass others. The final goal of activity reinforcements is to stimulate the single components of a group to improve themselves by continuously confronting each other (Fig. 1.8).

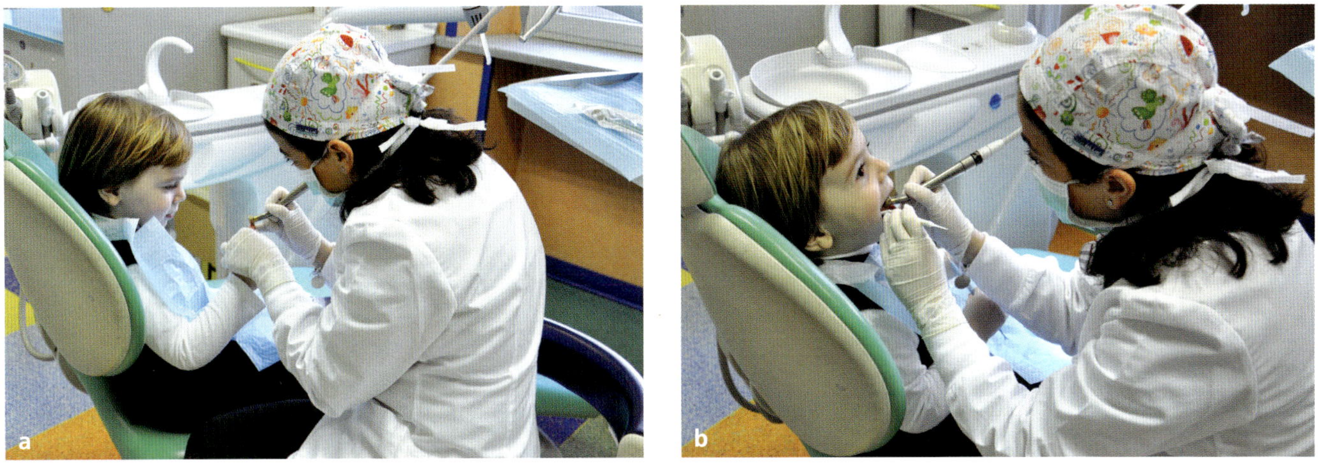

Figure 1.6 *Tell-show-do* technique. (**a**) Preliminary explanation to children about the operation of the instrument (turbine) and the feelings they might have. (**b**) Practical–clinical simulation and presentation of the use of the instrument presented to children.

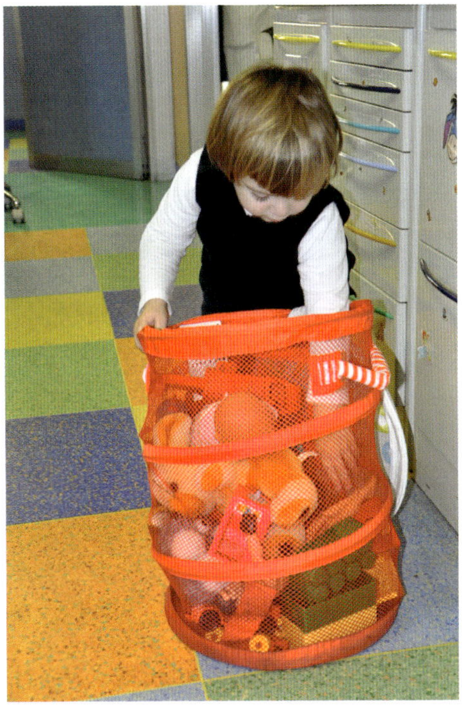

Figure 1.7 The material reinforcements are final prizes associated with the child's cooperation. Examples include toys chosen by the child at the end of a dental session.

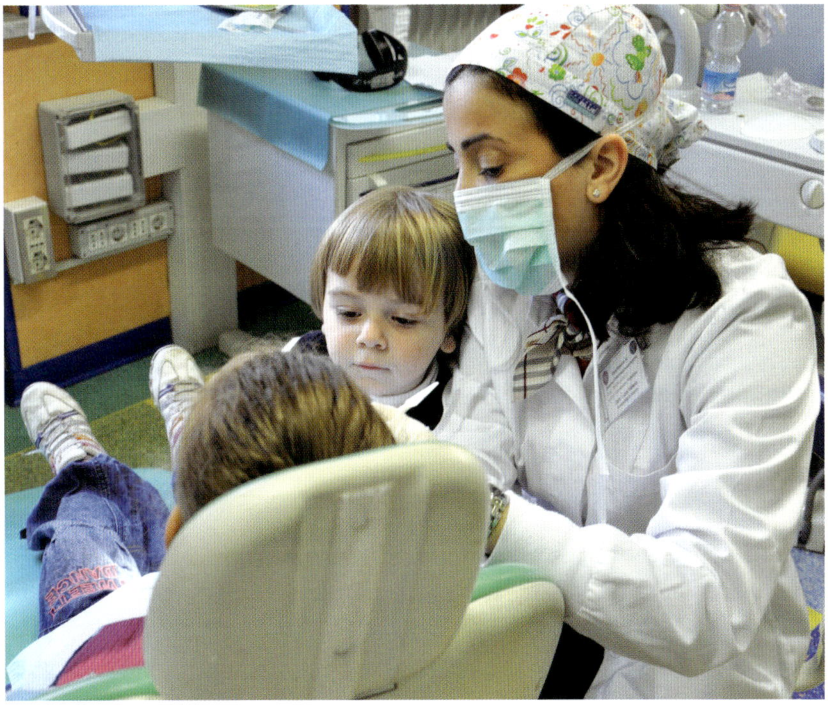

Figure 1.8 Activity reinforcements take advantage of the natural competitive tendency of an individual within a group: stimulated to surpass others. The goal: to stimulate the single group components to increase their cooperation through a continuous confrontation.

Behavior management techniques in the strict sense

The following methods used as approach techniques can be distinguished:
- slow approach method
- gradual approach method
- forced discipline method or "hand-over-mouth" method (HOM)

The slow approach method seeks to gradually obtain the acquisition of awareness of the dental treatment acceptability and allows the children to autonomously manage their own behavior.
The gradual approach uses the method of models and desensitization.
The method of models is commonly used with children facing their first dental experience and takes advantage of the mimetic instinct of a child to simulate a model that might be identified as a parent, a brother, or even a friend that undergoes a dental treatment without problems.
Desensitization is usually used for individuals aged more than 9-10 years; it involves inviting the patient to use the relaxation methods adequately learned to face situations that generate increasing levels of stress, such as the introduction of a syringe needle in the oral cavity.
The HOM method (Craig, 1971; Davis and Rombom, 1979) aims to solve the problem without causing permanent stress in the child and without prolonging the duration of the therapy. Usually, the first intervention involves firmly and softly positioning the hand over the child's mouth to muffle the screams. This is clearly applied in cases requiring a resolute therapeutic intervention, for example, during oral cavity drainage if the child is uncooperative. The advantage of this method is related to the mechanism by which children realize that their release only depends on themselves and, therefore, they are responsible for their own behavior. In the second intervention, the pediatric dentist gets closer to the child with the face and, with a calm and cold voice, explains that he/she "will free the mouth" only after he/she will stop screaming and that he/she only wants to look and count the teeth.
The most recent results regarding the application of child behavior management techniques in the dental setting (Adair, 2004; Ng, 2004; Farhat-McHayleh et al, 2009) indicate that the best outcome to reduce dental anxiety can be achieved with an adequate use of the model technique, particularly when the model involved is the parent. However, the *tell-show-do* method is still the most used technique in pediatric dentistry because of its easier implementation.

Appendix

Communication workshop: *learning from* experience

G. Pieragostini

In the appendix to the contribution regarding communication in the pediatric dentistry setting, it is very useful to include the experience of workshops on "subconsciousness in the dentist's room" within the scope of the master's degree in dentistry in developmental age at Sapienza University of Rome, established with the intention to offer an additional modality for both a theoretic and methodological approach in order to reflect on both the methods and places of therapy. The studies and researches found in the medical literature are usually confined to a scientific view, which prioritizes quantitative and descriptive data. Introducing a modality that refers to distant epistemological models might require an understanding effort, but at the same time, it might represent an alternative way of reading phenomena that interact with various professions and fields of knowledge.

Theoretical and methodological references

These workshops have had as theoretical reference framework the general *system theory* (von Bertalanffy, 1968), which defines the system itself as a complex of "related components," in which any change modifies every single part of the system. This theory allows understanding the circular aspects of communication, no longer intended unidirectionally but considered within the scope of the articulate reactions, both manifest and implicit or conscious and unconscious, that regard all the participants of the interaction.
The systemic orientation is integrated with a psychodynamic perspective of organizational analysis, as it is presented in the Tavistock Institut model (Hinshelwood and Skogstad, 2005; Obholzer and Zagier Roberts, 1999; Perini, 2007). This model, used in psychoanalysis, through the implementation of *group relations*, in addition to highlighting the unconscious group aspects, allows evaluation of the relationship with conflicts, the discomforts perceived, and the difficulties associated with achieving a task. Furthermore, it provides a coherent teaching (or rather counseling) methodology that consists of a "*learning from doing*" and "*use of self*" approach; the essential approach allows to test in the present what has been asserted in a continuous reference to the situation with patients. The work is done with the group considering the daily work setting and analyzing professional issues as they are actualized in the learning group dynamics. Moreover, apart from materials such as slides or literary passages, the prior knowledge of the students is primarily used, as well as their professional skills and the individual diversification of solutions. Because these frequently turn out to be students who are professionals with sound experience and great skills, a modality that allows a combination of various fields of knowledge is preferred rather than the passive learning approach of theoretical models.

Placing the workshop at the beginning of the master's degree course is not a random choice; in fact, it highlights the importance of the first encounter with the patient, the importance of the explicit and implicit communications that occur, and the importance of the necessity of welcoming and listening.
In terms of the importance of taking care of the setting in which the encounter with the patient occurs, transported on the experiential level of the workshop, this means ensuring that the encounter will occur in a setting that fosters mutual communication. Rather than in a usual room, the encounter takes place in a more personalized and cozier room, where it is possible to remain seated in a circle and face each other. Maintaining the schedule is carefully managed, and the attention given to each group component helps people to get to know each other better through the presentation of personal career paths and the expectations held in relation to the master.
Participants frequently have a personal motivation, in addition to a professional one, and the moment coincides with particularly significant stages of personal and professional life: the children have grown up and colleagues can significantly invest in their profession, the transition to another age group intended as a professional investment renewal, the emancipation from a particularly cumbersome fatherly figure, and the desire to confront oneself with professional issues and methods in a qualified setting.
If patients, in this case with their family, need to become the first care project collaborators to be informed on what is being done and why, also in the scope of the workshops, there will be moments of meta-communication on the theoretical and methodological prerequisites of what is shared.
Subsequently, the other aspects in which the profession of the dentist moves are explored, from the ethical–philosophical aspects to the division of knowledge and personal motivation. The communication aspects in the work setting are analyzed by considering the related department or surgery, both from the perspective of logistics and the perspective of rule implementation and the organization of the reception, waiting, and treatment places. The parameters considered include the facilitation of access, the wellbeing of the children, the practitioners, the exchange among colleagues, and the personalized communication with family members.
Activating awareness in the setting in which the encounter with the patient occurs means recording its characteristics from a communication perspective, in accordance with the first axiom of communication (Watzlawick, 1971), in which "*one cannot not communicate*," and it is impossible not to acquire awareness on how communication influences the success of a therapy with its times, methods, and spatial organization. Dentists always work in a material container, a hospital or private surgery, and becoming aware of the messages that pass through it means being in touch with perceptions and emotions, especially one's own and then those of others.

The relation in care relationship

As with concentric circles, from interviews with patients and their parents, it is possible to determine the reason of the encounter after establishing an environment of trust, and this applies in workshops too, where only after creating a container that is at the same time sufficiently reliable and elastic is it possible to work together on the task at hand.

If the goal in the dental setting can be defined as to treat a more or less severe dental pathology and, especially in patients in developmental age, to prevent malocclusions of several levels of severity, in the workshop, the task is defined as "*building a relationship that can convey and carry out the specific task of this profession*." As an introduction, it is useful to focus on some aspects never that are sufficiently discussed in the healthcare setting concerning the relational values of the doctor–patient relationship and the semiconscious and unconscious fantasies it provokes.

Desmond Morris, an ethologist and communication expert, defined a healthcare professional as a specialist of intimacy (1986), and by doing so he captured one of the most obvious and little-considered aspects regarding care relationship. This characteristic is linked to the uneven nature of this relationship, the condition of necessity in the patient, the involvement of the body, as well as the expectations and fears of damage associated with the treatment configuration (Tatarelli et al, 1998). In the dental setting, additional factors that can exacerbate the phantasmatic aspects involved in the relationship can be involved: the organ considered, the implications related to pain, the expectations related to self-image, and the reciprocal position between the caregiver and care receiver during the treatment.

The mouth, as an organ of communication, intimacy, aggressiveness, and pleasure, becomes a place of intrusion in the psyche-soma interaction during the treatment; furthermore, lying down with the caregiver in a predominant position can stimulate feelings of submission and helplessness. The use of necessary equipment that can be a source of pain fosters the feeling of danger and fragility. To these contextual data are added the expectations and fears associated with the outward appearance, the prior experiences, and the aspects of the individual personality evoked by the situation.

When it comes to the patient in a developmental age, the fantasies linked to the caregiver figure can be imbued with protective expectations as well as by threats of one's own bodily integrity and experience of physical pain. Since the report by Schilder (2002), the importance of the experiences related to the body in the construction of one's own identity is widely recognized; therefore, the caregiver should consider the criticality involved in each intervention, even more so if, as in the case of orthodontics and dentistry, it can have consequences on self-image.

The fragility of the growth processes intertwined with the events of narcissistic investments (Freud, 1977; Kohut, 1977) makes the professional operation in the developmental age intricate.

Furthermore, during the encounter, dentists will not only be subject to the reactions and communications of the child but will also find themselves in a relationship involving three persons, in which the parent (frequently the mother) plays a crucial role both in influencing the child's experience and in acting as a bearer of the anxieties and ghosts that characterize the family system. The presence of parental figures introduces elements of complexity in communication, as in the related expectations and fears, whether they are expressed or not, as it always happens when it comes to dealing with the health of children (Minuchin, 1980).

The caregiver as a subject of relationship and care

In theoretical and methodological presentations, even in those that focus on relations and in the caregiver's awareness, the position of the care receiver is often suppressed in the mind to hide the anxiety-causing situations as a defense mechanism: "*In the relationship with the patient, the caregiver has a series of emotional responses, which are frequently unconscious but have their own relevance in relation to the modifications in the patient's behavior they induce*" (Tatarelli et al, 1998). If care receivers, in their role as patients and identified in their organic syndrome, can be made insignificant in the level of communication, caregivers too can be considered only in relation to the specific medical actions and not as bearers of emotions and fantasies in the relationship with their patients and with their profession. Scientific evidence, both from an observational and experimental perspective, includes, as fundamental parts, both the observer and the context (Morin, 1993); therefore, talking about the anxiety of children should include the awareness of the model regarding the management of one's own feelings, a model introjected more or less consciously by the caregiver. Instead, caregivers are frequently confined by the collective imagination to an image of doctors wearing their white coats, a symbol of the diagram that should guarantee against inward and outward perturbations. If the pathology prevails over the patient as a person in the objectifying approach, it follows that the same caregiver is identified with functions and protocols. In this manner, the inevitable implicit subjectivity in each medical action is denied on the shared level to remain unheard both in its emotional values and in its clinical richness that it might represent.

In addition, in the current organization of the healthcare system, the avoidance of the doctor–patient relationship is by now validated by complex procedures, healthcare systems fragmentation, bureaucratization, and increasingly widespread technological systems (Virzì, 2007).

If it is true "*... that the only possible medicine is the one that takes into consideration the patient's emotional side, as the risk in the future will be to make too much "sterile" and impersonal what cannot be so by its very nature*" (Tatarelli et al, 1998), it is equally important to take into consideration the emotional needs of caregivers.

The so-called *burnout syndrome*, which defines the significant malaise of caregivers, in particular conditions and tasks, is currently the focus of evaluation studies and scales (Leiter and Maslach, 1988; Maslach and Leiter 2000; Leiter and Maslach, 2005). Additionally, groups of support, specific training, individual counseling dedicated to caregivers, and the attention to quality for the settings in which the healthcare and assistance operators work are just as important.

Fishbowl

Obviously, with the short lapses of time in workshops, it is not possible to explore the entire complexity of these topics, but it is possible to provide an experiential opportunity that activates the capacity of a group to observe what is obvious, in other words, what is never taken into consideration but that motivates behaviors in the professional setting.

A mother and her 8-year-old daughter with a severe upper jaw protrusion and with her thumb in her mouth show up. The mother throws a bag containing numerous damaged orthodontic devices on the table as a testimony of many failed care relationships. In that bag there is a help request and, at the same time, a gauntlet of challenge; on a conscious level, the dentist accepts the treatment request, on an unconscious level, he/she accepts the gauntlet of the challenge.

The relationship, despite the availability and competence, fails to meet the primary goal.
The *fishbowl* is a practical exercise proposed over the years in communication workshops. Participants sit in a circle; a volunteer is positioned at the center, within an inner circle, and presents the case to discuss and the colleagues chosen by him to be his interlocutors. During the presentation and discussion in the inner circle, the participants in the outer circle listen in silence and take notes, in accordance with a few parameters proposed by the consultant.

The group listens to what is being explained, observes the different attempts made, and notes the observations and advice of the interlocutors. However, the group primarily assesses the direction of communication and notes the tones of the voices, the postures, the repetition of key sentences, the attention to the context, and the compliance with the related times and tasks.

At the end of the established period of time, the components listen in silence to the comments and observations of colleagues, which they can then use in the next round of discussion. The round is ended by discussing together with those that led the experience.

In the present, the re-enactment of the same unconscious dynamic that has failed the task allows us to understand the emotional configuration of the care relationship and its phases, place the meaning of its failure, and hypothesize possible solutions.

At each time, the experience shows how crucial rules and contexts are in activating the capacity of reading the complexity of the cumulative phenomena and the emotional and relational meaning that they bear.
The cases discussed over time that were related to either the difficulties of a treatment underway or to the difficulties that led to its interruption, showed that it is not only the unconscious fantasies and conflicts that invade the pediatric dentist's room. If requests beyond the dental cure can hide claims of emotional compensations (displacement of emotional family conflicts), there can be expulsive temptations, collusions with the unconscious request, and slips from the specific care setting in the answer given to the caregiver.
In the present, the shared modalities and contents that contribute to increase the awareness experienced individually need a human container to develop. Reflecting on the profession, many relationships among participants were built, other possible group configurations were tested, and other latent group potentialities, as third elements in the learning process, were activated.

At the end of the encounter, the newly developed group identity is summarized, occasionally by a name and frequently by a final photo that becomes its symbol and testimony.

References

Adair SM. Behavior management conference panel I report – Rationale for behavior management techniques in pediatric dentistry. Pediatr Dent 2004;26(2):167-70.

American Psychiatric Association. Diagnostic and Statistical Manual of Mental Disorders. 5th ed. Arlington, VA: American Psychiatric Association, 2013. [Trad. it. Manuale Diagnostico e Statistico dei Disturbi Mentali, DSM-5®. 5 ed., Milano:Raffaello Cortina Editore, 2014].

Craig W. Hand over Mouth technique. J Dent Child 1971;38:387-9.

Davis MJ, Rombom HM. Survey of the utilization of and rationale for Hand-over-Mouth (HOM) and restraint in postdoctoral pedodontic education. Pediatr Dent 1979;1(2):87-90.

Farhat-McHayleh N, Harfouche A, Souaid P. Techniques for managing behaviour in pediatric dentistry: comparative study of live modelling and Tell-Show-Do based on children's heart rates during treatment. J Can Dent Ass 2009;75(4):283.

Frankl SN, Shiere FR, Fogels HR. Should the parent remain with the child in the dental operatory? ASDC J Dent Child 1962;29:150-63.

Freud S. Zur Einführung des Narzißmus. Jahrbuch der Psychoanalyse 1914. [trad. it. Introduzione al narcisismo. Torino: Bollati Boringhieri; 1977.]

Hinshelwood RD, Skogstad W, editor. Osservare le organizzazioni: ansia, difesa e cultura nei servizi sanitari. Torino: Ananke; 2005.

Holst A, Hallonsten AL, Schröder EKL et al. Prediction of behavior-management problems in 3-year-old children. Scand J Dent Res 1993;101:110-4.

Kendall PC, editor. Child and adolescent therapy: cognitive-behavioral procedures. 3rd ed. New York: The Guilford Press; 2006.

Klingberg G, Berggren U, Carlsson SG, Norén JG. Child dental fear: cause-related factors and clinical effects. Eur J Oral Sci 1995; 103:405-12.

Klingberg G, Broberg AG. Dental fear/anxiety and dental behaviour management problems in children and adolescent: a review of prevalence and concomitant psycological factors. Int J of Paediatr Dent 2007;17:391-406.

Klingberg G, Dahllöf G, Erlandsson AL et al. A survey of specialistic paediatric dental services in Sweden: results from 2003, and trends since 1983. Int J Paediatr Dent 2006; 16:89-94.

Kohut H. The analysis of the self. New York: International University Press; 1971. [trad. it. Narcisismo e analisi del Sé. Torino: Bollati Boringhieri; 1977.].

Kyritsi MA, Dimou G, Lygidakis NA. Parental attitudes and perceptions affecting children's dental behaviour in Greek population. A clinical study. Eur Arch Paediatr Dent 2009;10(1):29-32.

Leiter MP, Maslach C. Preventing burnout and building engagement. San Francisco: Jossey-Bass; 2000. [trad. it. OCS Organizational Checkup System. Come prevenire il burnout e costruire l'impegno. Firenze: OS Organizzazioni Speciali; 2005].

Leiter MP, Maslach C. The impact of interpersonal environment on burnout and organizational commitment. J Organ Behav 1988;9(4):297-308.

Maslach C, Leiter MP. The truth about burnout: How organizations cause personal stress and what to do about it. San Francisco: Jossey-Bass; 1997. [trad. it. Burnout e organizzazione: modificare i fattori strutturati della motivazione al lavoro. Trento: Erickson; 2000].

Milgrom P, Nanci L, King B et al. Origins of childhood dental fear. Behav Res Ther 1995;33(3):313-9.

Minuchin S, Rosman BL, Baker L. Psychosomatic families: anorexia nervosa in context. Harvard Univeristy Press 1978. [trad. it. Le famiglie psicosomatiche: l'anoressia mentale nel contesto familiare. Roma: Astrolabio; 1980.]

Morin E. Introduction à la pensée complexe. 1990. [trad. it. Introduzione al pensiero complesso. Milano: Sperling and Kupfer; 1993.]

Morris D. Intimate behaviour. 1971. [trad. it. Il comportamento intimo. Milano: Mondadori; 1986.]

Ng MW. Behavior management conference panel IV report – Educational issues. Pediatr Dent 2004;26(2):180-3.

Obholzer A, Zagier Roberts V. L'inconscio al lavoro: stress individuale e organizzativo nei servizi alla persona. Milano: Etas Libri; 1999.

Perini M. L'organizzazione nascosta: dinamiche inconsce e zone d'ombra nelle moderne organizzazioni. Milano: Franco Angeli; 2007.

Rosengren KE. Introduzione allo studio della comunicazione. Bologna: Mulino, 2001.

Scherer MW, Nakamura CY. A Fear Survey Schedule for Children (FSS-FC): a factor analytic comparison with manifest anxiety (CMAS). Behav Res Ther 1968;6:173-82.

Schilder P. The image and appearance of the human body. New York, 1935 [trad. it. Immagine di sé e schema corporeo. Milano: Franco Angeli, 2002.]

Smith RC. American College of Physicians 2004. Presentato al convegno "Rapporto medico-bambino malato, alleanza e cooperazione per la salute". Roma, 8 marzo 2005.

Tatarelli R, De Pisa E, Girardi P. Curare con il paziente. Metodologia del rapporto medico-paziente. Milano: Franco Angeli, 1998.

Virzì A. La relazione medico-paziente. Come riumanizzare il rapporto: un manuale introduttivo. Milano: Franco Angeli 2007.

von Bertalanffy L. General system theory. New York: Braziller, 1968. [trad. it. Teoria generale dei sistemi. Milano: Oscar Mondadori; 2004.]

Watzlawick P, Beavin JH, Jackson DD. Pragmatics of human communication. New York: WW Norton, 1967. [trad. it. Pragmatica della comunicazione umana. Roma: Astrolabio, 1971].

Winer GA. A review and analysis of children's fearful behavior in dental settings. Child Dev 1982;53:1111-33.

Chapter 2

Role and features of the environment in pediatric dentistry

G. Ierardo, C. Voglino, and A. Polimeni

Can the physical setting influence the behavior of children and support the psychological approach in pediatric dentistry?

Some results of interdisciplinary scientific research investigations are in favor of how *environmental conditions* can contribute to the therapeutic process and recovery, in addition to the technical, healthcare, and pharmacological aspects.

In the healthcare setting, physical-environmental, socio-relational, and architectonic aspects take on a therapeutic and strategic significance to achieve the goal of monitoring patients from a global perspective, taking into consideration their numerous and complex needs, including psychological ones.

Environmental psychology is a growing scientific field that deals with the interaction between people and their environment. A *sensitive and moral action* of the use of color in the environment had already been theorized at the beginning of the nineteenth century: the *theory of colors* by Goethe.

The understanding of spaces, relationships among objects, distances, as well as rules that govern the use of environments change during growth.

As far as environmental knowledge is concerned, children and adults differ in three main aspects:

- the level of understanding of environmental reality
- the role played by emotions on cognitive processes in relation to age
- the transformation of environmental preferences in relation to the various stages of life

The environmental vulnerability of children is larger:

- they are more exposed to negative environmental effects due to the immaturity of their physical and cognitive skills and, therefore, are more vulnerable than adults
- they depend on socio-physical environment features as they need an environment that suits their needs in order to develop correctly

Environmental stress, which is linked to an unsuitable setting, reflects itself in a negative way and can influence patient management in two ways:

- *directly*, by negatively influencing psychophysiological parameters and particularly delicate systems (cardiovascular, endocrine, gastrointestinal, and immune system), inducing states of anxiety and depression, and reducing cognitive performance and the compliance of the child
- *indirectly*, by acting on the performance of personnel (reducing the quality of the treatment provided and increasing the incidence of clinical errors) and family members (reducing assistance and social support and creating distrust)

In general, the factors that might be a *source of stress* in a healthcare facility can be distributed into the following critical areas:

- image of the facility
- sensory conditions
- physical discomfort
- risk of infection

There are other sources of stress in the pediatric setting:

- foreign environment
- sensorial hypo/hyperstimulation
- absence of child-friendly spaces
- absence of recreational areas
- environment unsuitable to the child's age
- crowding
- parents' attitude

The concept of a *healing environment* implies the design of space solutions aimed at satisfying the physical and psychosocial needs of all individuals within the environment, with the specific goal of positively influencing the clinical outcome.

Environmental Strategies

The environment of a pediatric dentistry clinic should be structured in such a way as to convey messages of reassurance and encouragement; the fact that the expectations of the children and those of the people that accompany them do not always coincide should be taken into consideration. Children in particular need a welcoming and familiar environment in which they can freely move and feel at ease; parents, in addition to the attention to detail and comfort of the environment, seek confirmation of competence and hygiene, which must be impeccable.
The environmental features and design strategies applied in a pediatric dentistry facility should therefore support the following points:

- sensorial conditions: colors, lights, spatial organization
- reassurance strategies: decorations, clothing of dental personnel, drawing board
- anxiety control strategies: play area, entertainment
- behavior management strategies; reinforcement, modeling
- information (leaflets and posters).

The objectives of these measures include

- a significant containment of anxiety in children and an increase in their compliance
- a reduction in treatment duration and, consequently, the possibility of treating a higher number of children
- an increase in the level of satisfaction and of the quality perceived by parents

For example, the environmental solutions adopted at the Pediatric Dentistry Unit at the Department of Odontostomatological and Maxillofacial Sciences of the Umberto I Hospital, Sapienza University of Rome are shown below.

Upon upgrading the department, in addition to the usual technical problems related to measurements, types of fittings, spaces, pathways, fixtures, and partitions, another two general issues were raised, whose solutions, one of many among the infinite possibilities, led the facility to assume the appearance that characterizes it today as it is experienced by its younger visitors.

The first question that was asked in relation to the healthcare setting concerned the identity of the environment and the expectations of patients; in this case, the children. Should pain and suffering necessarily be associated with the gloom, grayness, and uniformity of the surrounding facility?

Or rather, what is being proposed? Pain and suffering?

Or should a path be proposed, also and hopefully repeatable during the course of one's life, that focuses attention on the necessary steps toward wellbeing and health and that does not build a refusal whose support is fear?

The second question asked regarding the facility concerned its aspects of renewal and maintenance. The uniformity of the facility has traditionally proposed an initial "new, clean, and well-made" phase. It was realized that no sooner did new items become indispensable (repositioning of equipment, implementation of technologies, maintenance, repairs, etc.), the contrast between uniformity and renewal showed a rapid and premature aging of the facility that happened so suddenly to be able to show a collapse of what appeared to be just a moment before a new environment.

Therefore, will the prudent practitioners, who are aware of the new course characterized by very rapid advancements in the medical and healthcare sector, and as a consequence of their action, be able to accept the "resistance" of an environment that is hard to change?

Colors

Fifteen colors placed in different, repeating, and conflicting series were used.

Considerable importance was given to the chromatic characterization of the treatment environment.

Goethe's theory of colors states: "... *Colors occupy a very important position in the series of original natural manifestations* ..." It should not come as a surprise to learn that this exercises an action, in particular on the sense of sight, to which it evidently belongs, and, through it, on mood in its general elementary manifestations, without reference to the structure or shape of the material from whose surface it reflects. It can be said that this is a specific action when colors are considered on their own, whereas when in combination with others, it is also an action that appears partially harmonious, partially characteristic, and frequently non-harmonious too, but nevertheless always decisive and significant, linked to the moral aspect. This is the reason why colors, considered as an element of art, can be used as an element that cooperates for higher purposes.

In general, color gives man great pleasure. Eyes need them just as they need light. It is important to recall the relief one feels when the sun shines on a stretch of landscape, making its colors very visible on a hazy day.
The attribution of particular therapeutic virtues to precious colored stones can be explained by the depth of this inexpressible pleasure.
The consideration expressed over time by users about the service and facility was positive in the face of a varied audience (children of various ages, parents, and healthcare personnel); this was also determined by establishing a varied, cheerful, and stimulating environment.
The chromatic features affected all the environmental components: walls, floors, units, stools, and colored disposable materials in direct contact with children (mirrors, cotton rolls, covers, glasses, coats, and headphones) (Fig. 2.1–2.3).

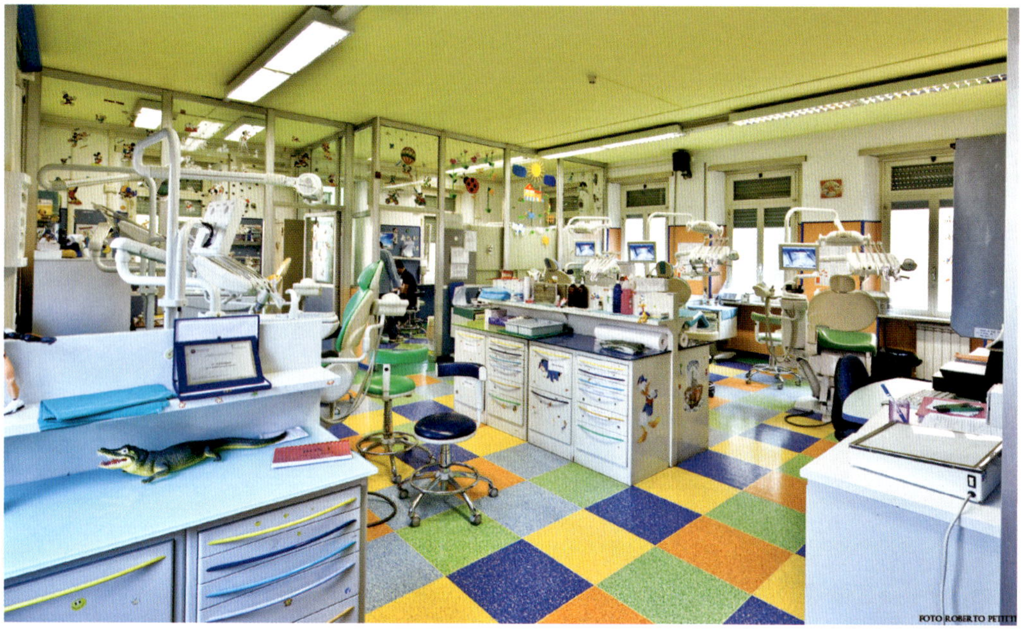

Figure 2.1 *Open plan* environment.

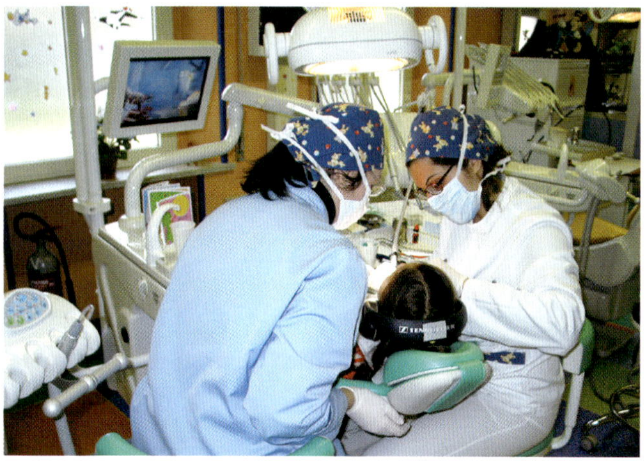
Figure 2.2 Operating phase on chair.

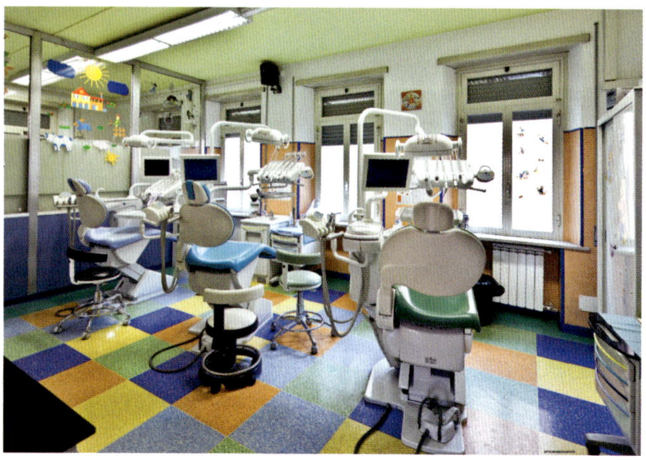
Figure 2.3 Detail of dentists' units.

Light

Adequate environmental brightness was guaranteed by a correct balance between natural and artificial light produced by the lamps inside the environments and units. Light influenced and enhanced the chromatic environmental features.

Decorations

In order to establish a familiar and friendly environment that is appropriate for children who visit the clinic, walls, movable surfaces, dividing walls, and window glasses were decorated with stickers of cartoon characters. The choice of characters from animation movies was determined by their popularity among children, who thus were able to find an element of continuity with their daily lives.

Staff Clothing

Although some studies found that there is no significant preference among patients, other researches proved that a fairly large number of children react unfavorably at the sight of a white coat. It is likely that the previous medical experiences of the children, during which they were restrained and traumatized, led them to identify and generalize the white coat with fear and pain in any medical setting, including the dental one. To break this ill-founded fear, colored coats, headphones, and masks were chosen for use; these were characterized by drawings and characters from cartoons.

Spatial Organization

The pediatric dentistry clinic was organized in an *open plan* with separate workstations; a separate sector was reserved to assist patients with special needs: patients with disabilities or with systemic pathologies and uncooperative children.

The *open plan* concept allowed *modeling* strategies to be applied, modified by applied psychology and based on imitation. Upon seeing another more cooperative child, an anxious child acquires the behavioral characteristics (learning from a model) of the latter by emulation.

One of the workstations was exclusively reserved for the first visit; this station was more comfortable in appearance, colorful, fun in its "strange" mechanized mobility, essential, and without a suction system and handpiece in order to offer a first impression to the child that is as calming as possible (Fig. 2.4).

The spaces allow the practitioner and the assistant to work together, "four-handed" or "six-handed" (the practitioner and two assistants); this is necessary if interventions need to be performed in a short space of time, but it is even more necessary within a facility that has the role of training future dentists.

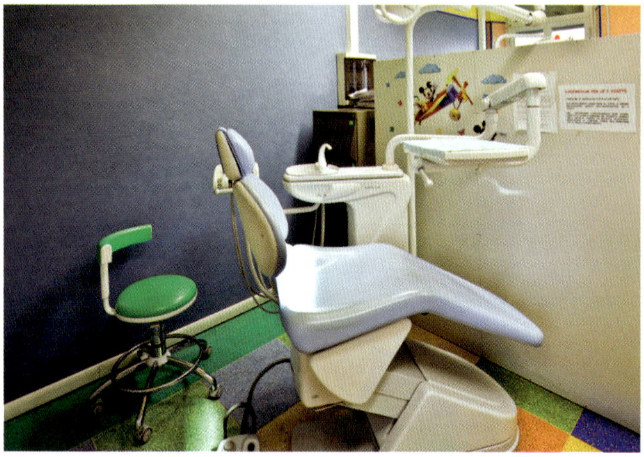

Figure 2.4 Chair used for the initial visit.

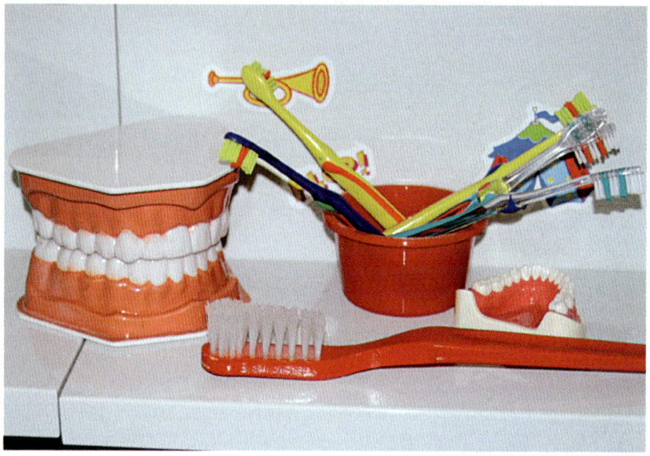

Figure 2.5 Objects to illustrate oral hygiene maneuvers.

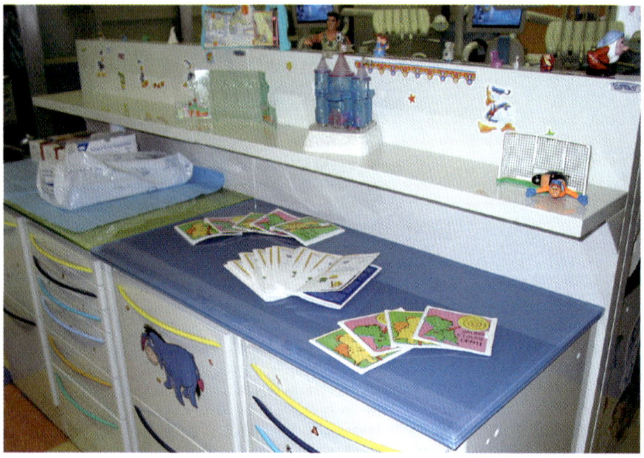

Figure 2.6 Decorations and brochures.

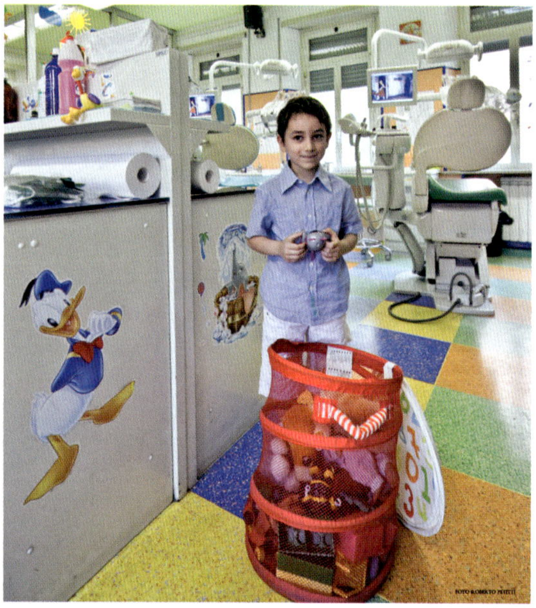

Figure 2.7 Example of positive reinforcement: prizes for children.

Objects

Workstations or shelves were furnished with materials and objects with captivating designs and shapes that attract the attention of children; during the training and motivational sessions for oral hygiene maintenance, models such as arches or colored toothbrushes were used (Fig. 2.5), as well as toys positioned near to the workstation or information material in the form of comics for children and brochures for parents (Fig. 2. 2.6).

It was useful to prepare a box or a basket with toys in order to support the differentiated behavior management technique of positive reinforcement (the related literature describes inhomogeneous behaviors toward tangible rewards as a useful approach for children in preschool age, whereas social reinforcements, such as praise and appreciation, can suffice with older children) (Fig. 2.7).

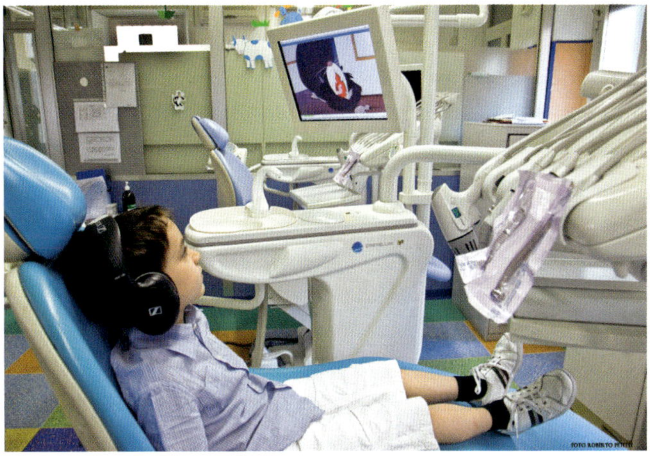

Figure 2.8 LCD monitor with wireless headphones.

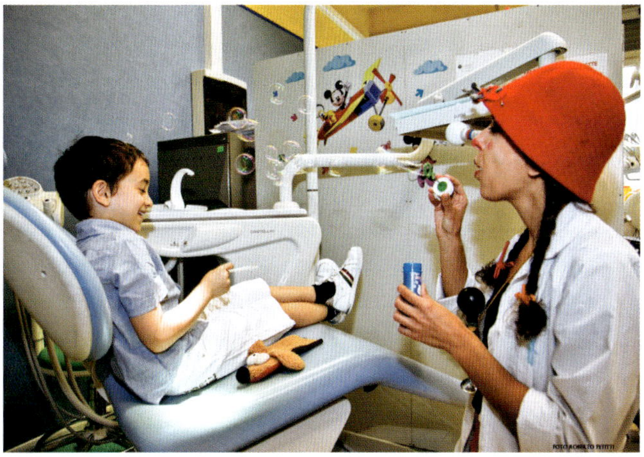

Figure 2.9 Clowns.

Distractions

Distraction represents a strategy to control stress and pain in pediatric dentistry. It was implemented by showing a video or with the interaction of clown entertainers.
A cartoon video projection system was installed, which consisted of an LCD monitor mounted on a movable support and wireless headphones connected to a central multimedia player in each station; attention is directed to the broadcast program so that stress during waiting times and pain perception during treatment can be reduced (Fig. 2.8).
The intervention of clown entertainers, initially intended as a distraction, sets in motion a psychophysiological mechanism, for which the emotional investment on external stimuli different from one's own body, such as soap bubbles or magic tricks, leads to a shift of attention; in other words, the focus of awareness on the imaginative and playful stimulus (Fig. 2.9).

Waiting Areas

Play and movement are important needs of children, as well as important coping resources.
An appropriate waiting area with several functions was established:

- to allow children to be distracted during waiting times and recover after treatment
- to calm parents, who then did not have to entertain their children
- to support the social interaction of children and parents

The setup was integrated with child-friendly furnishing (chairs and tables) and distractions such as monitors with cartoons, videogames, toys, comics, information brochures, drawing materials, and blackboards (Fig. 2.10).
The waiting room was equipped with a board with drawings that the children gave to the practitioners who had taken care of them. A child visiting for the first time will be

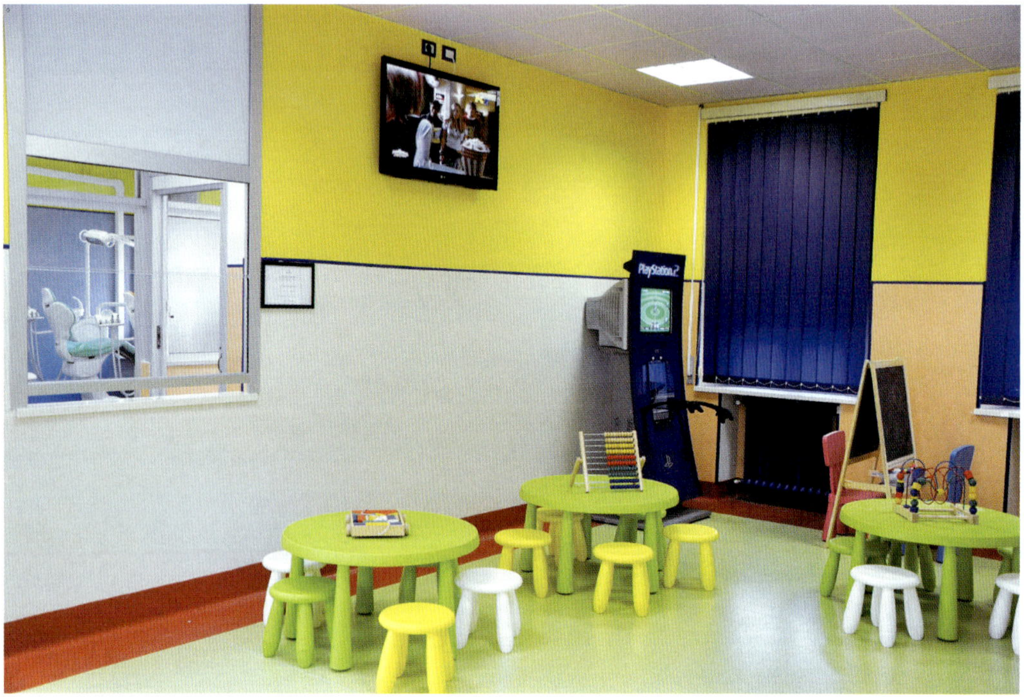

Figure 2.10 Dedicated waiting area.

able to observe that other children of the same age or younger faced and successfully overcame the same experience, as testified by the drawings.
At the same time, the drawings show the practitioner how a child perceived the dental experience and, in particular, focuses on the aspects that evoked the greatest level of apprehension.

References

Acredolo LP, Evans D. Developmental changes in the effects of landmarks on infant spatial behavior. Developmental Psychology 1980;16:312-8.

Assanthiany R, Kemeny J, Sznajder M et al. La salle d'attente du pédiatre: lieu d'education pour la santé? Archives de Pédiatrie 2005;12(1):10-5.

Bal Filoramo L, Gallo Vianzone G. Odontoiatria infantile e psicanalisi. Torino: Cortina, 1990.

Cohen HD, Eli I, Parush S. Behavioural and physiological effect of dental environment sensory adaptation on children's dental anxiety. European Journal of Oral Science 2007;115:479-83.

Greenbaum PE, Melamed BG. Pretreatment modeling. A technique for reducing children's fear in the dental operatory. Dental Clinics of North America 1988;32(4):693-704.

Ierardo G, Luzzi V, Vestri A et al. Evaluation of customer satisfaction at the Department of Paediatric Dentistry of "Sapienza" University of Rome. European Journal of Paediatric Dentistry 2008;9(1):30-6.

Horsburg CR. Healing by design. The New England Journal of Medicine 1995;333:735-40.

Klingberg G. Dental fear and behavior management problems in children: a study of measurement, prevalence, concomitant factors, and clinical effects. Swedish Dental Journal Supplement 1995;103:1-78.

McAndrew FT. Environmental psychology. Pacific Grove: Brooks/Cole; 1993.

Morgan PH, Wright LE, Ingersoll BD, Seime RJ. Children's perceptions of the dental experience. Journal of Dentistry for Children 1980;47(4):243-5.

Paglia L, Damia G, Caprioglio D, Toschi P. Psicologia in pedodonzia. Quaderni di Odontoiatria Infantile. Milano: Masson; 1993.

Shapiro M, Melmed RN, Sgan-Cohen HD et al. Behavioural and physiological effect of dental environment sensory adaptation on children's dental anxiety. European Journal of Oral Science 2007;115(6):479-83.

Shaw O. Dental anxiety in children. British Dental Journal 1975; 139(4):134-9.

Venham LL, Goldstein M, Gaulin-Kremer E et al. Effectiveness of a distraction technique in managing young dental patients. Pediatric dentistry 1981, 3(1):7-11.

Weinstein P, Getz T, Ratener P, Domoto P. The effect of dentists' behaviors on fear-related behaviors in children. Journal of American Dental Association 1982, 104(1):32-8.

Wright GZ, Alpern GD, Leake JL. The modificability of maternal anxiety as it relates to children's cooperative dental behaviour. Journal of dentistry for children 1973;40:265-71.

Zenter MR. Preference for colours and color-emotion combinations in early childhood. Developmental sciences 2001;4(4):389-98.

Chapter 3

The first visit in pediatric dentistry

A. Polimeni, M. Cordaro

The first visit, which is fundamental to start collecting the patient's clinical data, is even more important at the developmental age considering the practitioner–child relationship, which, from the start, should follow the principles of the pediatric dentistry approach. In pediatric dentistry, the clinical examination is the primary instance for diagnostic and therapeutic evaluation. Since the first time a child enters the treatment room, pediatric dentists should perform the first clinical evaluation with extreme care, which, together with the collection of medical history data, will direct them toward specialized clinical evaluation.

Medical History

The main points that should be noted in medical records are schematically listed below.

- family medical history
- physiological medical history
- pathological medical history
  - past
  - history of present illness

Family medical history. Its goal is to identify the presence of hereditary dental diseases, both systemic and specific:

- systemic:
  - hypertension
  - diabetes
  - coagulation disorders
  - allergic diathesis
- tooth number anomalies:
  - missing (agenesis)
  - extra (supernumerary)

Physiological medical history. Its goal is to collect information regarding the various stages of the patient's development:

- duration and course of pregnancy (drugs taken, rubella, etc.)
- type of delivery (eutocic or dystocic delivery) and term (at 39–40 weeks, full-term pregnancy)

- neonatal illness
- type of feeding (breastfeeding or bottle feeding)
- time of weaning (coinciding with tooth eruption)
- bad habits:
  - use of pacifier
  - thumb sucking
  - lower lip biting
  - habit of holding the tongue between the teeth
  - habit of keeping objects in the mouth
- psychophysical and motor development.

Past medical history. Its goal is to collect information regarding previous pathologies, from birth to the medical examination, excluding the reason for the visit:

- exanthematous diseases (they can cause symmetrical and hypoplastic enamel lesions)
- viral infections
- diabetes (especially for periodontal tissues)
- renal metabolic disorders
- hemorrhagic syndromes
- liver diseases
- allergic diseases
- heart diseases
- malabsorption syndromes (celiac disease)
- surgery (tonsillectomy, adenoidectomy)

History of present illness. The reason for the visit to the specialist is taken into consideration:

- reason for the visit
- presence of pain
- pain features
- other symptoms and their features

Past dental history. Its goal is to evaluate important information regarding the child's dental history:

- previous dental experiences
- traumas
- child's acceptance
- child's behavior
- fluoride intake and prescription

Pharmacological history. It is necessary to know if the child takes medications or suffers from allergies.

Clinical Examination

To perform the clinical examination appropriately, it is advisable to be methodical and systematic in data collection; accordingly, should be ensured that no element that might be key in establishing the diagnosis is neglected. Therefore, at the same time, it is necessary to maintain a schematic, complete, and well-organized clinical record in which it is possible to note observations.

In this chapter, a reference scheme is proposed that can also be modified by practitioners according to their own needs or those of the patient, provided that the same clinical evaluation criteria are followed.

Three phases of the clinical examination can be distinguished:

1. extraoral phase
2. intraoral phase
3. functional phase.

Extraoral Clinical Examination

The extraoral clinical examination starts with a general evaluation of the child's *facial appearance* during the phase of first approach and medical history recording. Subsequently, the clinical examination is performed on the dental unit. In this phase, it is important to maintain a correct chair position to maintain the reference planes for proper evaluation. The child should be positioned with the back of the chair perpendicular to the floor, the head with the eyes facing forward, and the Frankfurt plane (the line passing from the tragus to the nose wing) parallel to the floor; in this phase, it is necessary to use natural light rather than that of the dental unit so as to avoid false shadows that might alter the extraoral appearance (Fig. 3.1).

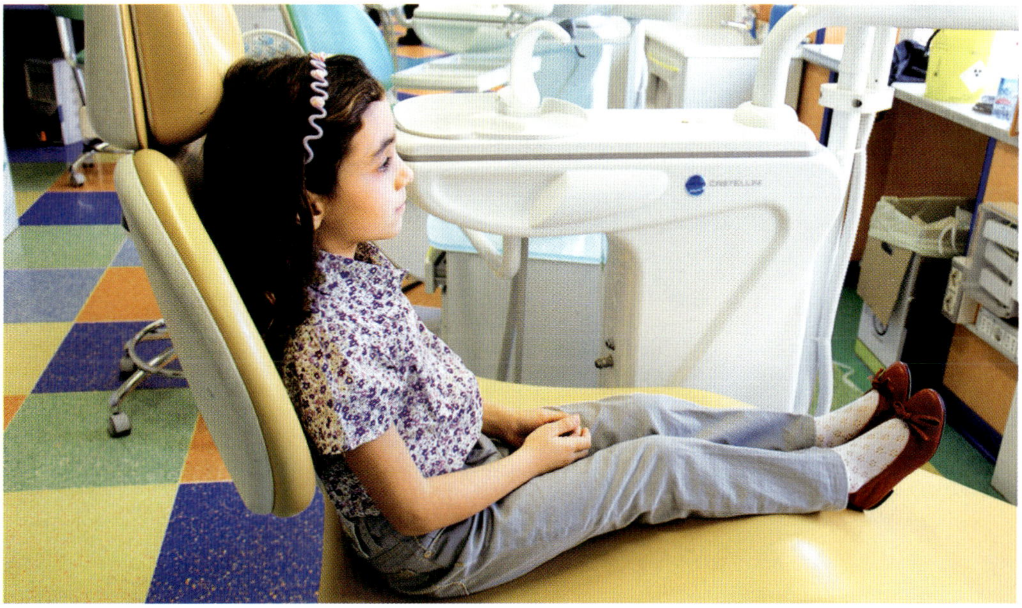

Figure 3.1 Position for extraoral examination.

The examination continues with the evaluation of the *general appearance of the skin*: color, trophism, presence of abnormalities such as moles, scars, herpetic manifestations, rhagades, previous traumatic lesions, cutaneous fistulas, allergic reactions, or presence of mouth breathing.
This is followed by *symmetrical facial* evaluation, considering that slight asymmetries can be considered perfectly normal. To perform this evaluation, the operator stands in front of the child and analyses symmetry according to the vertical and horizontal reference planes (Fig. 3.2).

- vertical line of symmetry
- horizontal superciliary line
- horizontal bipupillary line
- horizontal line of nose wings
- horizontal line of oral fissure

The *vertical line of symmetry* is an imaginary line passing through three reference points: glabella, subnasal point, and menton (Fig. 3.3).
Facial symmetry evaluation aims to raise the diagnostic suspicion on bone base or soft tissue abnormalities:

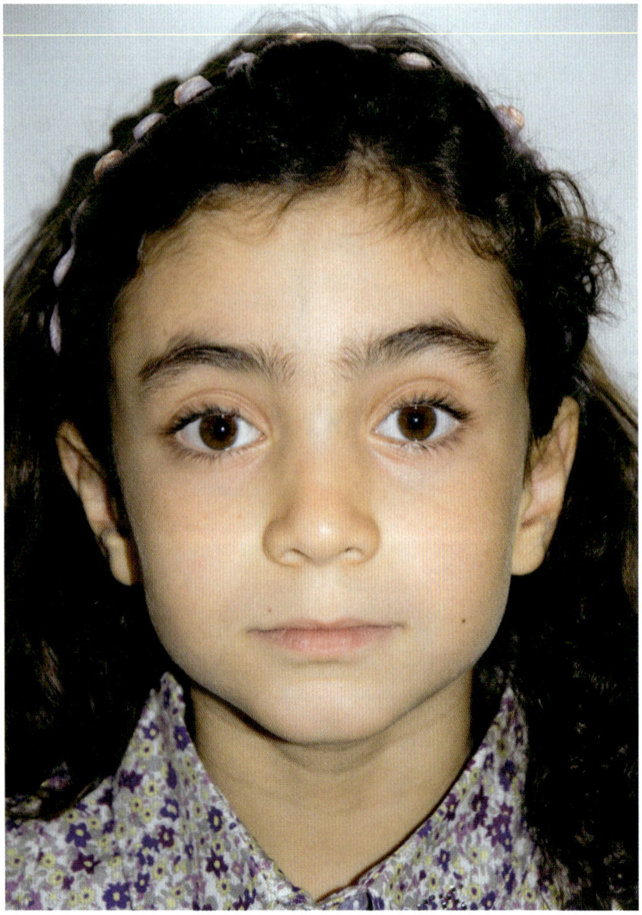

Figure 3.2 Frontal examination of child.

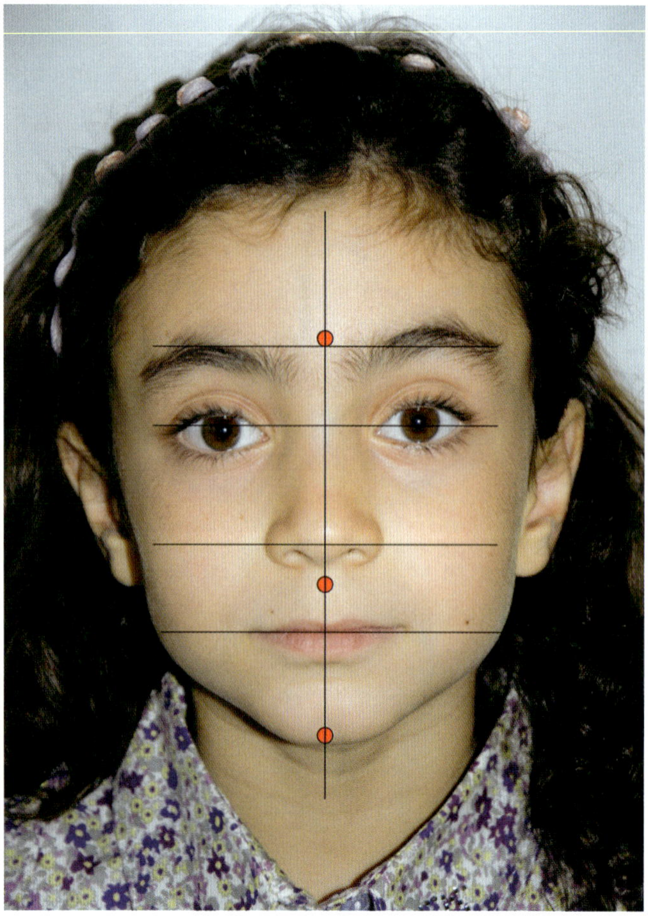

Figure 3.3 Facial symmetry lines.

- hypoplasia or hyperplasia of the jaw
- skeletal and condylar asymmetries
- mandibular lateral deviations
- swollen lymph nodes
- glandular swellings
- infectious swellings (abscess or phlegmon)
- neuromuscular abnormalities (facial nerve paralysis)

The abnormalities detected will be subsequently investigated and integrated with the medical history, intraoral examinations, and auxiliary investigations (x-ray examinations).
This is followed by the frontal examination of the child to evaluate the *facial type* and lip appearance. By comparing the vertical and diagonal facial dimensions, it is possible to classify patients as normofacial, brachyfacial, and dolichofacial.
In the first case, the facial growth is proportionate in both dimensions; in the second case, horizontal growth is prevalent and the face tends to be larger and shorter; in the third case, vertical growth is prevalent and the face tends to be longer and narrower. Furthermore, the facial type determines the different muscular typology that intervenes in growth. This evaluation should be taken into consideration in pediatric diagnosis and treatment planning.
It is important to evaluate *lip appearance*. In children, it is possible to find abnormalities in terms of posture, competence, tone, length, and particularly, bad habits; therefore, lip appearance is fundamental in diagnosis and treatment planning (Fig. 3.4).

It is necessary to take into consideration the following characteristics:

- general appearance
- color

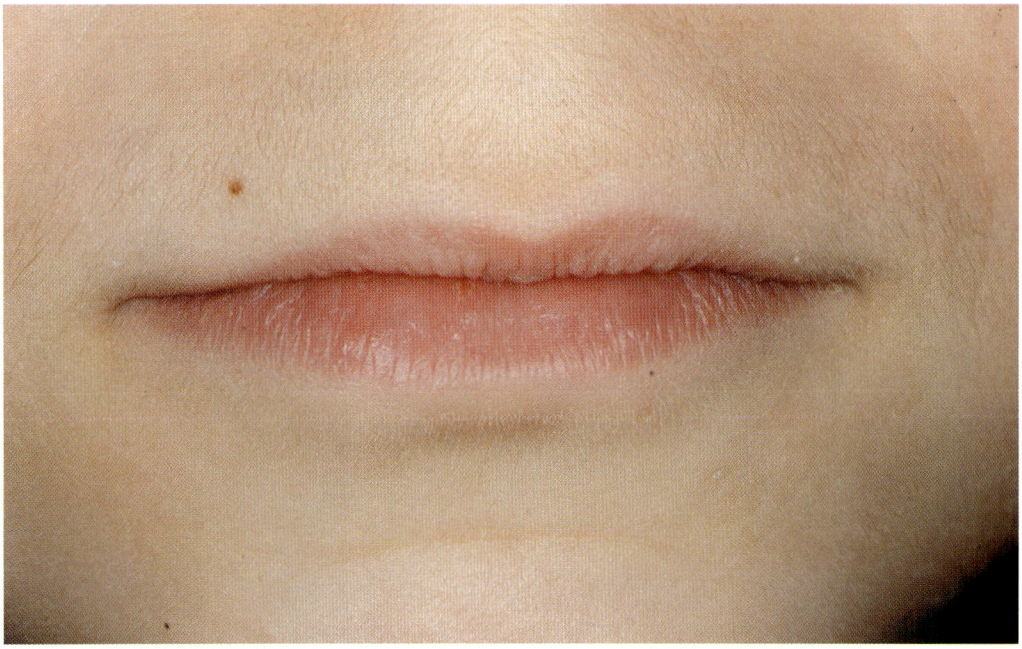

Figure 3.4 Lip examination.

- trophism
- length
- competence
- possible presence of rhagades at the commissures

Subsequently, the practitioner places himself/herself on the right and then on the left of the child to perform the *lateral facial evaluation*. It is possible to evaluate and confirm some elements already taken into consideration, such as facial type, by observing facial sizes and gonial angle appearance (narrower in the brachyfacial type, larger in the dolichofacial one).

Profile evaluation is fundamental for the identification of disharmonies in facial growth and esthetics (Fig. 3.5). The simplest and most direct method to perform this evaluation is to refer to an esthetic plan that passes from the tip of the nose to the most protruding point of the chin (Fig. 3.6). To make things easier, it is possible to use a mirror handle or a stretched thread between the reference points.

To perform the evaluation more accurately, it is possible to perform a real esthetic analysis using latero-lateral teleradiography of the skull or the lateral photography of the patient.

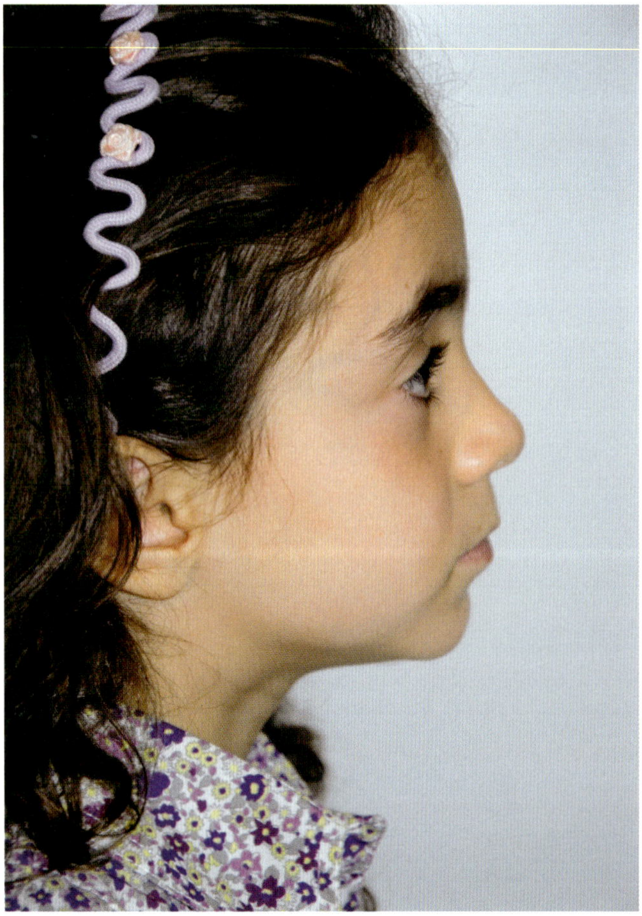

Figure 3.5 Lateral examination of child.

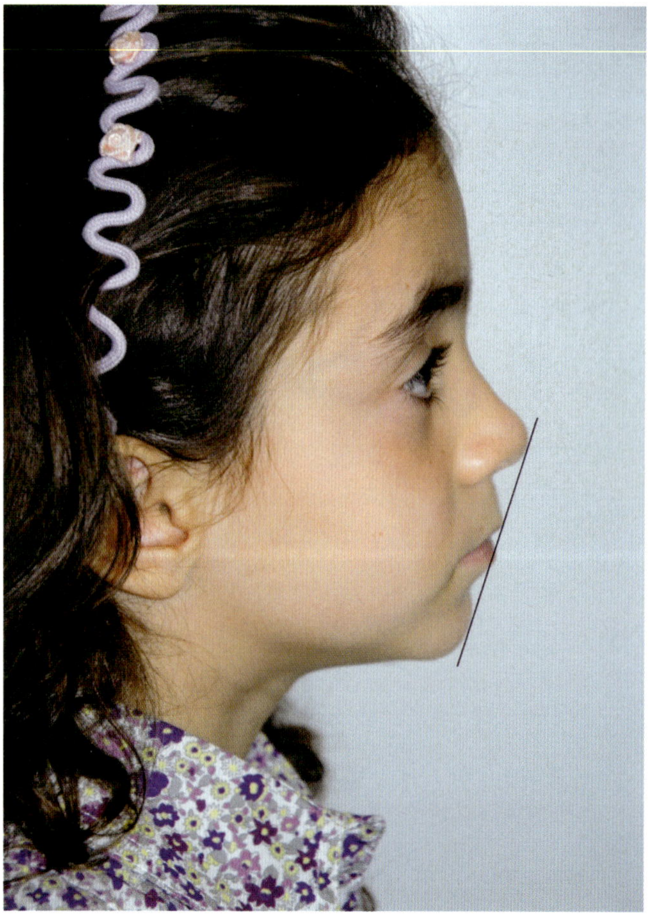

Figure 3.6 Profile esthetic line.

Physiologically, it is possible to distinguish several profile types:

- harmonious: the lips touch the plane or are 1–2 mm apart
- convex: it is characterized by a protrusion of the lips beyond the plane (Fig. 3.7)
- concave: the lips are positioned within the plane (Fig. 3.8).

The examination is completed with the palpation of the *lymph nodes* of the head and neck region (Fig. 3.9). To evaluate the symmetry of possible abnormalities, palpation should be performed bilaterally with both hands.

Therefore, it is necessary to take into consideration the following characteristics:

- symmetry
- volume
- mobility
- tenderness.

The involvement of multiple and symmetric lymph nodes indicates a systemic infectious origin; conversely, the involvement of a single and unilateral lymph node generally indicates a local infectious origin.

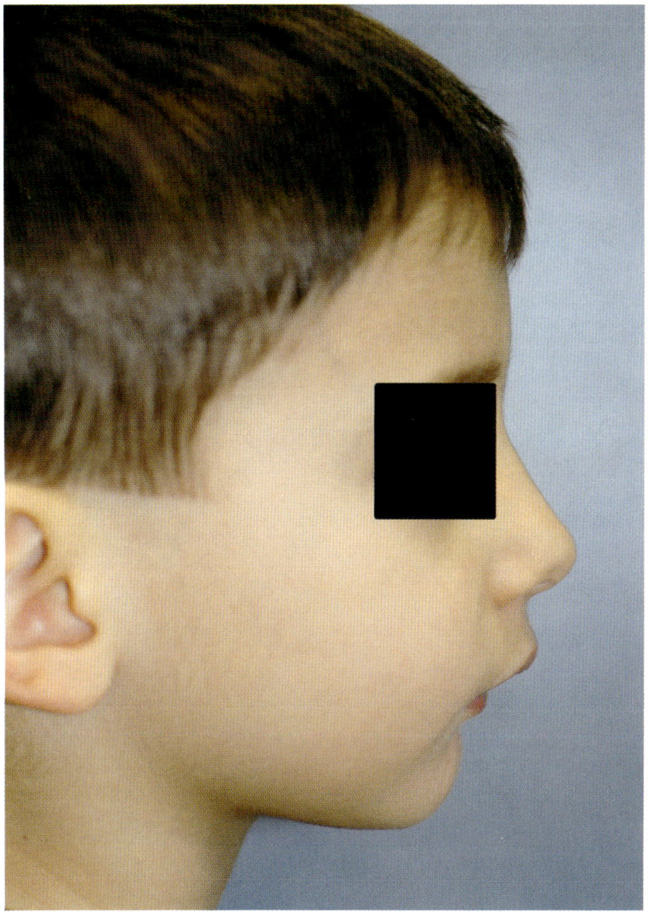

Figure 3.7 Convex profile.

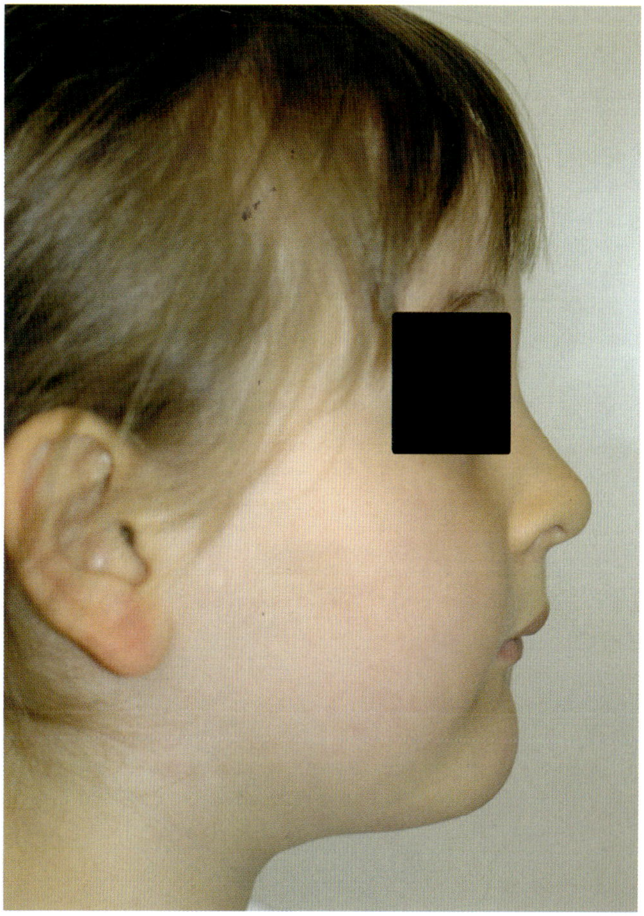

Figure 3.8 Concave profile.

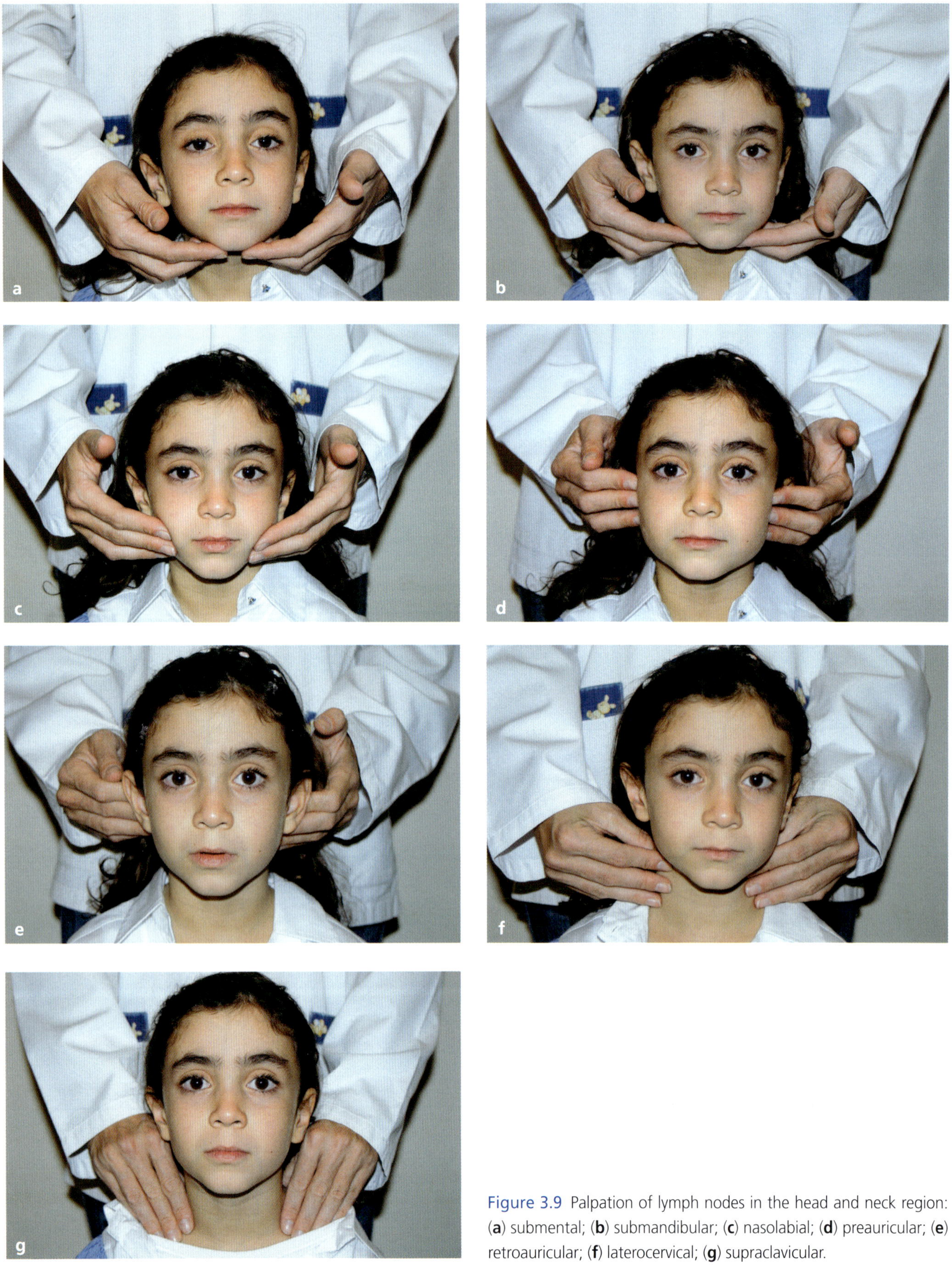

Figure 3.9 Palpation of lymph nodes in the head and neck region: (**a**) submental; (**b**) submandibular; (**c**) nasolabial; (**d**) preauricular; (**e**) retroauricular; (**f**) laterocervical; (**g**) supraclavicular.

Lymph node examination should be performed at the following locations:

- submental region
- submandibular region
- nasolabial region
- preauricular region
- retroauricular region
- laterocervical region
- clavicular region

The practitioner positions himself/herself behind the patient and performs palpation by following the procedure reported in the list. The following precautions should always be taken into consideration:

- during the palpation of submental and submandibular lymph nodes, it is necessary to ask the child to tilt his/her head slightly forward in order to relax neck muscles
- in order to identify the nasolabial lymph node, it is necessary to identify the anterior margin of the masseter muscle by asking the child to clench his/her teeth (as the lymph node is positioned in front of this margin)
- for the latero-cervical lymph nodes, it is necessary to rotate the child's head on the palpation side in order to relax the sternocleidomastoid muscle

Intraoral Clinical Examination

In order to perform the intraoral examination, it is necessary to maintain the correct positions on the chair. In this case, it is necessary to use the dental unit lamp.
For quadrants I and II, the child should be positioned with the chair reclining so as to keep the occlusal plane perpendicular to the floor; the practitioner positions himself/herself behind the child at the 11'clock position and performs the examination with indirect vision using the mirror (Figs. 3.10 and 3.11). For quadrants III and IV, the child should be positioned with the chair in the straight position such that the occlusal plane is parallel to the floor; the practitioner positions himself/herself at the 11 o'clock position and performs the examination with direct vision for quadrant III, moving along soft tissues using the mirror (Fig. 3.12); the practitioner positions himself/herself lateral to the child at the 9 o'clock position and performs the examination with a direct vision of quadrant IV (Fig. 3.13).
When examining a very young child (0–3 years) who does not cooperate during positioning on the chair, it is necessary to use another procedure that requires the parent's help: the so-called *knee-to-knee* position. The practitioner and parent sit facing each other with their knees in contact; the child, who is in the parent's arms, is positioned with the head on the practitioner's legs; the parent holds the child's arms; in this manner, the practitioner can proceed with the examination and the treatment maneuvers (Fig. 3.14).
This is followed by the evaluation of hard and soft tissues. In this case as well, the practitioner can choose the order to follow; it is recommended to be methodical and schematic: always repeating the same procedure ensures that no element is neglected.

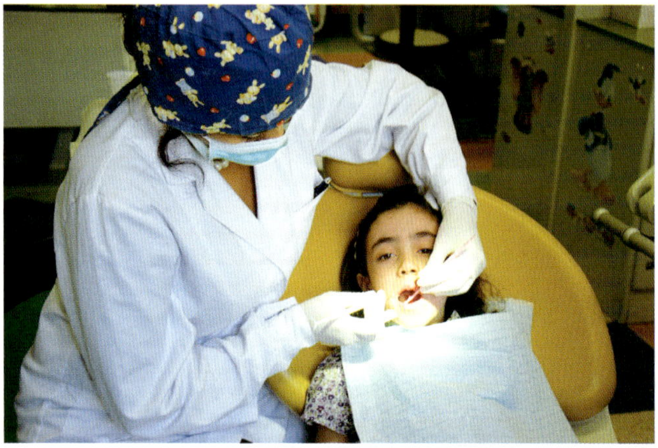

Figure 3.10 Assessment of quadrant I.

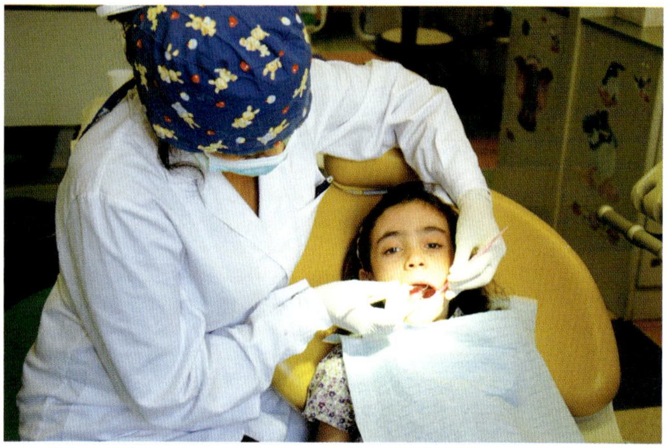

Figure 3.11 Assessment of quadrant II.

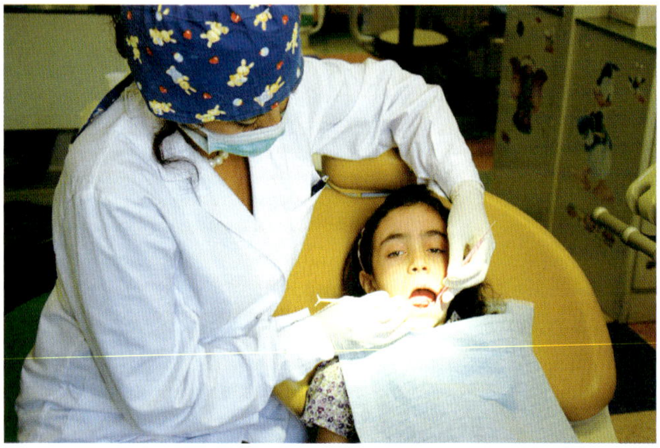

Figure 3.12 Assessment of quadrant III.

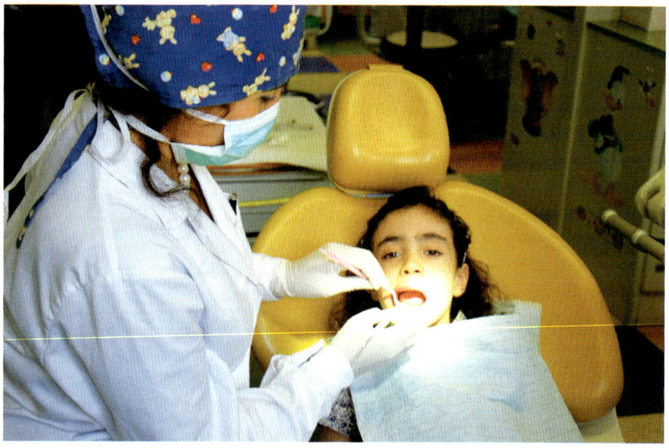

Figure 3.13 Assessment of quadrant IV.

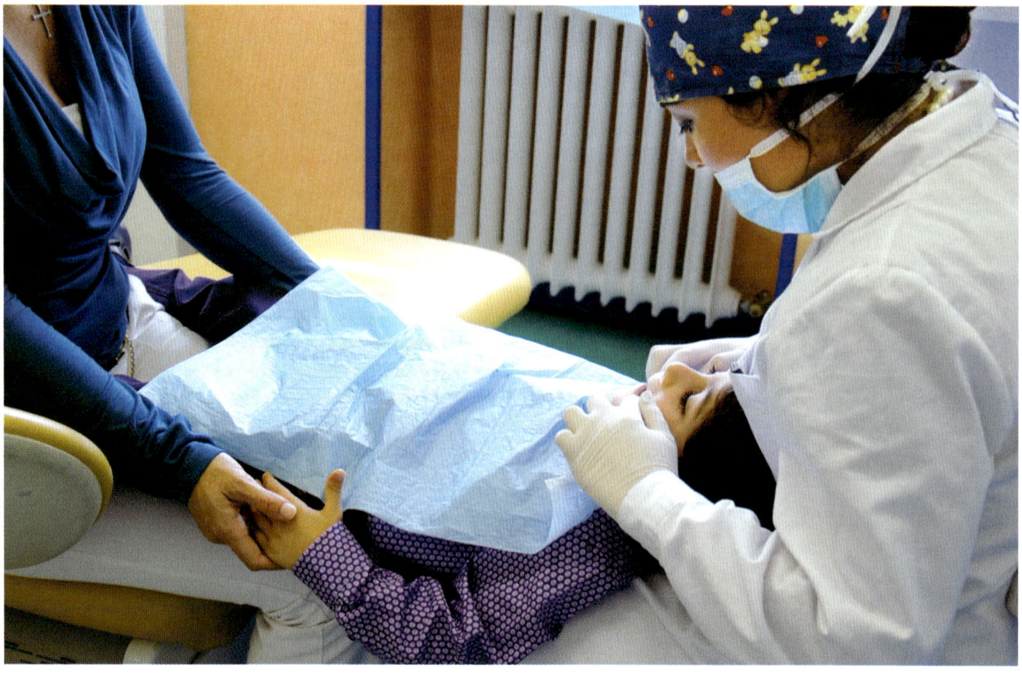

Figure 3.14 *Knee-to-knee* position.

Examination of hard tissues

The examination of arches should consider several characteristics. It is then possible to proceed with assessment of the teeth and specillation in search of carious lesions. It is possible to perform a general evaluation of arches initially and a more accurate intra-arch and inter-arch evaluation subsequently.

The arch shape should be analyzed and dental formula should be recorded using the WHO teeth numbering system (Figs. 3.15 and 3.16); subsequently, the presence of diastemas and dental anomalies in terms of number, shape, volume, structure, carious lesions, abrasions, enamel infractions or enamel fractures, discoloring and hypoplasia, is evaluated (Fig. 3.17).

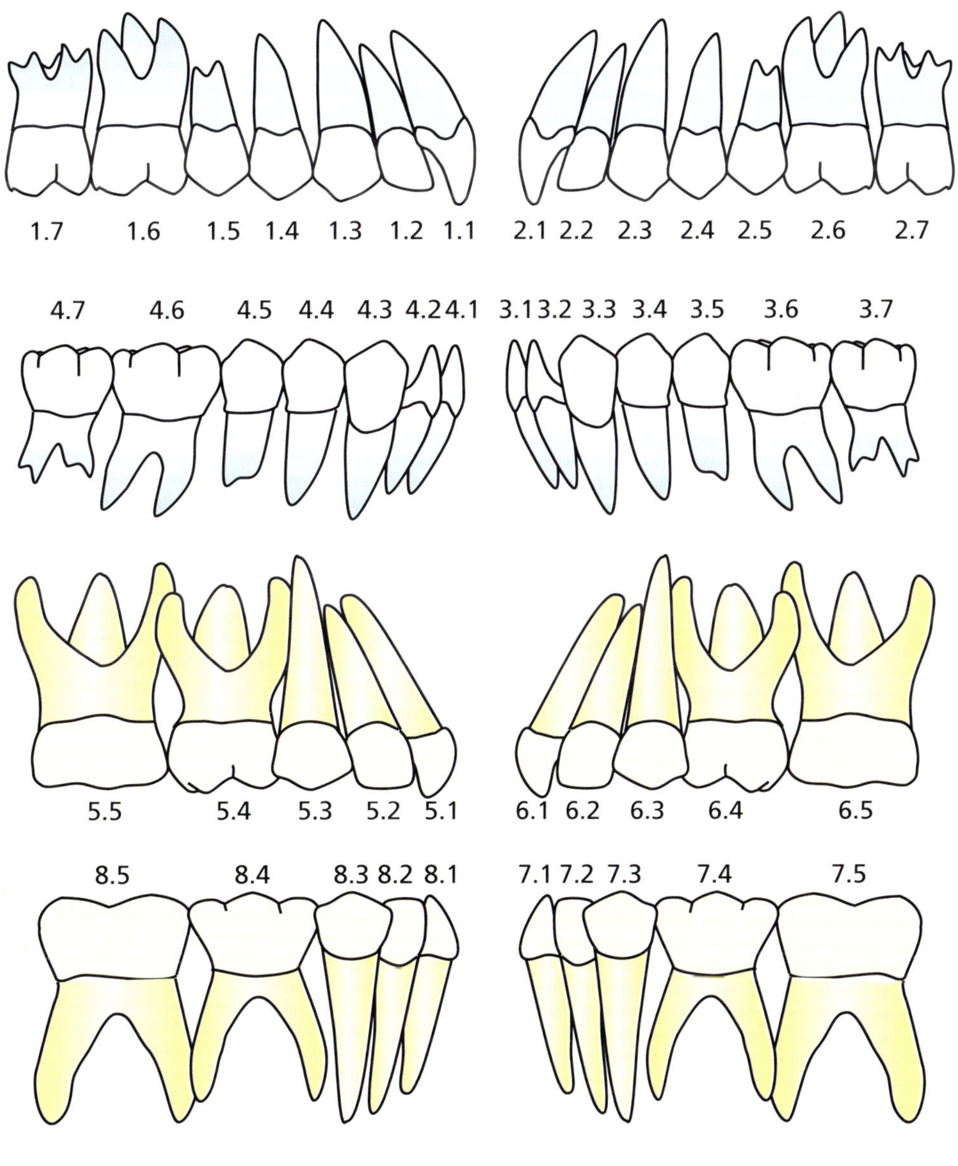

Figure 3.15 WHO dental formula of deciduous and permanent dentition.

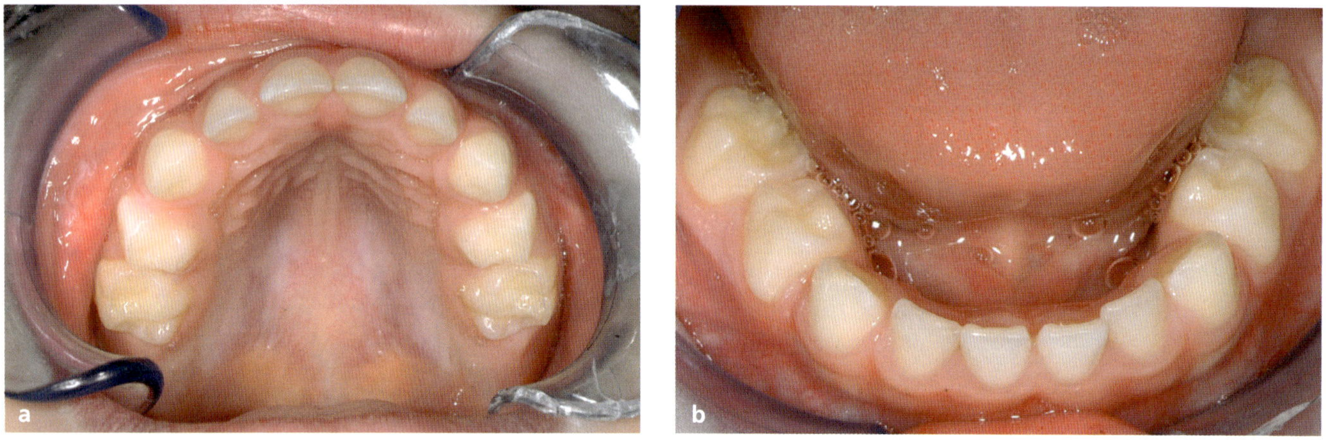

Figure 3.16 (**a**) Assessment of the upper deciduous arch. (**b**) Assessment of the lower deciduous arch.

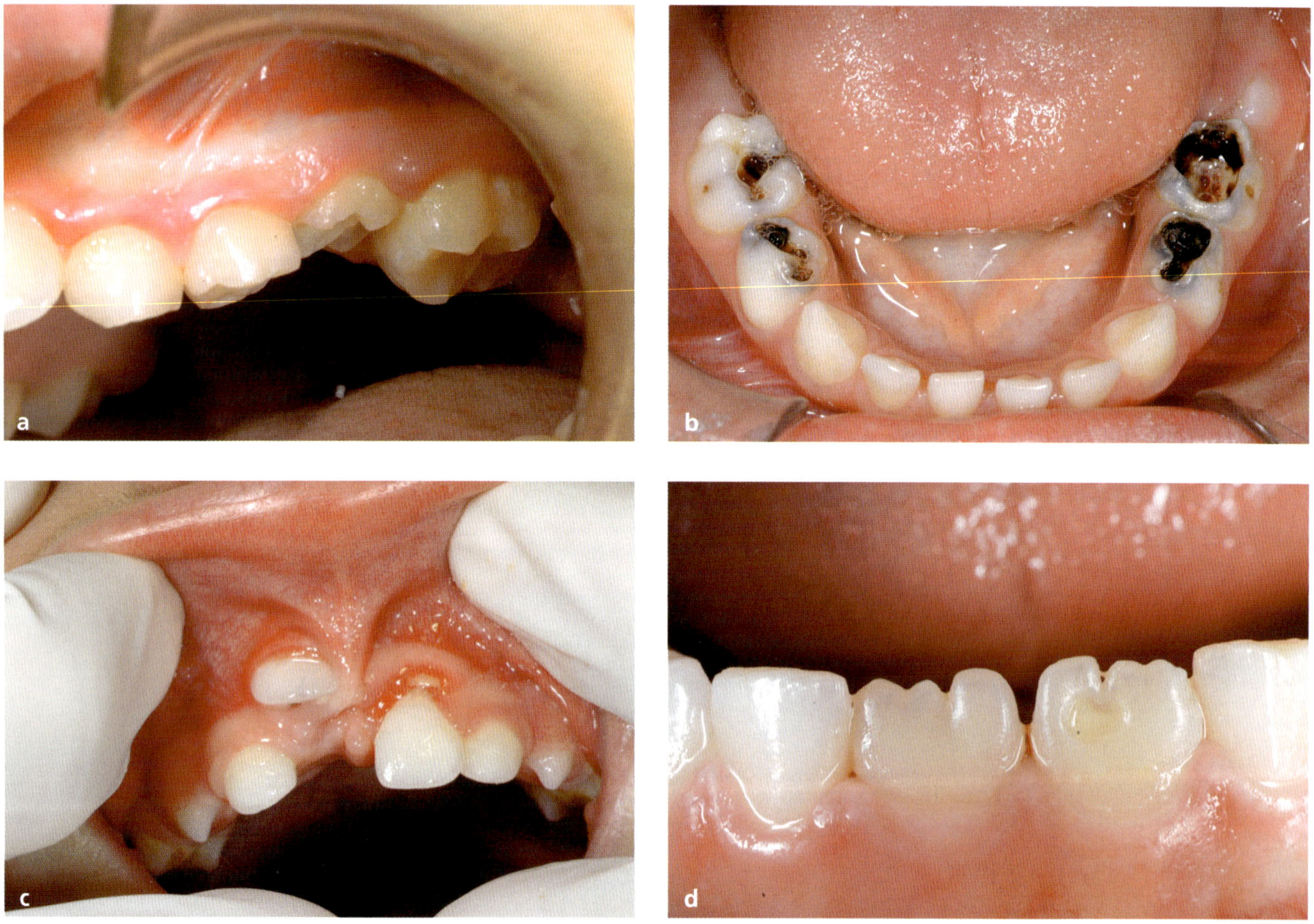

Figure 3.17 (**a**) Infra-occluded ankylotic deciduous element. (**b**) Carious lesions. (**c**) Intrusive trauma of 5.1. (**d**) Hypoplasia of 3.1 following trauma of the deciduous element.

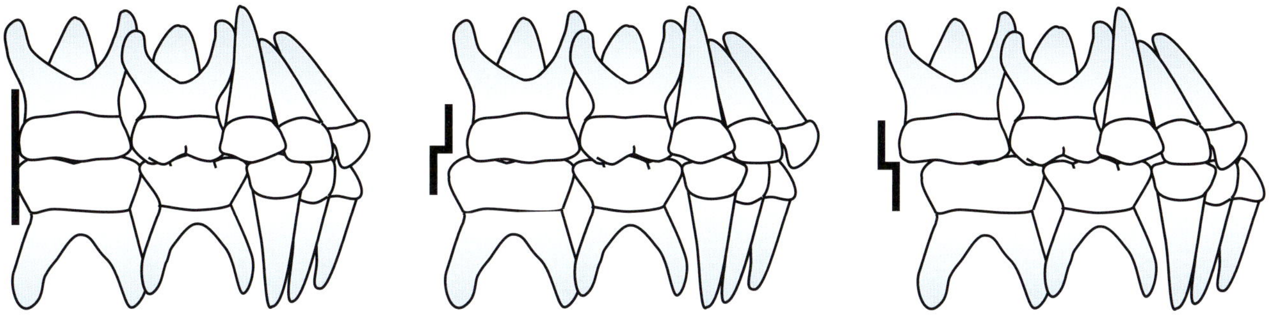

Figure 3.18 Ratios among deciduous second molars.

Subsequently, the inter-arch evaluation to assess the child's occlusal characteristics is performed. On the sagittal plane, overjet, canine ratio (deciduous or permanent), molar ratio (in the presence of first permanent molars), or terminal plane (in the presence of secondary deciduous molars only; Fig. 3.18) are identified and recorded. Overbite can be identified and recorded on the frontal plane, whereas physiological arch expansion can be identified and recorded on the transverse plane (Fig. 3.19–1.24). Other occlusal anomalies, such as crossbites (class II or III), increased overjets, deep bites, crowding, or space deficits, are identified and recorded on the three planes.

Examination of soft tissues

The examination of soft tissues aims to detect possible abnormalities in terms of color, trophism, shape, volume, and consistency, whether associated with pain symptomatology or not.

The procedure starts with the periodontal examination: general gum appearance, color, shape, gingival scaling, and orange peel appearance (Fig. 3.25). The presence of gingival phlogosis, localized or diffuse hyperplasia, plaque and tartar accumulations, gingival recessions, and pigmentations should be noted in the clinical record (Fig. 3.26).

A periodontal survey should be performed to identify any periodontal pockets or fistulas.

This is followed by the inspection of the buccal mucosa and fornices, moving the lips and cheeks aside using the mirror or fingers for better observation (Fig. 3.27–3.29).

In particular, it is necessary to examine the parotid duct outlet (in correspondence with the maxillary first molar) to identify inflammatory processes and the buccal mucosa to identify the presence of clinical signs associated with systemic infective pathologies.

This is followed by the examination of palatal mucosa and the oral floor (Fig. 3.30). For the latter, it is necessary to ask the child to lift the tongue or move it by pulling it with a piece of gauze; during the examination, check the outlet of sublingual glands (caruncles) and search for the presence of phlogoses and swelling.

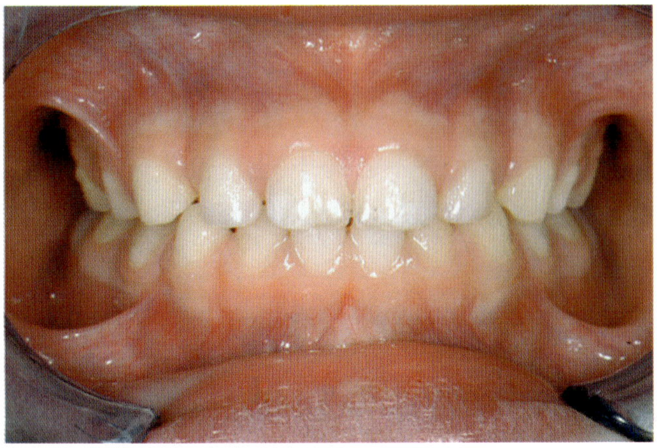

Figure 3.19 Assessment of frontal occlusion in the deciduous dentition.

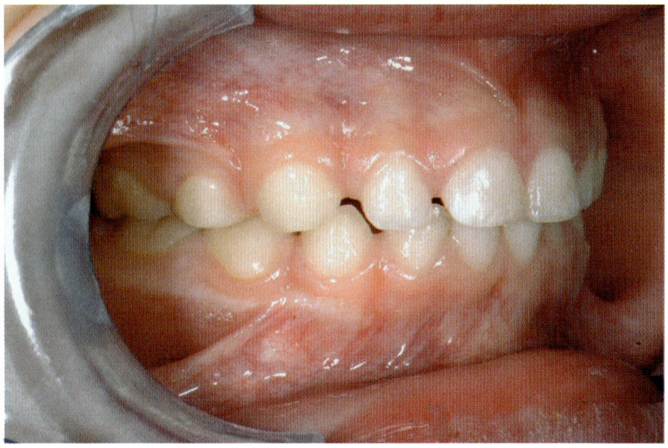

Figure 3.20 Assessment of lateral occlusion in the deciduous dentition.

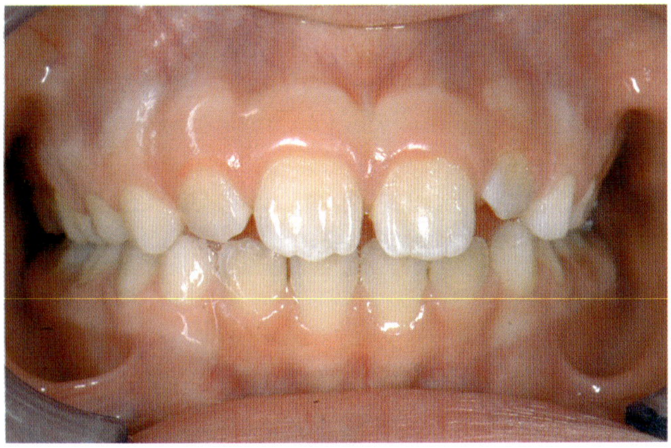

Figure 3.21 Assessment of frontal occlusion in the mixed dentition.

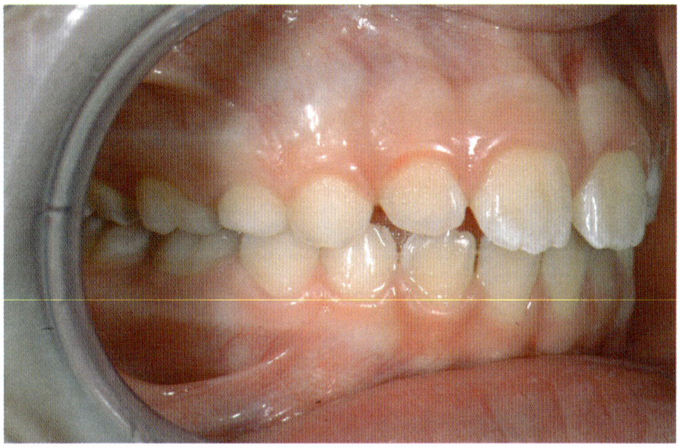

Figure 3.22 Assessment of lateral occlusion in the mixed dentition.

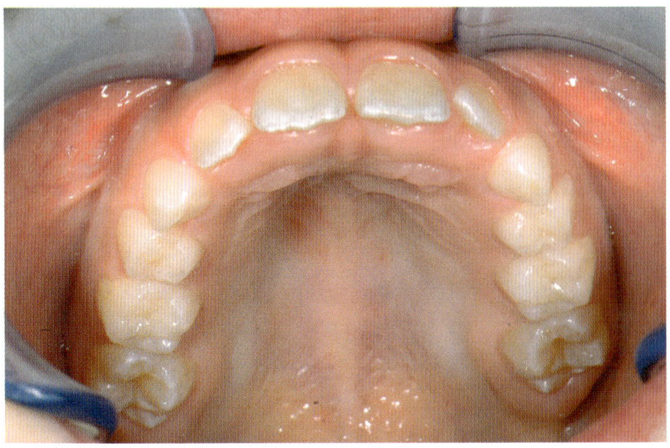

Figure 3.23 Assessment of upper arch in the mixed dentition.

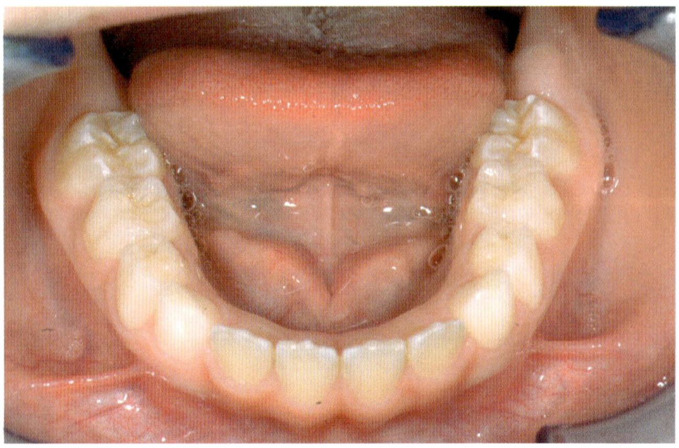

Figure 3.20 Assessment of lower occlusion in the mixed dentition.

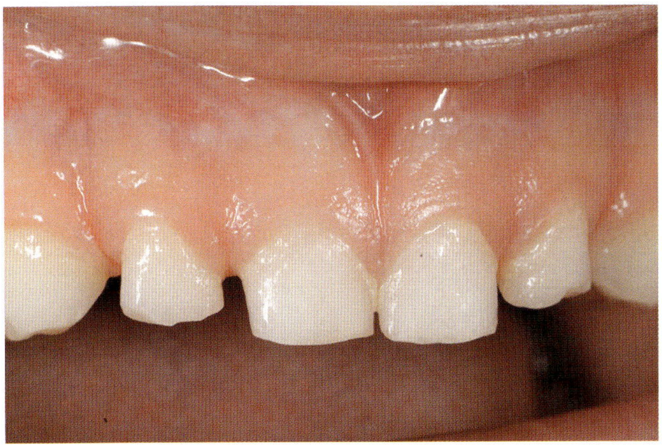

Figure 3.25 Periodontal examination.

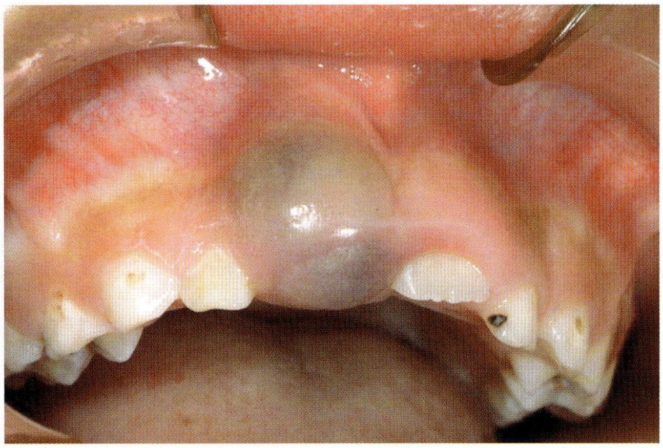

Figure 3.26 Eruption cyst.

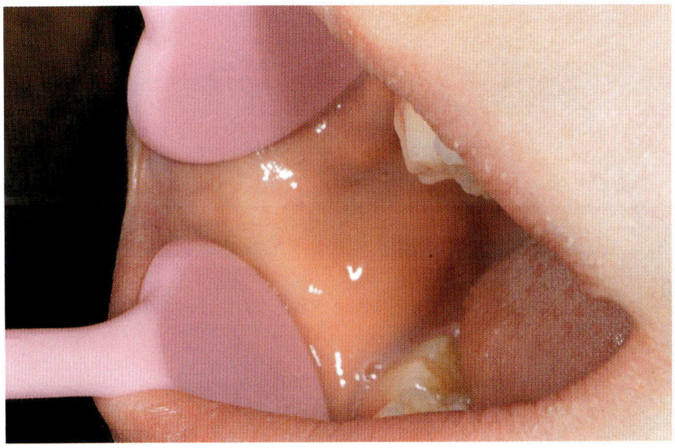

Figure 3.27 Examination of the buccal mucosa.

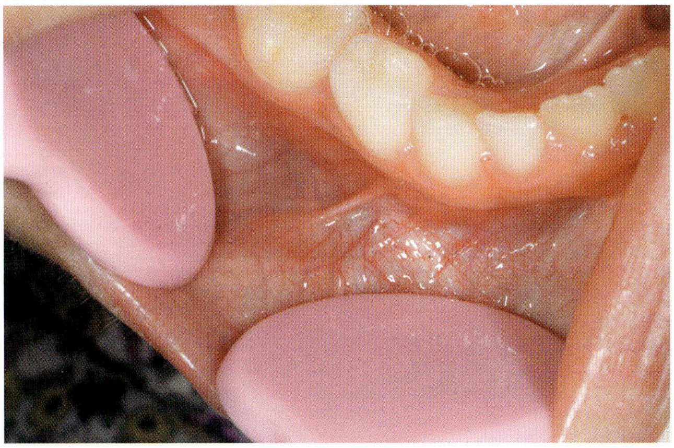

Figure 3.28 Examination of fornices.

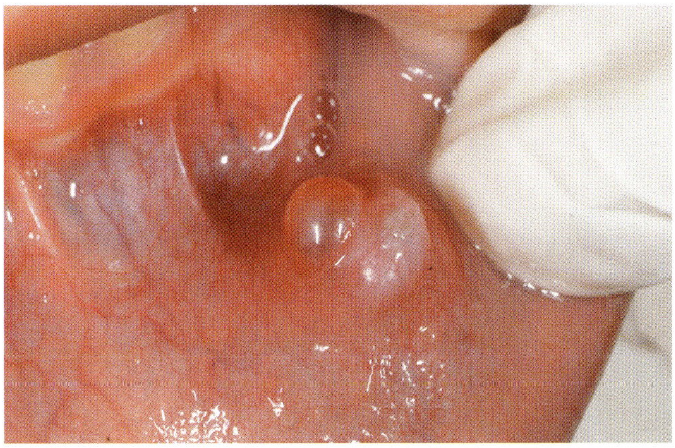

Figure 3.29 Cyst of the lip mucosa.

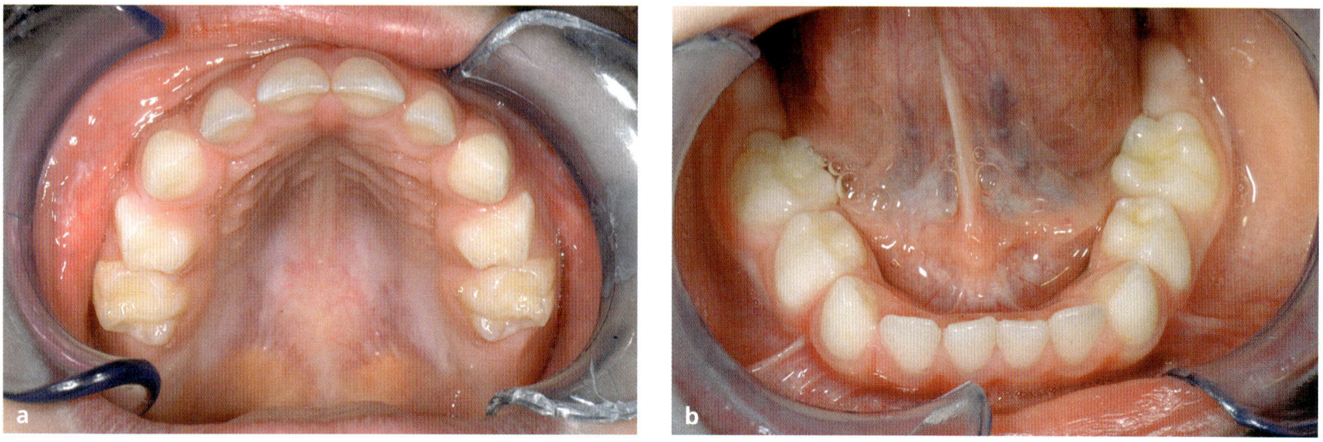

Figure 3.30 Examination of the (**a**) palatal mucosa and (**b**) oral floor.

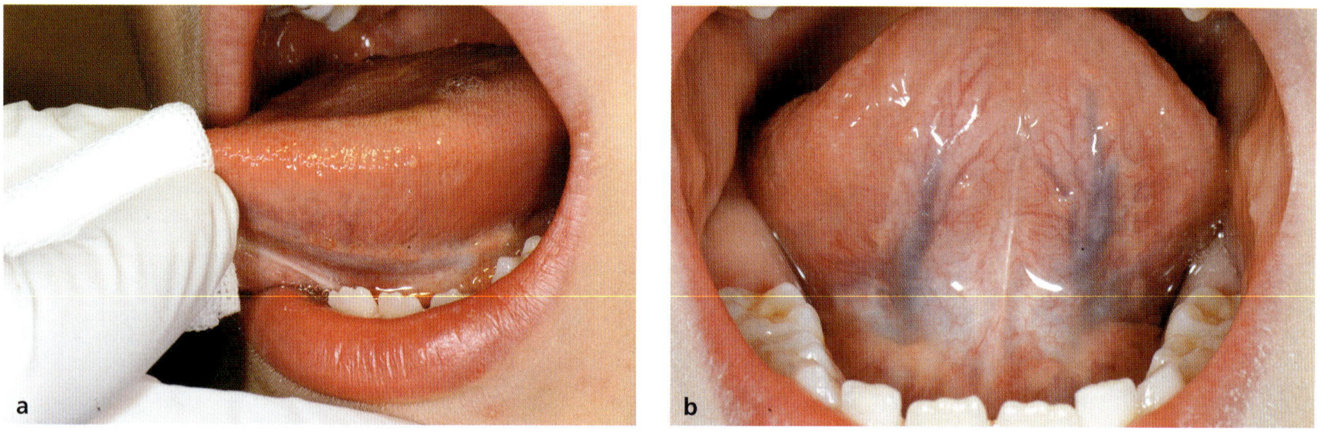

Figure 3.31 Examination of the (**a**) lingual margins and (**b**) lingual frenulum.

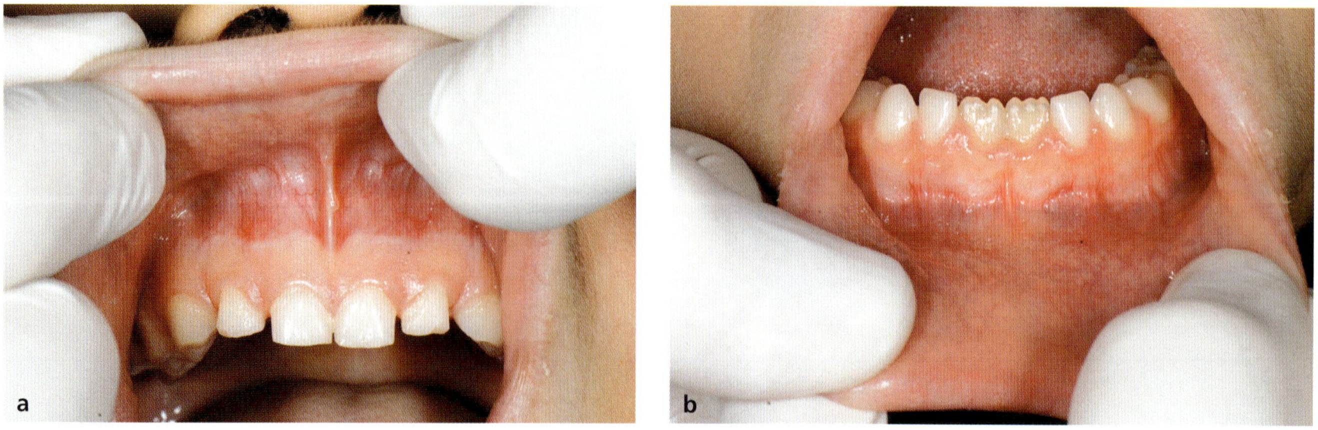

Figure 3.32 Examination of the (**a**) upper and (**b**) lower median frenulum.

Subsequently, the tongue should be examined by evaluating its shape, position, and length. The observation starts with the examination of the back, up to the circumvallate papillae, and ends with the examination of the margins. To correctly observe the lingual mucosa and margins, the practitioner can hold the tip of the tongue with a piece of gauze and gently move it outwards and sideways. It is possible to examine the lingual frenulum by asking the child to lift the tongue toward the palate in order to assess the size, length, and insertion to identify any ankyloglossia (Fig. 3.31).
Thereafter, it is possible to assess the size, length, and insertion of vestibular frenula via a pulling movement on the child's lips (Fig. 3.32). In particular, the short and fibrous median upper vestibular frenulum can be associated with a median diastema; in this case, the pulling of the upper lip and, therefore, of the frenulum will highlight an interdental papilla ischemization. The short and fibrous median lower vestibular frenulum can be associated with periodontal complications (pulling the frenulum) with the presence of gingival recession at the expense of the lower central incisors.

Functional Evaluation

Respiratory Evaluation

In children in whom a suspicion of mouth breathing arises from the analysis of medical history and clinical examination results, additional tests can be performed to confirm the suspicion. In any case, correct and complete diagnosis should be performed by an otolaryngologist.
There are three tests:

1. Gudin's nostril reflex test
2. Rosenthal's test
3. Glatzel mirror test.

The first test consists of compressing the nose wings using the fingers for 2 seconds, then releasing them, and checking for the presence of hypertension in the nose wings themselves. In mouth breathers, the outcome of this test is negative; in other words, no reflex can be detected as the child is not accustomed to balancing the small apnea with the nose.
The second test consists of instructing the child to take twenty breaths with the mouth closed, first using both nostrils and then using just one nostril, closing the left and right nostril alternately using a finger. If the child does not manage to finish the test, he/she should open the mouth to be able to breathe.
The third test can be performed using a Glatzel mirror or, alternatively, with a normal mirror. The test evaluates the areas reflected by the mirror under the child's nose. The Glatzel mirror has several concentric circles to measure these areas; usually, there should be symmetrical areas with a height of seven and a base of three. The mirror can identify monolateral or bilateral nasal obstructions.

Swallowing Examination

The analysis of swallowing modalities is very important because, following the principle of shape and function, the tongue serves as a real functional matrix for the correct development of the arches. In fact, these are included in the so-called "muscular corridor," which is defined externally by the perioral musculature (lips and cheeks) and internally by the lingual musculature. Muscle balance permits the harmonious and coordinated development of the two arches; any alteration of this balance is a risk factor for malocclusion, which frequently occurs as a result of bad habits. The swallowing pattern develops from the typical pattern of infants to that of adults, gradually passing through a series of stages, including neuromuscular development, weaning, tooth eruption, and phonetic development. In some children, atypical swallowing might persist, and this should be diagnosed and detected. Therefore, the practitioner should ask the child to swallow and look in front of the perioral musculature (Fig. 3.33).
In the presence of an atypical swallowing pattern, it is possible to assess the contraction of this musculature (lips and chin), which should balance the anterior lingual thrust to maintain the mouth seal. Usually, the perioral musculature does not contract during swallowing.
Subsequently, the lips should be distanced: the practitioner should hold the lips with the finger (thumb and forefinger), ask the child to swallow, and simultaneously spread the lips to observe the anterior and/or lateral lingual interposition (Fig. 3.34), which is a sign of atypical swallowing (Fig. 3.35).
The lingual frenulum evaluation should not be neglected in order to identify possible ankyloglossia, which should be detected early. In certain cases, it is possible to perform a more accurate evaluation using the Payne technique, which consists of marking the

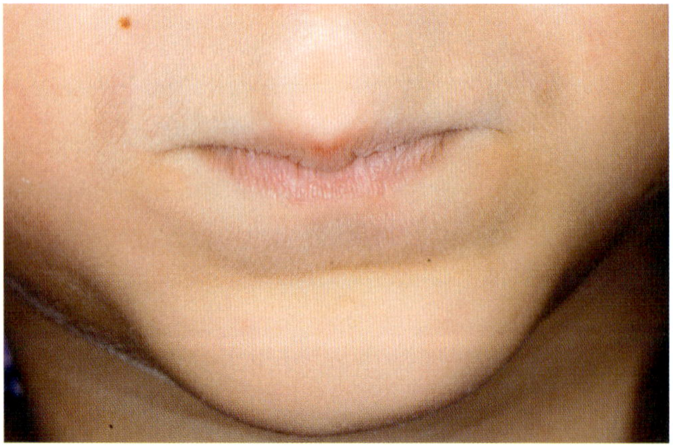

Figure 3.33 Contraction of the perioral musculature during swallowing.

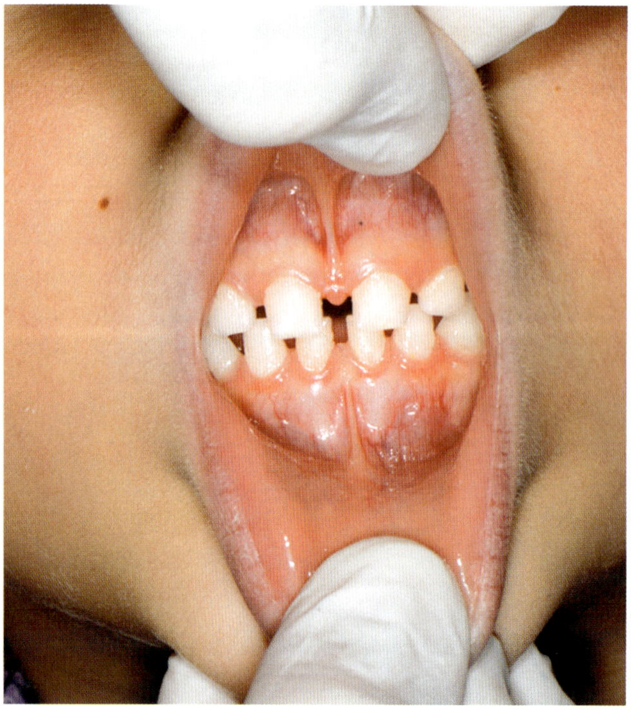

Figure 3.34 Separation of the lips.

tongue tip and margins with a fluorescent substance (fluorescein), asking the child to swallow, and observing the marked points on the palatal mucosa.

Vitality Test

This is a very important auxiliary test used to monitor dental vitality in the following cases:

- when examining traumatized teeth
- when making a treatment decision between pulpotomy and pulpectomy in case of deep caries
- when monitoring the success of conservative treatment over time
- when evaluating dental elements whose root has come into contact with elements such as impacted teeth, supernumerary teeth, or cysts

The practitioner can perform thermal or electrical tests. The simplest, most direct, and least invasive methodology is to perform the test in cold conditions using commercially available products based on tetrafluoroethane or other similar substances (Fig. 3.36).

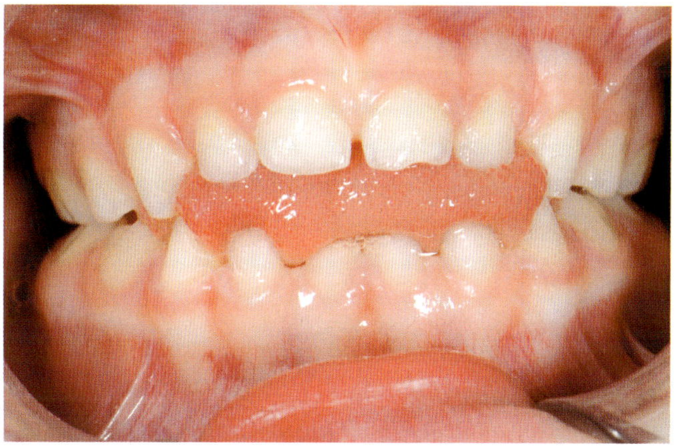

Figure 3.35 Atypical swallowing.

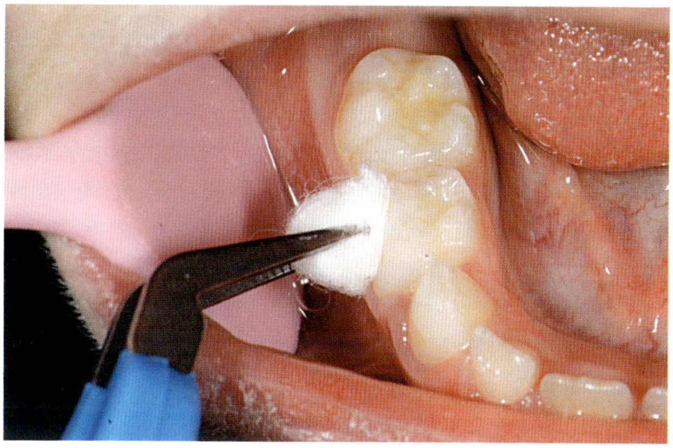

Figure 3.36 Vitality test.

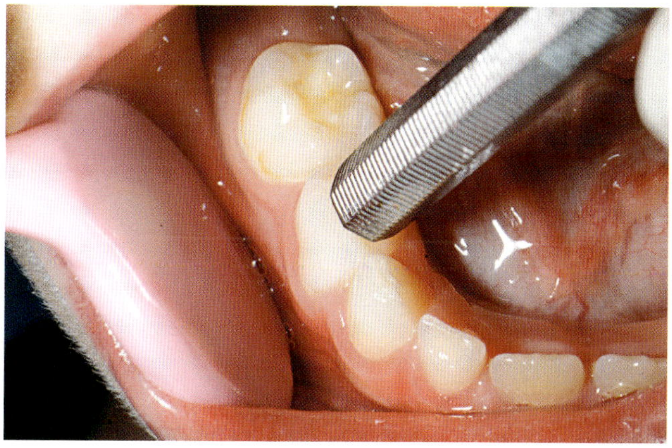

Figure 3.37 Percussion test.

These products, in the form of sprays, are applied on the concerned tooth using tweezers and cotton swabs. It is recommended to dry the surface before applying the product in cold conditions and to perform the test on teeth adjacent to the concerned tooth because the child may occasionally give false positive or negative answers.

Percussion

The percussion test is performed using the handle of a mirror on the concerned tooth (Fig. 3.37).
In this case as well, performing the test on adjacent teeth is recommended as the child may give false positive or negative answers.
The percussion test is used in the following cases:

- to assess tenderness in the case of apical periodontitis
- to assess noise in the case of ankylosed teeth.

In the latter case, as the tooth has lost periodontal support, it will emit a sound which is more muffled than the one emitted by a normal tooth. The diagnosis of ankylosis should, in any case, be confirmed using radiography.

Suggested Reading

American Academy of Pediatric Dentistry. Guidelines for management of the developing dentition in pediatric dentistry. Special issue: reference manual. Pediatr Dent 1998-1999;20:34-7.

American Academy of Pediatric Dentistry. Special issue: Reference manual 1998-99. Pediatr Dent 1998;20:72-4.

Andrews LF. The six keys to normal occlusion. Am J Orthod 1972;62:296-309.

Cameron AC, Widmer RP. Manuale di Pedodonzia. Milano: Masson; 2004.

Moskow BS, Barr CE. Examination of the patient. In: Goldman HM et al. Current therapy in dentistry, vol 4. St Louis: Mosby; 1970.

Okeson JP. Management of temporomandibular disorders and occlusion. 4th ed. St Louis: Mosby; 1993.

Staehle HJ, Koch MJ. Odontoiatria per l'infanzia e l'adolescenza. Milano: Masson; 1997.

Van Waes HJ, Stockli PW. Clinica Pedodontica. Milano: Masson; 2001.

Chapter 4

Characteristics and development of deciduous and permanent dentition

P. Cozza, E. Barbato, C. Chimenti

Regarding the development and emergence of permanent teeth, it is necessary to distinguish between two terms that are frequently used in dentistry: deciduous and permanent dentition. The term "*permanent dentition*" refers to a static period during which there is no modification in the number of dental elements present within the arch, whereas the term "*deciduous dentition*" refers to a dynamic situation during which there is emergence and subsequent eruption of dental elements within the arch.
Human dentition develops through distinctive and consecutive evolutionary phases (Fig. 4.1–4.3), leading to the appearance of the following elements:

- deciduous dentition: from 6 months to 6 years
- mixed dentition: from 6 to 12 years
- permanent dentition: from 12 years.

The deciduous dentition phase is followed by the mixed dentition phase, during which the dentition passes through an initial transition. The permanent dental elements that emerge in this phase include the central and lateral incisors and the first molars; the latter are monophyodont and therefore do not replace any deciduous element but erupt distally to the deciduous second molars.
The first transitional phase is followed by the physiological halting of development of dentition known as an "*intertransitional period*." This is a static period during which no changes occur within the oral cavity, which now comprises the central and lateral incisors, first permanent molars, canines, and first and second deciduous molars.

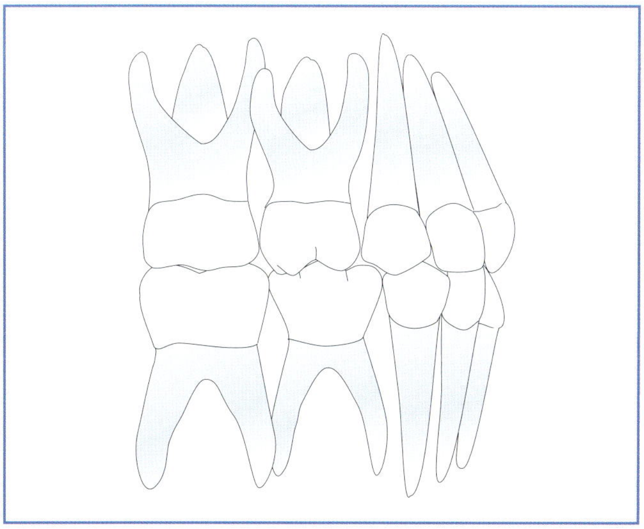

Figure 4.1 Dentition phases: deciduous dentition.

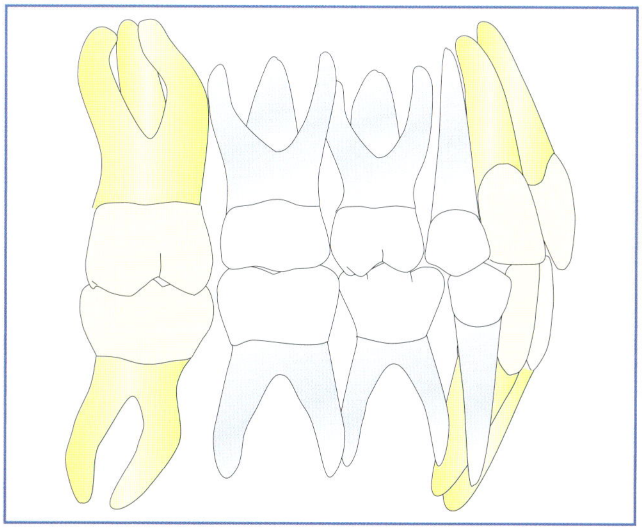

Figure 4.2 Dentition phases: mixed dentition.

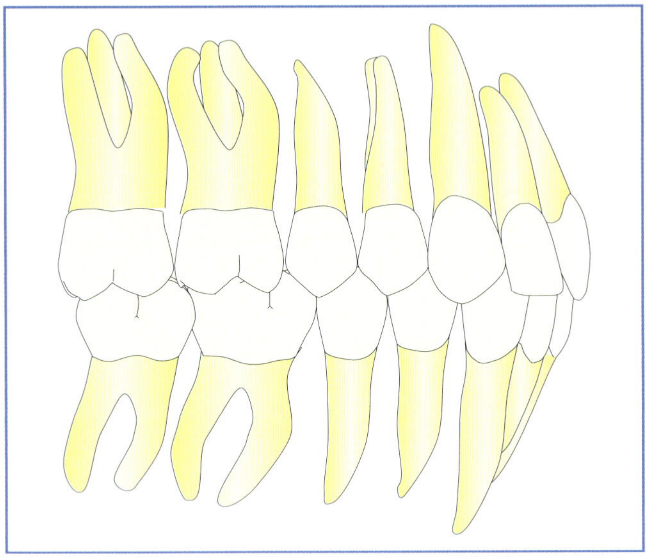

Figure 4.3 Dentition phases: permanent dentition.

This is followed by the second transitional phase during which exfoliation of the elements on the lateral arch regions occurs, and the canines and the first and second deciduous molars are replaced by canines and the first and second premolars, respectively. In this period, the second permanent molars erupt distally to the first than permanent molars to the complete dentition.
The precise moment of eruption of each tooth varies among individuals. A 6–8-month variability in the period of tooth eruption is considered normal.

Deciduous dentition

The deciduous dentition forms at approximately the sixth week of intrauterine life, whereas eruption initiates after birth at approximately 6 months of life and completes at approximately 36 months (Fig. 4.4).
This phase is generally characterized by considerable growth as well as morphological immaturity of all the craniomaxillofacial skeletal components (in particular, the jaw and temporomandibular joint). During this period, various functional elements represented by muscles, teeth, and bones, show a certain level of developmental instability so that growth-affecting factors may modify development. Therefore, the entire dentomaxillofacial complex is characterized by remarkable adaptability.

Eruption sequence of deciduous teeth

The first deciduous elements that erupt in the oral cavity include the lower central incisors (6 months), followed by the upper central incisors (10 months), the upper lateral incisors (11 months), and finally the lower lateral incisors (13 months). This eruption follows a typical "fountain-like pattern."

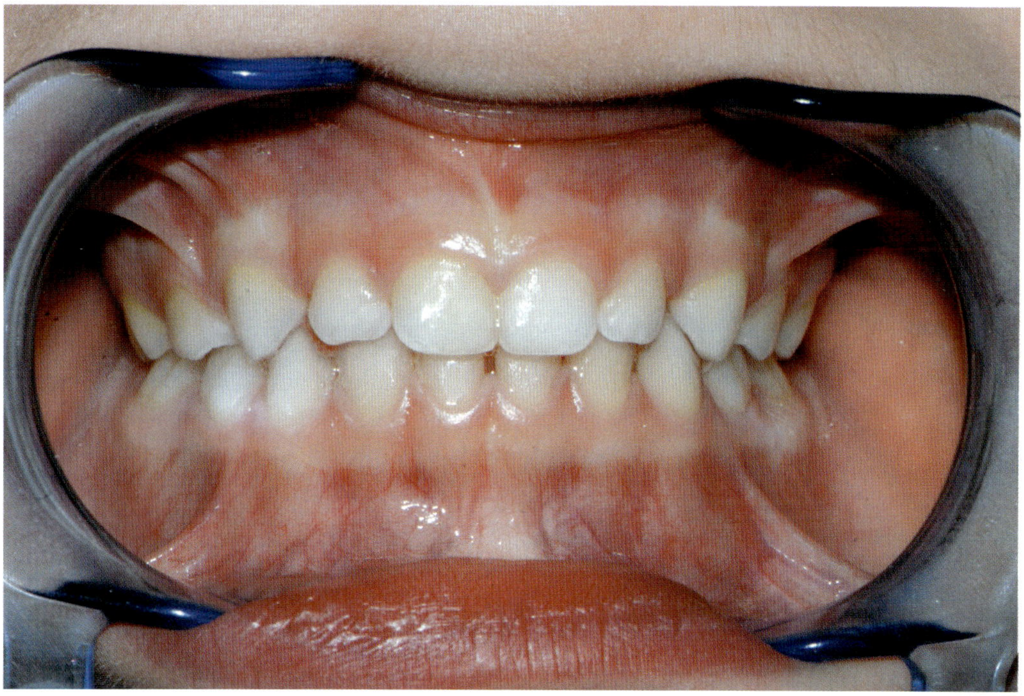

Figure 4.4 Deciduous dentition.

Subsequently, the eruption sequence progresses with the first molars (16 months), canines (20 months), and finally the lower (28) and upper (32 months) deciduous second molars.

From 36 months, upon the completion of the eruption phase of the deciduous dentition, to 6 years, no major changes can be observed in the deciduous dentition, and an initial static period defined as the *intertransitional period* is initiated. In fact, there are no changes in the number of elements; instead displacement of the teeth occurs particularly just before the exfoliation of the first deciduous elements because of the resorption of their roots by the permanent elements that are about to erupt.

Characteristics of deciduous teeth

Deciduous elements show certain characteristics that distinguish them from permanent elements.

Number. The deciduous physiological occlusion involves 20 dental elements belonging to three functional classes of teeth: incisors, canines, and molars.

Morphological groups. The primary dentition lacks the morphological group of premolars, which appear only in the secondary dentition to replace the deciduous molars.

Color. The reduced thickness and increased opacity of the enamel of the deciduous elements give them a typical milky color and therefore the name "milk teeth". This color the deciduous elements appears clearer compared with the yellowish to grayish appearance of the permanent elements. Usually, color is the first clear factor that differentiates a deciduous element from a permanent one; the only dental element that may be similar to the corresponding permanent one in terms of color and size is the deciduous canine.

Size. Generally, the mesiodistal dimensions of deciduous teeth are considered to be smaller those of permanent teeth; however, this is not true in all the arch regions. Undoubtedly, the deciduous teeth of the anterior region are smaller than the permanent ones that replace them. In fact, the mesiodistal diameters of the deciduous incisors and canines are approximately 75% and 85%, respectively, of the mesiodistal diameters of the corresponding permanent ones (Fig. 4.5 and 4.6). Conversely, the deciduous molars in the posterior region are larger than or almost equal to the premolars that replace them. The size of the first upper deciduous molar is essentially equal to that of the first premolar, whereas the size of the second upper deciduous molar and the first and second lower deciduous molars is mesiodistally 133%, 115%, and 138%, respectively, the size of the premolars that replace them (Fig. 4.7).

Crown morphology. The crowns of deciduous teeth are round and chunky with a marked narrowing at the neck. The type of contact established between two adjacent teeth is not identifiable at a single point, as is the case with permanent teeth except that the type of contact is characterized by a single surface because of the lower coronal convexity in the mesial and distal sides. The cusp height is reduced both in terms of constitution and physiological abrasion.

Root morphology. The roots of deciduous teeth are thin with pointed apices, and the size of their crowns is proportionally larger than that of the roots of permanent teeth. Furthermore, molar roots diverge starting from the cervical area to the dental follicles of permanent teeth (Fig. 4.8).

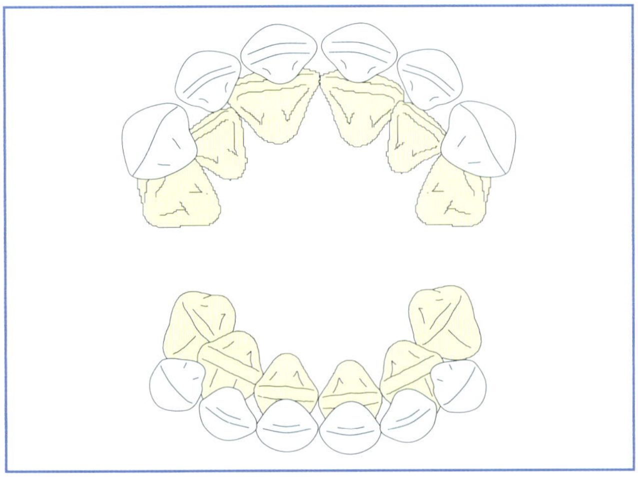

Figure 4.5 Differences in the sizes of deciduous incisors/canines and permanent incisors/canines.

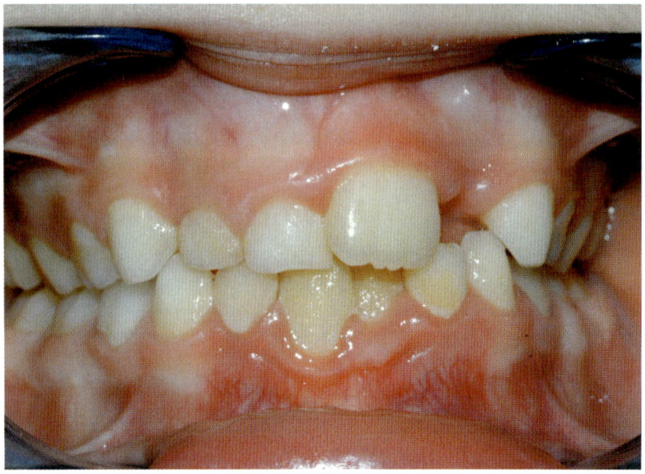

Figure 4.6 Differences in the sizes of deciduous and permanent incisors.

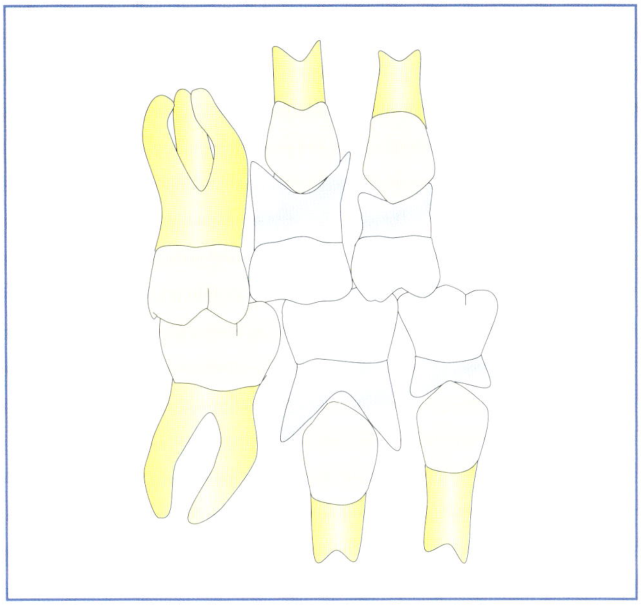

Figure 4.7 Differences in the sizes of deciduous molars and premolars.

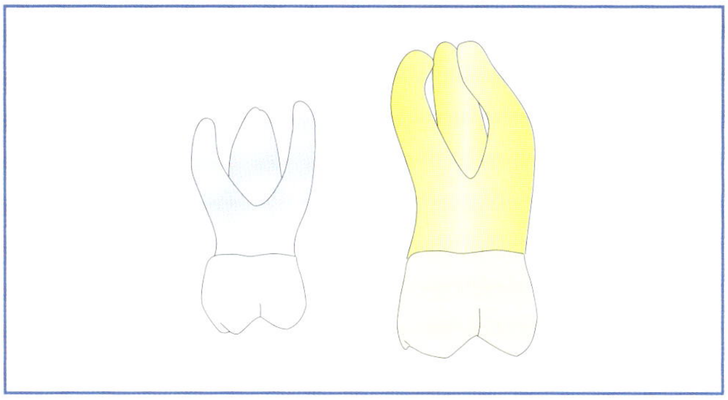

Figure 4.8 Shape of the crowns and roots of deciduous and permanent elements.

Thickness of dental tissues. The reduced thickness and hardness and the increased permeability of hard tissues lead to deciduous teeth having a less resilient structure permanent teeth. Therefore, they are more easily exposed to destructive carious processes.

Pulp chamber. The pulp anatomy is broad in terms of the crown size, and the superficiality of the pulp chamber easily exposes deciduous elements to pulpitis following carious processes.

Eruption sequence. The eruption sequence of deciduous elements substantially differs from that of permanent ones. The position of dental follicles is highly superficial, and they are close to the top of the bone crest. Therefore, the intraosseous eruption sequence is usually short and fairly smooth. Consequently, dental malpositioning such as rotation or inversion is scarce, and the alignment is generally regular. On the other hand, other types of dental anomalies such as supernumeraries and geminated or fused elements, are more frequent observed.
There are two dynamic physiological phenomena that affect the roots and crowns of deciduous elements but do not affect the permanent ones.

Physiological root resorption. Root resorption of a deciduous element allows exfoliation of the element itself; it is a concomitant process associated with the eruption of the corresponding permanent tooth. However, these two processes do not always occur in a coordinated manner. The most frequent cause of failed root resorption is dental ankylosis, which most frequently affects the deciduous molars, especially those in the lower arch. The pathogenic mechanism underlying the fusion between the dental cementum and alveolar bone involves direct ossification caused by an altered local metabolism in the periodontal membrane. A similar condition leads the permanent tooth to deviate from the eruption pathway or remain impacted.

Abrasion. The abrasion of deciduous elements affects all surfaces involved in occlusion, i.e., the incisal margins of the incisors and the cusps of the canines and molars. This phenomenon induced by the structure of mineralized substances, is considered physiological during the deciduous dentition phase and is directly related to bruxism, a "parafunction" identified in this period and justified by the morphological immaturity of the articular skeletal components. In fact, the rotatory movements of the jaw promote the remodeling and development of the temporomandibular joint to achieve occlusal stability, which can only occur at the moment of eruption and occlusal contact between the first permanent molars, a period beyond which bruxism must be considered a real pathological parafunction.

Elements of occlusion in the deciduous dentition

At birth, the upper and lower alveolar processes covered by gum pads are in contact in almost all the points of the circumference of the arch, while a "bite" cannot be yet. Once all the deciduous elements have erupted, it is possible to identify a series of peculiar occlusal features that distinguish between the arches and occlusion of the deciduous elements and those of the permanent ones.

Dental implantation in relation to bone bases

Deciduous teeth are positioned with an implantation that is almost perpendicular to the bone bases represented by the upper and lower jaws. Conversely, permanent teeth are always tilted in relation to the reference planes of the maxillary skeletal bases. This is derived from the position of the dental follicles of deciduous teeth, which lie immediately below the bone crests without encountering any obstacle and directly teeth in the oral cavity without any dental inclination (Fig. 4.9).
The absence of inclination allows deciduous occlusion to always truly reflect the skeletal relationships between the upper and lower jaw on the sagittal plane. Instead, permanent teeth can mask or *camouflage* skeletal pathologies because of the balance they can create by modifying their inclination during eruption.

Shape of the dental arches

Physiologically, both the arches in the deciduous dentition are round, smooth, and almost semicircular (Fig. 4.10).
In cases of any bad habits or lifestyle (after 2.5 years of age), the arches change particularly in the anterior portion. In cases of remarkable adaptability of muscular, dentoalveolar, and skeletal components in this growth phase, the arches and occlusion can easily recover once the bad habits or lifestyle are stopped.

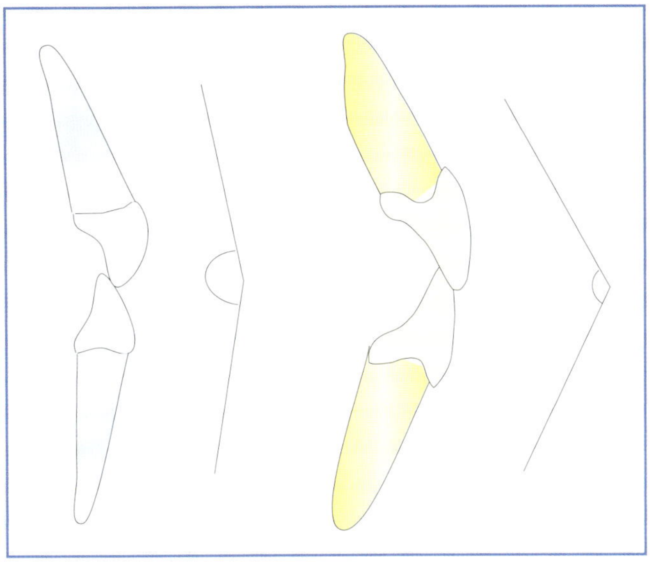

Figure 4.9 Inclination of deciduous and permanent teeth in relation to bone bases.

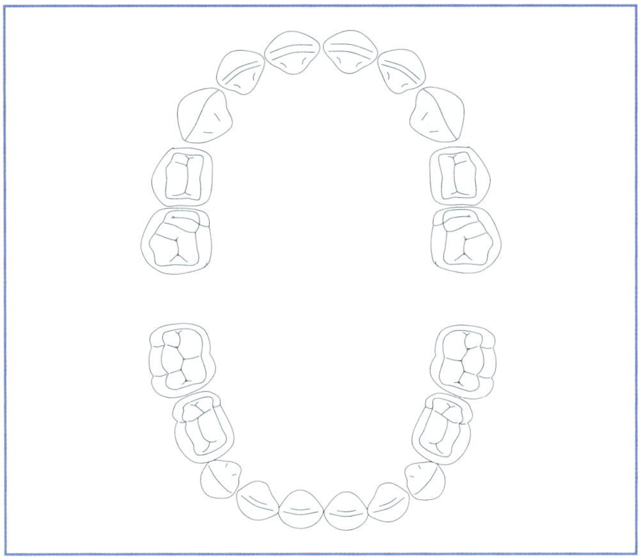

Figure 4.10 Shape of the arch in the deciduous dentition.

Diastemas

Diastemas, the spaces between adjacent teeth, are a typical aspect of deciduous arches and can be distributed more or less uniformly or only in the canine region, where they are called "primate diastemas" because they can be identified in some lower primates (Fig. 4.11). In the lower arch, a diastema is called "*postcanine*" because it is situated between the canine and the first deciduous molar, whereas in the upper arch, the diastema is called "*precanine*" because it is situated between the lateral incisor and the canine.

Generally, all diastemas constitute space retainers and have a functional significance associated with the need for space for the eruption of permanent teeth with a mesiodistal size greater than that of deciduous teeth.

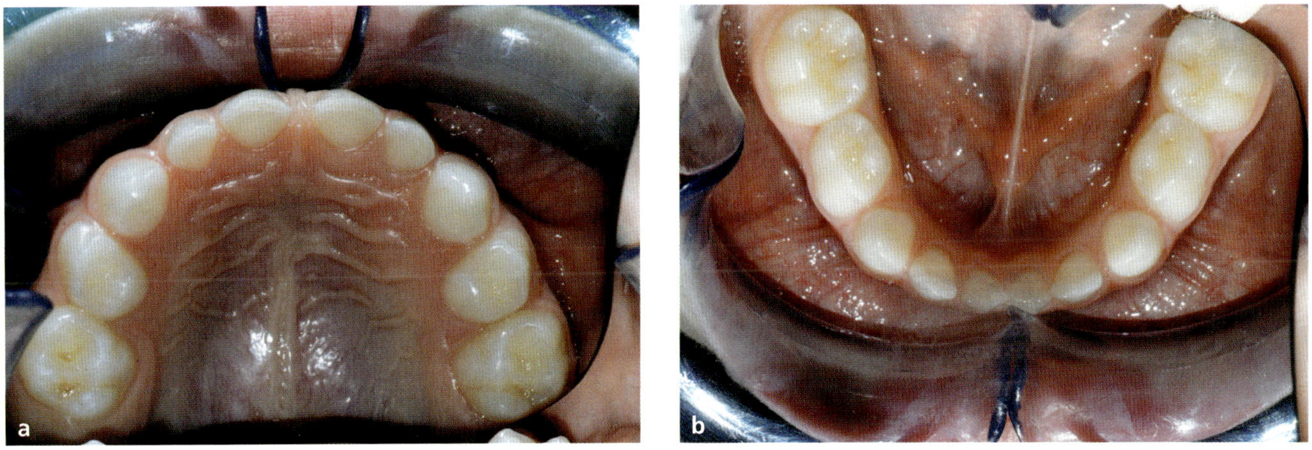

Figure 4.11 Diastemas in the deciduous dentition: (**a**) in the upper and (**b**) lower arches.

Contact surfaces

All the teeth in deciduous dentition do not present diastemas; there is a mandatory contact between the distal surface of the first deciduous molar and the mesial surface of the second deciduous molar. Because of the low convexity of the interproximal walls of the molars in the deciduous dentition, this contact does not comprise a single point but a more or less extended area.

Interarch relationships

The relationships between the upper and lower arches define the occlusion, and similar to that in permanent dentition, they are considered in terms of the three arch regions:

- anterior regions: interincisor relationship
- middle regions: intercanine relationship
- posterior regions: intermolar relationship.

Interincisor relationship. In the deciduous dentition, the incisors show poor over-occlusion on the vertical and sagittal planes, given that their position reflects the position of the dental follicles on the bone bases: the overbite and overjet are approximately 1 mm in size in the deciduous and 2.5 mm in the permanent dentition (Fig. 4.12).

Intercanine relationship. The physiological intercanine relationship identifies the "canine key," wherein the cusp of the upper canine occludes between the lower deciduous canine and the first molar. When the lower canine is situated in the distal position in relation to the canine key relationship, class II malocclusion occurs, whereas when the lower canine is situated in the mesial position, class III malocclusion occurs (Fig. 4.13).

Intermolar relationship. The intermolar deciduous relationship is classified according to the sagittal relationship between the terminal planes tangent to the distal surfaces of the upper and lower second deciduous molars.

Neutrocclusion is defined as the relationship between the second deciduous molars that produces a vertical terminal plane with a mesial step (Fig. 4.14). In the vertical terminal plane, the terminal planes of the upper and lower second deciduous molars

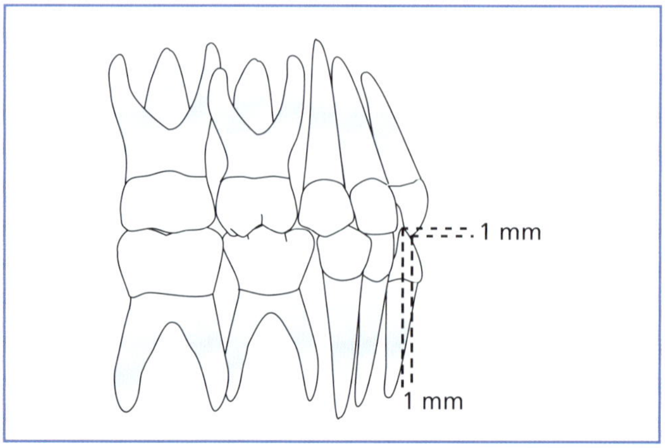

Figure 4.12 Deciduous occlusion: interincisor relationship.

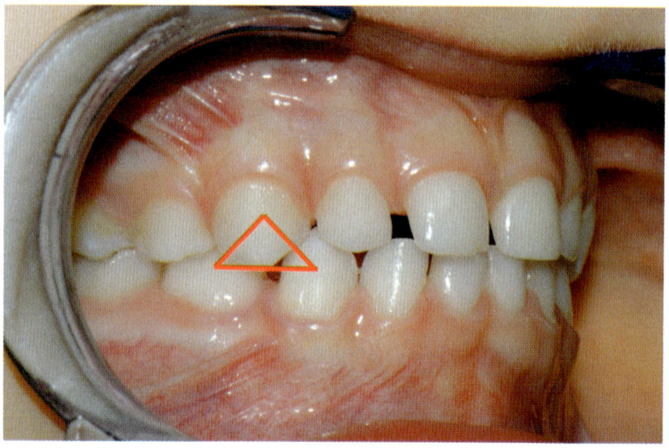

Figure 4.13 Deciduous occlusion: canine key factor.

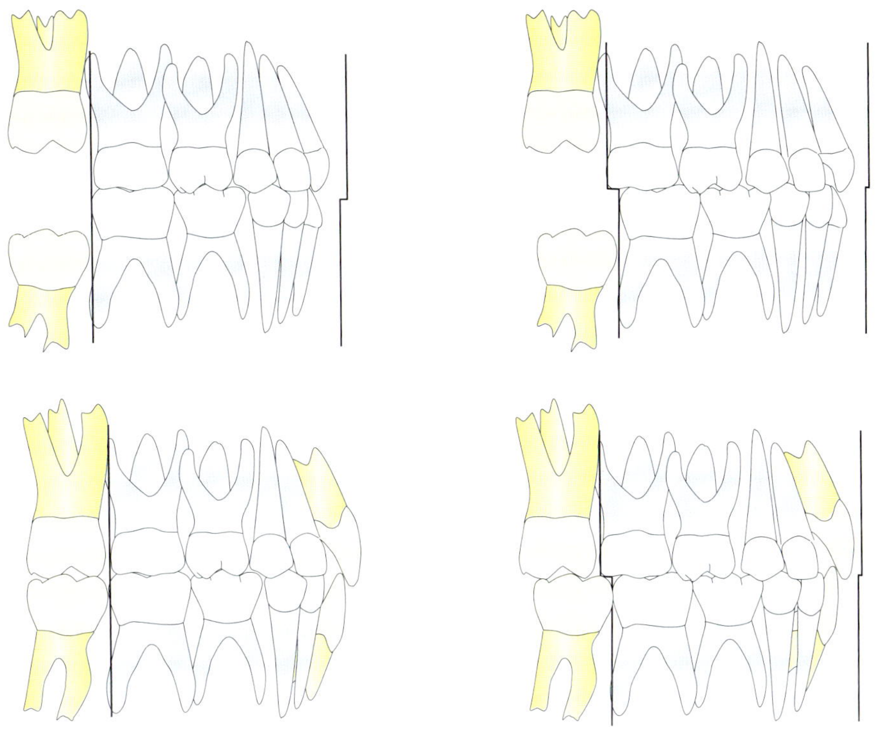

Figure 4.14 Molar relationship in deciduous dentition: vertical terminal plane with a mesial step.

correspond to such an extent that they are aligned. In the relationship with a *mesial step*, the lower second deciduous molar is mesially displaced compared to the upper second deciduous molar.

This condition of the vertical terminal plane will lead to the development of class I molar in permanent dentition possibly because of the difference in the mesiodistal diameters of the deciduous molars in relation to those of the premolars replacing them; in cases in which the mesiodistal diameters of the deciduous molars are larger, the *leeway space* is physiologically used by the first permanent molars to mesialize and acquire the class I molar relationship.

The condition of the mesial step stabilizes the class I molar relationship into mixed dentition.

The deciduous intermolar relationship with a *distal step*, in which the lower second deciduous molar is distally situated in relation to the upper one, is instead considered pathological. In such cases, a class II malocclusion will develop in the permanent dentition.

Occlusal plane

In physiological deciduous occlusion, the occlusal plane is flat (Fig. 4.15), unlike that in permanent dentition, in which the occlusal plane is characterized by two balancing curves: the curve of Spee (on the sagittal plane) and the curve of Wilson (on the frontal plane).

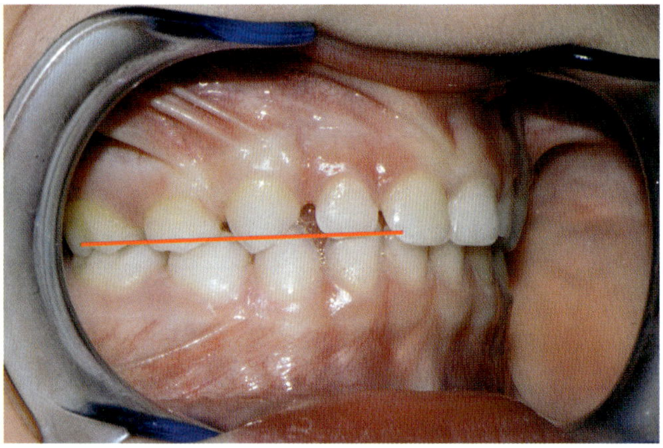

Figure 4.15 Flat occlusal plane in the deciduous dentition.

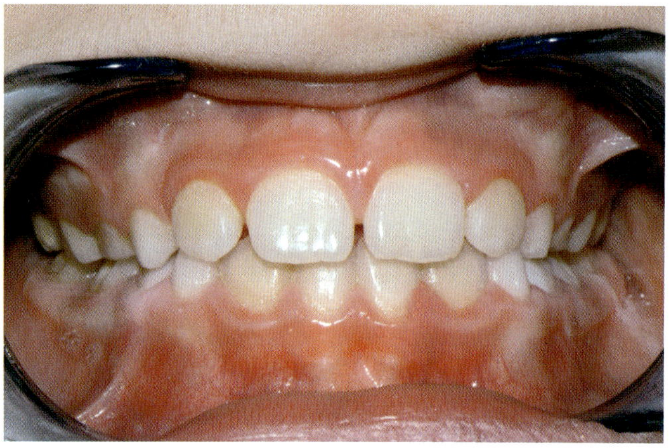

Figure 4.16 Mixed dentition.

The flattening of the occlusal plane is a consequence of several factors such as poor incisor over-occlusion, reduced height of cusps, insufficient and poorly differentiated development of alveolar processes, and physiological abrasion of dental enamel, which can affect various arch regions.

Mixed dentition

Mixed dentition is the phase in which the oral cavity is characterized by the simultaneous presence of both deciduous and permanent elements. Therefore, it involves the transition toward permanent dentition (Fig. 4.16).

The formation of dental follicles in permanent teeth is initiated in the final phases of intrauterine life and continues even after birth (Tab. 4.1). The eruption of permanent teeth is initiated and completed on average between 6 and 12 years of age, with a significant variability in terms of time and sequence (Tab. 4.2).

Eruption sequence of permanent teeth

The exfoliation of deciduous elements and their replacement by permanent ones occur progressively, usually in a very similar manner as their eruption. The first deciduous teeth to erupt are also the first ones to exfoliate.

The most common eruption sequence of permanent teeth is as follows:

- upper and lower first molars
- lower and upper central/lateral incisors
- lower canines and first upper premolars
- first lower premolars and second upper premolars
- upper canines and second lower premolars
- upper and lower second molars
- third molars

Table 4.1 Formation times of permanent dental elements

	First sign of calcification	Enamel completion
First lower molar	At birth	2.5–3 years
First upper molar	At birth	3–4 years
Incisors	3–4 months	4–5 years
First premolar	1.5–2 years	5–6 years
Second premolar	2–2.5 years	6–7 years
Second molar	2.5–3 years	7–8 years
Canines	4–5 years	6–7 years
Third upper molar	7–9 years	12–16 years
Third lower molar	8–10 years	12–16 years

Source: Ash MM. Wheeler's Atlas of the dental morphology. Milan: Dental Science and techniques international editions; 1991.

Table 4.2 Eruption and root completion times of permanent dental elements

	Eruption	Root completion
First upper molar	6 years	9–10 years
First lower molar	6–7 years	9–10 years
Lower central incisor	6–7 years	9 years
Lower lateral incisor	7–8 years	10 years
Upper central incisor	7–8 years	10 years
Upper lateral incisor	8–9 years	11 years
Lower canine	9–10 years	12–14 years
First upper premolar	10–11 years	12–13 years
First lower premolar	10–12 years	12–13 years
Second upper premolar	10–12 years	12–14 years
Second lower premolar	11–12 years	13–14 years
Upper canine	11–12 years	13–15 years
Second lower molar	11–13 years	14–15 years
Second upper molar	12–13 years	14–16 years
Third molar	17–21 years	18–25 years

Source: Ash, *op. cit.*

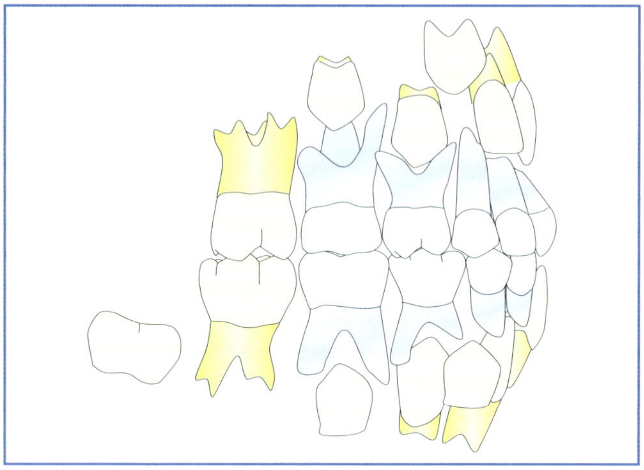

Figure 4.17 Mixed dentition: first transitional period.

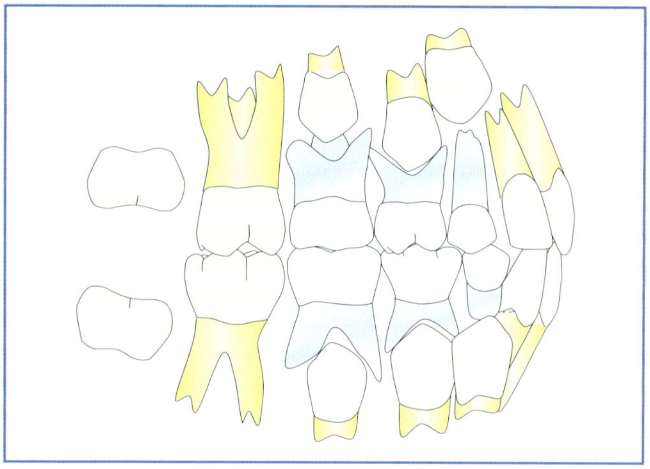

Figure 4.18 Mixed dentition: intertransitional period.

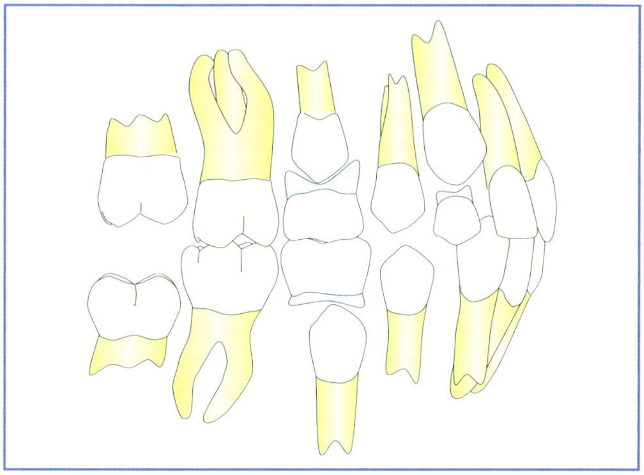

Figure 4.19 Mixed dentition: second transitional period.

Although the first molars are generally the first permanent elements to erupt in the arch, they reach occlusal contact with the antagonist only after complete eruption of the lower central incisors.

In the lateral regions, a particular phenomenon known as "jumping" of the upper canine can be observed; the lower canine is the first tooth to erupt in the arch, whereas the upper canine is the last.

Because the mixed dentition phase covers a fairly long period, lasting from 6 to 12 years of age, it is useful to subdivide the development of dentition into three periods:

- First phase or *first transitional period* (6–8 years): this covers the exfoliation of the deciduous incisors and the eruption of the first molars and the central and lateral permanent incisors (Fig. 4.17)
- *Intertransitional period* (8–10 years): a period of physiological halting during which no changes occur in the permanent incisors, first permanent molars, deciduous canines, and molars in the arch (Fig. 4.18)
- Second phase or *second transitional period* (10–12 years): a period that covers the exfoliation of the deciduous canines and molars and the eruption of the canines, first and second premolars, and second permanent molars (Fig. 4.19).

Transition from deciduous to permanent dentition

The transition from deciduous to permanent dentition is a long and complex process that involves several intervening factors to ensure completion of the eruption of permanent teeth.

Position of the dental follicles of permanent teeth within the alveolar bone

The position of the dental follicles of permanent teeth within the alveolar bone depends on several factors, such as their primitive morphogenetic position, the size and position of the crowns of deciduous teeth, and the size of the "apical region," which is defined as the portion of alveolar bones in which the roots and crowns of deciduous and permanent elements are contained in different periods.

Depending on the *position*, it is possible to distinguish an anterior apical region, two medial regions, and two posterior regions for each arch. The anterior region is bordered by the mesial surfaces of the crowns, roots, and root apices of the canines depending of the stage of dentition. Medial regions are bordered anteriorly by the anterior apical region and posteriorly by the mesial surfaces of the crowns, roots, or root apices of the first permanent molars. The posterior apical regions are posteriorly situated in relation to the medial apical regions.

Depending on the *size*, the apical region can be defined as large, medium, or narrow.

The apical region is considered large when there is sufficient space to contain the tooth as well as dental roots for tooth development. Only in this condition can dentition occur in a normal manner, dental alignment be ensured, no diastema persist, and the arch achieve a harmonious arrangement.

The apical region is considered average in size when there is sufficient space and the various mechanisms involved in tooth replacement can work favorably. In this condition, dentition can occur in a normal manner, no diastema will persist, and the arch can achieve a harmonious arrangement.

The apical region is considered narrow when there is not enough space to allow the dental elements and the already formed roots to conveniently settle. In this condition, dentition occurs abnormally, leading to dental malpositioning and overcrowding.

Within the apical region, the special relationships among the dental follicles of permanent elements and the dental follicles and roots of deciduous elements vary across the various regions of the arch (Fig. 4.20).

Incisors. The position of the dental follicles of the incisors depends on the size of the anterior apical region and its relationship with the size of dental elements.

Originally, the crowns of the permanent incisors are situated lingually in relation to the roots of the corresponding deciduous elements.

In particular, the crowns of the lower central incisors are closer to the occlusal plane than those of the lateral incisors situated in a more lingual position; their mesiodistal orientation is almost perpendicular in relation to the occlusal plane. The crowns of the lateral elements are covered by central elements at an extent varying from one-fourth to one-third of its mesiodistal size.

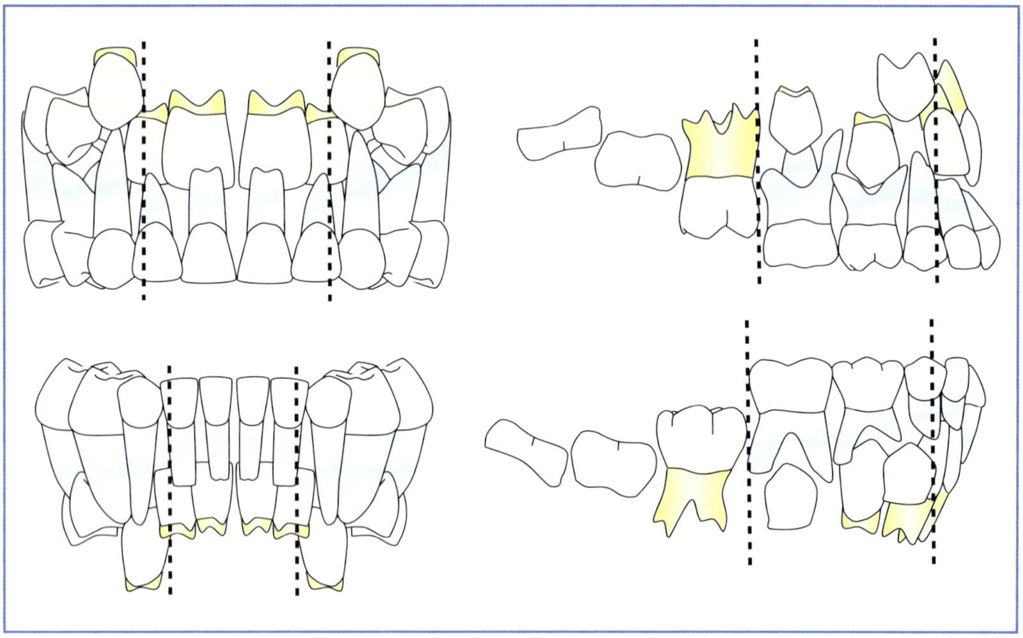

Figure 4.20 Anterior, median, and posterior apical regions of the upper and lower arch.

The upper central permanent incisors are situated proximal to the anterior wall of the floor of the nasal cavities on the sides of the intermaxillary suture in the vestibular position in relation to the lateral permanent elements. The distal angle of the central permanent element is in contact with the mesial surface of the roots of the lateral deciduous elements. The lateral permanent incisors are situated closer to the occlusal plane than the central ones, unlike that observed in the lower arch.

Canines. The lower canines are the furthest elements from the occlusal plane because they are positioned in proximity to the inferior margin of the mandibular body. They are oriented in a moderate lingual manner, and their cusps are lingually situated in relation to the roots of their deciduous counterparts.
The upper canines are situated at the sides of the pyramid-like nasal base in the area adjacent to the piriform incisure at a deep level in relation to the bone site where the dental follicles of the permanent incisors are situated. They are the furthest elements from the occlusal plane. The upper canines show slight mesiovestibular inclination, and their cusps are lingually situated in relation to the roots of their deciduous counterparts. The coronomesial portion of the canines is frequently in close contact with the roots of the upper lateral incisor and is frequently covered by the vestibular side.

Premolars. The dental follicles of the upper and lower premolars lie closer to the occlusal plane than the canines and form among the roots of the deciduous molars. Of all the elements, the first premolar is the closest to the lateral region, whereas the second premolar occupies an intermediate position between the canine and the first premolar.
In the sagittal direction, the size of the upper median apical region is smaller than that of the lower one; therefore the first upper premolar is not generally situated distally to the upper canine but underneath it, where it is partially covered; furthermore, it is situated in a vestibular position in relation to the second premolar.

Molars. The dental follicles of permanent molars are distally situated in relation to the roots of the teeth, which are mesially situated.

Pre-eruptive phase and root resorption of deciduous teeth

Tooth displacement toward occlusion starts as soon as crown formation is completed and continues for the entire period of root extension as long as the root apex remains dilated.

The pre-eruptive phase is the path that a tooth follows inside the alveolar bone from its initial position at the dental follicle stage until it reaches the oral mucosa. The progressive movement is accompanied by alveolar bone resorption in the direction of eruption.

The *initiation of dental eruption* coincides with the completion of crown and root formation. In fact, this mechanism is not yet completely understood, although it seems clear that tooth progression during eruption occurs because of the pressure developing from the open dental pulp at the extremity of the forming root or from the subapical connective tissue via vascular congestion phases. In particular, the eruption potential derives from the activity of the periodontal membrane at the apical level.

The *direction of tooth eruption* is always directly dependent on root orientation, although the path can be modified by two factors, namely, the contact with adjacent teeth during eruption and the size of the maxillary apical region where eruption occurs.

The *eruption sequence* reflects the order in which the adjacent erupting elements actually undergo their pre-eruptive phases. This clearly depends on the initial position of dental follicles and the maxillary space conditions in which eruption occurs.

Incisors. The lower central incisors are the first to initiate eruption, which occurs according to their intramandibular orientation and progressively reduces lateral overcrowding. When the central elements reach the occlusal plane, the lateral incisors, whose path remains in the lingual position in relation to the path of the central elements themselves initiate eruption. Therefore, at the moment of eruption, the incisal margin of the lateral elements is situated further back compared with that of the central elements. The contact between the crowns of the erupting lateral elements and the roots of the adjacent deciduous canines causes the ejection of the deciduous canine itself, which in turn will occupy the lower postcanine diastema, thereby modifying the size of the arch via an increase of the intercanine deciduous distance.

The first elements to erupt in the upper arch are also the central incisors, surpassing the crown of the lateral permanent elements after eruption by sliding along the roots of the lateral deciduous elements and partly ejecting the crown. The upper lateral incisors follow a more vestibular eruption direction than the central ones to ensure that they reach the correct position within the arch. When the available space is insufficient, the tooth modifies the eruption pathway by acquiring a palatine position in relation to the central element.

Canines. In the lower arch, the canine precedes the first premolar, which is initially situated closer to the occlusal plane. In fact, the area of the apical region in the lower arch is larger than the space that the elements occupy within the arch once they have erupted, enabling the teeth to move more freely within the alveolar process.

In the upper arch, the morphology of the apical region generally makes the canine the last tooth to erupt in the lateral region. The canine initiates eruption by initially coming in contact with the root apex of the lateral incisor. Subsequently, the coronomesial portion of the canine comes in contact with the root of the lateral permanent incisor already present within the arch. The canine initiates eruption by moving mesially toward the occlusal plane and gradually straightening along the roots of the lateral permanent elements, which functions as a guide.

In this phase of intraosseous eruption, the thrust exerted by the canine toward the lateral elements causes the latter to undergo distovestibular rotation, thus causing the teeth to tilt, which in turn causes the formation of a diastema between the central and lateral elements. This temporary phase is characterized by the anomalous tilt of the lateral incisor and is termed *"ugly duckling" stage*. This is actually a frequently detected physiological phase, which can spontaneously correct itself with the eruption of the permanent canine.

If there is sufficient space in the arch, the upper canine follows a vestibular eruption direction In relation to that the roots of the lateral elements; however, if the spatial conditions are not favorable, the canine follows its palatine eruption direction or remains impacted.

Premolars. In the lower arch, the first premolar is preceded by the canine, which initially is further away from the occlusal plane, whereas the second premolar is generally the last element of the lower arch to erupt.

Conversely, the teeth situated in the medial apical region in the upper arch are contained within a space that is narrower than that available in the arch. Therefore, the tooth closest to the occlusal plane is the first one to erupt. The most frequent eruption sequence in the upper arch is as follows: first premolar, second premolar, and canine.

Molars. The space available in the arch for eruption of molars is ensured by bone remodeling occurring along the anterior margins of the ascending mandibular ramus and in the posterior side of the upper jaw.

During craniofacial growth, the mandible develops because of resorption of the anterior margin of the mandibular ramus and bone apposition occurring on its posterior margin and at the level of the condyle head. In this manner, the length of the jaw and particularly of the mandibular body increases. Similarly, the upper jaw extends sagittally because of the bone apposition occurring in the area of tuberosity. Through these remodeling processes, the space available for accommodating the molars in the lower and upper jaw increases.

The molars follow an eruption direction of an arc with greater concavity for the lower elements, transitioning from the distal to mesial side, and with a lower concavity for the upper elements, transitioning from the distal to medial side.

Sometimes, the crown of a molar may remain impacted against the distal root of the

molar that is mesial to it during eruption, with consequences affecting both elements. In particular, it is possible to observe a difficulty in eruption until the retention–inclusion of the distal elements and resorption of the roots of the mesial elements, resulting in early loss of the element itself in the case of the second deciduous molar. In these conditions, the permanent molars erupt mesially compared with their original position, resulting in a consequent lack of space for eruption of the second premolar.
During dentition, eruption of the permanent tooth is associated with root resorption of the corresponding deciduous tooth.
Clearly, the modalities of root resorption vary among teeth depending especially on the position of the crowns of the erupting permanent teeth compared with the roots of deciduous elements.
Incisors and canines mainly resorb their palatolingual face and the apex owing to the position of the crowns of permanent incisors and canines. Exfoliation frequently occurs much earlier than the emergence of the corresponding permanent tooth in the arch.
Conversely, root resorption of the deciduous molars occurs when the premolars approach their roots. Deciduous teeth remain in situ until the inner part of their crowns is resorbed. In fact, the replacing premolars frequently emerge even before exfoliation of the corresponding tooth.

Eruptive phase and occlusal contact

The eruption phase is the final stage of dental follicle development; it comprises the emergence of the elements in the oral cavity until they come in occlusal contact with the antagonist teeth. Only at this moment is eruption completed.
During the eruption phase, the pathway followed by the tooth is conditioned by the presence of certain muscular conditions that are typical of the oral cavity structures and that affect the position of the tooth both on the sagittal and transversal planes.
On the sagittal plane, the lower incisors are guided along their eruption pathway from the tongue, consequently allowing the dental follicles of the permanent elements, which are lingually positioned in relation to the roots of deciduous teeth, to reach the alveolar process by exerting a centrifugal force, thus maintaining the vestibular tilt typical of their pre-eruptive pathway. Despite the presence of the postcanine diastema as an important space retainer and the fact that the incisor eruption direction is vestibular, the space for incisor alignment is frequently insufficient in this dentition phase; an extent of overcrowding varying from 1 to 3 mm is considered physiological.
Unlike the lower incisors, the upper ones are anteriorly positioned in relation to that of the vestibular surfaces of deciduous teeth owing to their original vestibular orientation. The contact with the upper lip causes a change in the axial tilt of the erupting permanent incisors, limiting their vestibular progression. Eruption stops at the moment of incisal contact with the antagonist teeth and the lower lip.
The vestibulolingual tilt of the canines after eruption mostly depends on the space conditions found within the arch; the forces exerted by the tongue and the perioral musculature play an entirely secondary role, contrary to that observed for incisors and molars. The vertical position of canines is also barely influenced by the occlusal contact with the antagonist teeth because their relationships are poorly defined.

The vestibulolingual position of lower premolars depends on the contact with antagonist elements and their eruption direction, particularly the first premolar, shows a slight tendency to erupt in the vestibular direction, whereas the second premolar erupts in the lingual direction. The mesiodistal position of the lower premolars instead depends on the eruption sequence, the space found within the arch and finally their contact with adjacent elements. In particular, the first premolar shows slight tendency to erupt in the mesial direction, whereas the second premolar erupts in the distal direction.
The upper premolars erupt in the occlusal direction and are "centered" in the coronal area of the deciduous molars to be replaced. The eruption sites of the upper premolars depend more on their pre-eruptive position than their eruption direction, which cannot change much owing to the limited size of the upper median apical region.
In a narrow medial apical region, the first premolar tends to erupt in the vestibular direction, whereas the second premolar tends to erupt in the palatal direction.
Finally, the vertical position of the premolars is strongly influenced by their occlusal contact with the antagonist teeth that precede them during dentition, whereas the role of the forces exerted by the tongue and the perioral musculature is entirely secondary in determining their final position.
The eruption pathway of the upper and lower molars after their emergence within the arch is conditioned by the balance between the centrifugal force exerted by the tongue and the centripetal force exerted by the buccal musculature. When the tongue keeps its position at the top laying over the palate, this balance of forces is preserved. Conversely, in cases of atypical deglutition or mouth breathing wherein the tongue is positioned at the bottom over the oral floor, the centripetal forces exerted by the cheeks modify the correct tilting of the upper molars during eruption.
Similarly, molars maintain their eruption pathway in the vertical direction until they come in contact with the antagonist teeth.

Space retainers

Space retainers are physiological mechanisms that allow permanent teeth to replace deciduous ones, thereby establishing a harmonious alignment in permanent dentition. These mechanisms include the following:

- diastemas
- increase in intercanine distance
- eruption direction of permanent incisors
- *leeway space*.

Diastemas. The presence of diastemas in deciduous dentition ensures further space for eruption of permanent teeth, which are smaller than the deciduous ones (where diastemas are mostly found) in the anterior region of the arches.
Increase in intercanine distance. The upper precanine diastema represents a space retainer for accommodating the central and lateral incisors, which are considerably larger than the deciduous ones. The lower postcanine diastema allows a physiological increase in the deciduous intercanine distance owing to the distal migration of the deciduous canines because of the pressure exerted by the crown of the erupting lateral permanent

incisors against the roots of the deciduous canines themselves. The increase in the intercanine distance occurring toward the end of the first dentition phase involves an increase in the transverse diameter of the lower arch, which represents the last moment of growth for the lower arch and is considered unchangeable after 9 years of age (Fig. 4.21).

Eruption direction of permanent incisors. Due to their lingual position in relation to the roots of deciduous elements during the developmental stage of dental follicles and the thrust of the tongue, permanent incisors erupt in the vestibular position compared with deciduous ones and create an arc with a greater diameter, thus increasing the arch perimeter.

Leeway space. It constitutes the difference in the mediodistal diameters of deciduous molars and the premolars that replace them. The upper *leeway space* is approximately 0.9 mm for each hemiarch, whereas the lower *leeway space* is approximately 1.7 mm for each hemiarch. From a physiological viewpoint, the leeway space is occupied by the mesialization of the first permanent molar to reach the first occlusal molar relationship because the difference in the mediodistal diameters of the deciduous and permanent elements is greater in the lower arch (Fig. 4.22).
However, *leeway space* constitutes a space retainer that must be orthodontically managed in case of crowding in the anterior arch.

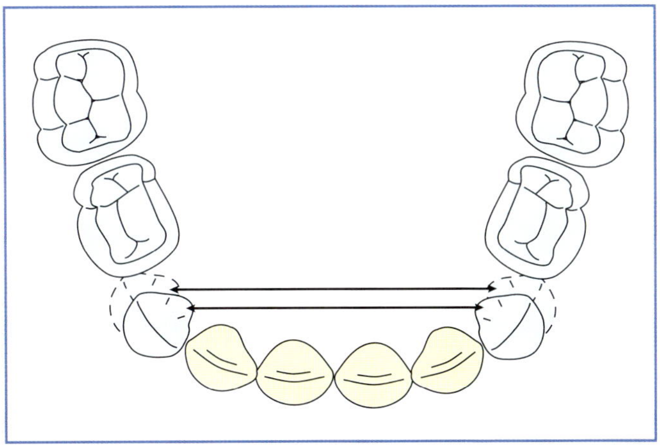

Figure 4.21 Increase in intercanine distance.

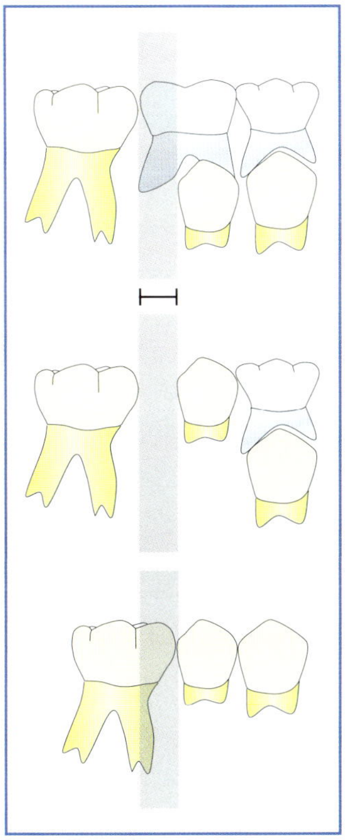

Figure 4.22 *Leeway space.*

Permanent dentition

Approximately at the age of 12 years with the eruption of the second permanent molar, it is possible to identify the definitive dentition of all the deciduous elements. Therefore, a permanent dentition of 32 elements is established after the eruption of the third molar (Fig. 4.23).

Elements of occlusion in permanent dentition

Similar to deciduous dentition that possesses peculiar occlusal characteristics, permanent dentition is also characterized by parameters that define the ideal physiological occlusion.

Shape of the arch

After eruption of all the permanent elements, the arch is generally elliptical, unlike that observed in deciduous ones (Fig. 4.24). This shape already appears in the first phase of mixed dentition with eruption of the molars and increase in the perimeter of the anterior arch, thus coinciding with the dentition of incisors.
Several arch shapes can be identified in permanent dentition (oblong, oblong and narrow, normal, ovoid, and ovoid and narrow) depending on the facial type, i.e., brachyfacial, mesofacial, or dolichofacial.
During permanent dentition, physiological occlusion has traditionally been defined in a very simple manner by E.H. Angle exclusively based on the relationships between the first upper and lower molars. This classification, which is still in use, is clearly incomplete. In 1972, L.F. Andrew proposed *six key factors for normal occlusion*,

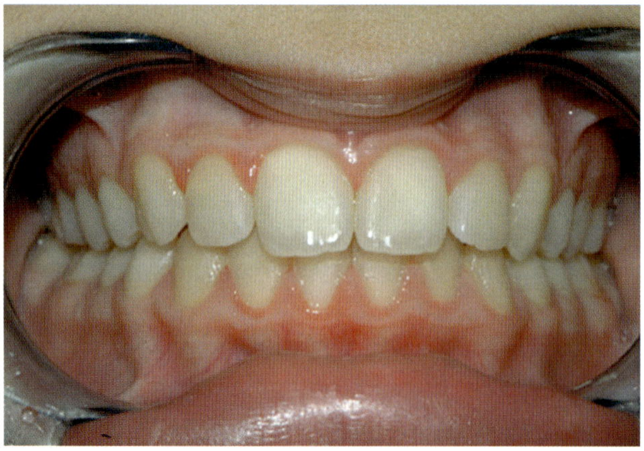

Figure 4.23 Permanent dentition.

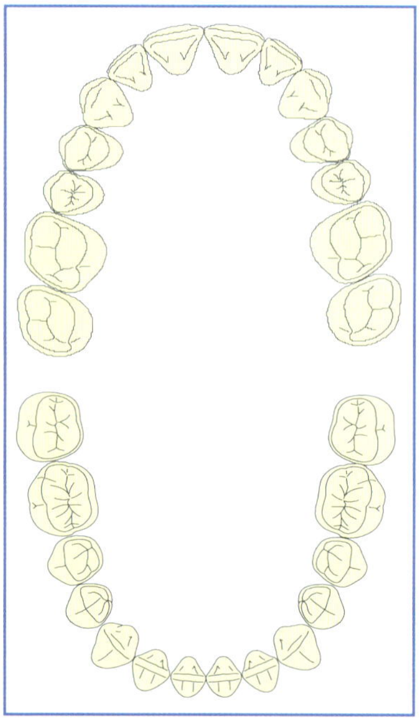

Figure 4.24 Shape of the arch in deciduous dentition.

which were fundamental for designing his preprogrammed orthodontic equipment in a more complete way and which defined the characteristics constantly identified in physiological occlusion.

First key factor for normal occlusion: interarch relationships

Interarch relationship defines the relationship between the upper and lower arch in various arch regions.

Molar relationship

The first characteristic that defines the relationship between the first molars corresponds perfectly to the definition of the class I molar relationship, as described by E.H. Angle: "*The mesiovestibular cusp of the first upper molar occludes in the sulcus between the mesial and medial vestibular cusps of the first lower molar*" (Fig. 4.25).
According to E.H. Angle, this is the "*conditio sine qua non*" for a correct occlusion, whereas according to L.F. Andrews, this condition alone is not sufficient to define a correct molar relationship. Despite the presence of an acceptable molar relationship, as described by E.H. Angle, it is frequently not possible to achieve a close relationship among the molar cusps. Therefore, L.F. Andrews introduced the following two concepts further:

- the marginal distal ridge of the first upper molar occludes with the marginal mesial ridge of the second lower molar (Fig. 4.26)
- from an occlusal viewpoint, the mesiolingual cusp of the first upper molar occludes within the central fossa of the first lower molar (Fig. 4.27).

Premolar relationship

Furthermore, similar to E.H. Angle's definition, the posterior interarch relationships described by L.F. Andrews also involve premolars both on the vestibular and occlusal sides. In fact, the vestibular cusps of the upper molars in normal occlusion show a relationship between the cusps and their point of contact with the lower premolars (Fig. 4.28), whereas the lingual cusps of the upper premolar show a relationship between the cusp and the fossa with lower premolars (Fig. 4.29).
In an optimal posterior occlusion, each tooth of the mandibular arch occludes with the antagonist and the adjacent mesial one (Fig. 4.30). In this manner, the relationship between one tooth and two teeth contributes to a more homogeneous distribution of occlusal forces. In particular, there are two possible positions for the cusps in relation to the antagonist teeth as follows:

- the relationship between the cusp and interproximal space, also termed "one-tooth-to-two-teeth" relationship, in which the upper tooth is distovestibularly situated in relation to the lower antagonist. All the lower vestibular cusps occlude the interproximal space of the upper teeth, except the distovestibular cusps of the first and second lower molar, which come in contact with the central fossa of the first and second upper molars
- the cusp–fossa relationship, also termed the "tooth-to-tooth" relationship, in which the cusps of the upper and lower elements are situated in the fossae of the antagonist teeth.

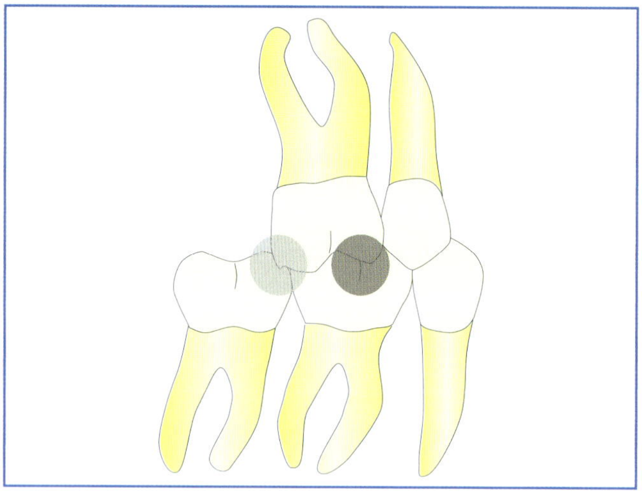

Figure 4.25 Molar relationship between the first upper molar and the first lower molar.

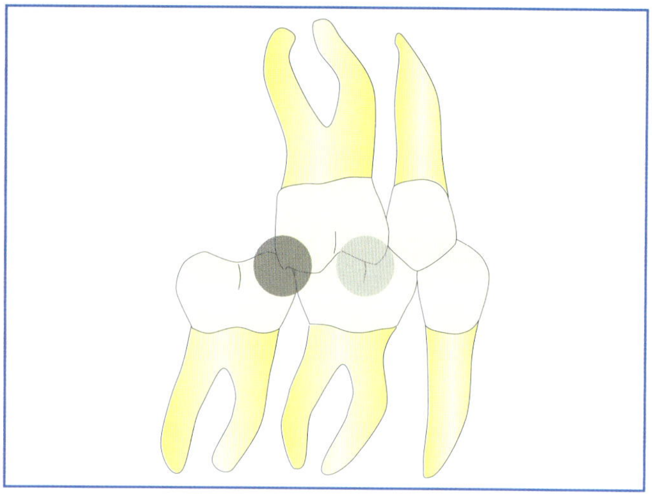

Figure 4.26 Molar relationship between the first upper molar and the second lower molar.

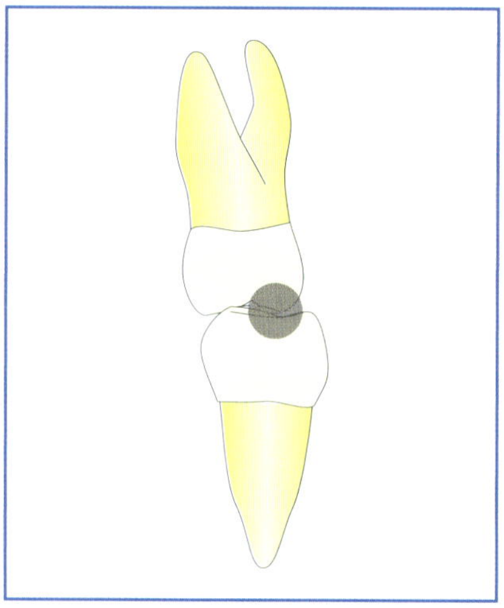

Figure 4.27 Molar relationship between the first upper molar and the first lower molar in the lingual view.

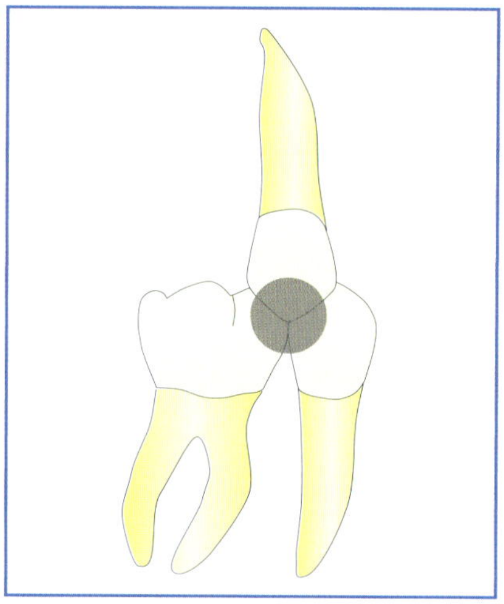

Figure 4.28 Relationship between the upper and lower premolars in the vestibular view.

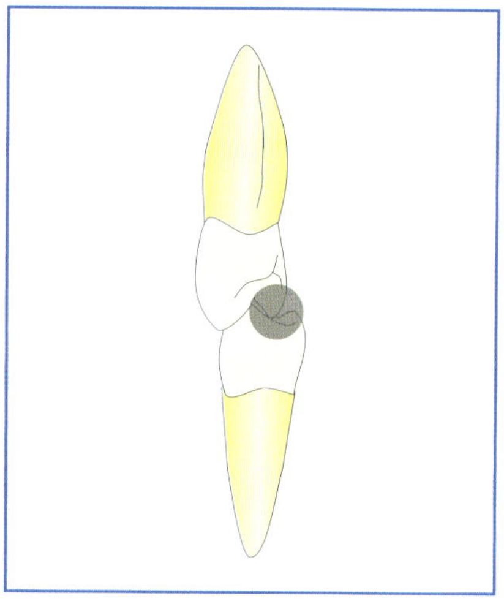

Figure 4.30 Interarch relationships: molar and premolar relationship.

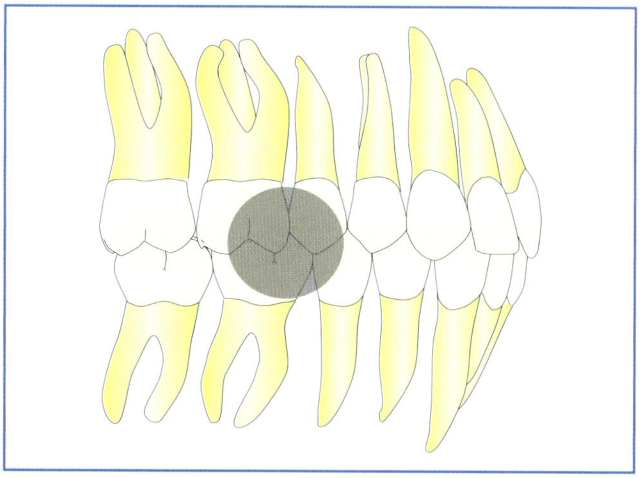

Figure 4.29 Relationship between the upper and lower premolars in the lingual view.

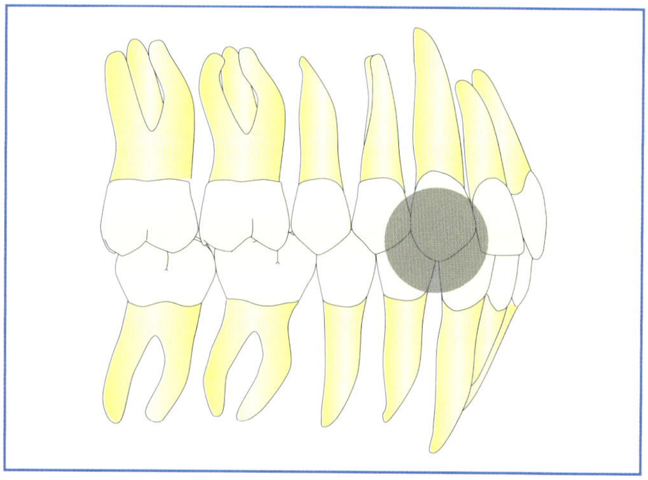

Figure 4.31 Interarch relationships: canine relationship.

Canine relationship

The upper canine shows a "cusp to point of contact" relationship with the canine and the first lower premolar. The apex of the canine cusp has a slightly mesial position in relation to the point of contact (Fig. 4.31).
This relationship is usually defined as class I canine and is completely similar to the relationship of the canine key factor identified in physiological deciduous dentition.
An optimal canine occlusion allows the canine to disocclude by separating all the posterior teeth and thus ensuring a *canine-guided* eccentric lateral mandibular movement.

Incisor relationship

The upper incisors exceed the lower ones and the medial lines of arches coincide. The exact relationship of the anterior teeth is defined by overjet and overbite relationships. Overjet is defined as the distance between the incisal margin of the upper incisor and the incisal margin of the lower incisor on the sagittal plane. Normally, overjet is approximately 2.5 mm, which is equal to the sagittal thickness of the incisal margin of the upper incisor.
Overbite is defined as the distance between the incisal margin of the upper incisor and the incisal margin of the lower incisor on the vertical plane. Normally, overbite is also approximately 2.5 mm, which is equal to one-third of the vestibular surface of the lower incisor covered by the upper one (Fig. 4.32).
An optimal incisive occlusion, determined by the contact of the incisal margins of anterior teeth, guarantees *anterior guidance* for protrusive mandibular movements and a posterior disocclusion. The anterior guidance determined by overjet and overbite defines posterior disocclusion.

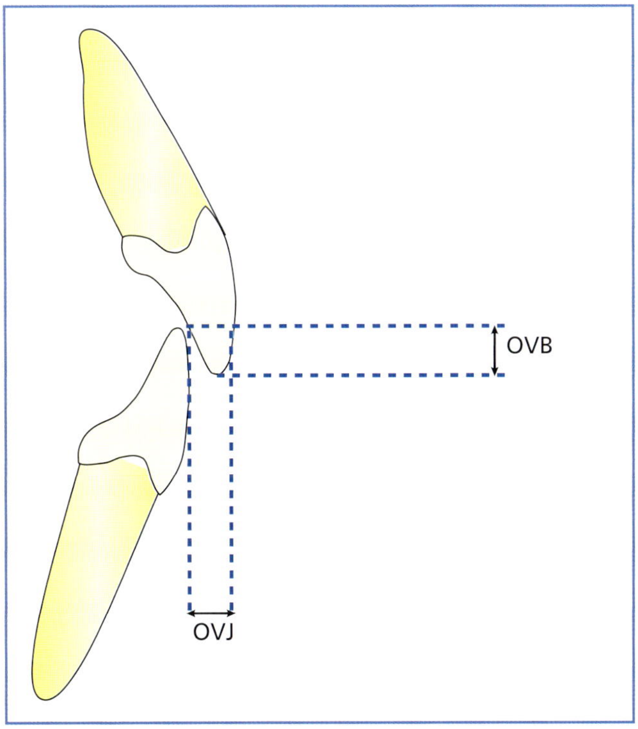

Figure 4.32 Interarch relationships: incisor relationship. OVB: overbite; OVJ: overjet.

Second key factor for normal occlusion: crown angulation

Crown angulation corresponds to the position of the tooth crown in the mesiodistal direction; it is incorrectly indicated with the term "*tip*."

In optimal occlusion, the crowns of all the dental elements have positive angulation (in other words, the occlusal portion of the crown is placed in the mesial position in relation to the gingival one), which varies among elements (Fig. 4.33).

All the upper arch elements have higher angulation values than the lower arch elements because they must occupy relatively more space.

The upper canines have high angulation values because they must only come in contact with the cusp of the lower one in the lateral direction. The upper canines that appear "too straight" interfere with the first lower molars and do not allow an adequate posterior disocclusion.

Finally, the upper molars have higher angulation values than the antagonist teeth to satisfy the first key factor for occlusion and allow the distal marginal ridge of the first upper molar to occlude with the mesial marginal ridge of the second lower molar to stabilize the class relationships.

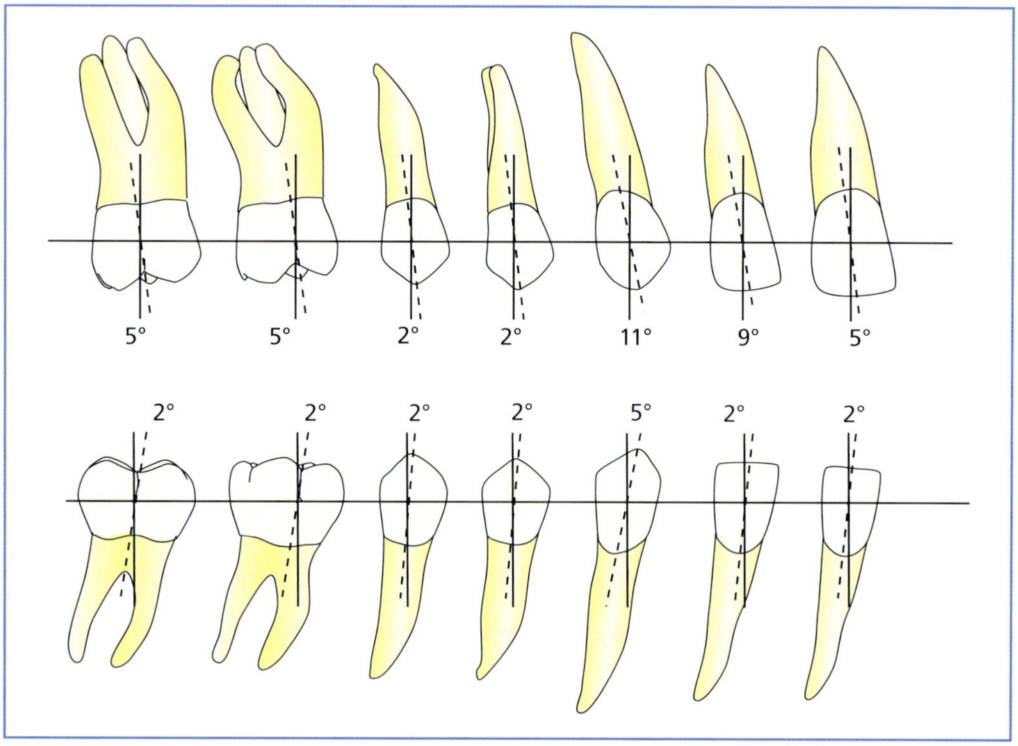

Figure 4.33 Crown angulation of single dental elements. (From: Andrews e Straight, 1993.)

Third key factor for normal occlusion: crown inclination

Crown angulation corresponds to the position of the tooth crown in the vestibulolingual direction; it is incorrectly indicated using the term "*torque*."

In normal occlusion, all the elements have negative crown inclinations (in other words, the occlusal crown portion is in the lingual position in relation to the gingival one), with the exception of the upper incisors, which have positive crown inclinations (in other words, the occlusal crown portion is in the vestibular position in relation to the gingival one) (Fig. 4.34).

Crowns with marked inclination increase the length of the arch. In fact, the inclination values of the upper arch elements are higher than those of the lower arch elements. In particular, with respect to the inclinations of the incisors, these elements must have the correct inclination in agreement with the angles of articular eminences to be able to regulate the mandibular protrusion. In fact, during protrusive movements, the contact with incisors determines the incisive guidance, whereas the condylar path determines the condylar guidance. Furthermore, the inclinations of the incisors and eminences determine the posterior disocclusion.

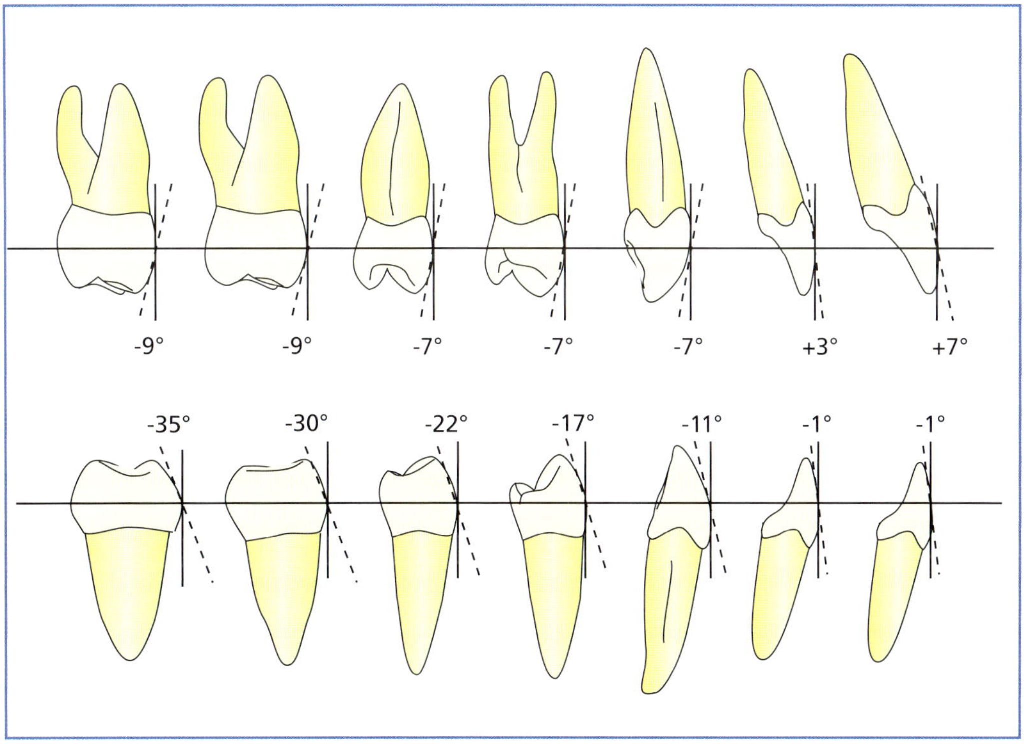

Figure 4.34 Crown inclinations of single dental elements. (From: Andrews e Straight, 1993.)

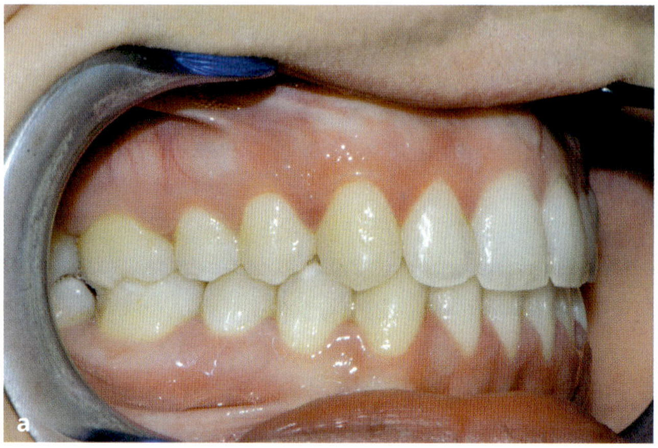

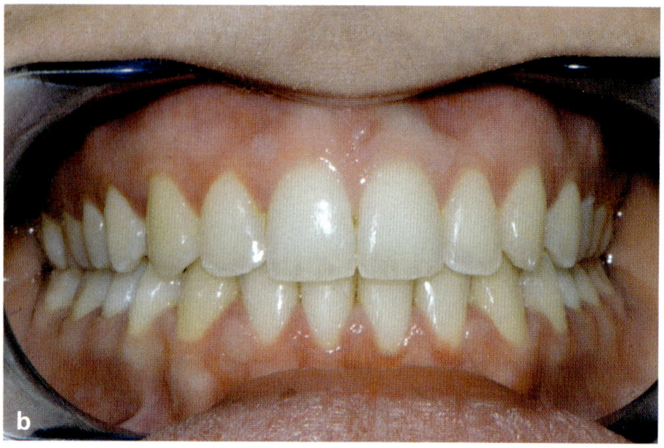

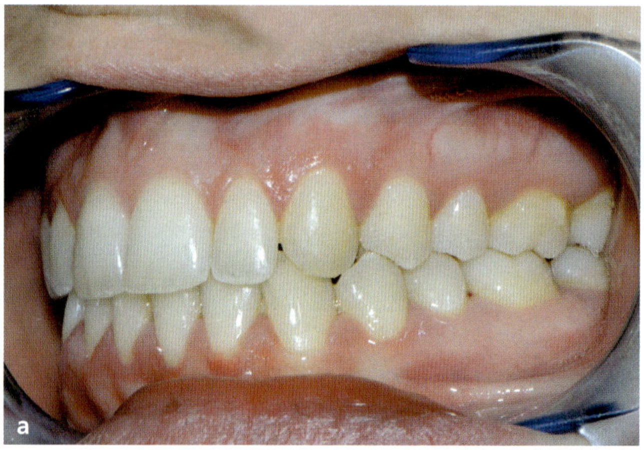

Figure 4.35 Permanent occlusion in the (**a**) right lateral, (**b**) frontal, and (**c**) left lateral view with the upper arch closing as if it was a "box lid" over the lower arches.

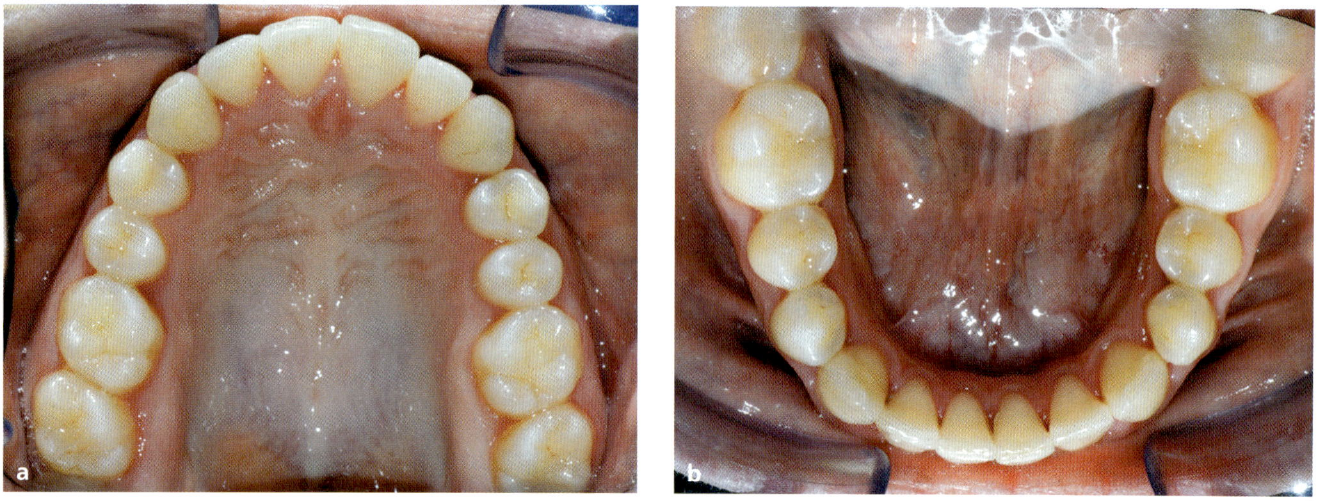

Figure 4.36 Absence of rotations and close points of contact in the upper (**a**) and (**b**) lower arches.

The correct angulation and inclination, along with the size of the crowns, are indispensable factors for the upper arch teeth to occupy more space than that occupied by the lower arch teeth, thereby allowing the maxillary arch to be "greater" and to form a seal over the mandibular one (similar to a box lid) and including all the dental elements within the arch perimeter (Fig. 4.35).

Fourth key factor for normal occlusion: rotations

In optimal occlusion, there are no dental rotations (Fig. 4.36).
The term "rotation" refers to the malposition of the dental element around its own greater axis. In other words, a tooth is considered to be rotated when the axis linking its ideal points of contact is not parallel to the axis representing the arch shape.
Dental rotations alter the correct static occlusal relationships between the upper and lower arch elements. In fact, rotated incisors and canines occupy less space within the arch, whereas rotated premolars and molars occupy more space within the arch.
The presence of dental rotations can generate occlusal interferences in lateral and protrusive mandibular movements, thereby creating alterations in dynamic occlusions.
Finally, the presence of rotations, particularly the anterior arch regions, can significantly compromise the esthetics of the smile.

Fifth key factor for normal occlusion: close contacts

Once the teeth have erupted within the arch, a proximal contact relationship (mesial and distal) between two adjacent teeth is established; this is incorrectly indicated by the term "*point of contact*." In reality, some teeth have points of contact with adjacent elements in young individuals only because the surfaces of contact preserve unaltered curves. Therefore, it is generally more correct to define this relationship based on the areas of contact.
In optimal occlusion, the close points of contact between two adjacent teeth within the arch should be maintained. The only exception admitted is the presence of an inverse dentoalveolar discrepancy, in which the sum of the teeth sizes is lower than the length of the arch. In such cases, the ubiquitous presence of diastemas is confirmed and considered physiological.
The proximal contact between adjacent teeth ensures stabilization of the dental arches subjected to masticatory forces through the combined anchoring of all the teeth, thereby contributing to normal arch alignment. In fact, the alveolar bone and gingival fibers surrounding the teeth exert a functional response during mastication, resulting in a thrust of the teeth toward the midline in the mesial direction.

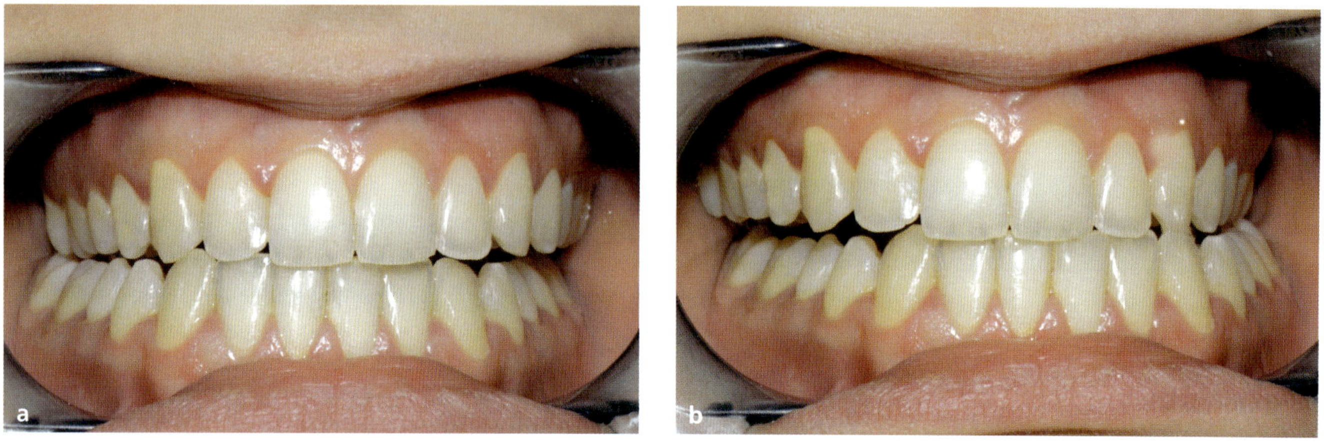

Figure 4.37 Compensation curves in the permanent dentition (curve of Spee and curve of Wilson) allowing eccentric movements of the mandible in (**a**) the right laterality and (**b**) the left laterality.

Sixth key factor for normal occlusion: occlusion curves

Unlike the flat deciduous occlusal plane, the permanent occlusal plane follows a curvilinear pattern both on the sagittal and frontal planes. In fact, this is characterized by two curves termed "compensation curves" (Fig. 4.37).

- The curve of Spee: this has an upward-facing concavity, and it develops in the anteroposterior direction visible from the sagittal viewpoint. It initiates with the cusp of the lower canine, follows the vestibular cusps of the premolars and molars, and continues up to the anterior margin of the mandibular ramus. If the curved line continued to progress, it would ideally form an arch passing though the condyle.
- The curve of Wilson: this has an upward-facing concavity, and it develops in the frontal direction. It comes in contact with the apices of the vestibular and lingual cusps from one side of the arch to the other and can be considered the result of coronal lingual inclination of the posterior teeth of the lower arch.

The curvature of the occlusal plane results from variations in the axial alignment of the lower arch teeth, which in turn depends on the eruption direction of dental elements. In optimal occlusion, the curve of Spee is slightly concave and has a maximum depth of 2.5 mm, whereas a greater depth of the curve indicates crowding within the arch. All mandibular movements are produced by the right and left temporomandibular joints, which rarely make the same movements synchronously; a flat occlusal plane would not allow a simultaneous functional contact in more than one area of the arch. The curvature of the occlusal plane allows the maximum use of dental contact and permits disocclusion of the posterior teeth during mandibular protrusion movements. The curve of Wilson also has a functional significance such that the coronolingual inclination of the lower molars is related to the dominant direction of the force exerted by muscles on them. In fact, the lower molars are aligned parallel to the internal pterygoid muscles to achieve optimal resistance to functional stresses. Furthermore, the

coronolingual inclination of the lower occlusal plane during mastication allows direct access of food from the lingual area with no interference created by the lingual cusps. The curve of Wilson favors disocclusion of the lower vestibular cusps in relation to the upper ones in lateral mandibular movements.
The arrangement of permanent elements in compliance with the six keys factors described by L.F. Andrews allows occlusion to be stable and to protect the health of the temporomandibular joints in conditions of maximum intercuspidation, particularly in eccentric movements. In fact, the six key factors allow occlusion to have centric stops on all the posterior teeth as well as come in contact with all the anterior teeth in the *static phase* of maximum intercuspidation, whereas in the *dynamic phase*, they also allow protrusive anterior guidance and canine guidance in the lateral direction accompanied by bilateral posterior disocclusion. Occlusion with these characteristics is defined as "mutually protected occlusion," which functions without damaging the articular structures.

References

Andrews LF. Straight wire. Basi teoriche e applicazioni pratiche. Milano: Masson; 1993.

Ash MM. Atlante della morfologia dentale di Wheeler. Milano: Scienza e tecnica dentistica edizioni internazionali; 1991.

Gianelly AA. Tecnica bidimensionale teoria e pratica. Milano: Orteam SPA; 1999.

Graber TM e Vanarsdall RL. Ortodonzia. Principi e tecniche attuali. Padova: Piccin; 1998.

Langlade M. Diagnosi ortodontica. Milano: Scienza e tecnica dentistica edizioni internazionali; 1983.

McNamara Jr JA, Brudon WL. Trattamento ortodontico e ortopedico in dentatura mista. Milano: Masson; 1998.

Moyers RE. Manuale di ortodonzia. Milano: Scienza e tecnica dentistica edizioni internazionali; 1991.

Okeson JP. Management of temporomandibular disorders and occlusion. 4th ed. St. Louis: Mosby; 1993.

Proffit WR. Ortodonzia moderna. 3th ed. Milano: Masson; 2008.

Rakosi T, Jonas I. Diagnostica ortognatodontica. Milano: Masson; 1992.

Salzmann JA. Ortodonzia oggi. Padova: Piccin; 1986.

Tollaro I, Antonini A, Bassarelli V et al. La fase della dentatura decidua. Quaderni di Odontoiatria infantile. Milano: Masson; 1990.

Van der Linden FPGM, Wassemberg HJW, Bakker PJMR. La permuta nella dentizione umana – Parte I. Dental Cadmos 1985:6:19-45. Parte II. Dental Cadmos 1985:7:19-46. Parte III. Dental Cadmos 1985:9:17 AM-55. Parte IV. Dental Cadmos 1985:11:15 AM-43.

Chapter 5

Radiology in pediatric dentistry

F. D'Ambrosio

In pediatric radiodiagnostic assessment, it is necessary to subdivide the available methodologies into first- and second-level investigations:

- first-level investigations include *panoramic X-ray*, *intraoral radiography*, and *skull teleradiography*
- second-level investigations include computed tomography (CT) and three-dimensional (3D) *cone beam* computed tomography (CBCT)

All investigations performed by dentists are digitalized; this allows the reduction of radiation doses administered to pediatric patients. Furthermore, it also allows the modification of images in cases of under- or over-exposure.

Panoramic X-Ray (Orthopantomogram)

In the diagnostic procedures used by pediatric dentists, panoramic X-ray is an indispensable tool for formulating an accurate diagnosis. This is a methodology based on rotary tomography, which requires correct head positioning by the patient who is asked to stand still.

There are numerous advantages of this radiographic examination. First, undoubtedly, there is an ease with which the examination is performed, and this is linked to the opportunity of highlighting numerous anatomical structures on a single film. Furthermore, panoramic X-ray is associated with a low radiation dose, and the examination can be repeated during follow-ups over time.

The disadvantages include higher costs of the equipment than those of the equipment needed for intraoral radiographic examination, need for space to install it, and long exposure time, with possible motion artifacts obtained with noncooperative pediatric patients. Furthermore, it generates a geometric enlargement, which might result in distortions and poor images.

The radiographic anatomy as observed via panoramic X-ray provides an overview of the main anatomic structures. In fact, only radiographic examination can highlight the upper and lower jaws, alveolar processes, and temporomandibular joints on one single film and can provide an overview of the periodontal apparatus.

Panoramic X-ray provides a complete view of the alveolar bone architecture. In the mixed and permanent dentition of growing individuals, the alveolar bone shows a reticular arrangement, with large meshes of bone trabeculae arranged regularly. The orientation of lines is parallel to the occlusal forces and follows the direction of growth forces. Conversely, alveolar cancellous bone shows a fine and intertwined arrangement and has a heterogeneous orientation. Furthermore, it provides information related to the presence of possible congenital or acquired defects of the deciduous or permanent dentition, such as anomalies of number, site, position, development, shape, eruption, and structure as well as carious processes, cysts, and tumoral pathologies. Moreover, in pediatric dentistry, panoramic X-ray allows the detection of general development conditions related to dentition, development phases, and eruption path of permanent teeth. It is also possible to highlight the root resorption of deciduous teeth and the root formation of permanent teeth.

Digital panoramic X-ray

The advantage of digital panoramic X-ray in pediatric patients is not the radiation dose provided, which is slightly lower than that provided with analog panoramic X-ray, but the fact that the procedure need not be repeated even in cases of incorrect provision of data. In such cases, it is possible to reprocess the image using the control panel (Tab. 5.1; Fig. 5.1-5.3).

Table 5.1 Digital orthopanoramic X-ray dosage

I	62 kV	8 mA	Up to 6 years
II	64 kV	8 mA	Up to 14 years
III	69 kV	15 mA	Up to 18 years

These data are indicative and related to the latest generation of digital machines. Indicated values may vary according to the manufacturer.

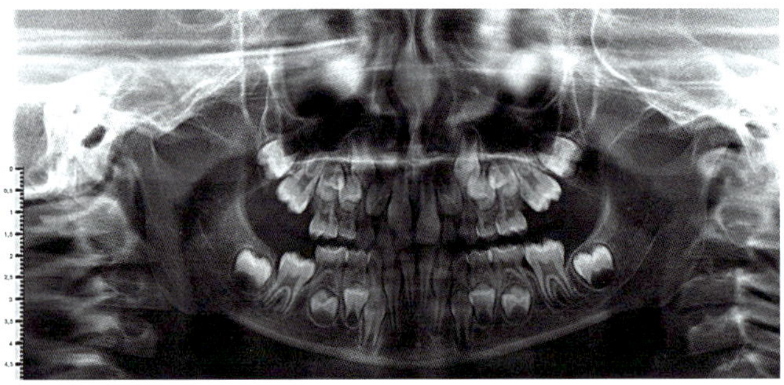

Figure 5.1 Digital panoramic X-ray: check in mixed dentition (7 years).

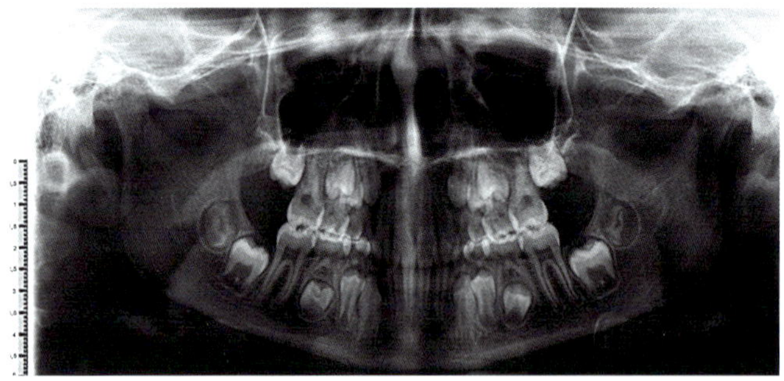

Figure 5.2 Digital panoramic X-ray: check in mixed dentition (11 years).

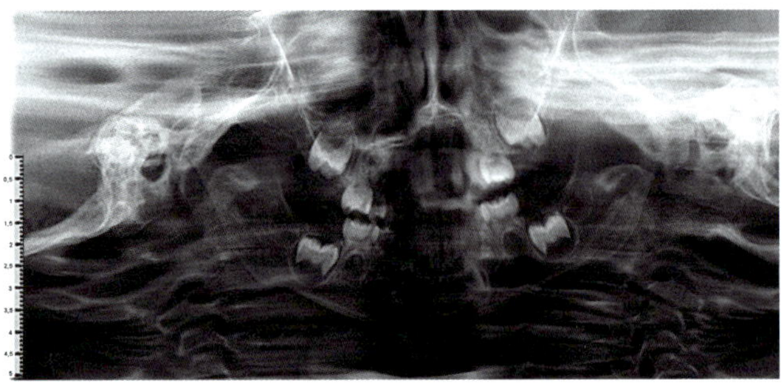

Figure 5.3 Digital panoramic X-ray: motion artifacts.

Intraoral radiography

Periapical, *bitewing*, and occlusal intraoral radiographs are used in pediatric dentistry. While obtaining these, it is better to protect the patient with an apron and a collar to reduce exposure to radiation (Fig. 5.4).

Periapical intraoral radiographs are obtained to examine a specific region and allow the diagnosis of dental caries, radicular and periapical pathologies, bone defects, and impacted or supernumerary teeth. Furthermore, they are indicated in traumatic lesions of teeth and jaws as well as for observing resorption modalities in deciduous teeth and the development of permanent teeth (Fig. 5.5-5.8).

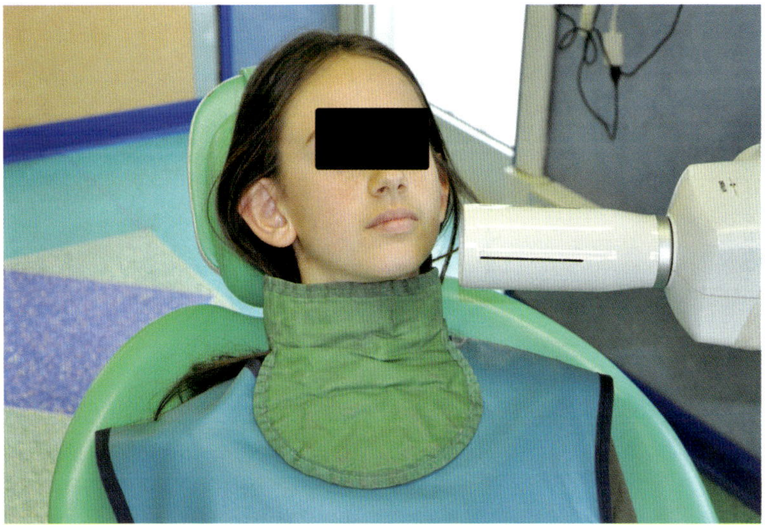

Figure 5.4 Devices for pediatric radioprotection: apron and collar.

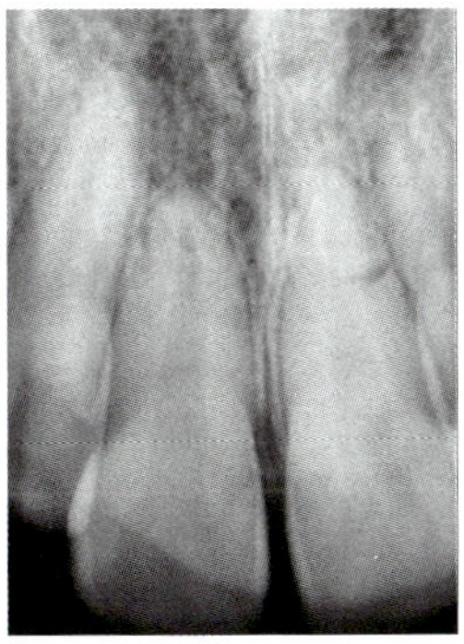

Figure 5.5 Intraoral radiography: presence of traumatic apical fracture of 22.

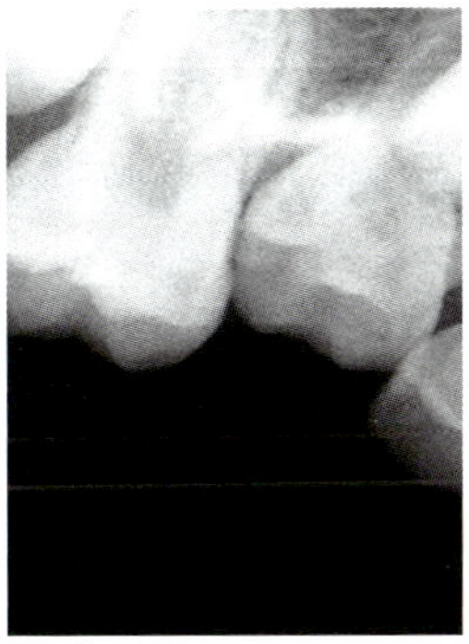

Figure 5.6 Intraoral radiography: presence of deciduous anchylotic element 55 in infraocclusion.

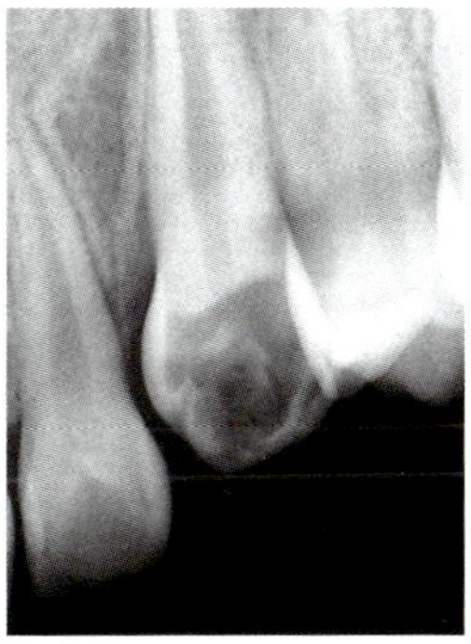

Figure 5.7 Intraoral radiography: presence of anomaly in the coronal structure of 23.

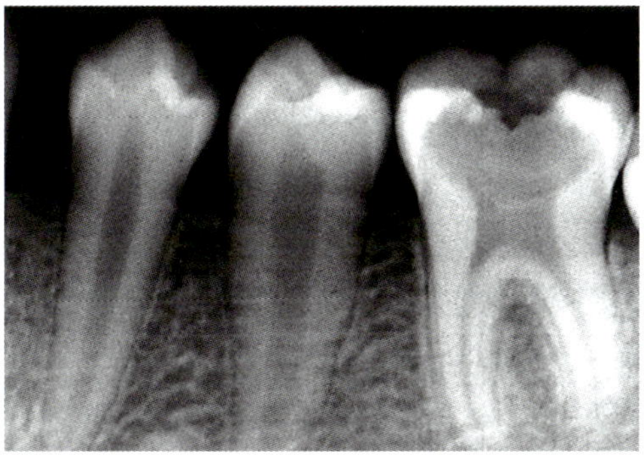

Figure 5.8 Intraoral radiography: presence of destructive caries of 46.

Bitewing radiographs are specifically obtained for the diagnosis of small carious lesions and, in particular, for the diagnosis of lesions under formation because they provide precise details of pathologies involved even in youngest children (Fig. 5.9).
Occlusal radiographs are obtained particularly for the diagnosis of impacted teeth, when it is necessary to establish the site of vestibular or palatolingual impaction to diagnose supernumerary elements and to control the median palatine suture opening in case of rapid expansion of the palate.
In clinical practice, they increasingly tend to be replaced, especially for assessing the localization of impacted teeth, by 3D *CBCT* scans for obtaining better anatomical information (Fig. 5.10; Tab. 5.2).

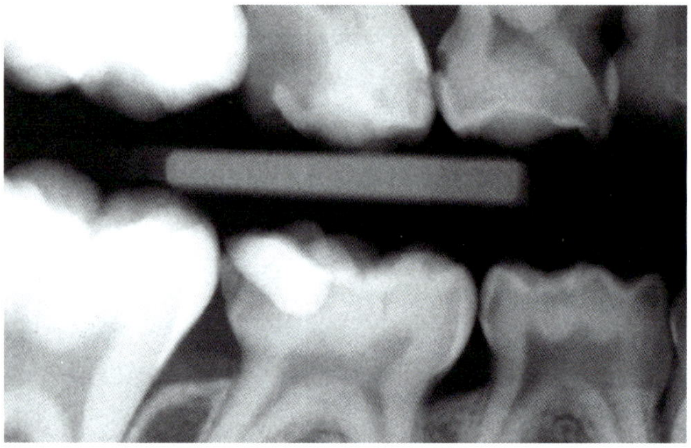

Figure 5.9 *Bitewing* radiography. Investigation of interproximal caries presence.

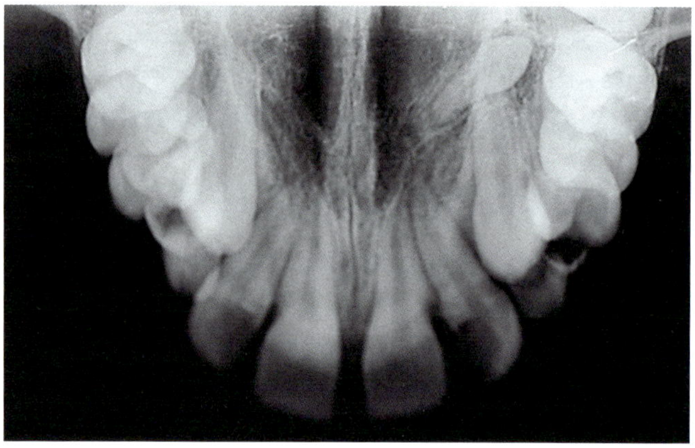

Figure 5.10 Upper occlusal radiography with the presence of supernumerary element.

Table 5.2 Digital intraoral X-ray dosage

Molars		Premolars/Canines		Incisors		Occlusal
Upper	Lower	Upper	Lower	Upper	Lower	
0.08	0.06	0.06	0.04	0.05	0.03	0.10

70 kV, 7 mA (fixed values: only the exposure time varies).
These data are indicative and related to the latest generation of digital machines. Indicated values may vary according to manufacturers. The values are expressed in msec.

Latero-lateral teleradiography

Latero-lateral teleradiography is a standard radiographic procedure for assessing skull and soft tissues and is performed by complying with some parameters, which are as follows: the Frankfurt plane must be parallel to the floor, whereas the medial sagittal plane must be parallel to the radiographic plate and perpendicular to the radiogenic source, which is placed at a distance of 1.50 m. Latero-lateral teleradiography allows the quantification of sagittal and vertical discrepancies of skeletal bases as well as the analysis of the profile of soft tissues in pediatric patients. Furthermore, it is possible to control the nasopharyngeal area, any calcifications or focal lesions of the skull, and the size and shape of the sella turcica (Fig. 5.11 and 5.12; Tab. 5.3).

Posteroanterior teleradiography

This is a fundamental radiographic methodology for formulating an accurate orthodontic diagnosis in pediatric patients, when the detected anomaly involves the vertical and transverse plane. It is indicated in cases of malocclusion characterized by asymmetries and allows diagnoses to be made in cases of lateral deviation or laterognathia. Furthermore, it is possible to compare the latter in time using radiographic images of the same individual to assess the progress as well as response to an orthodontic therapy (Fig. 5.13).

Table 5.3 Digital laterolateral telecranial X-ray dosage

I	70 kV	15 mA	14.9 sec	Up to 5 years
II	73kV	15 mA	14.9 sec	Between 5 and 15 years
III	77 kV	15 mA	14.9 sec	Up to 18 years

These data are indicative and related to the latest generation of digital machines. Indicated values may vary according to manufacturers.

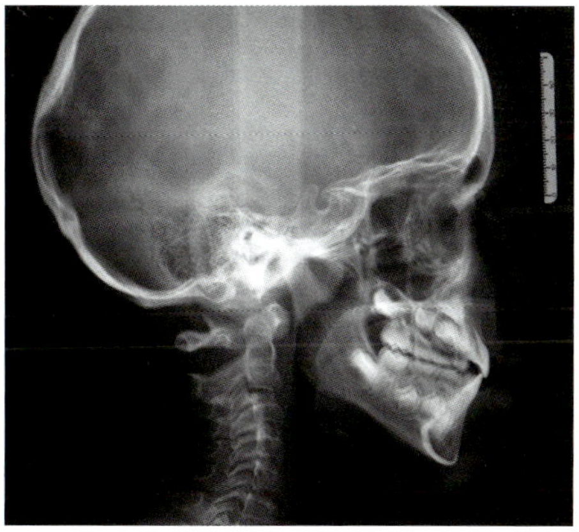

Figure 5.11 Latero-lateral teleradiography.

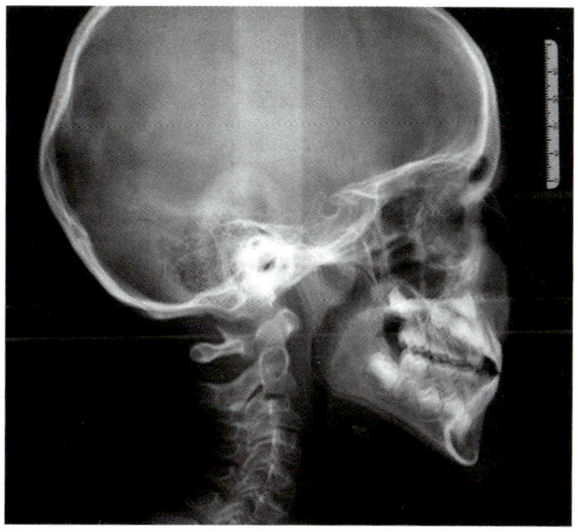

Figure 5.12 Latero-lateral teleradiography, incorrect intercuspidation.

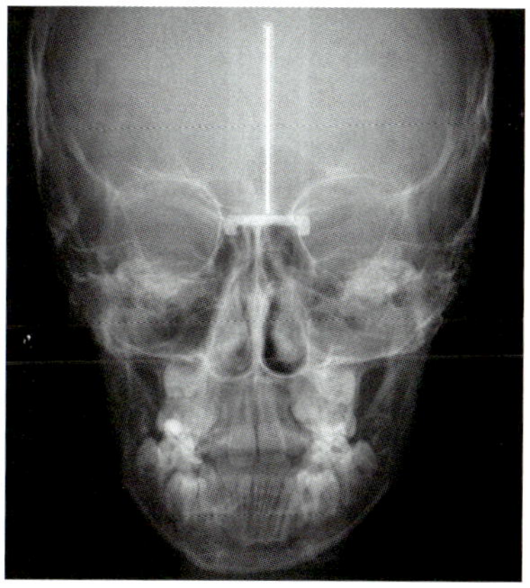

Figure 5.13 Posteroanterior teleradiography.

CT Dentascan

This examination is performed with a specifically dedicated reconstruction software that involves the use of volumetric acquisitions in axial incidence, with a thickness of 0.5–1.0 mm, is performed for high reconstruction with a window specifically dedicated to bones. The examination is performed using a multidetector equipment with an acquisition time of a few seconds, which can vary depending on the number of detectors included in the device. Although this assessment delivers a radiation dose higher than that delivered by 3D *CBCT*, in some cases, it is indispensable to eliminate motion artifacts in children aged <5 years. Obviously, it is necessary to assess the cost–benefit ratio in each case; therefore, the radiation dose absorbed by the patient will be justified in cases of serious pathologies.

3D *cone beam* CT

This methodology allows the entire volume of the upper and lower jaws to be visualized, with radiation doses lower than those used for obtaining CT scans. Acquisitions are performed through *cone beam* rotation with a device that rotates around pediatric patients, with acquisition times slightly longer than those needed for CT Dentascan. Therefore, patient cooperation is critical. The position assumed by the child is vertical and not supine, as in the case of CT scan, and is therefore less comfortable. In this type of methodology, it is impossible to get help from family members to restrain the child's movements owing to the rotation of the tube around the head (Fig. 5.14-5.23).

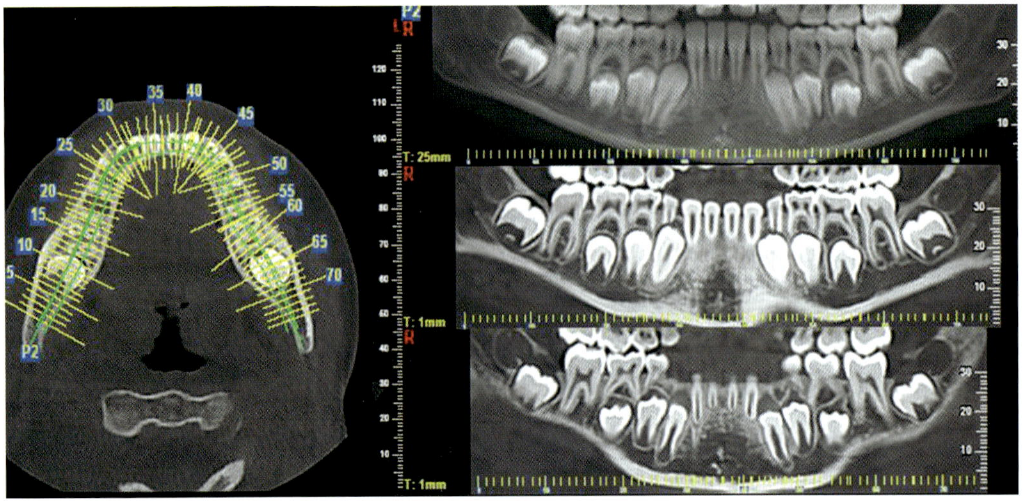

Figure 5.14 3D *cone beam* CT: Control in mixed dentition (axial and Panorex).

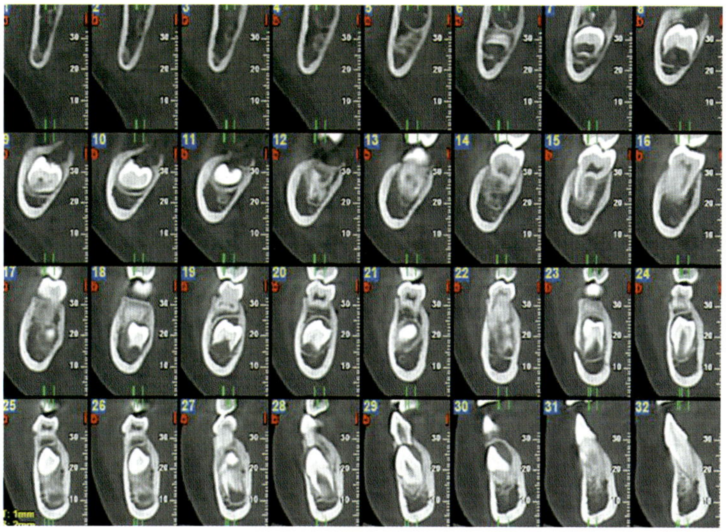

Figure 5.15 3D *cone beam*: check in mixed dentition (cross reconstructions)

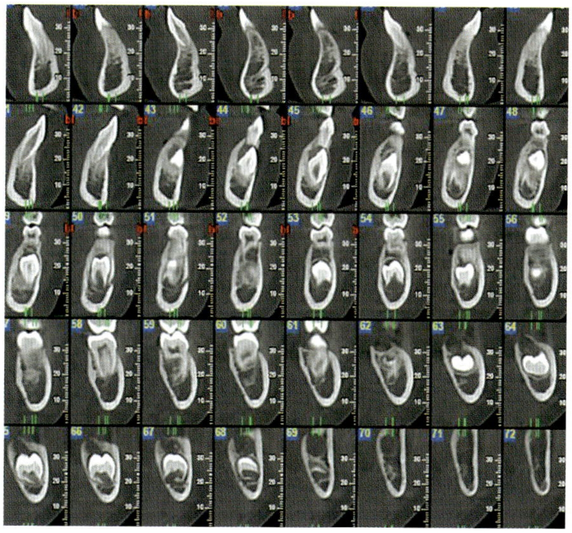

Figure 5.16 3D *cone beam*: check in mixed dentition (cross reconstructions)

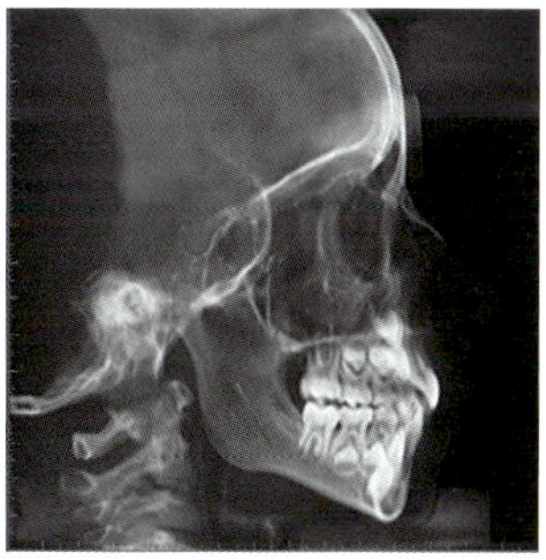

Figure 5.17 Latero-lateral teleradiography through *cone beam* reconstruction.

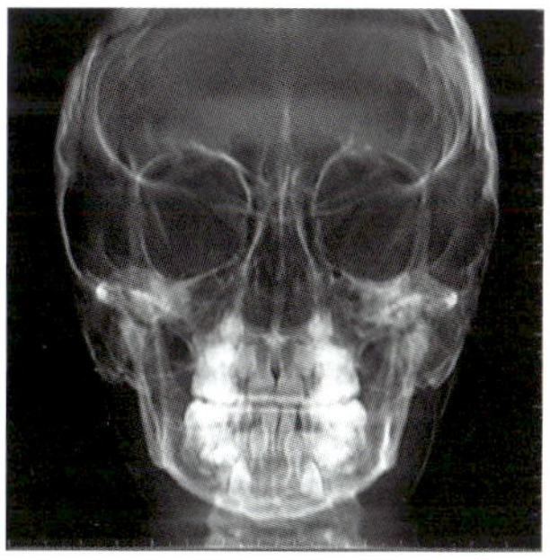

Figure 5.18 Posteroanterior teleradiography through *cone beam* reconstruction.

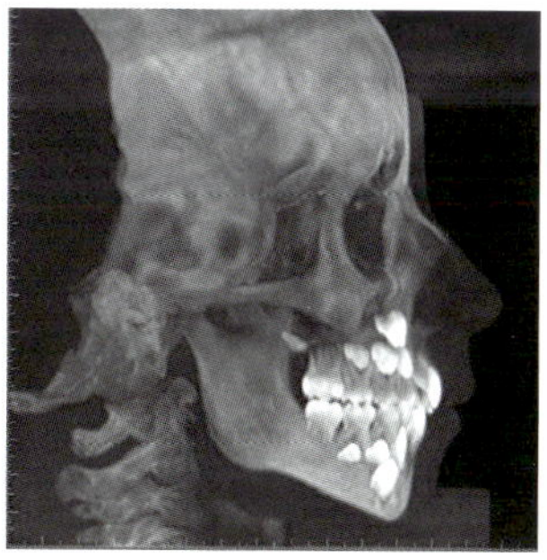

Figure 5.19 Latero-lateral 3D through *cone beam* reconstruction.

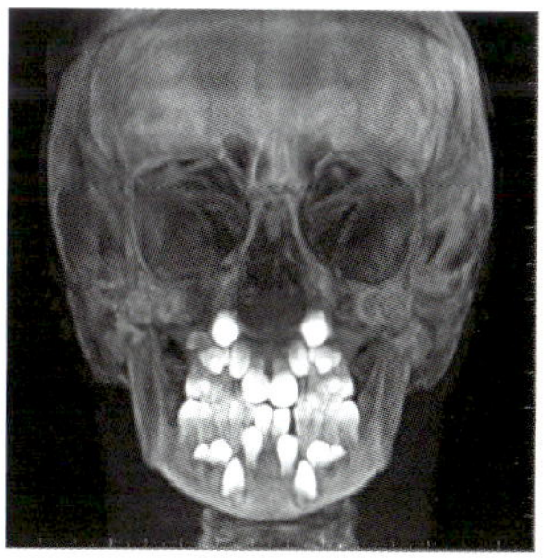

Figure 5.20 Posteroanterior 3D through *cone beam* reconstruction.

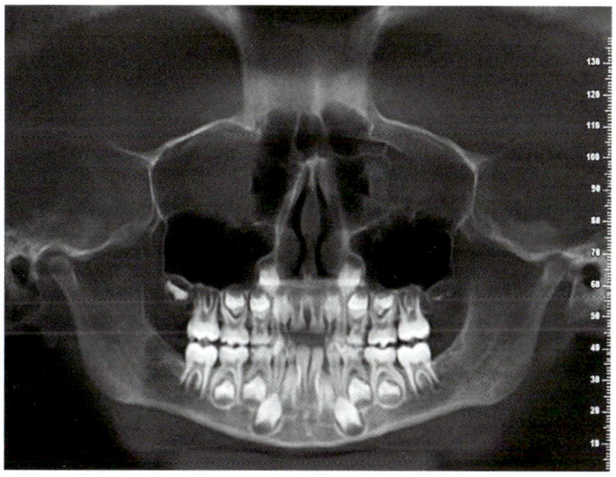

Figure 5.21 Digital panoramic X-ray through *cone beam* reconstruction.

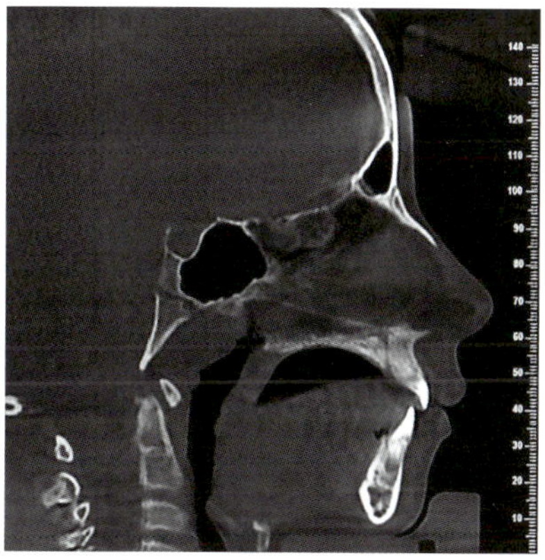

Figure 5.22 Mid-sagittal plane in *cone beam* reconstruction.

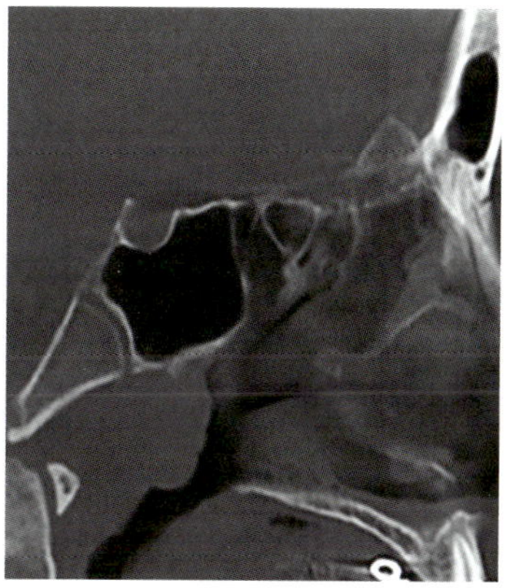

Figure 5.23: View of adenoid vegetation through *cone beam* reconstruction.

Table 5.4 Comparison between CT Dentascan and 3D *cone beam*

CT Dentascan	3D *cone beam*
High radiation dose	Low radiation dose
Supine patient position	Vertical patient position
Short acquisition time	Long acquisition time
Patient may be restrained	Patient is on its own

Both CT Dentascan and 3D *cone beam* provide more information in terms of the opportunity to visualize the alveolar bone two- and three-dimensionally. They are also useful for revealing the relationship of any existing dental anomalies with the surrounding anatomical structures (Tab. 5.4).

Pediatric pathologies

Caries

From a radiographic viewpoint, it is possible to identify an area of radiolucency localized on the crown, on the collar, or at an interproximal level between two adjacent dental elements. Caries can be observed only when it reaches the dentin. Conversely, in lesions that are at an initial stage, it is possible to identify only a shadow below the amelodentinal junction. A possible assessment error is the so-called "*mach band*," which is owing to a line of increased density above or below the occlusal enamel. There are three severity levels of caries, which are as follows:

- superficial, if it only involves the superficial dentin
- average, if it involves the enamel and dentin but not the pulp
- deep, if it also involves the pulp, and this stage might evolve into pulpitis (Fig. 5.24 and 5.25)

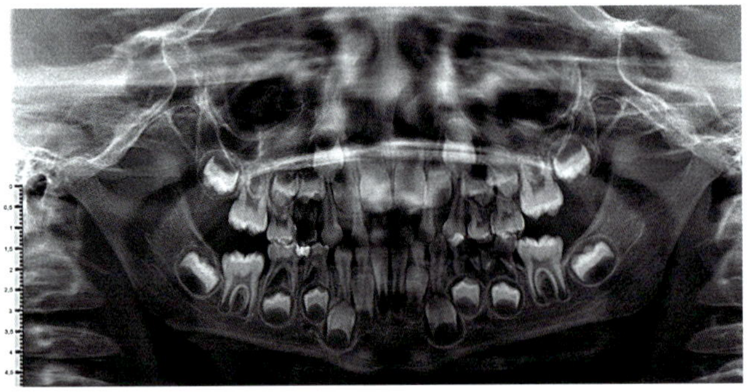

Figure 5.24 Digital panoramic X-ray: caries of 84.

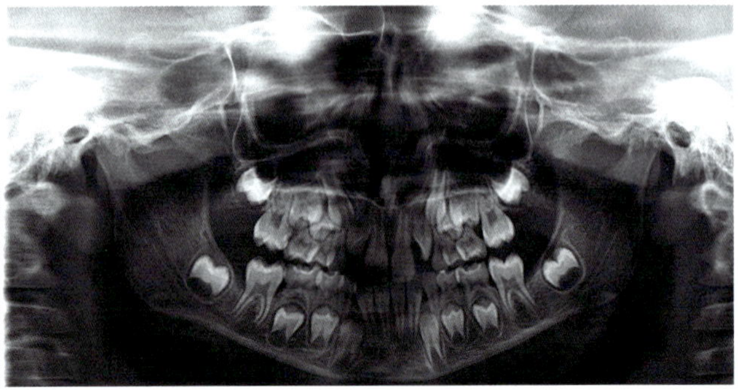

Figure 5.25 Digital panoramic X-ray: destructive and interproximal caries of 74-75 and destructive caries of 54.

Cysts

Cystic lesions are considered as a closed and round cavity of epithelial origin. Via traditional radiography, they appear as distinct translucent areas, whereas on CT or 3D *cone beam* scans, they appear as hypodense images, with somewhat regular margins. Because they are lesions detected most frequently in pediatric dentistry, radicular and follicular cysts are indicated below.

Follicular or dentigerous cysts These most frequently involve the third lower molar or the upper canine and often appear at the site of an unerupted tooth. The cyst wraps the crown of the retained tooth and originates from the dental follicles. This makes the cysts easily detectable during radiological examinations. For differential diagnosis, it is important to remember that the same appearance as that of a follicular cyst can be seen in a magnified dental follicle (to make the diagnosis, the rule that a follicular cyst should have a greater axis of at least 3-4 mm is followed). Ameloblastoma and keratocysts are among the pathologies identified through differential diagnosis.

Radicular cysts. These are characterized by a constant relation with the roots of one or more dental elements. They are frequently associated with dental caries and develop from a previous apical granuloma. On radiological examination, they appear as areas of osteolysis with clear margins that include the root apexes. The most affected sites are the lateral upper incisors. (Fig. 5.26-5.32).

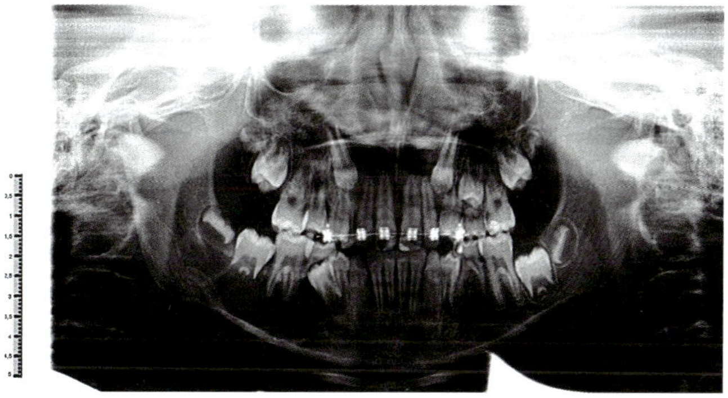

Figure 5.26 Digital panoramic X-ray: right hemimandibular cyst.

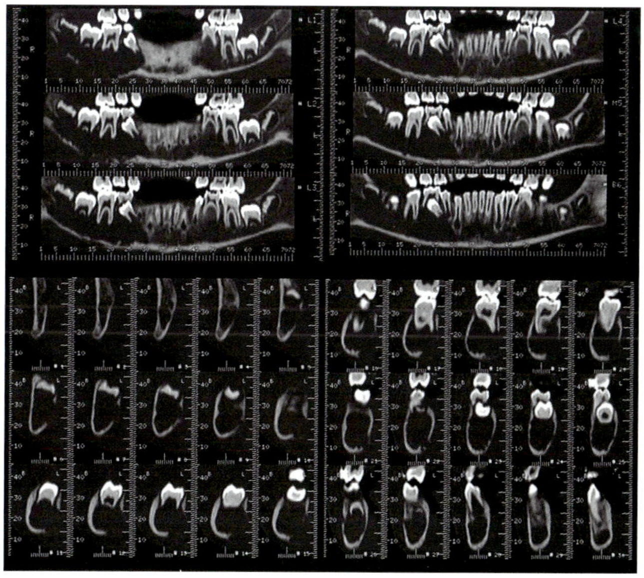

Figure 5.27 CT Dentascan: right hemimandibular cyst (panorex and cross reconstruction).

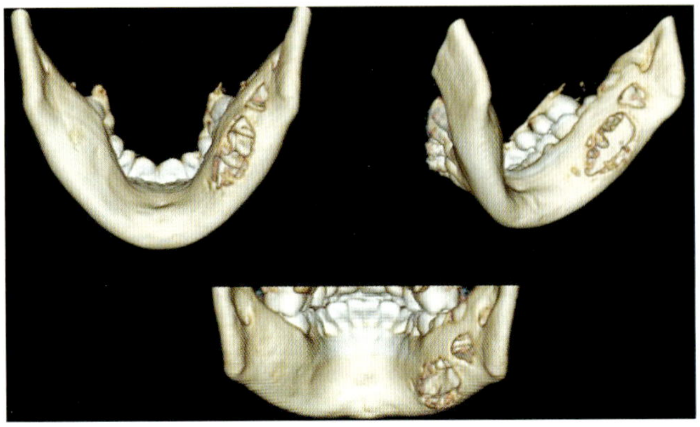

Figure 5.28 CT Dentascan: right hemimandibular cyst.

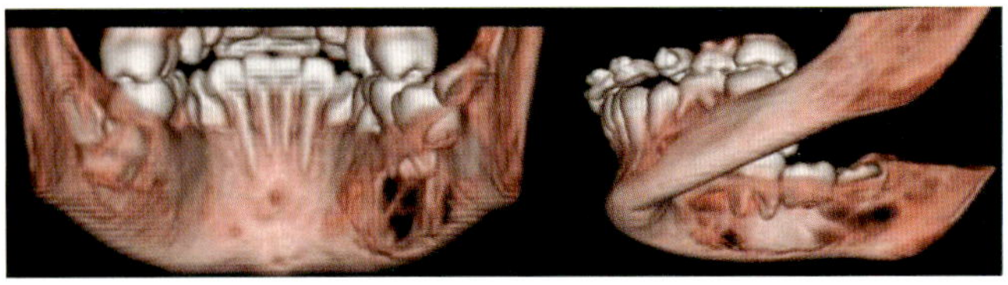

Figure 5.29 CT Dentascan: right hemimandibular cyst.

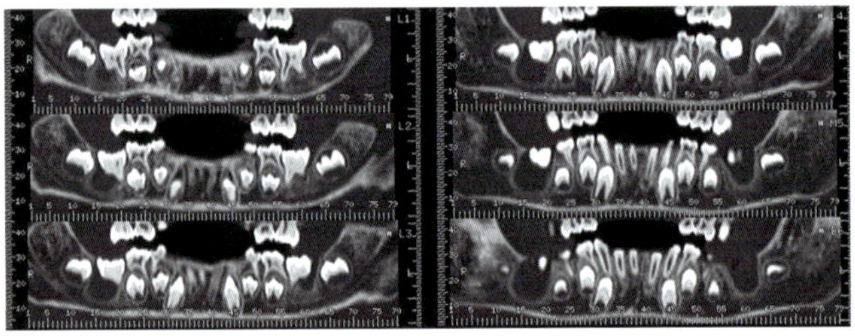

Figure 5.30 CT with panorex reconstruction: bilateral cyst.

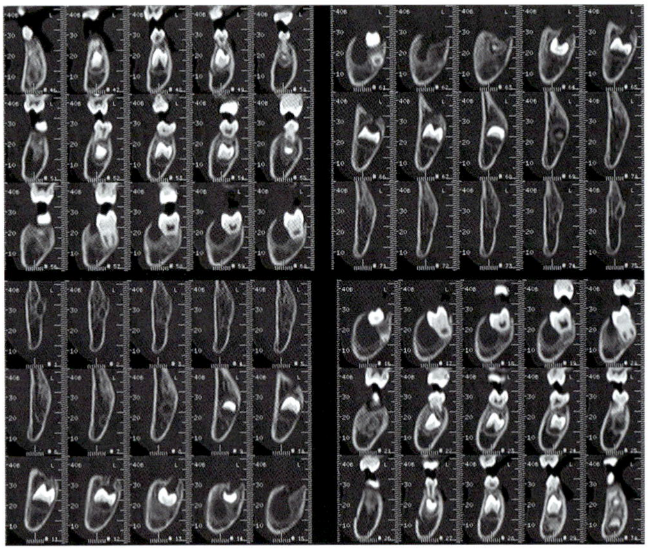

Figure 5.31 CT with cross reconstruction: bilateral cyst.

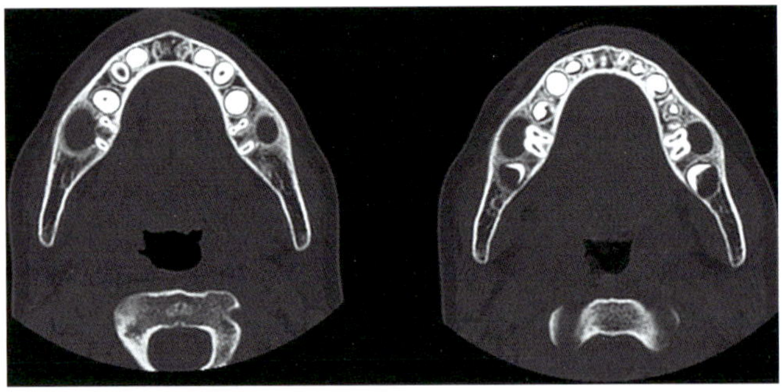

Figure 5.32 Computed axial tomography: bilateral cyst.

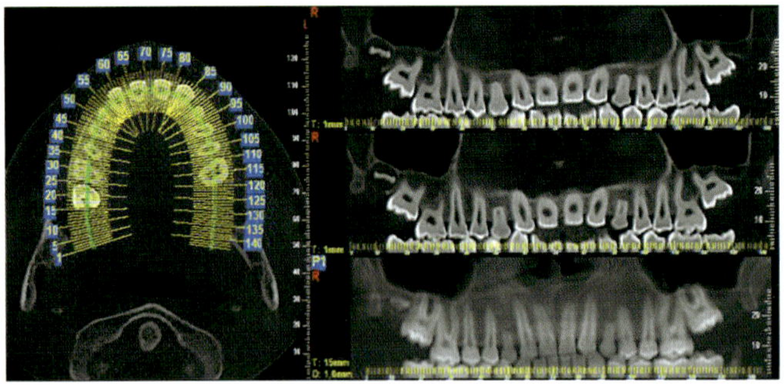

Figure 5.33 *Cone beam*: agenesis of 13 and 23 (axial and panorex).

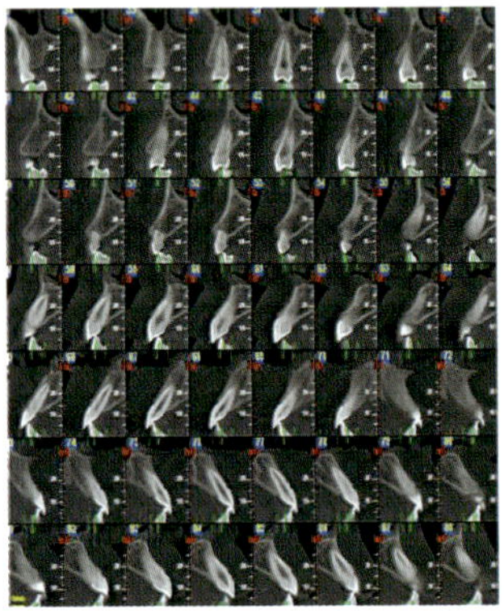

Figure 5.34 *Cone beam*: agenesis of 13 and 23 (cross reconstruction).

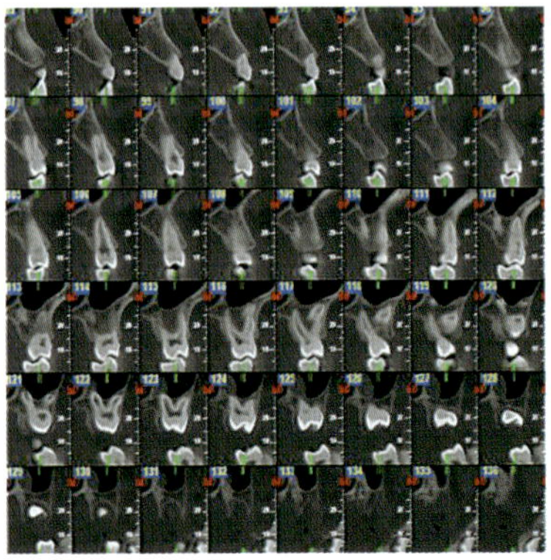

Figure 5.35 *Cone beam*: agenesis of 13 and 23 (cross reconstruction).

Dental anomalies

Dental development in children can be affected by numerous malformations and anomalies. Particularly, it is important to remember the anomalies of number (rounded up or rounded down), position, and eruption.

Dental agenesis

Agenesis refers to the absence of one or more dental elements. In terms of frequency, teeth that are most frequently involved are the third molar, second lower premolar, lateral upper incisor, second upper premolar, upper canine, and central lower incisor. In most cases, a first-level investigation, such as orthopanoramic or intraoral radiography, is sufficient (Fig. 5.33-5.35).

Agenesis can be subdivided as follows:

- *hypodontia*, that is, when one or more dental elements are missing, and lateral incisors are the most frequently involved
- *oligodontia*, that is, when numerous dental elements are missing
- *anodontia*, that is, when all dental elements are missing

Supernumerary teeth and transposition

In this case, first-level investigations cannot be performed to assess spatial relations with surrounding structures; therefore, the two-dimensionality offered by second-level investigations becomes extremely useful for accurate diagnostic and surgical evaluations. Second-level investigations are also indispensable with regards to impacted teeth, particularly for impacted canines, to assess eruption modalities and establish the exact dental position, that is, whether they are vestibularly or palatally located in relation to adjacent elements.

Supernumerary teeth. This condition is believed to be hereditary. These teeth are classified as *mesiodens* (supernumerary tooth interposed between upper incisors), paramolars (if they erupt in the molar area), distomolars (distally to the third molar), and supernumary central incisors.

Transposition. This occurs when there is an incorrect order of dental elements within the arch, that is, when the position of dental elements within the same quadrant is switched. The occurrence of ectopic eruption is an essential condition to be discussed in transposition. The most frequently affected site is the maxilla and in particular, canines, which are usually transposed with first premolars and less frequently with lateral incisors (Fig. 5.36 and 5.41).

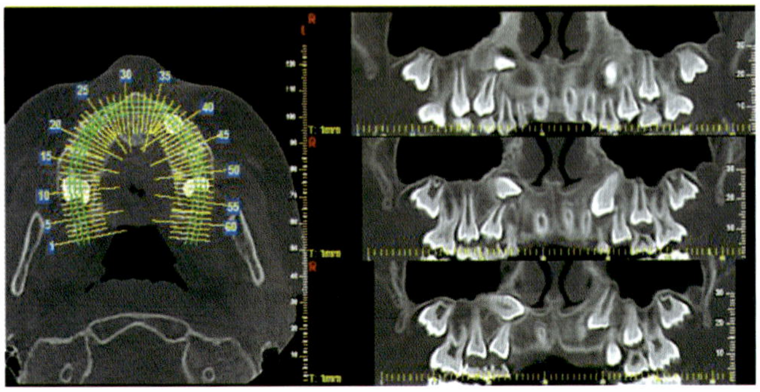

Figure 5.33 *Cone beam*: impacted canines (13) - axial and panorex.

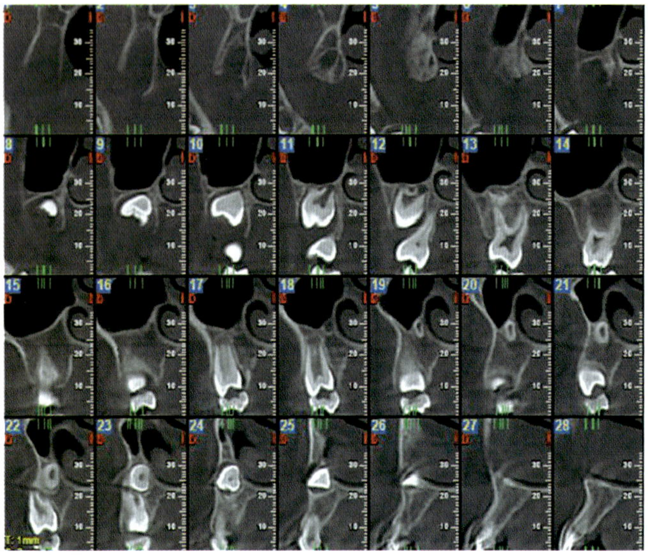

Figure 5.37 *Cone beam*: impacted canines (13) - cross reconstruction.

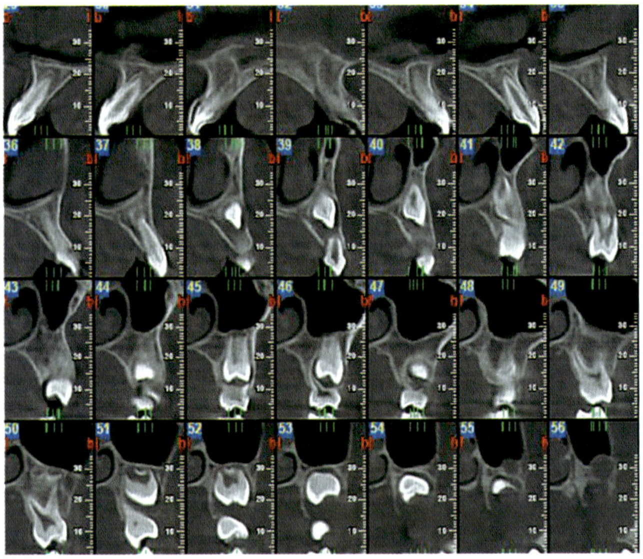

Figure 5.38 *Cone beam*: impacted canines (13) - cross reconstruction.

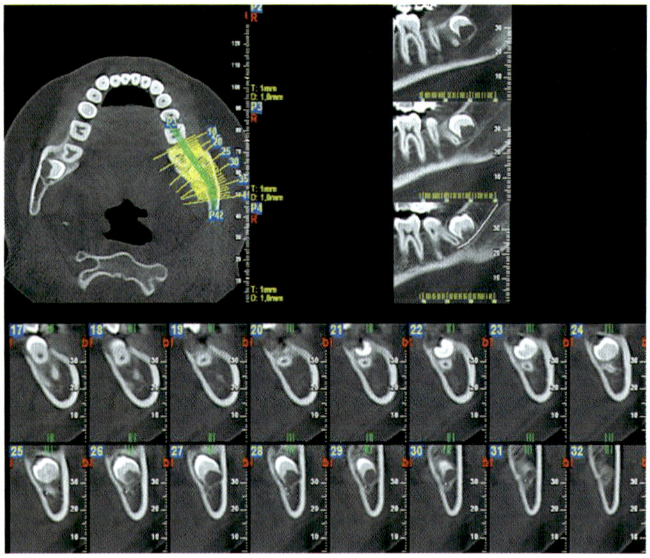

Figure 5.39 *Cone beam*: Impacted 38 (axial with panorex and cross reconstruction).

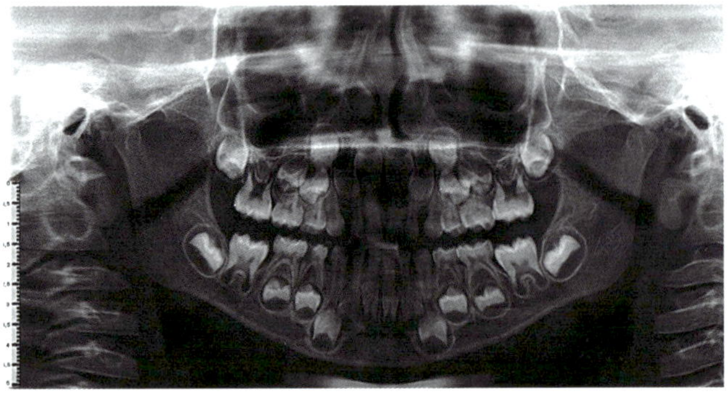

Figure 5.40 Digital panoramic X-ray: 22 rotated.

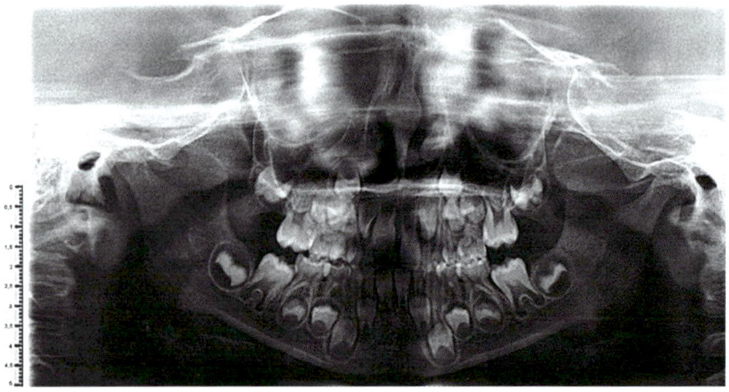

Figure 5.41 Digital panoramic X-ray: crowding in 14-15.

Tumoral lesions

Tumoral lesions in pediatric patients warrant special mention because although rare, they need to be immediately identified and treated. According to the 2005 WHO universal classification, odontogenic tumors are classified as lesions deriving from epithelial, ectomesenchymal, or mesenchymal elements of the tooth formation apparatus, radiologically characterized by osteolytic and osteoblastic areas. Many neoplasias indicated in the aforementioned classification occur during adulthood and therefore do not fall within the subject discussed here, whereas some, fortunately just a few, predominantly affect pediatric patients, and these include ameloblastic fibroma, ameloblastic odontoma, odontoma, melanotic neuroectodermal tumor of infancy, myxoma, and adenomatoid odontogenic tumor.

Ameloblastic fibromas

This is a type of tumor with mixed origin affecting children and adolescents, with a maximum peak of onset at 5–20 years of age.
It mostly affects the lower jaw, particularly in the molar–premolar region. It is generally asymptomatic because it occasionally presents with a painless swelling. It is characterized by slow growth and often tends to recur locally, despite surgical excision of the primary lesion. Radiologically, it appears as a unilocular or multilocular radiolucent area with slightly irregular margins and is associated with affected teeth in 90% of cases.

Ameloblastic odontomas

This is a benign tumor that affects children and adolescents (6 months–15 years) and mostly occurs in the molar–premolar region without evident distinction between the upper and lower jaws. It is hard and occasionally presents with painful swelling, which radiologically appears as a unilocular or multilocular radiolucent area similar to a cyst, containing radiopaque sections attributable to calcifications or impacted teeth. This also tends to recur locally after surgical excision owing to the presence of tumoral residues within the surgical cavity that continue to proliferate.

Odontomas

This is a benign tumor that includes the following two variants:

- *Complex odontoma*: In this, it is possible to identify dentin, enamel, and sometimes cementum. It most frequently affects females. This tumor mostly involves the lower jaw, at the site of the first or second molar. It appears as a structure comprising amorphous calcified masses.

- *Compound odontoma*: It is characterized by dental elements of different shapes and volumes. It tends to affect males slightly more frequently and mostly appears at the level of the premaxilla at the site of an unerupted canine.

This tumor affects patients of all ages, although it tends to appear more frequently in young adults, with a maximum peak onset at the age of approximately 20 years. Clinically speaking, this too is frequently asymptomatic because it is characterized only by a slight swelling in the affected area and by a failed tooth eruption. Radiologically, it appears as a unichambered or multichambered radiopaque area with smooth or irregular margins (Fig. 5.42-5.52).

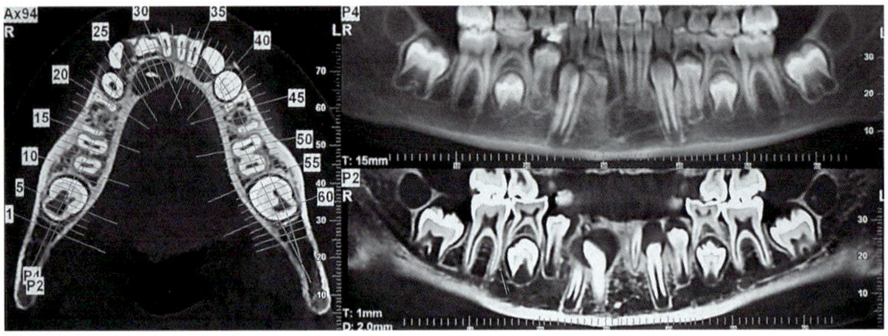

Figure 5.42 *Cone beam*: odomtoma (axial and panorex)

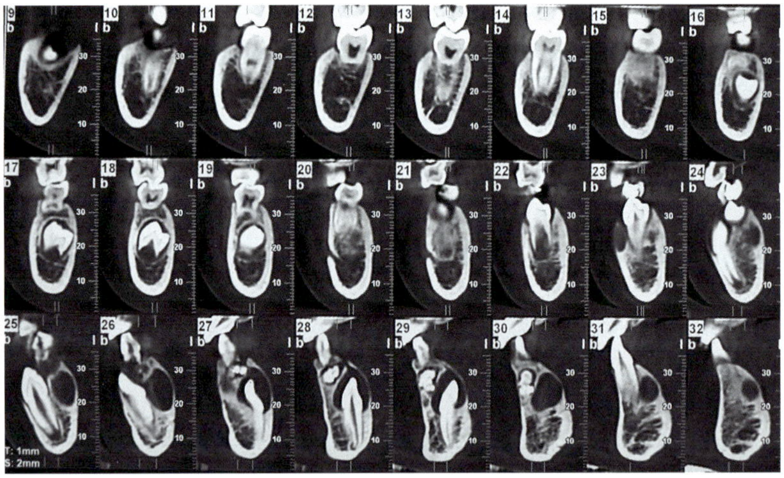

Figure 5.43 *Cone beam*: odontoma (cross reconstruction from 27 to 30).

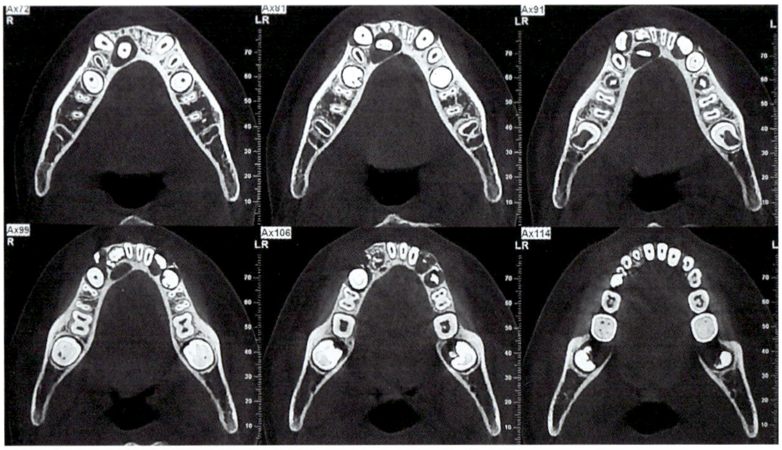

Figure 5.44 *Cone beam*: odontoma (axial reconstruction).

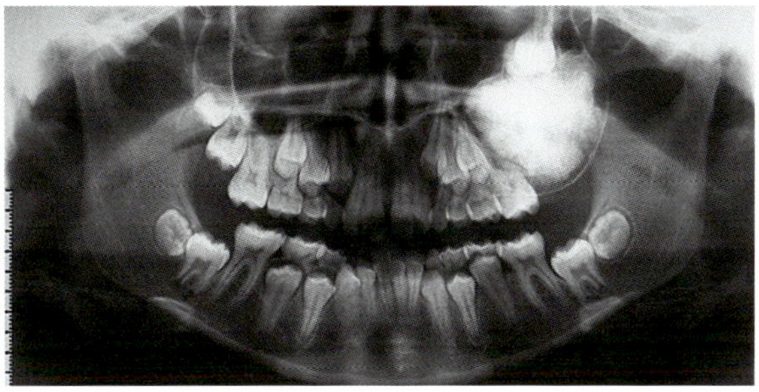

Figura 5.45 Digital panoramic X-ray: ameloblastic odontoma.

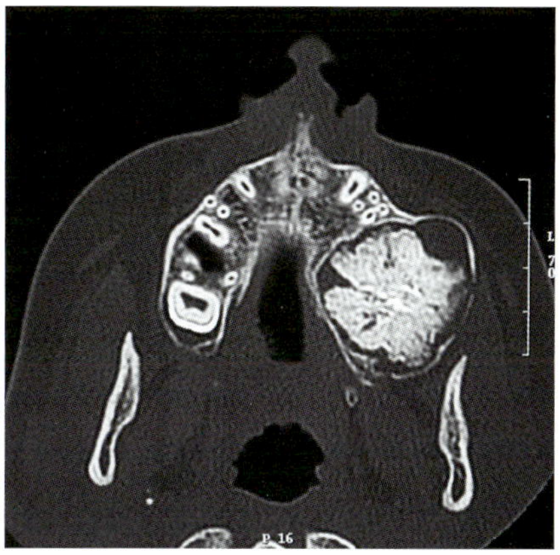

Figure 5.46 Computed axial tomography: ameloblastic odontoma.

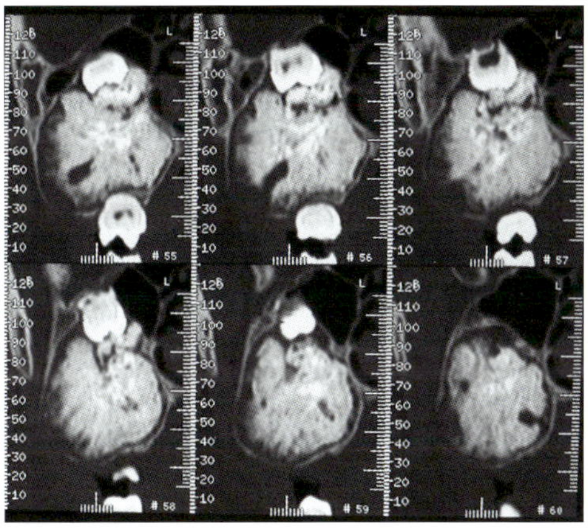

Figure 5.47 CT with cross reconstruction: ameloblastic odontoma.

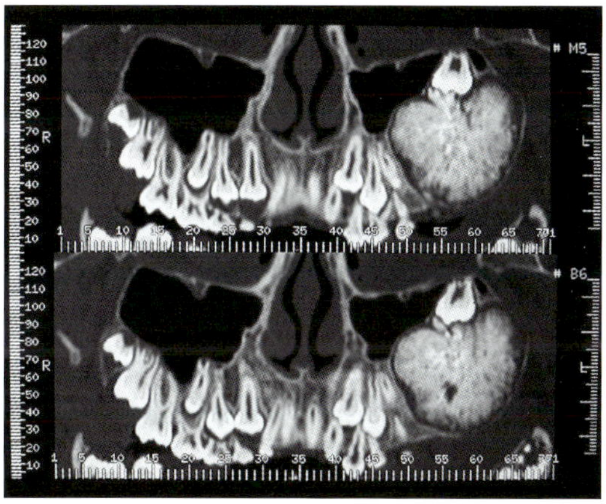

Figure 5.48 CT with panorex reconstruction: ameloblastic odontoma.

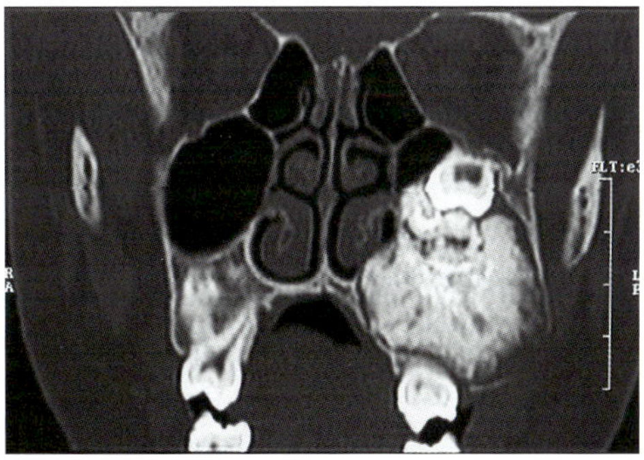

Figure 5.49 CT with coronal reconstruction: ameloblastic odontoma.

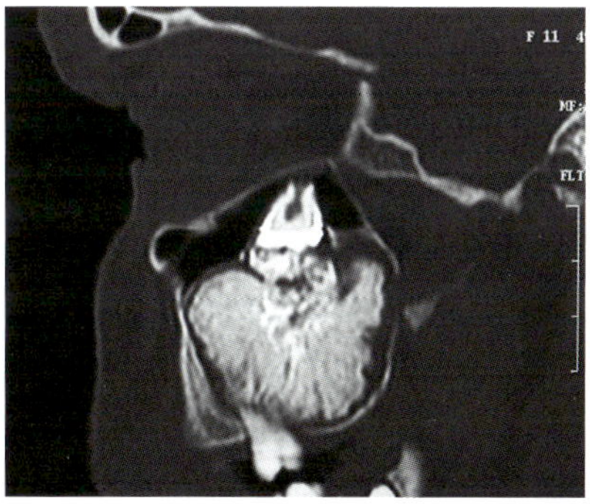

Figure 5.50 CT with sagittal reconstruction: ameloblastic odontoma.

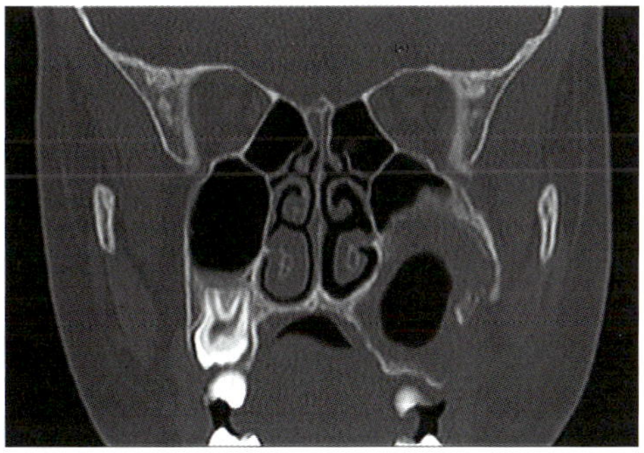

Figure 5.51 CT with coronal reconstruction: residual fragment observed after postoperative check.

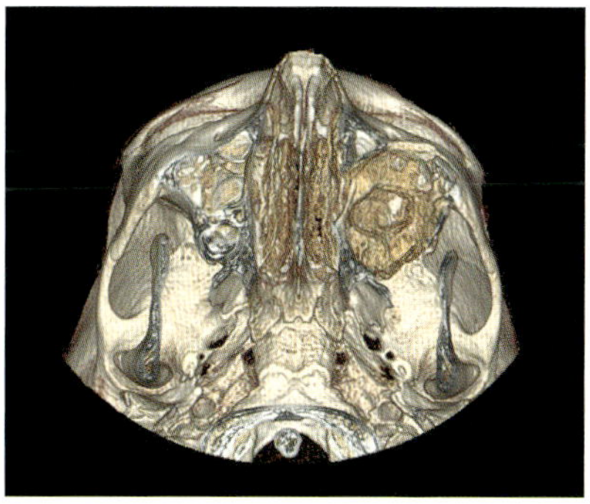

Figure 5.52 3D reconstruction, postoperative check 3D: ameloblastic odontoma.

Myxomas

This is a tumor belonging to the relatively frequent mesenchymal type, which affects patients of all ages, including children, adolescents, and young adults, with a maximum peak onset at the age of approximately 30 years.
It has no preferential site of onset, and it can appear in equal measure in the upper and lower jaws; in this case, it particularly appears in the posterior quadrants.
Its growth is slow and is frequently associated with unerupted teeth or dental agenesis.
Radiologically, it appears as a radiolucent area with indistinct limits and numerous chambers, which give it a typical "soap bubble" or "honeycomb" appearance; it might be associated with impacted or missing teeth.
This too tends to recur locally after surgical excision.

Melanocytic neuroectodermal tumors of infancy

This is a rare tumor that particularly affects children aged 0–12 months, with a maximum peak onset at around 6 months, mostly appearing in the upper jaw.
It is characterized by rapid growth and appears as a lesion with blurred and indistinct margins on radiological examination.
Its treatment is exclusively surgical, with the possibility of local recurrence in approximately 20% patients.

Adenomatoid odontogenic tumors

This is an infrequent benign pathology of the upper jaw affecting young adults, particularly women, with a maximum peak onset at the age of 20–30 years.
The site is usually between the level of canines and lateral incisors.
Radiologically, it might appear as a well-circumscribed mass with cystic areas or internal calcifications. This lesion often surrounds the crown of the tooth involved, and the teeth affected sometimes appear divergent.

Adenoameloblastomas

This is a rare tumor affecting young adolescents of approximately 16 years of age and has a higher prevalence in females.
It is possible to identify two histotypes, one with central development, further subdivided in a follicular and an extrafollicular variant, and one with peripheral development.
It usually occurs in the upper jaw and frequently affects unerupted canines.

Conclusions

Imaging plays an important role in the radiological diagnostics of pediatric patients. It should be performed by specialists to establish an accurate diagnostic assessment and involve the use of the most appropriate technique with a limited radiation dose. Furthermore, it should be remembered that self-referentiality of this assessment, as prescribed and performed in many dental clinics, is causing overexposure of pediatric patients owing to poor dosimetric and radiodiagnostic knowledge of dentists.

References

Watanabe H, Honda E, Tetsumura A, Kurabayashi T. A Comparative study for spatial resolution and subjective image characteristics of a multi-slice CT and a cone-beam CT for dental use. Eur J Radiol 2011;77(3):397-402. Epub 2009 Oct 9.

Abanto J, Carvalho TS, Mendes FM et al. Impact of oral diseases and disorders on oral health-related quality of life of preschool children. Commun Dent Oral Epidemiol 2011;39(2):105-14.

Barnes L, Eveson JW, Reichart P, Sidranski D. Pathology and genetics of Head and Neck tumours. World Health Classification of Tumours, Lyon, 2005.

Becker A, Chaushu S, Casap-Caspi N. Cone-beam computed tomography and the orthosurgical management of impacted teeth. J Am Dent Assoc 2010;141(Suppl 3):14S-8S.

Dudic A, Giannopoulou C, Leuzinger M, Kiliaridis S. Detection of apical root resorption after orthodontic treatment by using panoramic radiography and cone-beam computed tomography of super-high resolution. Am J Orthod Dentofacial Orthop 2009;135(4):434-7.

Estrela C, Bueno MR, De Alencar AH et al. Method to evaluate inflammatory root resorption by using cone beam computed tomography. J Endod 2009;35(11):1491-7.

Fujiwara T, Nakano K, Sobue S, Ooshima T. Simultaneous occurrence of unusual odontodysplasia and oligodontia in the permanent dentition: report of a case. Int J Paediatr Dent 2000;10(4):341.

Gisler V, Enkling N, Zix J et al. A multidisciplinary approach to the functional and esthetic rehabilitation of amelogenesis imperfecta and open bite deformity: a case report. J Esthet Restorative Dent 2010;22(5):282-93.

Grauer D, Cevidanes LS, Styner MA et al. Accuracy and landmark error calculation using cone-beam computed tomographygenerated cephalograms. Angle Orthod 2010;80(2):286-94.

Greer RO Jr, Johnson M. Botryoid odontogenic cyst: clinicopathologic analysis of ten cases with three recurrences. J Oral Maxillofac Surg 1988;46(7):574-9.

Haiter-Neto F, Wenzel A, Gotfredsen E. Diagnostic accuracy of cone beam computed tomography scans compared with intraoral image modalities for detection of caries lesions. Dento Maxillo Fac Radiol 2008;37(1):18-22.

Haney E, Gansky SA, Lee JS et al. Comparative analysis of traditional radiographs and cone-beam computed tomography volumetric images in the diagnosis and treatment planning of maxillary impacted canines. Am J Orthod Dentofacial Orthop 2010;137(5):590-7.

Hassan B, van der Stelt P, Sanderink G. Accuracy of three-dimensional measurements obtained from cone beam computed tomography surface-rendered images for cephalometric analysis: influence of patient scanning position. Eur J Orthod 2009;31(2):129-34. Epub 2008 Dec 23.

Huybrechts B, Bud M, Bergmans L, Lambrechts P, Jacobs R. Void detection in root fillings using intraoral analogue, intraoral digital and cone beam CT images. Int Endod J 2009;42(8):675-85.

Jaeggi T, Lussi A. Prevalence, incidence and distribution of erosion. Monogr Oral Sci Review 2006;20:44-65.

Kapila S, Conley RS, Harrell WE Jr. The current status of cone beam computed tomography imaging in orthodontics. Dento Maxillo Fac Radiol Review 2011;40(1):24-34.

Katheria BC, Kau CH, Tate R et al. Effectiveness of impacted and supernumerary tooth diagnosis from traditional radiography versus cone beam computed tomography. J Pediatr Dent 2010;32(4):304-9.

Kressin NR, Nunn ME, Singh H et al. Pediatric clinicians can help reduce rates of early childhood caries: effects of a practice based intervention. Med Care 2009;47(11):1121-8.

Loubele M, Bogaerts R, Van Dijck E et al. Comparison between effective radiation dose of CBCT and MSCT scanners for dentomaxillofacial applications. Eur J Radiol 2009;71(3):461-8. Epub 2008 Jul 18.

Ludlow JB, Ivanovic M. Comparative dosimetry of dental CBCT devices and 64-slice CT for oral and maxillofacial radiology. Oral Surg Oral Med Oral Pathol Oral Radiol Endod 2008;106(1):106-14. Epub 2008 May 27.

McWhorter AG. Treatment planning for the pediatric patient. Tex Dent J 2010;127(12):1275-80.

Merrett SJ, Drage NA, Durning P. Cone beam computed tomography: a useful tool in orthodontic diagnosis and treatment planning. J Orthod 2009;36(3):202-10.

Metzger Z, Teperovich E, Zary R, Cohen R, Hof R. The self-adjusting file (SAF). Part 1: respecting the root canal anatomy-a new concept of endodontic files and its implementation. J Endod 2010;36(4):679-90.

Nordgarden H, Jensen JL, Storhaug K. Oligodontia is associated with extra-oral ectodermal symptoms and low whole salivary flow rates. Oral Dis July 2001;7(4):226-32.

Ramos-Gomez F, Crystal YO, Ng MW, Tinanoff N, Featherstone JD. Caries risk assessment, prevention, and management in pediatric dental care. Gen Dent 2010;58(6):505-17; quiz 518-9.

Ramos-Gomez FJ, Crystal YO, Ng MW, Crall JJ, Featherstone JD. Pediatric dental care: prevention and management protocols based on caries risk assessment. J Calif Dent Assoc 2010;38(10):746-61. Erratum in: Ramos-Gomez FJ, Crystal YO, Ng MW, Crall JJ, Featherstone JD. J Calif Dent Assoc 2010;38(10):746-61.

Schorer-Jensma MA, Veerkamp JS. A comparison of paediatric dentists' and general dental practitioners' care patterns in paediatric dental care. Eur Arch Paediatr Dent 2010;11(2):93-6.

Suomalainen A, Kiljunen T, Käser Y, Peltola J, Kortesniemi M. Dosimetry and image quality of four dental cone beam computed tomography scanners compared with multislice computed tomography scanners. Dento Maxillo Fac Radiol 2009;38(6):367-78. Erratum in: Suomalainen A, Kiljunen T, Käser Y, Peltola J, Kortesniemi M. Dento Maxillo Fac Radiol 2009;38(6):367-78.

Szczawinska-Poplonyk A, Gerreth K, Breborowicz A, Borysewicz-Lewicka M. Oral manifestations of primary immune deficiencies in children. Oral Surg Oral Med Oral Pathol Oral Radiol Endod Review 2009;108(3):e9-20. Epub 2009 Jul 12.

Tyndall DA, Rathore S. Cone-beam CT diagnostic applications: caries, periodontal bone assessment, and endodontic applications. Dent Clin North Am 2008;52(4):825-41, vii.

van Vlijmen OJ, Bergé SJ, Bronkhorst EM et al. A comparison of frontal radiographs obtained from cone beam CT scans and conventional frontal radiographs of human skulls. Int J Oral Maxillofac Surg 2009;38(7):773-8. Epub 2009 Apr 14.

Viswanathan K. Infant oral exam and first dental home. Tex Dent J 2010;127(11):1195-205.

Walker L, Enciso R, Mah J. Three-dimensional localization of maxillary canines with cone-beam computed tomography. Am J Orthod Dentofacial Orthop 2005;128(4):418-23.

Chapter 6

Dental prevention in pediatric dentistry

L. Ottolenghi, L. Strohmenger, L. Mazzucchelli

Concept of health and prevention in dentistry

Definitions

The concept of health formulated by the World Health Organization (WHO) in 1948 is still considered the basis of the official definition of "health." The definition formulated by the WHO has, for more than 50 years been, as follows: "*Health is a state of complete physical, mental, and social well-being and not merely the absence of disease or infirmity.*"
Subsequently, the process of promoting health began in 1984 and was defined as "*the process of enabling people to increase control over, and to improve, their health.*"
In 1978, to stimulate the commitment of national health services, the WHO declared the *goals of oral health* for the year 2000, which was subsequently renewed for the year 2020 (Tab 6.1).
In 2007, the WHO General Assembly included oral health among the priority elements for achieving general health, defining the areas of priority of action for public health interventions in dentistry (Tab. 6.2) (Poul, 2008; Poul, 2005).
Preventive intervention is organized into three levels depending on the state of health of the persons treated:

- primary intervention
- secondary intervention
- tertiary intervention

Primary intervention. This consists of promotion and maintenance of health among the healthy population. Its goal is to prevent the onset of diseases and improve quality of life. It uses the assessment of the risk conditions of the individual or population concerned.

Secondary intervention. This consists of implementation of measures for the early identification of diseases in order to implement a treatment intervention that stops or at least slows down the disease course.

Tertiary intervention. This can be defined as the prevention of complications related to an existing disease. The main goal of tertiary intervention is damage mitigation and rehabilitation.

Table 6.1 WHO global oral health goals for 2000 and 2020

2000	2020
50% of 5–6-year-old subjects caries-free	95% of 5–6-year-old subjects caries-free
DMFT < 3 at 12 years	DMFT < 0.7 at 12 years
85% of 18-year-old subjects having all dental elements present	95% of 18-year-old subjects having all dental elements present
75% of 35–45-year-old subjects with at least 20 dental elements	75% of 35–45-year-old subjects with at least 20 dental elements
50% of the population aged >65 years with at least 20 dental elements	50% of the population aged >65 years with at least 20 dental elements

Table 6.2 WHO priority areas of action for the overall improvement of oral health

- Effective use of fluoride
- Healthy diet and nutrition
- Tobacco control
- Oral health of children and young people through health promotion in schools
- Improvement of oral health among elderly people
- Oral health, general health, and quality of life
- Healthcare systems
- HIV/AIDS and oral health
- Information systems, scientific evidence, health policy, and setting of goals
- Oral health research

Table 6.3 Caries index. Decay-Missing-Filled Teeth/Surfaces (DMFT/S)

Calculus		Explanation
DMF(T/S)/dmf(t/s)	$\frac{\Sigma\,(D+M+F)}{\text{n of subjects}}$	Number (individual) or average number (population) of teeth with caries experience
Need for treatment	$\frac{D}{DMF \times 100}$	Percentage of untreated active caries
Treatment provided	$\frac{F+M\ DMF}{\times 100}$	Percentage of treatment received (a high percentage of M may mean delayed treatment or extraction)

Table 6.4 Community Periodontal Index (CPI)

0: healthy

1: bleeding, observed directly or using a mouth mirror, after probing

2: calculus observed on probing, although the entire black section of the probe is visible

3: pocket depth = 4–5 mm (gingival margin on the black section of the probe)

4: pocket depth ≥6 mm (black section of the probe not visible)

X: excluded sextant (<2 teeth present)

9: not recorded

Source: WHO, 1997.

Standard investigations according to WHO epidemiological indicators (Oral Health Surveys Basic Methods, 1997)

WHO developed a standardized system for oral health examination that uses methods and indicators suitable for the epidemiological detection of oral and dental diseases in the framework of community dentistry.
The WHO system can be accessed on the website of the Oral Health Database Country/Area Profile Project at the following link: www.mah.se/CAPP/Methods-and-Indices/for-Measurement-of-dental-diseases/.
The main indicators for the detection of caries and periodontal diseases [decay-missing-filled (DMF) and community periodontal index (CPI)] are listed below.

Decay-Missing-Filled. **DMF** is a descriptive epidemiological indicator that is used to quantify the severity of caries by counting the number of carious elements and surfaces that are subsequently reconstructed or extracted. It can be calculated in permanent teeth (upper-case letters: DMF), excluding 18, 28, 38, and 48, and in deciduous teeth (lower-case letters: dmf) for 28/20 teeth (DMFT/dmft: decay-missing-filled-teeth) or 128/88 surfaces (DMFS/dmfs: decay-missing-filled-surfaces). A DMFT of 28 indicates that all permanent dental elements of an individual or a population are or have been affected by caries. The main advantage of DMFT is that it allows standardization of detection modalities for dental caries and, therefore, comparison of different epidemiological studies at a global level. DMF indicators have different derivatives, as explained in Table 6.3.

Community Periodontal Index. The **CPI**, an initiative of WHO, was developed in 1982 as an epidemiological indicator with the aim of detecting individual or group conditions related to the assessment of tissue inflammation levels, the amount of calculus both at the supragingival and subgingival levels, and the presence of periodontal pockets of varying degrees. The principles of this index can be summarized as follows:
- dentition is divided into six sextants (Fig. 6.1)
- through surveys, assessments are performed around all the dental elements of a sextant, to which is a score is assigned (the highest score obtained for each sextant)
- a WHO probe is used for the assessment, which is characterized by a working tip 0.5 mm in diameter with reference markers to facilitate the measurement of periodontal pocket depths
- each sextant is assessed a score varying from 0 to 4 (Tab. 6.4). For individuals aged under 15 years, the score varies from 0 to 2

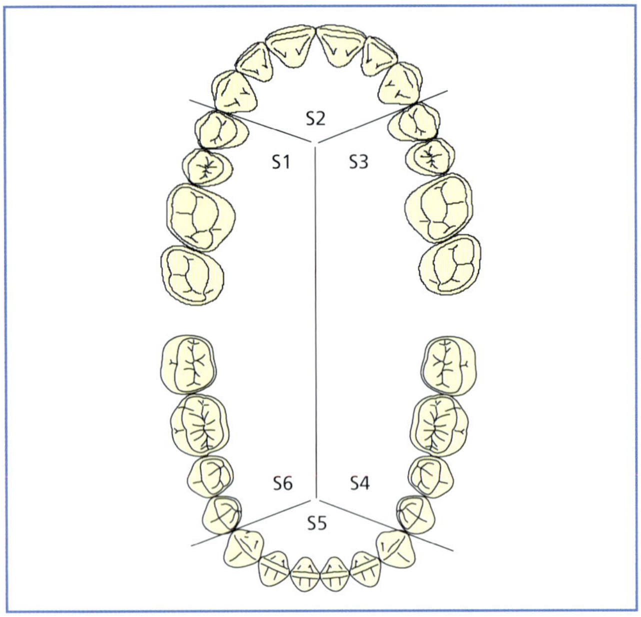

Figure 6.1 Division of the oral cavity into sextants.

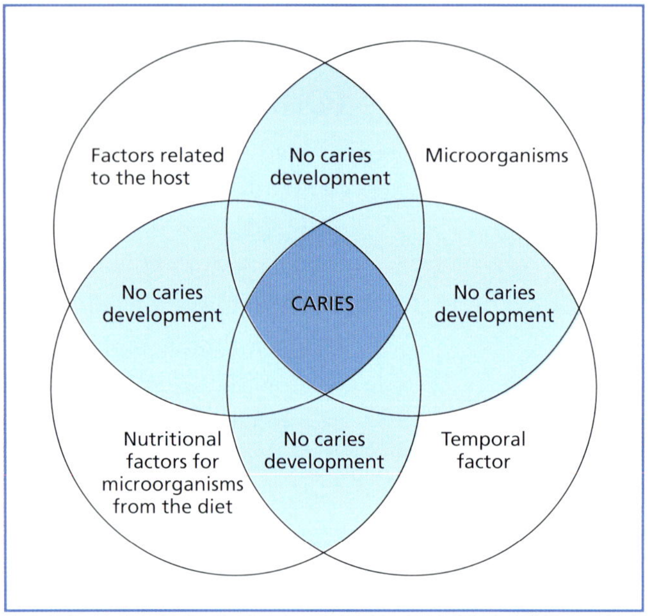

Figure 6.2 Cariogram of Keyes.

Caries in patients in the developmental age

Definition, epidemiology, and diagnosis

Dental caries is a chronic degenerative infectious disease with multifactorial etiology that affects hard dental tissues. Currently, it represents one of the most widespread pathologies, both in the general and pediatric population, despite the fact that over the last 30 years, a clear decline in this pathology has been observed due to prevention measures implemented on an increasingly larger scale (Campus et al, 2007; Bratthall, 2005; Hobdell et al, 2003). In 1960, Keyes proposed his cariogram, which consisted of three intertwining circles (subsequently brought to four after the addition of time) that represented different risk factors (bacterial plaque, diet, and individual susceptibility); overlapping of these circles identifies dental caries (Fig. 6.2). In industrialized countries, despite the increased consumption of cariogenic foods, the decrease in caries did not actually occur following precise and predictable patterns. The decrease is attributable both to the consumption of fluoride products and the improvement in oral hygiene habits. Therefore, each prevention program cannot ignore the implementation of educational campaigns dedicated to the correct oral and food hygiene standards.

Diagnosis

The traditional diagnosis of caries is clinically performed based on the loss of tissue and discoloration of lesions. This type of diagnosis assumes that the lesions lie in visible and accessible areas.

Radiological examinations are performed particularly for the diagnosis of caries lying in less accessible areas (interproximal spaces). Importantly, diagnosis using a sharp-tipped probe is still considered a subject of debate. In fact, there is a possibility of causing early carious lesions on enamel that is only demineralized, which may subsequently remineralize. Furthermore, it is believed that the sensitivity of this tool is limited as the probe cannot enter very narrow fissures to reach the caries (Staehle and Kock, 1997).

On the other hand, intraoral radiology is not effective for the diagnosis of occlusal caries, although it is very useful for the diagnosis of interproximal caries.

Notably, the process of caries development in occlusal molar surfaces seems to be mutated: the caries becomes more insidious (*hidden caries*) as the depth of the occlusal sulci is underestimated, and only later does the process itself become clinically evident in the most superficial portion.

See chapter 11 for further information about the diagnostic criteria and thresholds used for caries assessment.

Nutrition and prophylaxis

Many authors have clearly shown that frequent and prolonged exposure to certain carbohydrates is fundamental to caries activity.

Dental plaques use mono- and disaccharides as a substrate for producing energy, and acids are a product of sugar metabolism. Consequently, following the intake of these substances, the acidity of the plaque can decrease to such a point that it can induce demineralization of dental hard tissues.

The extent of demineralization depends on the absolute reduction of the pH value and the period during which the pH value of the enamel remains under the harmless level.

Studies conducted in the 1950s and 1960s demonstrated that high carbohydrate content in the diet increases carious lesion activity, the extent of which is associated more with high frequency of carbohydrate intake rather than the total quantity of carbohydrates consumed; it is associated with frequent demineralization without an opportunity to remineralize.

Furthermore, pediatricians point out that a diet that is harmful for the teeth is harmful for general health as well: in fact, foods that contain large quantities of sugar are low in essential nutrients and are at the top of the food pyramid (to be taken in small quantities and infrequently).

Instructions regarding food hygiene, which will be explained later, must be proposed to parents by considering the fact that family eating habits are always deep-rooted and, therefore, can be assimilated at different periods depending on the patient concerned.

During the first years of life, faulty eating habits that compromise dental health are frequent, such as the consumption of sugary drinks through baby bottles (see subsequent paragraph).

In children aged between 3 and 6 years, the frequent consumption of snacks and sweet drinks is harmful for the teeth.

In this age group, the risk consists of the establishment of a vicious circle: the child does not eat much, and because of the fear of not feeding them enough, they are frequently fed fruit juices and snacks, which cover a part of their daily energy needs; therefore, they do not eat during main meals. This pattern, if not identified early, continues even in the 6–12-year age group, and bad lifestyle and dietary habits become rooted.

In adolescents aged 13–18 years, esthetics and personal image compared with those of other people become increasingly important: in particular, girls frequently consume foods such as yogurt; fruit juices (possibly without added sugars); or in general, "light" foods without considering that even small quantities of sugar can trigger bacterial metabolism.

Another typical aspect of this age group is the decreased opportunity to brush the teeth after eating due to the increased frequency of having meals outside of the home.

Early Childhood Caries (ECC): Peculiarities and prevention

ECC is a pathology with multifactorial etiopathogenesis affecting deciduous dentition. It manifests as a consequence of incorrect dietary habits: prolonged consumption, even at night, of sugary drinks (for example, sweetened herb-infused drinks or fruit juices) from a very early age through baby bottles and pacifiers imbued with sugar-containing substances to provide a soothing effect.

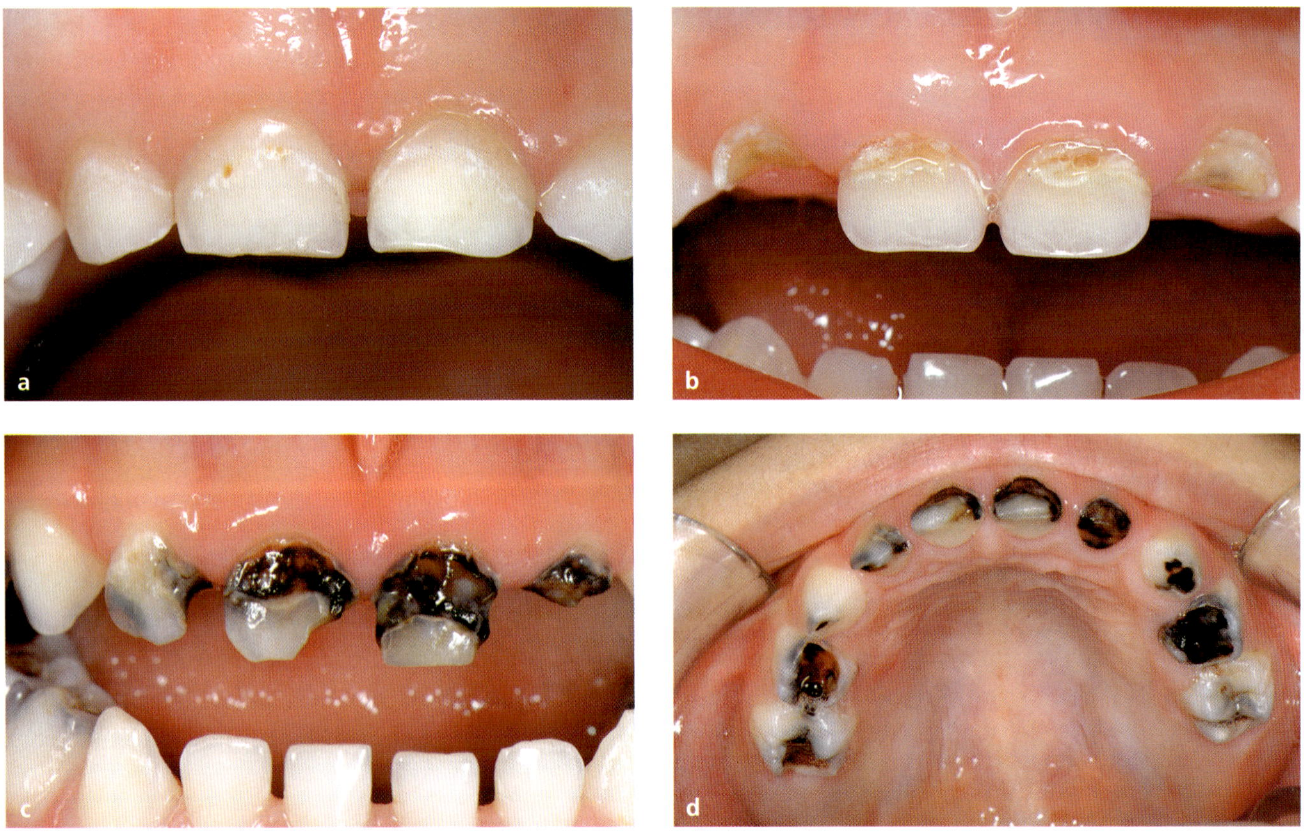

Figure 6.3 Early childhood caries.

Initially, it manifests as the demineralization of the gingival third of the upper incisors: these rapidly turn into small cavities that subsequently converge and form larger lesions that are prevalently located in the upper anterior region (Fig. 6.3). These teeth frequently fracture, sometimes even before the involvement of other teeth in the caries process. Regarding the eruption sequence, the teeth usually involved in this process are the first deciduous molars following the upper incisors. The lower incisors are the last to be damaged despite being exposed for a long time to cariogenic liquids; in fact, they are protected by the cleansing effect of saliva that is secreted through the Wharton's duct and the tongue during suction. ECC is distinguished, based on the clinical and topographical characteristics as well as the patient's age, as ECC and S-ECC (severe form) (Tab. 6.5). For the prevention of ECC, the American Academy of Pediatric Dentistry has highlighted the importance of some preventive measures (Tab. 6.6).

Table 6.5 Early childhood caries (ECC): clinical and topographic features

ECC Classification	Description
ECC (Early Childhood Caries) in children aged <6 years	• Presence of one or more decayed (non cavitated or cavitated lesions), missing (due to caries), or filled surfaces in deciduous teeth
S-ECC (Severe Early Childhood Caries) in children aged <3 years	• Any sign of smooth surface caries
S-ECC (Severe Early Childhood Caries) in children aged 3–5 years	• Presence of one or more smooth decayed (cavitated), missing (due to caries), or filled surfaces in the anterior deciduous maxillary or mandibular teeth • DMFS score (decayed, filled, or missing surfaces in deciduous teeth) ≥4 (3 years), ≥5 (4 years), or ≥6 (5 years)

Table 6.6 Guidelines of the American Academy of Pediatric Dentistry

- Children should not fall asleep with milk bottle.
- Parents should encourage the child to drink from a cup from the first year of life and to lose the habit of using the baby bottle around 12–24 months of age.
- Drinking fruit juices from bottles, including baby bottles, should be avoided, the use of a cup being preferable.
- Oral hygiene should be observed with greater care after the eruption of the first deciduous molar.
- A dental examination between 6 and 12 months of age is recommended following the eruption of the first deciduous tooth to educate parents and provide early guidance regarding the prevention of periodontal diseases.
- Salivary *Streptococcus mutans* levels of the mother or whoever has contact with the infant should be controlled and reduced to prevent bacterial transmission and reduce the risk of caries development.

Prevention problems associated with chronic drug intake for pediatric use

The prolonged and frequent use of drugs sweetened with saccharose or acids can cause carious and erosive lesions; in particular, drugs to be administered to children typically have a sweet flavor and an acidic pH so that they are more pleasant and, therefore, more easily taken by younger patients. They are frequently sold as syrups or effervescent tablets, which act for a long time in the oral cavity.
At present, in Italy, saccharose is added to most pediatric syrups increasing the risk of caries development in children; therefore, this risk must be better controlled and children must be protected against it. Furthermore, according to a study conducted in 2010 in Brazil on 23 drugs for pediatric use, only 2 had basic pH, i.e., a pH value that is not corrosive to the enamel (Neves et al, 2010). In particular, it was observed that effervescent vitamin C tablets and chewable acetylsalicylic acid tablets typically have marked acidity and cause dental erosion, especially if frequently consumed and left in contact with the teeth for a long period of time.
Other drugs can cause caries and dental erosion because of their ability to reduce salivary flow; in fact, they reduce mechanical cleansing and the buffering action and hinder the formation of acquired pellicles, which would act as a semipermeable membrane preventing a direct contact between acids and dental surfaces, thereby protecting the teeth.

Erosion in the developmental age

Definition, epidemiology, and diagnosis

Dental erosion is characterized by a progressive and irreversible loss of dental hard tissue through a chemical process under the influence of acids with extrinsic or intrinsic **non** bacterial origin (Wright, 2010).
Depending on the cause and dental surfaces involved, it is possible to note the progressive loss of physiological morphology in hard tissues that gain a concave, smooth, and hard appearance with the possibility of dental hypersensitivity and occlusal abnormalities, leading to difficulties in eating, to the point of pulp exposure and abscess formation in the most serious cases.
This phenomenon easily affects deciduous teeth as they typically have a thin and less mineralized enamel; in particular, the surfaces of deciduous teeth in which this phenomenon most frequently occurs include the occlusal surfaces of the molars and the incisal/palatal surfaces of the upper incisors.
As individuals with erosion of deciduous teeth are at high risk to develop them on permanent dentition too, prevention and early diagnosis from an early age are particularly indicated (Tab. 6.7).

Table 6.7 Intrinsic and extrinsic causes of erosion: preventive strategies

Acidogenic source	Pathogenic mechanism	Localizations	Preventive strategies
Intrinsic			
Stomach acid produced by parietal cells of the stomach pH = 1–1.5	• Gastresophageal reflux, eating disorders (bulimia, anorexia, or *binge eating*)	• Palatal and lingual surfaces of the upper dentition and occlusal surfaces in posterior sextants	• Treatment of reflux and vomiting • Avoid brushing teeth immediately after contact with gastric juices (wait 1 for hour) • End the meal with calcium- and potassium-rich foods such as cheese or milk • Topical application of remineralizing substances (e.g., fluoride) • Avoid hard or highly abrasive toothbrushes
Extrinsic			
	• Acidic foods and drinks • Acidic medicinal products • Bad habits • Occupational causes	• Vestibular surfaces in particular • Cervical surfaces of the upper dentition and occlusal surfaces in posterior sextants • In case of prolonged sucking of citrus fruits or other sources of acid, localization depends on the means of consumption.	• Avoid hard or highly abrasive toothbrushes • Stimulate salivary flow using chewing gums • Avoid keeping acidic foods and drinks in the mouth for prolonged periods • Avoid sipping acidic drinks; use a straw • End meals with calcium- and potassium-rich foods, such as cheese or milk • Topical application of remineralizing substances (e.g., fluoride)

Source: Holbrook, 2003; Lussi, 2006.

Dental erosion is presently considered a common occurrence in pediatric patients; according to a review of the literature in 2010, the prevalence of dental erosion in children varies from 10% to 80% depending on the study considered.
Recently, the Basic Erosive Wear Examination index was introduced, which allows performing a standardized screening of dental erosion (Tab. 6.8) (Bartlett, 2010).

Table 6.8 Criteria for assessment of erosive lesions

Score	Features
0	No erosive lesions
1	Initial loss of hard tissue
2	Well distinguishable defect, loss of hard tissue involving <50% of the surface
3	Loss of hard tissue involving >50% of the surface

Periodontal pathology in the developmental age

Definition, epidemiology, and diagnosis

Gingivitis and periodontitis are inflammatory pathologies of the supporting tissues of the teeth and are characterized by an essentially bacterial multifactorial etiology with the interaction of three main cofactors: host susceptibility, environmental factors, and behavioral factors.

In fact, despite being a necessary condition, plaque is affected by the indispensable role of the interaction with the host, so much so that the same quantity and quality of bacterial flora in different individuals cause different reactions.

Among the risk factors that might favor the onset of gingivitis, it is important to consider smoking (important during adolescence), drugs, systemic pathologies, and some oral conditions that cause salivary gland hypofunction and, therefore, facilitate plaque accumulation.

It has been shown that the prevalence and extent of gingivitis increase with age; inflammation can affect gingiva up until the eruption with the first elements of deciduous dentition and can reach its peak during puberty. Subsequently, the prevalence of gingivitis decreases during adolescence and gradually increases during adulthood (William, 2000).

According to a study conducted in 2009 on 913 Italian adolescents, one-third of the sample showed a healthy periodontium, whereas 34.9% had bleeding on probing and 37.9% had calculus (Campus et al, 2009; Jasim et al, 2000).

The classification of periodontal diseases in developmental ages is shown in Table 6.9.

Alterations associated with the eruption and transition of dental elements occur during puberty. These abnormalities are physiological and are not to be confused with the manifestations of gingival diseases. They can be clinically recognized as follows: pre-eruptive gingival swelling, edematous and protruding gingival margin as a consequence of the complete eruption of the dental element concerned, and normal protuberance of gingival margins during mixed dentition period. Traumatic alterations of the

Table 6.9 Classification of periodontal disease

Features		Etiology
Chronic marginal gingivitis	• Surface color reddish with swelling	• Presence of plaque and calculus • Gingivitis due to the eruption of partially exfoliated and mobile deciduous teeth • Tooth in malocclusion • Puberty gingivitis
Localized gingival recession	• The gingiva may be healthy or inflamed	• Labial inclination of the teeth • Rotated teeth • Open bite
Primary herpetic gingivostomatitis	• Presence of blisters on lip vermilion	• Complication from upper respiratory infection
Candidiasis	• White film easily removable	• *Candida albicans* mycotic infection
Ulcerative necrotic gingivitis	• Severed and ulcerative interdental papillae	• Trisomy 21 • Malnutrition

Source: Armitage, 1999.

weakened periodontal tissues of deciduous teeth can occur during the physiological transition of deciduous elements (Bernick and Freedman, 1954).
Some infectious diseases (such as chicken pox or measles) present specific signs of alterations of the oral mucosa and gingival tissue.

Tools for prevention of oral diseases

Fluoride in caries prevention

The importance of fluoride in the prevention of caries originates from the publication of the *Denti di Chiaie* (*Chiaie teeth*) report in 1901 on Public Health Reports by J.M. Eager, an assistant surgeon of the US Navy hospital service serving at the port of Naples and in charge of the medical visits by immigrants embarking for the United States. Eager described the *"frequency of a dental peculiarity common among the inhabitants of the Italian littoral* [...] *person with blackened teeth with inscription on their surface"* (as these discolorations on the tooth surfaces resembled writings). In 1938, McKay and Dean analyzed the waters in the areas affected by these enamel discolorations in the United States and finally determined that the lesions were caused by the presence of fluoride in the water.
The sources of fluoride are listed in Table 6.10.

Table 6.10 Fluoride sources

Natural	Artificial
• Drinking water • Food • Drinks • Air (suspension pollution from fluoride dust around glass, aluminum, and steel industries)	• Water additives • Milk • Medicinal products • Pharmaceutical preparations: tablets, fluoridated solutions, oral hygiene products (toothpaste, mouthwash, dental floss) • Dental products (gels and topical varnishes, restoration materials)

Mechanisms of fluoride action

Fluoride exerts preventive actions against different determining factors of caries via several mechanisms of action, which can be classified as "minor injuries" and "major defenses." This feature makes it invaluable for primary and secondary prevention. It can be administered both in the pre- (systematically) and post-eruption (topically) phases.

Remineralization. This mechanism of action has recently acquired importance in the prevention of caries.
The decrease in the prevalence of caries, in fact, does not appear to differ between countries that have adopted policies of artificial fluoridation and those that have not. The main element responsible for this phenomenon is probably the use of fluoride toothpastes on a large scale, which is supported by other sources in the literature that show the efficacy of post-eruption fluoroprophylaxis in caries prevention in populations already subjected to pre-eruption fluoroprophylaxis, and this trend includes persons aged over 12 years.
At the sites of carious demineralization, fluoride favors the precipitation of calcium and phosphate ions in the form of apatite rather than water-soluble calcium phosphates, and this, in turn, causes remineralization at the primary site of caries.
The remineralization of the initial enamel caries [white spot lesion (WSL), ICDAS scores 1 and 2] depends on two elements: the concentration of fluoride in the material used and the frequency of fluoride application. WSL remineralization is facilitated by low concentrations of F^- and high frequencies of use. Post-eruption (topical) application at low frequency and high power, instead, shows a remineralization effect preferably on the superficial layer of the lesion.

Replacement. This mechanism occurs during the enamel remineralization process and particularly during the maturation phase, replacing hydroxide ions [OH−] and converting hydroxyapatite into fluorapatite. This mechanism, called the replacement mechanism, exploits the pre-eruption administration (systemic) of fluoride during

amelogenesis, which occurs between 0–12 years of age, a period during which the enamel mineralization of the third permanent molar is completed.
The presence of fluoride to replace one or more hydroxyl groups gives stability to the crystalline enamel structure because of the stronger ionic bond with the adjacent calcium ions of apatite crystals. From the chemical perspective, this can be explained on the basis of the fact that the critical pH (acidity value below which enamel becomes saturated with electrolytes compared with saliva, thereby causing enamel demineralization) of fluorinated apatite (3.5) is lower than that of hydroxyapatite (5.5). Fluorapatite is more resistant to demineralization but is not exempt from it.

Mechanisms of bacterial inhibition. Fluoride acts as a true "cellular toxin" against bacteria. In fact, it inhibits the main enzymatic systems of glycolysis, decreases the production of pyruvate, and lowers salivary pH. Furthermore, this mechanism lowers ATP production, leading to the reduction of transmembrane transport and, in general, bacterial cell metabolic activity.
Among the processes that are inhibited by fluoride is the production of extracellular polysaccharides that work as a supporting structure for bacterial plaque stratification and interfere with bacterial adhesion because of the competition from plaque matrix surface proteins.

Information on fluoride metabolism

Fluoride is electively absorbed in the acidic environment of the stomach. After ingestion, plasma fluoride levels peak within 20–60 min. Fluoride clearance through the kidneys and skeletal tissues decreases fluoremia. During growth, only a very small fraction (approximately 1%) of the ingested fluoride reaches the enamel matrix under formation, whereas the rest is distributed across the other tissues of the organism or eliminated via feces or urine.

Fluoride toxicity

The acute or chronic toxic reactions associated with fluoride depend on the concentration, extent, duration, and frequency of intake, as well as on the physiopathological state of a person, such as age or weight.

Acute toxicity. Acute fluoride intoxication causes symptoms varying from excessive salivation, nausea, abdominal pain, vomiting, and diarrhea to neuromuscular symptoms, convulsions, ventricular fibrillation, and cardiorespiratory failure.
The minimum dose that can cause signs of toxicity [probable toxic dose (PTD)] was calculated to be 5 mg F/kg of body weight (Whitford, 1987). For prompt identification of toxicological risk, one must be aware of the average weights of the pediatric population (for example, the average weight of a 1-year-old child is 10 kg, whereas that of a 5–6-year-old child is 20 kg). If an individual ingests a quantity equal to or greater than the PTD, immediate intervention is necessary. In fact, some materials used for outpatient and/or home-based fluoroprophylaxis contain high fluoride concentrations, and their use must be thoroughly considered. In fact, 5 ml of fluoride gel can reach

Table 6.11 Phases of treatment of acute fluoride poisoning

1. Monitoring and support of vital signs, including cardiac monitoring
2. Gastric lavage, if no emesis has occurred
3. Monitoring of serum electrolytes and calcium and magnesium levels
4. Treatment of hypocalcemia, hypomagnesemia, and hyper- or hypokalemia
5. Administration of milk, calcium salts, aluminum, or magnesium antacids to bind fluorine
6. Consider hemodialysis in patients with severe toxicity
7. Treatment of arrhythmias, especially in the presence of refractory hyperkalemia
8. Consult a poison control center for the recommended treatment

the toxic dose in individuals who have a medium weight and are aged less than 6 years (Tab. 6.11) (Whitford, 1992).

Chronic toxicity. Chronic systemic intake of excessive amounts of fluoride during amelogenesis can cause dental fluorosis. The minimum dose that causes fluorosis was found to be 0.08–0.1 mg/kg/day. Intake of fluoride prevalently occurs through drinking water. Fluoridated water (>1.5 mg/L) is prevalently found in areas of volcanic origin. In Italy, regions with endemic fluorosis are found in the northern part of Lazio, in the areas surrounding Mount Vesuvius and Mount Etna, and in some areas of Sardinia. Clinically, dental fluorosis is characterized by the presence of patches or bands whose colors vary from chalky-white to brown. Fluorosis prevention is performed by using alternative sources of drinking water during the first 48 months of life and during the amelogenesis of esthetically relevant permanent teeth (upper incisors).

Fluorosis classification. Fluorosis has been classified over the years based on clinical and histological evidence. The first scientist to propose a classification was H.T. Dean; he proposed a classification system in 1934, that was subsequently modified in 1942 (Fig. 6.4). His proposal is still adopted by WHO (Tab. 6.12) (Dean, 1934).

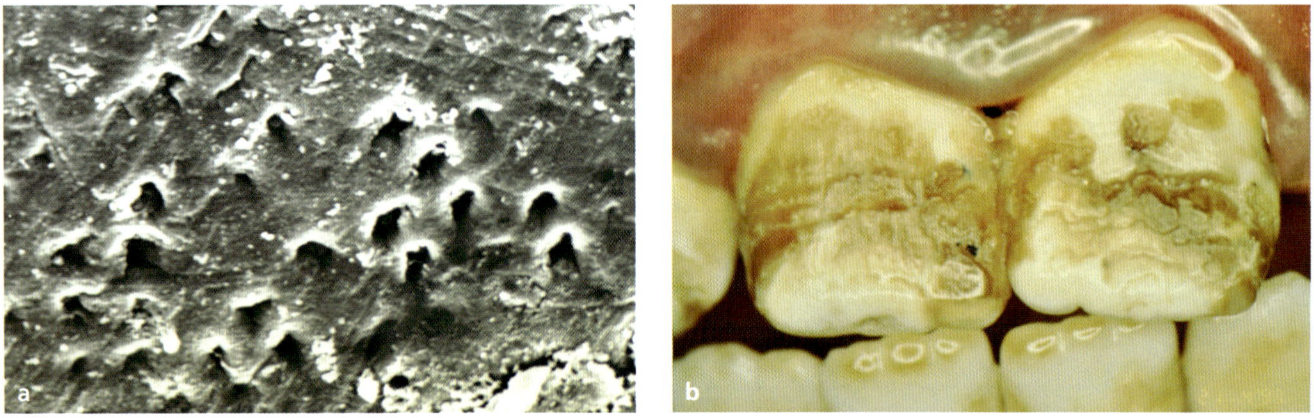

Figure 6.4 (**a**) Microscopic aspect of fluorotic enamel; (**b**) severe fluorosis (courtesy of Professor G. Goracci).

Pre-eruption fluoroprophylaxis

The dose that is considered ideal, under which "almost all" people exposed are at no risk, is calculated to be 1 mg/day or 0.05 mg/kg/day for individuals with a weight lower than 20 kg (for temperate climates, an average water intake of 1 l/day is considered, with an ideal concentration of approximately 1 ppm or mg/l).

One of the main advantages of artificial fluoridation in aqueducts is the reduction of disparities in the incidence of caries across social classes, especially in children of preschool age. Disadvantages and aversions are essentially associated with the imposition of a particular method and the freedom of choice by individuals regarding their health. Furthermore, the dosage turns out to be approximate because of the individual variation in daily water consumption.

The use of fluoride toothpastes is the most recommended method to date and has shown efficacy practically worldwide, although with feasibility issues in many developing countries. For this reason, water fluoridation is a matter of heated debate in the international scientific community. Alternative systemic administration sources (salt; milk; bottled fruit juices; tea; carbonated beverages; and fluoride-rich foods, such as fish and marine crustaceans or cereals for infants) provide the advantage of being freely chosen by consumers.

Table 6.12 Fluorosis classification by Dean's index (1942)

Type	Score	Criteria
Normal	0	Enamel surface is smooth and glossy and usually shows a creamy-white color.
Questionable	0.5	The enamel has slight alterations of translucency compared with the normal enamel, varying from small patches to sporadic white spots. This classification is applied when the word "normal" is not fully applicable.
Very mild	1	Small opaque white areas unevenly distributed over <25% of the vestibular surface of the tooth
Mild	2	The opaque white areas on the enamel are more extensive but cover <50% of the vestibular surface of the tooth.
Moderate	3	The enamel surface shows evident areas of wear, with brown blemishes being frequently present.
Severe	4	All enamel surfaces are affected, and hypoplasia is so marked that the general tooth shape may be altered. There are worn or hollowed out areas and diffuse brown spots on the tooth surface; the teeth often have a corroded appearance.

Source: Dean, 1942. As shown in "Health Effects of Ingested Fluoride" National Academy of Sciences, 1993. pp 169.

The use of fluorinated tablets, commercially available in the preparations of 0.25 and 1.00 mg, is the most widespread method of individual fluoroprophylaxis. An advantage of fluoridated tablets compared with the artificial fluoridation of aqueducts is the possibility to choose whether or not to use them. The dose should be calculated based on the weight of the individual and on the daily fluoride *intake* (calculation from potential sources of systemic fluoride such as water, food, or drugs).

Fluoride in pregnancy

There is substantial uncertainty regarding the systemic use of fluoride during pregnancy as a preventive measure against caries in unborn children.
The national guideline for the promotion of oral health and prevention of oral pathologies in developmental ages by the Ministry of Health (2008) substantially considers that systemic fluoroprophylaxis in prenatal ages and during breastfeeding is not adequately supported by scientific evidence. However, fluoride can have an important role in the care and control of oral health in pregnant women and unborn children through its topical administration and the care of maternal oral health. In fact, a decrease in the maternal bacterial titer lowers the probability of the oral transmission of cariogenic bacteria between mother and child (in particular, *Streptococcus mutans*), i.e., the mechanism underlying the risk of caries in early childhood. Fluoroprophylaxis protocols for pregnant women are the same as those found in the standard recommendations.

Post-eruption fluoroprophylaxis

This type of fluoroprophylaxis mainly exploits the mechanism of remineralization and bacterial inhibition. With various indications of use and dosages, it is administered via the following:

- toothpastes: low concentration, home application
- mouthwashes: low concentration, home application
- gels: high concentration, professional application
- varnishes: high concentration, professional application

It should be noted that these products have fluoride concentrations varying from 500 to 20,000 ppm, and their inappropriate use can cause acute and/or chronic intoxication. The proficiency of the administration protocols for minimizing the risk of overdose is indispensable.

Fluoride toothpastes. The Centers for Disease Control and Prevention (2001) states that "[...] *the predominant effect of fluoride is the post-eruptive and topical one* [...] *the presence of fluoride in the right quantity, in the right place, and at the right moment* [...] *small quantities constantly present in the oral cavity. For this reason, not just children but adults too benefit from topical fluoroprophylaxis, as was previously considered.*"

Fluoride mouthwashes. Fluoride mouthwashes are solutions for oral rinses that contain variable quantities of fluoride that are proposed as alternatives or aids to toothpastes. They are effective in several cases, such as in the primary and secondary prevention of carious pathologies, prevention and limitation of enamel erosion, and dental hypersensitivity. They are frequently used for their refreshing and antiseptic properties.

Fluoride gels. Fluoride gels are substances with high fluoride concentration that are mainly produced for professional purposes and outpatient applications.
The indications for the use of fluoride gels are as follows:

- age more than 4 years
- widespread initial carious demineralization (ICDAS 1, 2, or 3)
- high risk of caries
- decreased saliva production
- dentin sensitivity

These gels can reach concentrations up to 20,000 ppm of fluoride; thus, it is necessary to strictly abide by the rules of application of fluoride gels to minimize the risk of accidental ingestion (Fig. 6.5).

- first, test perforated *trays* and select the one that appears to be the most suitable based on the size of the patient's arches (this does not apply if a customized *tray* is being used)
- add a small quantity of gel into the applicator
- seat the patient in an orthostatic position with the head slightly tilted forward
- place the trays with the gel on both arches simultaneously
- place a surgical aspirator between the arches
- place a container under the patient's chin and ask him or her to drain the saliva
- wait for 4 min
- remove the *trays*
- aspirate the residual gel from the mucosa and teeth
- remove saliva for 30 s
- do not rinse
- do not let the patient consume foods or drinks for 30 min after the end of treatment

The professional application of fluoride gels requires a booster every 3, 6, and 12 months depending on the risk of caries for individual patients.

Fluoride varnishes. Fluoride varnishes are lacquers that are mostly based on natural rosin containing 5% NaF. They are part of products that have high power and low frequency. Fluoride varnishes are indicated for infants or people with disabilities who show a high risk of caries with the presence of *white spots* (ICDAS 1, 2, or 3); these varnishes must be professionally applied. The risk of accidental ingestion is lower than that for other fluoride-based compounds. The recommended application frequency is two biannual applications repeated for 2 years. The application of fluoride varnishes is simple and does not imply the cleansing of dental surfaces; after drying tooth surfaces with cotton gauzes, the arch should be isolated using cotton rolls and the varnish should be applied on all dental elements using a small brush. The varnish quickly hardens on coming in contact with saliva. The child can rinse but not brush the teeth for 24 h.

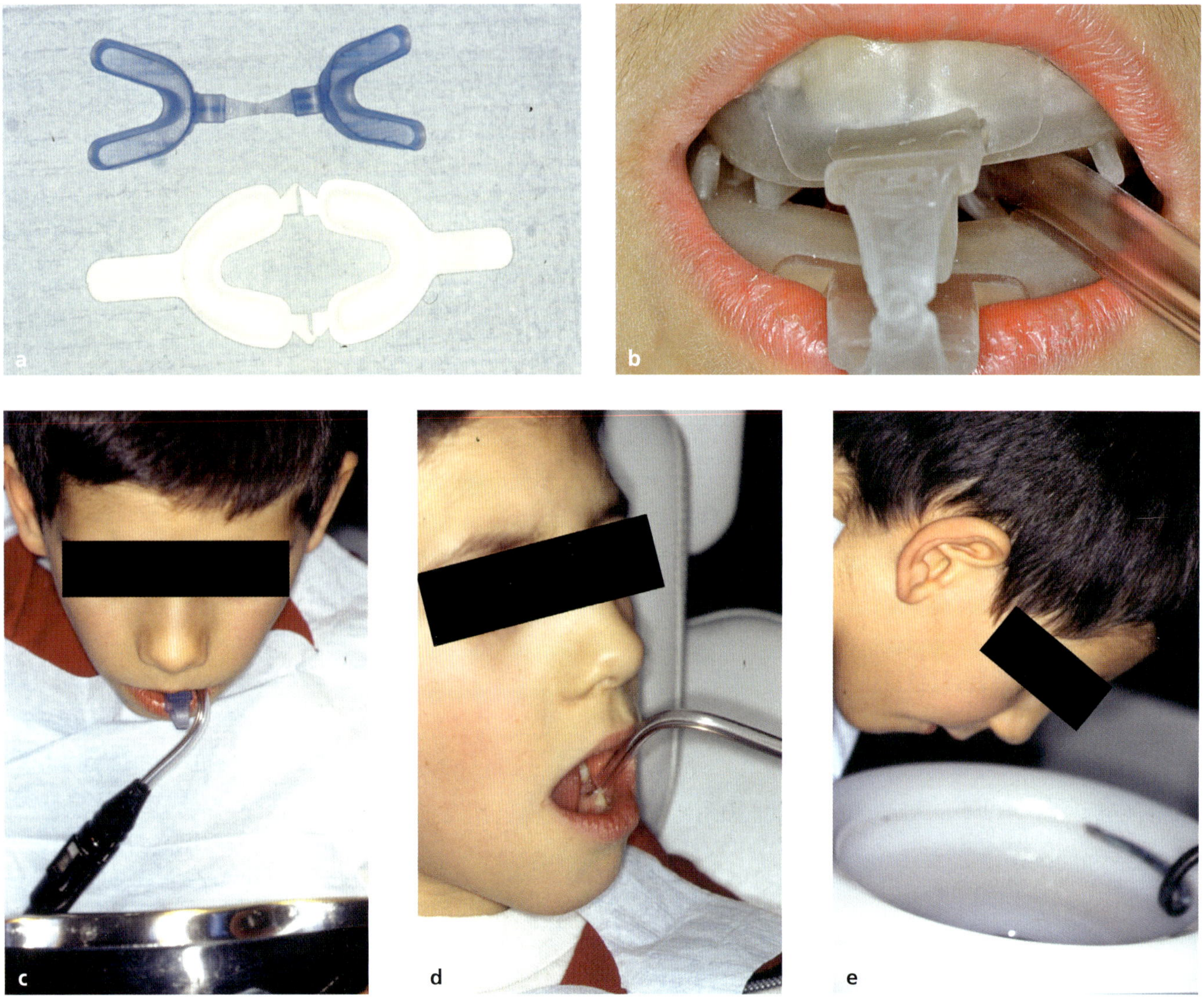

Figure 6.5 (**a**) Gel application; (**b**) applicator in the mouth; (**c**) bucket for saliva control; (**d**) aspiration of gel residues; (**e**) elimination of excess saliva.

Recommendations and guidelines for fluoroprophylaxis. Table 6.13 shows the recommendations by the Ministry of Health regarding the use of fluoride.

In 2009, the European Academy of Pediatric Dentistry defined its guidelines, which outline the details (Tab. 6.14) regarding the correct use of toothpastes in children.

Recently, the American Academy of Pediatric Dentistry (2009–2010) introduced the concept of *smears* associated with toothpastes in order to further minimize the risk of accidental ingestion by children aged less than 2 years.

In any case, the duration of brushing should never exceed 1 min, and children should be encouraged to spit out excess toothpaste and avoid or minimize rinsing.

Table 6.13 Recommendations for fluoride use

Topic	Description	Occurrence grade	Recommendation strength
Fluoride prophylaxis	Fluoride prophylaxis should be recommended for all individuals of developing age.	1	A
Fluoride prophylaxis	Topical fluoride administration via low-fluoride toothpastes (500 ppm) is recommended from 3 to 6 years of age, twice a day. After 6 years, the use of a toothpaste containing at least 1000 ppm fluoride twice a day is of fundamental importance in caries prevention and may be the only form of administration.	1	A

Source: Italian Ministry of Health.

Table 6.14 Recommendations on the correct use of toothpaste in children

Age	Fluoride concentration	Daily use	Quantity to be used
6 months–2 years	500 ppm	Twice daily	pea-size
2–6 years	1000 (+) ppm	Twice daily	pea-size
≥6 years	1450 ppm	Twice daily	1–2 cm

Source: European Academy of Paediatric Dentistry.

Integrated use of fluoroprophylaxis strategies. In terms of systemic use, fluoridated milk and fluoride salt are not adequately supported by scientific studies and evidence (Espelid, 2009).

On the contrary, fluoride tablets and topical fluoroprophylaxis with gels or varnishes are considered on an individual basis for children with a high risk of caries, including those with disabilities and/or special needs.

Home oral hygiene

Correct oral hygiene: tools, timing, manual skills, and techniques

The main goal of oral hygiene is daily disintegration of bacterial plaque. Bacterial plaque is a generic term that indicates a biofilm or a microbial (mainly bacterial) aggregate present on dental surfaces integrated with a polymeric matrix of salivary and bacterial origin. It is naturally deposited on the tooth, with stratification starting from the acquired pellicle, a glycoprotein layer of salivary origin. Maintenance of this dental pellicle within the physiological quantitative and qualitative limits does not allow bacterial plaque to stabilize and the ensuing colonization by pathogenic bacteria. Starting from this point, the importance of a correct and regular home oral hygiene routine in all ages can be understood.

The areas of prevention that involve oral hygiene are as follows:

- primary prevention (health education and promotion, oral hygiene instructions, home oral hygiene, and periodic visits to receive professional oral hygiene interventions)
- secondary prevention (monitoring and self-care, daily application of products dedicated to the remineralization of incipient caries, early diagnosis of dental pathologies, professional oral hygiene, and periodic checks)

The tools of oral hygiene are classified as follows:

- mechanical tools, such as manual and mechanical toothbrushes or tools for interdental oral hygiene
- chemical tools, such as plaque detectors, mouthwashes, or toothpastes
- psychological and organizational tools, such as motivation or periodic visits

The correct oral hygiene requires the following phases and tools:

- visualization and awareness: plaque detectors
- materials: toothbrushes, dental flosses, interdental brushes, electrical toothbrushes
- oral hygiene techniques
- motivation

Plaque detectors. Plaque detectors are coloring substances that are marketed as tablets or solutions that highlight bacterial pellicle accumulations, making them more easy to eliminate via oral hygiene procedures. Another advantage offered by plaque detectors is the self-monitoring of patients' oral hygiene technique as a means of oral hygiene self-learning and optimization (Fig 6.6 and Tab. 6.15).

An ideal plaque detector has the following features:

- easy to use
- water-soluble
- non toxic
- motivating (unpleasant aspect)
- easy to eliminate

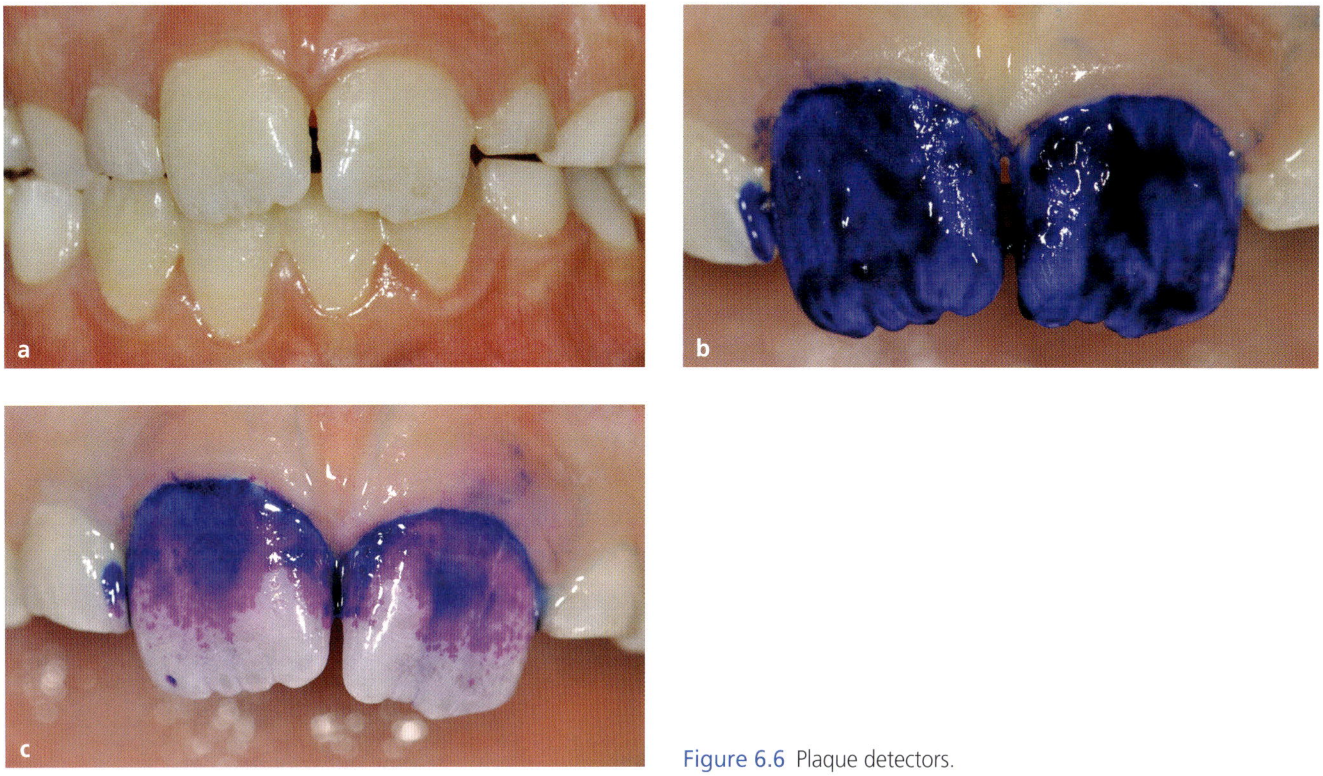

Figure 6.6 Plaque detectors.

Table 6.15 Colored agents used for dental plaque detection

Bitonal (two color shades)	They allow the differentiation of the newly formed plaque from the less recently formed one (erythrosine red for the most recent plaque)
Methylene blue	A blue dye for dental plaque
Bismarck brown	Dyes the acidic mucin yellow-brown
Eosin	A fluorescent red dye
Sodium fluorescein	Fluorescein is only evidenced via the visual-photographic detection of the fluorescence emitted after illumination with a specific light (Wood light, blue light with a wavelength of 490 nm)
Fuchsin	A red to violet dye composed of (hydrochloric or acetate) rosaniline and pararosaniline salts
Sanguinarine	A red coloring, alkaloid extract that is a component of *Sanguinaria canadensis* and has antiplaque properties
Tartrazine	A yellow synthetic azo dye, *not recommended for pediatric use*. In Europe it is banned in Norway and Austria

Toothbrushes. Historically, plant fibers, for example, Arak roots, animal bristles, or whatever nature had to offer, were used to clean teeth. The first toothbrushes were made of precious materials such as metals, woods, or ivory and natural bristles. With the advent of artificial fibers (1950), production costs substantially decreased, allowing the use of more regular and effective oral hygiene measures on a vast scale.

The ideal requisites of a toothbrush are listed below:
- a handle that facilitates easy handling: this aspect is very important, particularly for persons with difficulties in grasping, such as those with disabilities, elderly people, and neurological patients
- a head size that allows access to all dental elements: it is necessary to consider the difficulties involved in accessing the lingual surfaces of the molars (vomit induction) and the vestibular surfaces of the upper molars
- possible curve at the neck level in order to enhance flexibility and ease of handling
- size, shape, and materials that meet the specific necessities of dental and gingival tissues
- effective and non traumatizing brushing surfaces: the bristles should be artificial and with a rounded end in order to avoid injury to gingival tissues and dental enamel
- waterproof, easy to clean, and rot-proof
- durable and economical
- esthetically pleasant
- easily recognizable

Electric toothbrushes. The first electric toothbrushes with a vertical arch movement mimicking the movement of manual toothbrushes were developed in the 1960s. The main difficulties include feeding and brushing effectiveness. The first electric toothbrush with a quarter-turn oscillatory motion was produced in 1991.
There is substantial scientific evidence to support the use of electric toothbrushes and to show its greater effectiveness in removing dental plaque compared with manual toothbrushes.
The main advantages include greater brushing effectiveness considering equal brushing durations, a reduced head size that allows access to all dental surfaces (posterior regions and lingual surfaces of molars), a greater effectiveness in patients with mobility and grasping difficulties, and a substantial motivational improvement in children and neglected people.

Brushing techniques. There is no ideal brushing technique. Before providing the oral hygiene instructions, it is important to observe the characteristics of the brushing technique already used by the patient. If these are adequate, it would be sufficient to apply the necessary corrections without radically changing the patient's methods and facilitate the gradual implementation of correct practices.

The characteristics of an ideal technique are listed below:
- effective: it should help remove bacterial plaque from all dental surfaces

- repeatable: it should be simple to use for patients so that they can repeat and apply it on a daily basis
- not harmful: it should not injure the enamel or gingival tissues

Horizontal technique. It can cause abrasive lesions on vestibular tooth surfaces. It is correct only for the brushing of occlusal surfaces (Fig. 6.7).

Vertical technique. This too is incorrect as it is not very effective and is potentially harmful, involving movements that may push the plaque into the gingival sulcus rather than removing it (Fig. 6.8).

Rolling technique. This technique is acceptable, with discrete effectiveness and limited damage. It involves rotating the bristles from the gingival to the occlusal margin, imparting a rotatory motion to the toothbrush. The rolling technique can be easily used by children and people with disabilities; in children in particular, it can be used as an intermediate step toward learning a more complete method (for example, the Bass technique) (Fig. 6.9).
The cervical–occlusal brushing direction can be easily explained using the phrase "from red to white" because of the ease of understanding; the technique can be adapted to both arches just as easily without any misunderstanding.

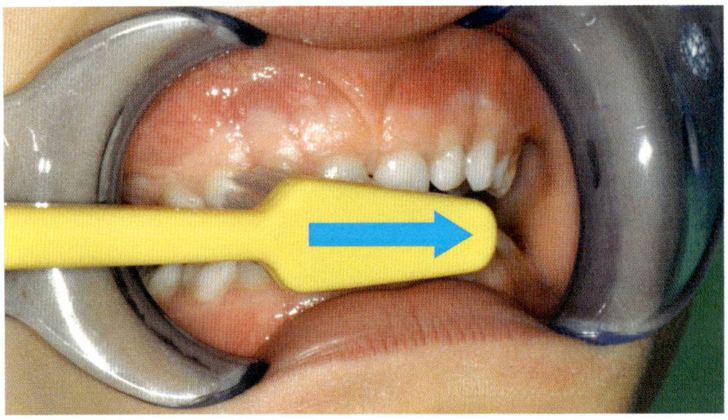

Figure 6.7 Horizontal brushing technique, incorrect.

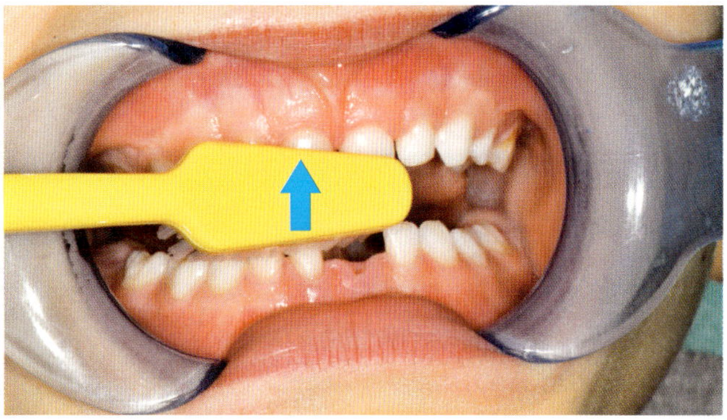

Figure 6.8 Vertical brushing technique, incorrect.

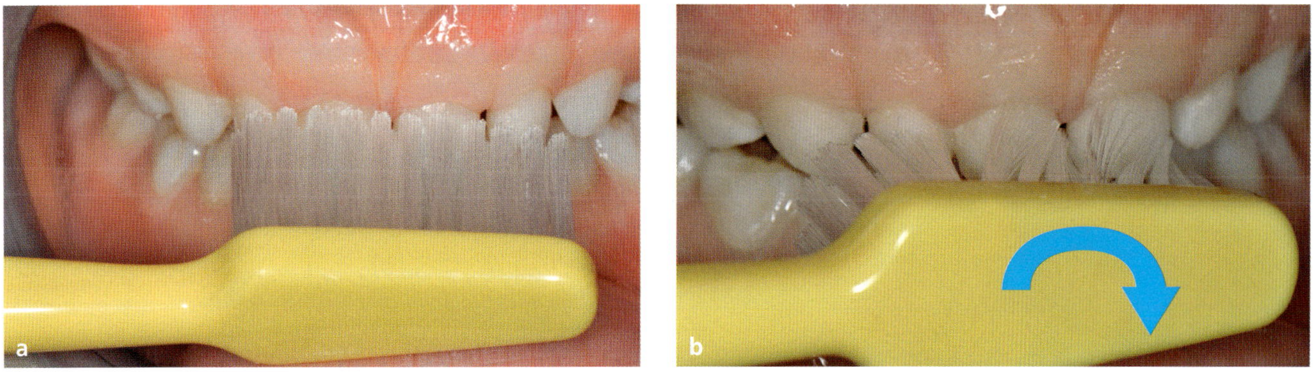

Figure 6.9 Rolling brushing technique.

Modified Bass technique. This consists of combining a slight vibration movement of the bristles in the gingival sulcus (45° direction) with the rolling technique. Thus, it is possible to disintegrate the plaque adhering to the sulcus and apply an effective removal method. The Bass technique requires the use of artificial bristles with medium hardness, a first phase using a dry toothbrush and subsequently the application of toothpaste (Fig. 6.10).

Brushing contraindications. The following occurrences represent contraindications to the use of toothbrushes due to the risk of local and/systemic complications:

- acute necrotizing ulcerative gingivitis
- inflammatory reactions in irradiated patients
- gingival diseases of leukemic origin
- use in the initial days after a traumatic event
- after difficult avulsion, with uncovered alveolus

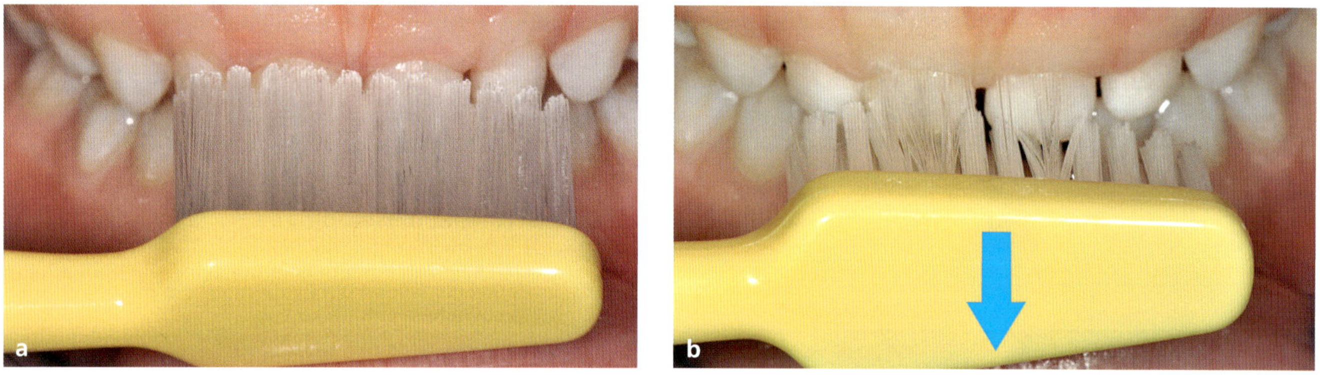

Figure 6.10 Modified Bass technique.

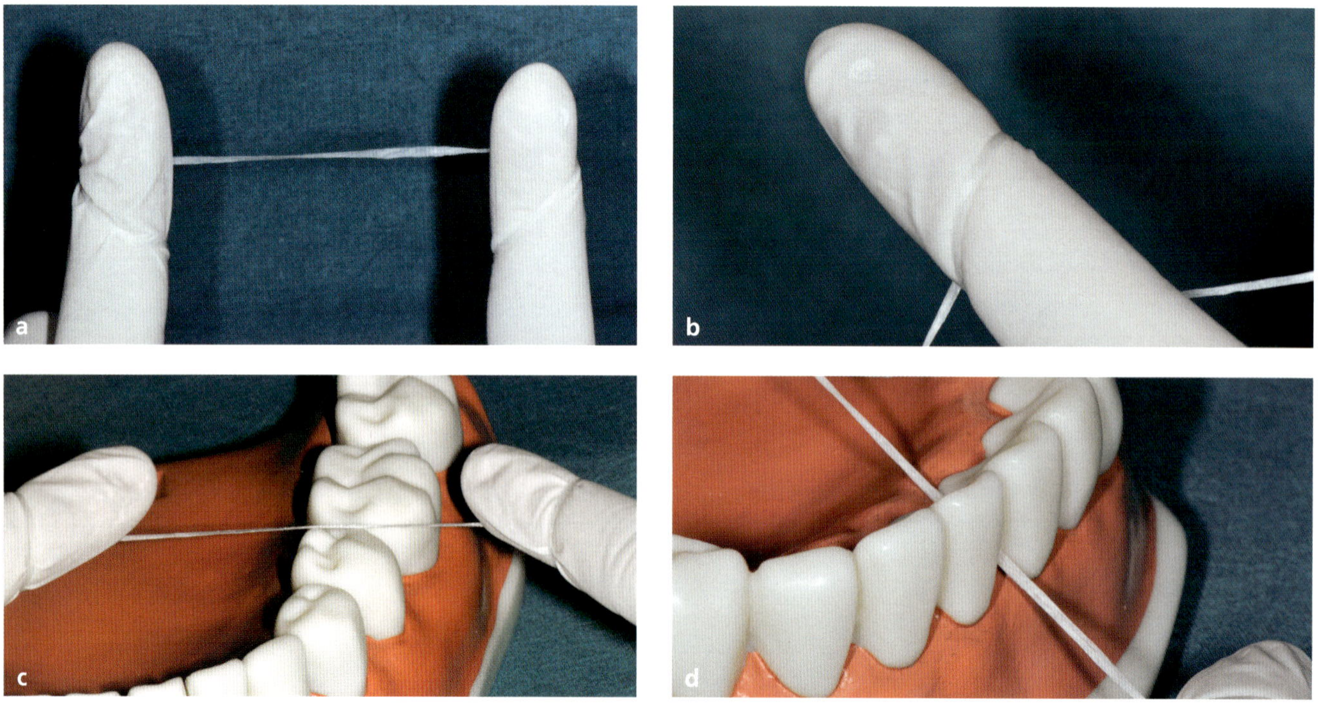

Figure 6.11 Use of dental floss (*continued*).

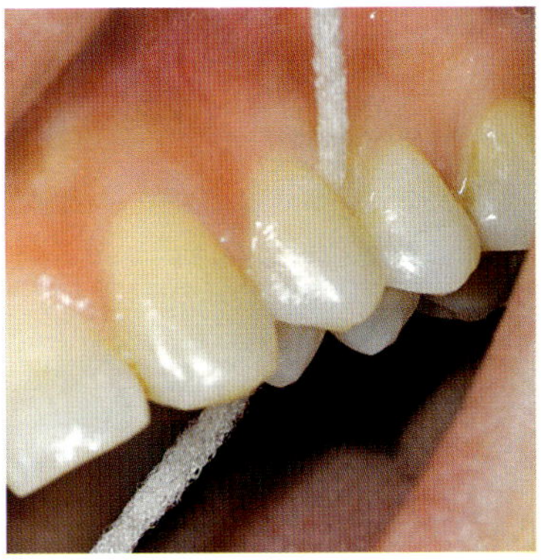

Figure 6.12 Flossing technique.

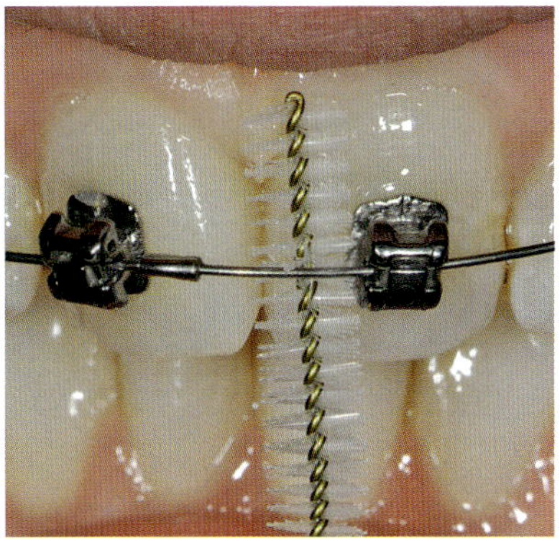

Figure 6.13 Interdental brushes.

Dental flosses and tapes. Two products are available to maintain the hygiene of interproximal surfaces: dental flosses and tapes. Tapes can comprise many fibers that come in contact with the dental surface, whereas flosses are made of a simpler and more manageable fiber.

Flosses and tapes can be simple, waxed (easier to use in case of particularly tight contact points), or fluoridated (for preventing interproximal caries) (Fig. 6.11).

In case of inaccessibility of the contact point (for example, patients with fixed orthodontic equipment), there are special flosses with rigid ends that work as "threading devices," a spongy section (through which active ingredients can be carried, e.g., antiplaque or demineralizing solutions), and a section with waxed floss (Fig. 6.12).

Interdental brushes. The dental floss cannot completely remove the plaque from anatomic concavities on interdental surfaces. To meet this necessity, interdental brushes were developed; these are made of an intertwined metallic thread and bristles that unfold from it in a radial fashion. These brushes can adapt to the brushing surface of the tooth anatomy.

If interdental carioreceptivity is present, patients are advised to immerse their toothbrush/brush/floss in a fluoride mouthwash or gel. Interdental brushes are useful for cleaning orthodontic *brackets* (Fig. 6.12).

Motivation

Motivation is an unconscious act and is typical of a person who develops a spontaneous interest for a particular task.

The motivational intervention of the dentist/hygienist is, in reality, an intervention of persuasion according to the science of advertising. In this case, the "product" to be advertised is *oral health*. To persuade people, it is necessary to make proposals, reinforcements, and stimuli that work on unconscious behaviors through hearing and sight. The persuasion capacity improves with a greater comprehension of the psychological problem.

It should be noted that motivating a new patient is easier: therefore, it is important to begin a new motivational routine cycle since the first visit with all patients. This is all the more true in cases of pediatric patients: an adequately motivated child will probably become an adult who is more aware of the importance of oral health and its professional as well as home maintenance.

References

Albandar JM, Tinoco EM. Global epidemiology of periodontal diseases in children and young persons. Periodontol 2000 2002;29:153-76.

American Association of Paediatric Dentistry (AAPD). Reference Manual 2009-2010;31(6):128-31.

Armitage GC. Development of a classification system for periodontal diseases and condition. Ann Periodontol 1999;4:1.

Bartlett D. A proposed system for screening tooth wear. Br Dent J 2010;208:207-9.

Bernick S, Freedman N. Microscopic studies of the periodontum of the primary dentition of monkeys. II. Posterior teeth during the mixed dentition period. Oral Surg Oral Med Oral Pathol 1954;7:322.

Bratthall D. Estimation of global DMFT for 12-year-olds in 2004. Int Dent J 2005;55:370-2.

Campus G, Cagetti MG, Senna A et al. Differences in oral health among Italian adolescents related to the type of secondary school attended. Oral Health Prev Dent 2009;7(4):323-30.

Campus G, Solinas G, Cagetti MG et al. National pathfinder survey of 12 year-old children's oral health in Italy. Caries Res 2007;41:512-17.

CDC. Recommendations for using fluoride to prevent and control dental caries in the United States. MMWR 2001;50.

Dean HT. Classifications of mottled enamel diagnosis. J Am Dent Assoc 1934,21:1421-6.

Espelid I. Caries preventive effect of fluoride in milk, salt and tablets: a literature review. Eur Arch Paediatr Dent 2009 Sep;10(3):149-56.

Hobdell M, Petersen PE, Clarkson J et al. Global goals for oral health 2020. Int Dent J 2003;53: 285-8.

Holbrook WP, Árnadóttir IB, series editor, Kay EJ. Br Dent J 2003;195:75-81.

Lussi A, editor. Dental erosion: from diagnosis to therapy. Basel: Karger; 2006. p. 77-87.

Ministero della Salute. Linee guida nazionali per la promozione della salute orale e la prevenzione delle patologie orali in età evolutiva (2008). (http://www.salute.gov.it/sorrisoSalute/documenti/Linee_guida_approvate_10_ott_2008.pdf)

Neves BG, Farah A, Lucas E et al. Are paediatric medicines risk factors for dental caries and dental erosion? Community Dent Health 2010;27(1):46-51.

Panetta F, Dall'Oca S, Nofroni I et al. Early childhood caries. Oral health survey in kindergartens of the 19th district in Rome. Minerva Stomatol 2004;53(11-12):669-78.

Petersen PE. Priorities for research for oral health in the 21st Century: the approach of the WHO Global Oral Health Programme. Community Dent Health 2005;22:71-4.

Petersen PE. World Health Organization global policy for improvement of oral health – World Health Assembly 2007. World Health Organization Geneva, Switzerland. Int Dental J 2008;58:115-21.

Staehle HJ, Kock MJ. Odontoiatria per l'infanzia e l'adolescenza. Milano: Masson; 1997.

Taji S, Seow WK. A literature review of dental erosion in children. Aust Dent J 2010;55:358-67.

WHO (World Health Organization). Oral Health Surveys: Basic Methods. Geneva: WHO, 1997. (www.mah.se/CAPP/Methods-and-Indices/for-Measurement-ofdental-diseases/).

Jenkins WM, Panos N. Epidemiology of periodontal disease in children and adolescents. Periodontol 2000 2001;26:16-32.

Wright JT. Defining the contribution of genetics in the etiology of dental caries. J Dent Res 2010;89(11):1173-4.

Chapter 7

Dental anomalies in pediatric dentistry

L. Franchi, T. Baccetti†, E. Defraia

Dental anomalies occurring during the developmental age can affect both the deciduous and permanent dentition. This chapter explores dental anomalies in the deciduous dentition and the resultant consequences on the permanent dentition. Dental anomalies in the deciduous dentition involve the following risks, which may lead to clinical progression rather than a pathological situation:

- possible repetition in the permanent dentition
- problems at the orthodontic level, such as the formation of diastemas, dental crowding, reduction in dental arch length, and midline deviation
- increased risk of caries formation
- possible esthetic problems during preschool age (Marinelli et al, 2012)

Data in the literature show that dental anomalies in the deciduous dentition are either less frequent than those in the permanent dentition or are less frequently detected in clinical settings because of the physiological transitory nature of the deciduous dentition, as long as there are no sequelae in the permanent dentition that can be traced back to the anomalies in the deciduous dentition.

Dental anomalies in the deciduous dentition can be classified according to Vichi (Tollaro et al, 1990) as shown in Table 7.1.

Table 7.1 Dental abnormalities in deciduous dentition according to Vichi

Eruption	Number	Shape
• Impaction • Re-impaction	• Deficiency • In excess	• Simple: – of the crown – of the root • Complex: – fused teeth – geminated teeth

Source: Tollaro, 1990; modified.

Clinical Case 1 – Inclusion of deciduous canine

L.L., female child of 3 years and 6 months of age during the first medical visit, showed failed eruption of the right upper deciduous canine. Orthopantomography (OPT) revealed the presence of a large complex odontoma responsible for the displacement of the right upperdeciduous canine and that of the follicle of the corresponding permanent element, in a veryhigh position within the bone structure of the maxilla and with a distal displacement of the first right upper premolar (Fig. 7.1a). Given the young age of the patient and to ease the surgical intervention, trusting in a favorable evolutive dynamism of the dental elements involved, it was decided to remove only the odontoma (Fig. 7.1b). During the subsequent period of monitoring, and precisely 2 years later, spontaneous eruption of the deciduous canine within the arch was observed (Fig. 7.1c). OPT also highlighted a more favorable intraosseous position for the permanent canine, whereas the first premolar still appeared significantly displaced. After 2 years, the subsequent radiographic control highlighted a radicular resorption of the deciduous canine due to the corresponding permanent element, that terminated the physiological eruption after 1 year and 3 months. At the same time, it was observed that the second right upper premolar freed the eruption path for the first premolar, as it had undertaken its normal eruptive process. At the age of 17, the patient showed a complete permanent dentition (Fig. 7.1d) with the eruption of all the permanent teeth that had taken place spontaneously.

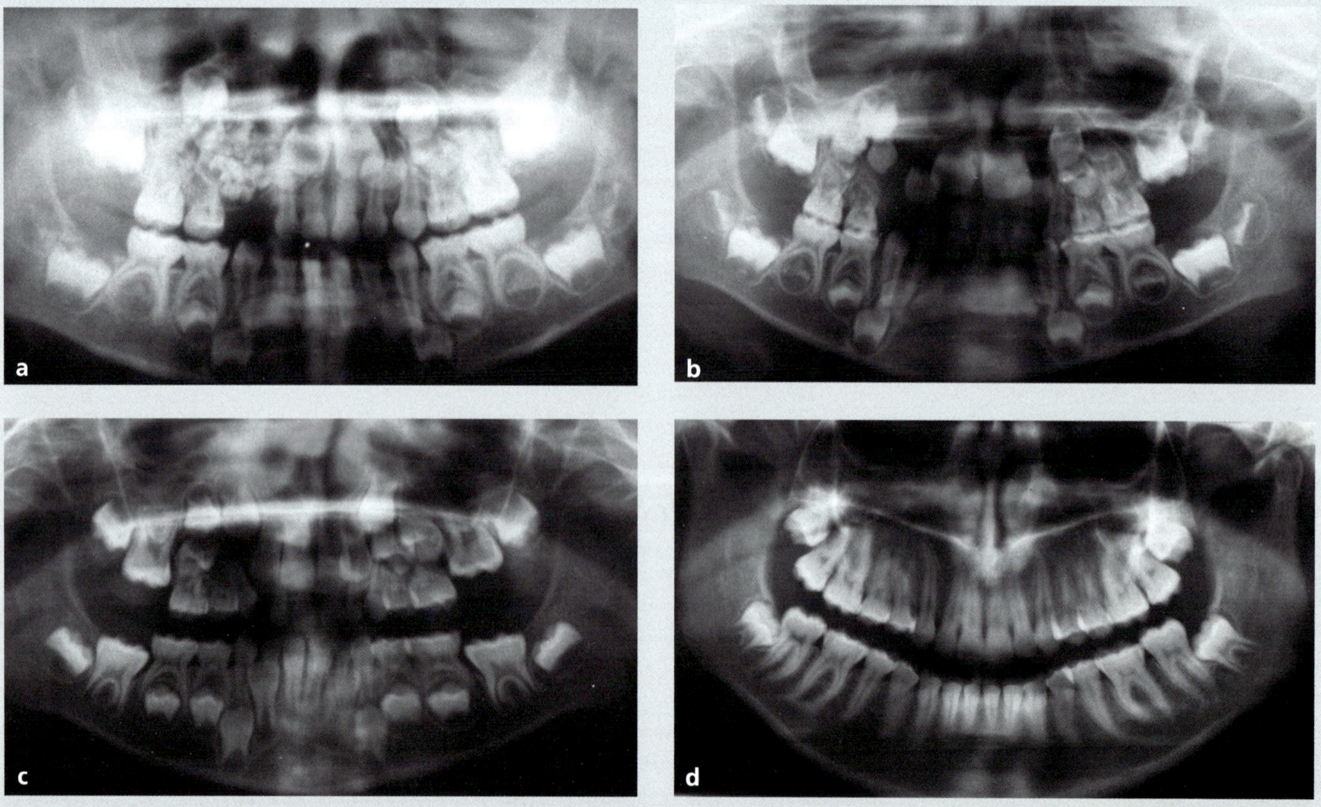

Figure 7.1 (**a**) OPT showing the presence of a large odontoma. (**b**) OPT after odontoma removal. (**c**) OPT 2 years after odontoma removal. Note the spontaneous eruption of the deciduous canine. (**d**) OPT of the same patient at the age of 17 years: complete permanent dentition.

Eruption anomalies in the deciduous dentition

Dental impaction

Analysis of the relevant literature (Yassin, 1999; Cildir et al, 2005) and related clinical investigations show that, except in a small number of cases, tooth impactions in the deciduous dentition appear to be always affecting the upper canine. This points to a diagnosis of impaction if one of the deciduous upper canines is missing, considering that the agenesis of this dental element is a very rare occurrence (Clayton, 1956).
The literature shows that the impaction of the upper canines is linked to the presence of simple and composite odontomas (Sheehy et al, 2004).
See clinical case 1 shown in Figure 7.1.
Another clinical condition that can be identified in the deciduous dentition is the impaction of the deciduous molars, which must be considered in the differential diagnosis of *reimpaction*.

Reimpaction

The reimpaction of the deciduous molars represents a rare clinical event that can be found in the mixed or permanent dentition. Reimpaction is considered to be a sign of other pathologies, including ankylosis, retention, infraocclusion, and hypotrusion of the deciduous molars.
Clinically, reimpaction manifests as one or more deciduous molars not reaching the occlusal level of adjacent teeth (Fig. 7.2). The hypotrusion of the molars has been classified based on the distance between the masticatory surface of the molar and the occlusal plane (Tollaro et al, 1990). The highest hypotrusion level (fourth degree) manifests as a dental element deeply rooted in the bone structure and covered by mucosa (Fig. 7.3).

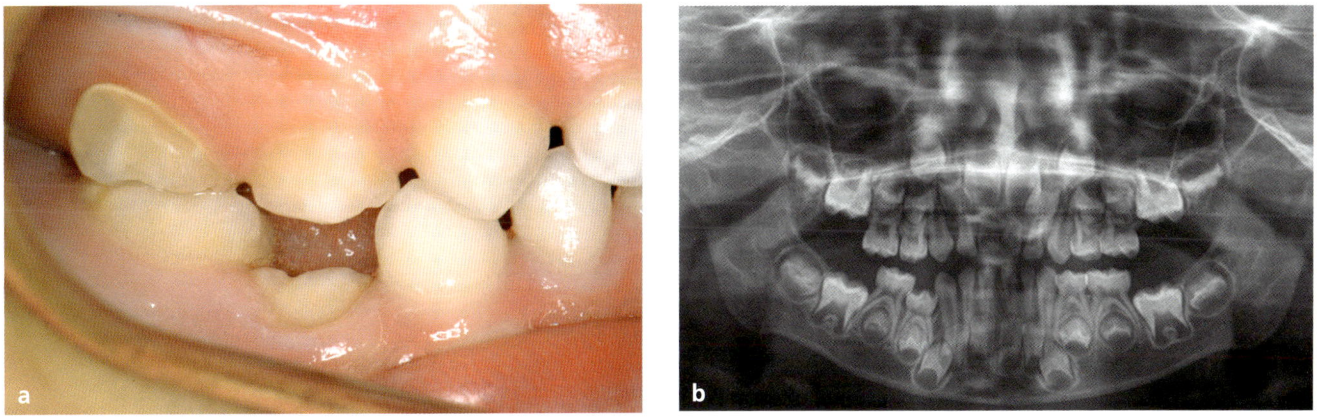

Figure 7.2 (**a**) Clinical evidence of reimpaction. (**b**) OPT.

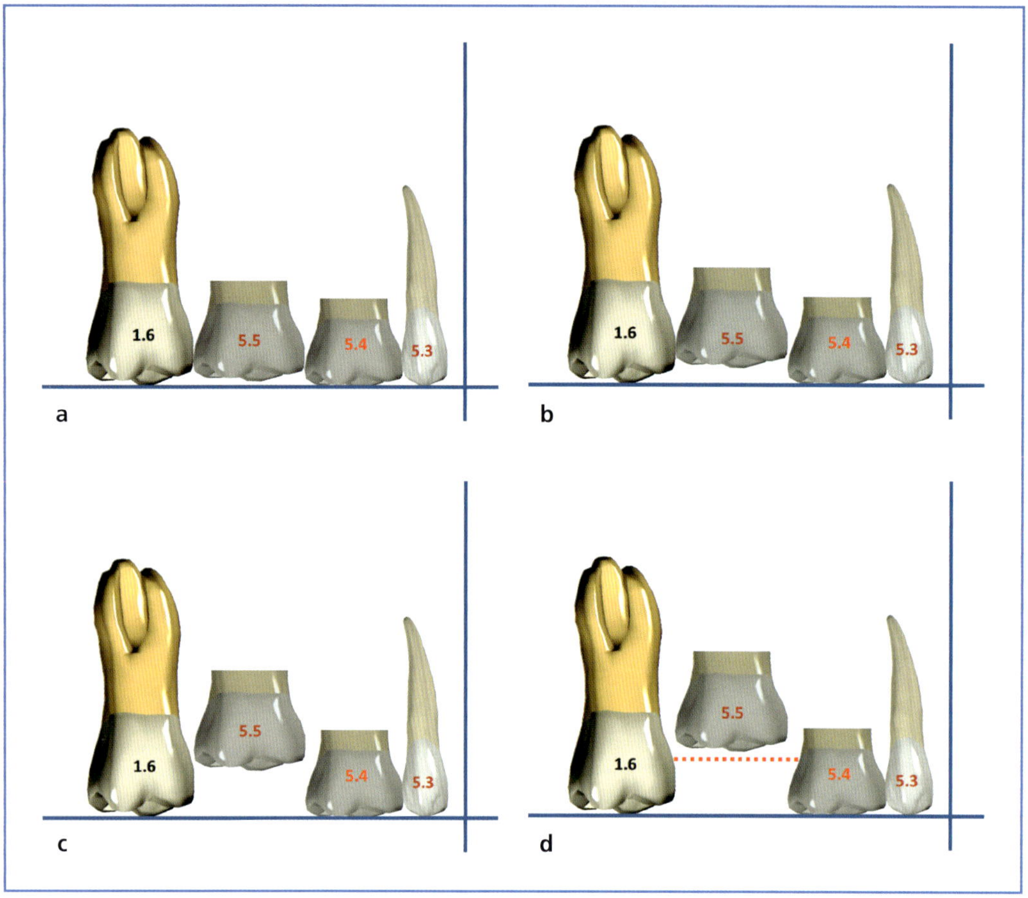

Figure 7.3 (**a**) First-degree hypotrusion, not beyond the equator of the adjacent teeth. (**b**) Second-degree hypotrusion, beyond the equator of the contiguous teeth. (**c**) Third-degree hypotrusion, at the level of the neck. (**d**) Fourth-degree hypotrusion, beyond the neck, deep in the bone structure (reimpaction).

Table 7.2 Prevalence of re-impacted deciduous molars in a case study of 29 dental elements

Enamel completion	Prevalence of re-inclusion of the first and second molars
55 or 65	55.17%
85 or 75	27.58%
54 or 64	10.34%
84 or 74	6.89%

Source: Tollaro, 1990; modified.

It should be noted that it is difficult to highlight a primitive reimpaction. In most clinical cases, a secondary reimpaction is observed. If reimpaction of a healthy dental element is clinically detected, a primitive reimpaction may have occurred. The situation is different in the case of reimpacted dental elements detected using conservative treatment. This differential diagnosis is exclusively speculative because the clinical approach and the related treatment remain the same.
As shown in Table 7.2, the second upper molars are the dental elements most affected by this eruption anomaly.
Considering the importance of the differential growth of the alveolar processes in the clinical manifestations of hypotrusion and reimpaction, the higher incidence detected in the deciduous upper molars can be explained by the various developmental characteristics of the alveolar processes in the upper and lower arches, particularly in the lateroposterior regions (Enlow and Hans, 2008). These authors state that the vertical growth of alveolar processes is quantitatively greater in the upper arch than in the lower arch. This condition occurs because of a compensating effect of the upper jaw to counterbalance the vertical growth of the spheno-occipital structure and the condyle, which are supported by the growth of the maxillary bone basis and the dentoalveolar processes.
Considering the possible clinical consequences, it is important to note that early detection of reimpaction can help clinicians avoid unfavorable effects at the expense of the definitive dental elements. There are essentially two conditions:

- The possibly significant displacement of dental elements replacing the impacted tooth (Fig. 7.4): this clinical occurrence can be detected via a three-dimensional analysis [computed tomography (CT) or *cone-beam* CT] to assess the reciprocal relationships at an intraosseous level between the reimpacted deciduous element and the impacted permanent element. This investigation provides a greater precision for a prognostic assessment of the possibility of permanent tooth eruption. Furthermore, it provides important elements to define the surgical intervention. Surgical avulsion can be difficult owing to the possible presence of ankylosis between the roots of the deciduous tooth and the surrounding bone tissue. Furthermore, it should be noted that the permanent dental elements always undergo a developmental interruption, which may result in impaction if the reimpacted deciduous element is not removed in time
- The inclination of the dental elements adjacent to the reimpacted one (Fig. 7.5): this can facilitate the impaction of the permanent elements that replace the deciduous elements. In such cases, clinicians should recover the space to facilitate permanent tooth eruption

See clinical case 2 shown in Figure 7.6.

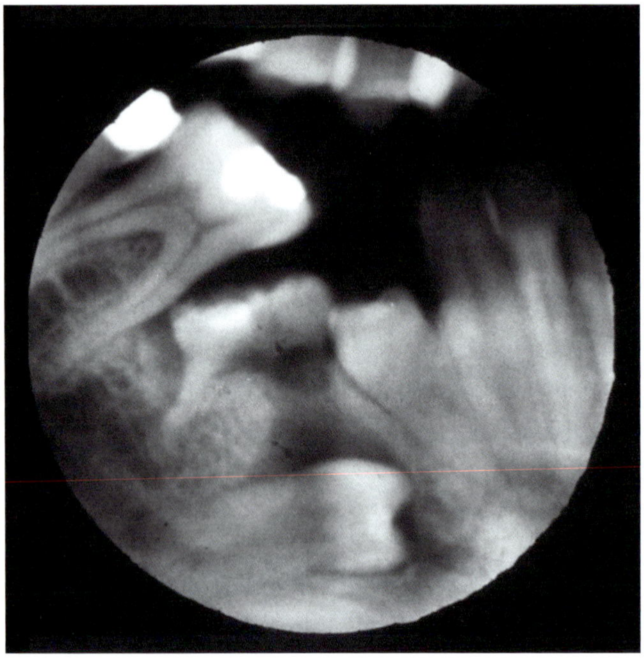

Figure 7.4 Severe dislocation of 45.

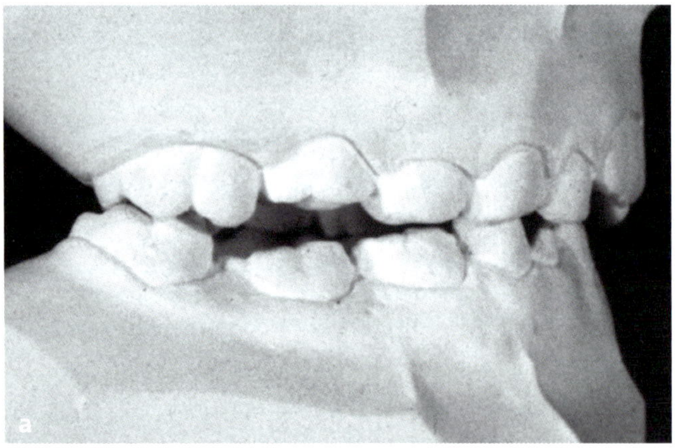

Figure 7.5 (**a**) Example of reimpaction. (**b**) Example of reimpaction with inclination of dental elements adjacent to the reimpacted tooth. (**c**) OPT.

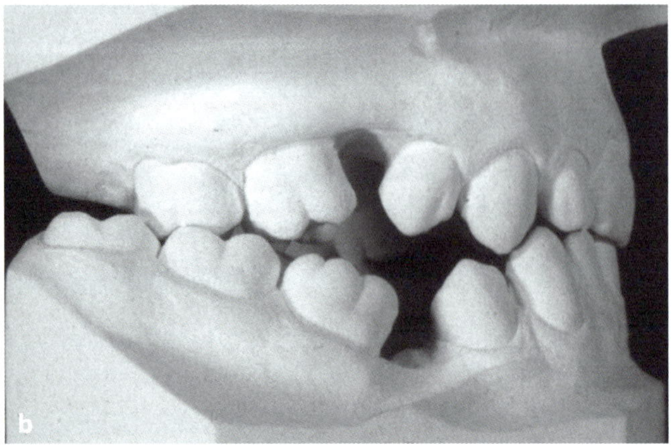

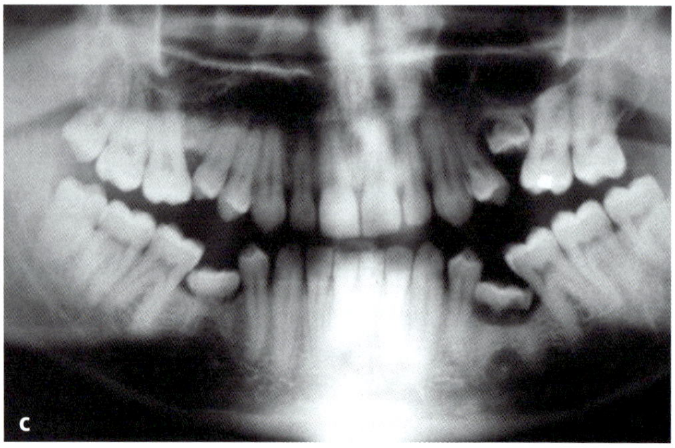

Clinical Case 2 – Reimpactation

S.S., a 9-year-old girl with reimpaction of the left upper deciduous molar. In this case, the clinician attempted to stop the development of the dental element (Fig. 7.6 a, b) by analyzing the cephalometric tracing (Fig. 7.6 c) of the patient against the standard described by Broadbent et al. (1975). For this purpose, the skull base line, Bo-N, was used as the line for superimposition together with the *registration point* (Fig. 7.6 c). The superimposition of the images of the two molars shows the related topographic position, which suggests that the interruption of dental element eruption must have occurred at approximately 3 years of age. Considering the individual variability in the eruption sequence, it is plausible to diagnose the failure of second molar eruption.

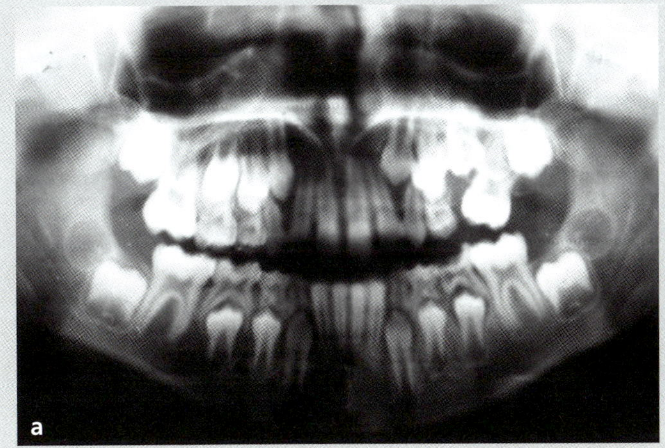

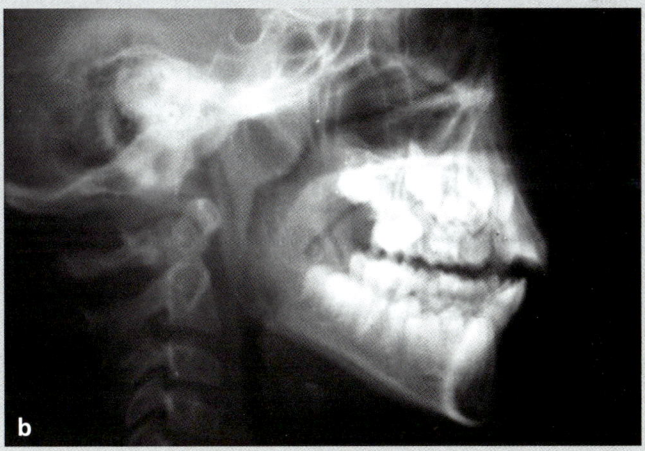

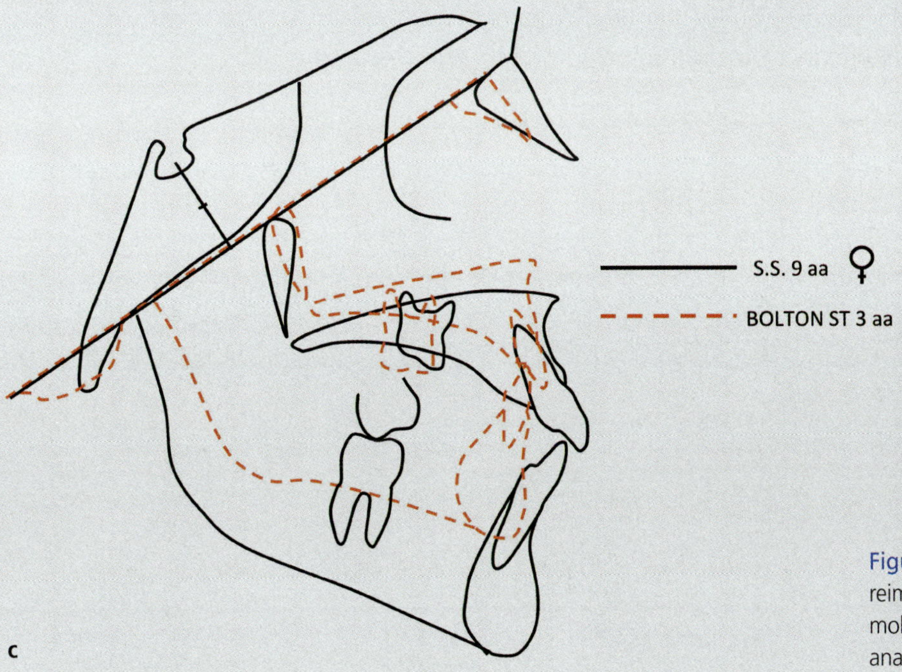

Figure 7.6 (**a**) OPT of a 9-year-old girl, with reimpaction of the left upper second deciduous molar. (**b**) Teleradiography. (**c**) Cephalometric analysis.

Tooth number anomalies

Absent teeth

Dental agenesis, i.e., the lack of one or more dental elements, has a prevalence of 0.4%–0.9% in the European population (Magnusson, 1984) and is higher in individuals of oriental origin (2.4%) (Yonezu et al, 1997). In the deciduous dentition, the prevalence is approximately 0.3%–0.8% (Ravn, 1971).

A recent study conducted at our school (Marinelli et al, 2012) analyzed the repetitiveness of dental anomalies of the deciduous dentition in the permanent dentition. In this study, 189 subjects (100 boys and 89 girls) affected by dental anomalies in the deciduous dentition, such as agenesis, supernumerary teeth, fusions, and gemination, and with an average age of 5 years and 7 months ± 13 months were evaluated. Intraoral images, plaster models of dental arches, and panoramic radiographs were available for all the subjects. All the subjects were analyzed again in the permanent dentition phase (average age, 11 years and 2 months ± 14 months). This experimental group was compared with a control group of 271 subjects (123 boys and 148 girls) who exhibited no dental anomaly in the deciduous dentition (average age, 5 years and 2 months ± 9 months). All the subjects in the control group were analyzed again in the permanent dentition phase (average age, 11 years and 5 months ± 13 months) to assess the presence of dental anomalies in the permanent dentition.

The study showed that compared with agenesis in the deciduous dentition, agenesis in the permanent dentition occurs almost systematically (95.6%), with a few exceptions (Tab. 7.3). The authors of the study reported a repetitiveness of 100% in the case of agenesis of the central deciduous incisors, upper deciduous canines, and lower deciduous molars. In accordance with the results reported in previous studies (Clayton, 1956; Grahnen and Granath, 1961), the deciduous dental elements more frequently affected by agenesis are the upper lateral incisors, both mono- and bilaterally. Agenesis

Table 7.3 Presence of deciduous and permanent dentition agenesis in the experimental and control groups*

	Agenesis in permanent teeth	Absence of agenesis in permanent teeth	Total
Agenesis in the deciduous teeth	43	2	45
Absence of agenesis in the deciduous teeth	12	259	271
Total	55	261	316

* Numbers refer to dental elements. Source: Marinelli et al, 2011; modified.

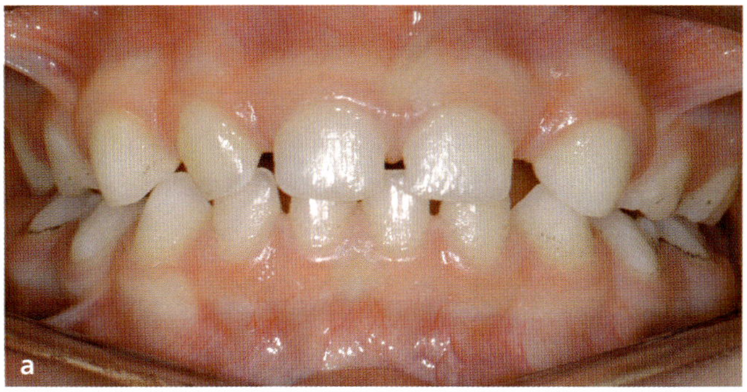

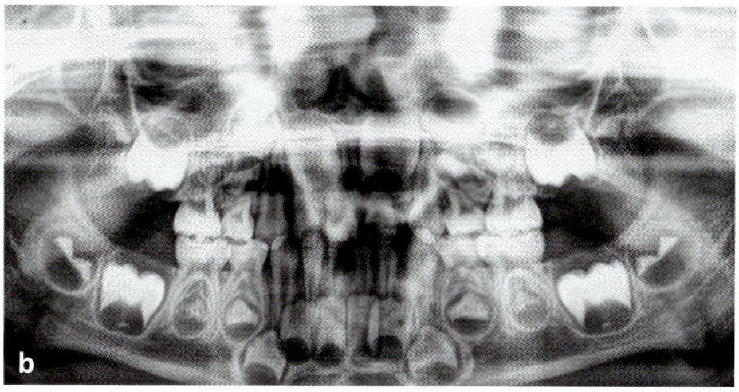

Figure 7.7 (**a**) Agenesis of 62 in the deciduous dentition. (**b**) OPT showing agenesis of 12 and 22.

was also found at the level of the lower incisors, albeit with a lower incidence rate. Regardless of the agenesis site, the most important aspect is that in almost 100% of the cases, the anomaly is repeated in the permanent dentition period. This condition appears to be normal because the germ of the permanent dental element is derived from that of the related deciduous one. Consequently, agenesis of a deciduous tooth, which is a rare event and is not repeated at the level of the permanent tooth, appears to be difficult to interpret.

The longitudinal study by Marinelli et al. (2012) shows an important aspect of the anomalies regarding the number of absent teeth. In addition to the appearance of the dental anomaly in both the deciduous and permanent dentition, two additional events were detected at the clinical level:

- agenesis in the deciduous dentition, not followed by agenesis in the permanent dentition (4.4%)
- agenesis in the permanent dentition with the presence of the corresponding deciduous element (Fig. 7.7)

These two rare events can be explained by the embryonic development of deciduous and permanent dentition. Deciduous and permanent dentition are derived from different regions of the general lamina (lateral and successional, respectively) (Avery, 1992). As illustrated in Figure 7.8, it can be hypothesized that a defect in the general lamina, which is apparently very frequent, causes agenesis of both the deciduous and permanent teeth. The specific defects of the lateral or successional lamina, which are much rarer, might cause agenesis of only the deciduous or permanent element.

An important clinical aspect to note in such cases is that the permanent tooth not preceded by the corresponding deciduous one is characterized by early maturation and eruption (Ranta, 1983). From an orthodontic perspective, there is a high risk of class III malocclusion in cases of agenesis of the upper lateral deciduous and permanent elements.

The authors report the case of a patient with multiple agenesis requiring orthodontic intervention, which, in turn, will be followed by a prosthetic phase at the end of the development period (Fig. 7.9).

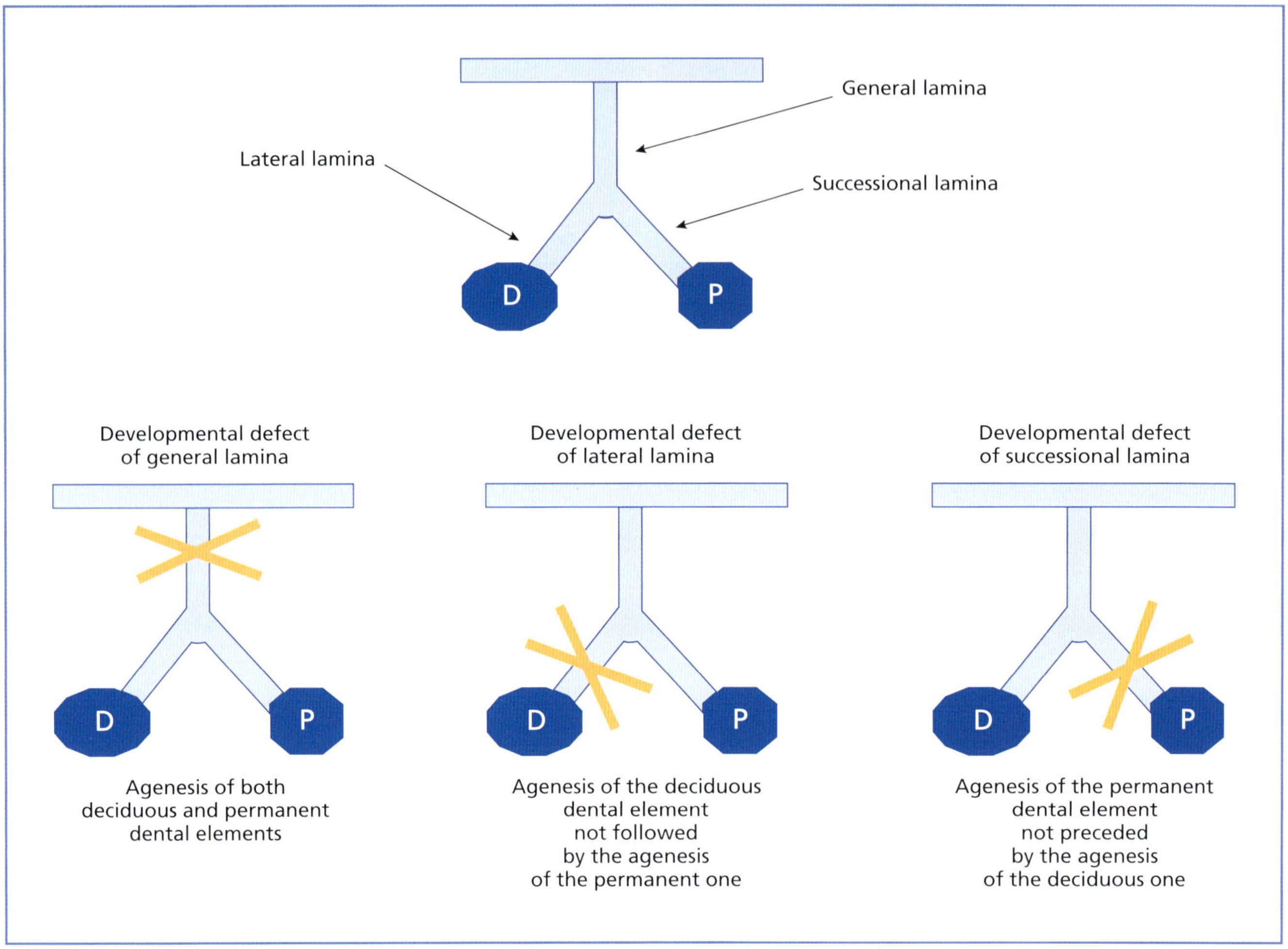

Figure 7.8 Diagram showing the relationship between the lamina defect and tooth agenesis.

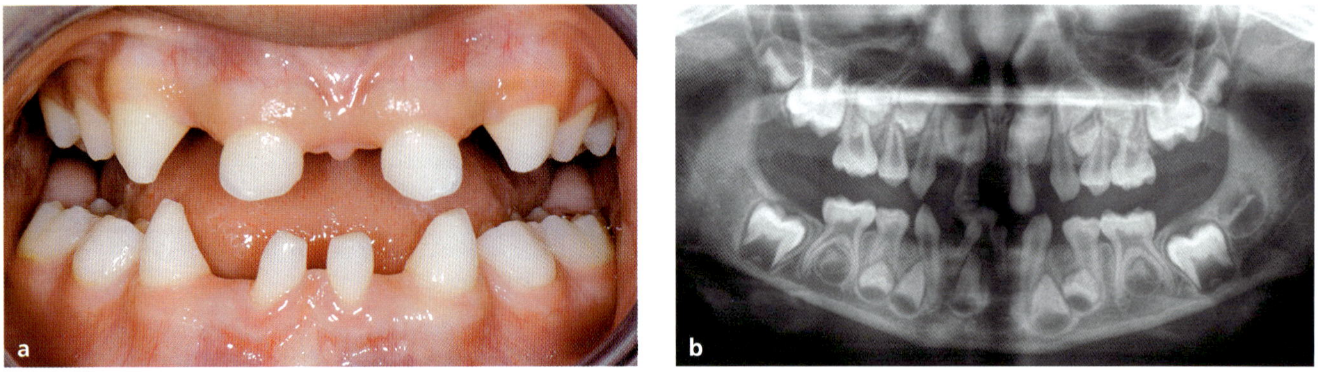

Figure 7.9 (**a**) Multiple agenesis. (**b**) OPT.

Table 7.4 Presence of deciduous and permanent supernumerary teeth in the test and control groups*

	Supernumerary teeth in the permanent dentition	Absence of supernumerary teeth in the permanent dentition	Total
Supernumerary teeth in the deciduous dentition	54	35	45
Absence of supernumerary teeth in the deciduous dentition	15	256	271
Total	69	291	360

* Numbers refer to teeth. Source: Marinelli et al, 2012; modified.

Extra teeth

This type of anomaly shows marked site selectivity in the upper lateral incisors, and the incidence is also confirmed by previous studies (Plaetschke, 1938; Menczer, 1955; Magnusson, 1959; Bolender, 1964; Magnusson et al, 1985). The detection of supernumerary teeth in the deciduous dentition poses no risk for the repetition of this dental anomaly in the permanent dentition (Marinelli et al, 2012); supernumerary teeth in the deciduous dentition showed repetition in the permanent dentition in 60.7% of cases (Tab. 7.4). By evaluating the clinical and practical aspects, clinicians should manage the presence of supernumerary monolateral teeth to avoid deviations from the upper interincisive line. An early assessment of the anomalies of excess tooth numbers in the permanent dentition, suggested by the presence of supernumerary deciduous elements, allows avoiding the complications of alignment or impaction of the dental elements adjacent to the supernumerary ones through a timely avulsion (Fig. 7.10).

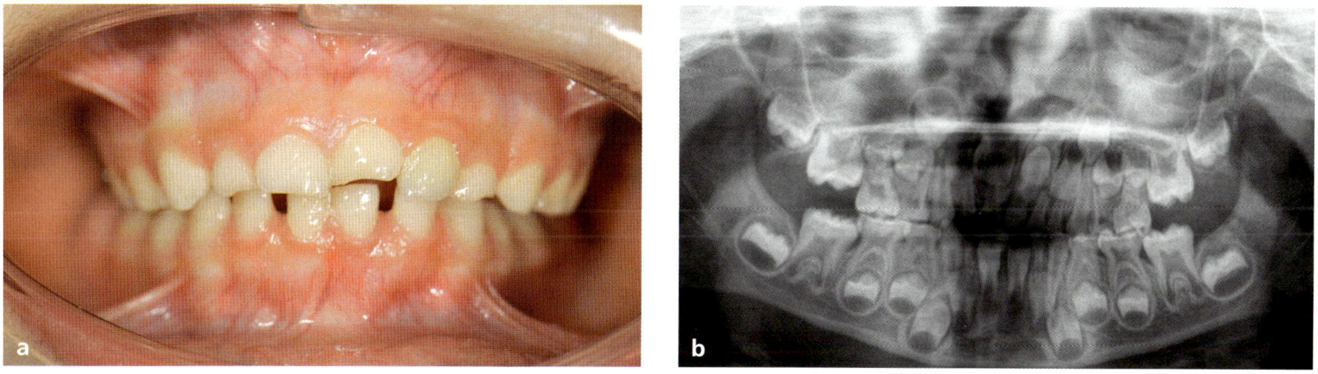

Figure 7.10 (**a**) Supernumerary tooth at the level of 62. (**b**) OPT showing a supernumerary tooth at the level of 21 (with reverse polarity).

Shape anomalies

Simple

Simple shape anomalies can occur at two locations:
- the crown (Fig. 7.11)
- the root (Fig. 7.12).

Complex

Complex shape anomalies are represented by the following forms:
- fused teeth
- geminated teeth.

English-speaking authors define double tooth as both gemination and partial separation of a single tooth bud and the fusion of two teeth or the partial union of two different tooth buds.
An in-depth analysis of the related literature shows that complex anomalies, such as fused teeth and geminated teeth, occur more frequently at the expense of the deciduous dentition (0.5%–09%) than at the expense of the permanent dentition (01%–0.2%) (Boyne, 1955; Castaldi et al, 1966).
Clinically, the differential diagnosis between fusion and gemination is often difficult.

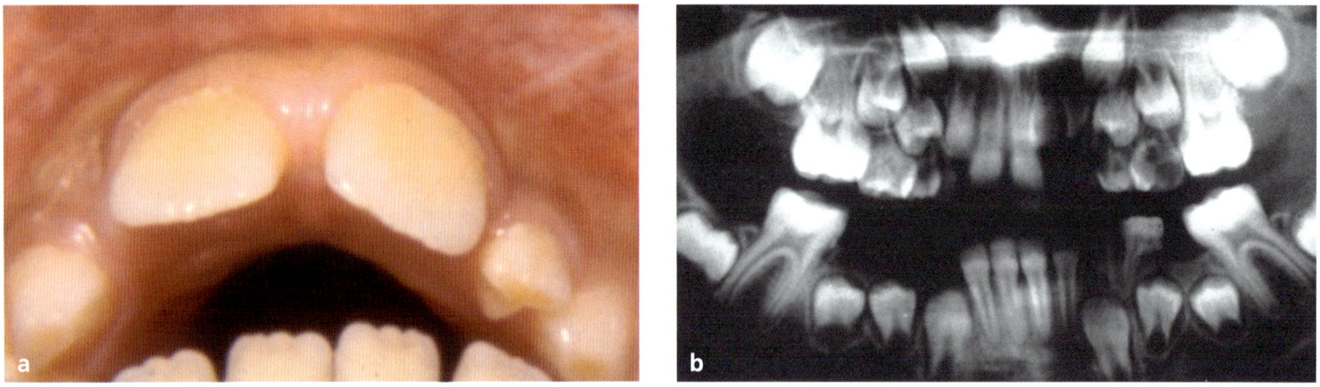

Figure 7.11 (**a**) Simple anomalies of the crown of 62. (**b**) OPT showing a supernumerary tooth at the level of 22.

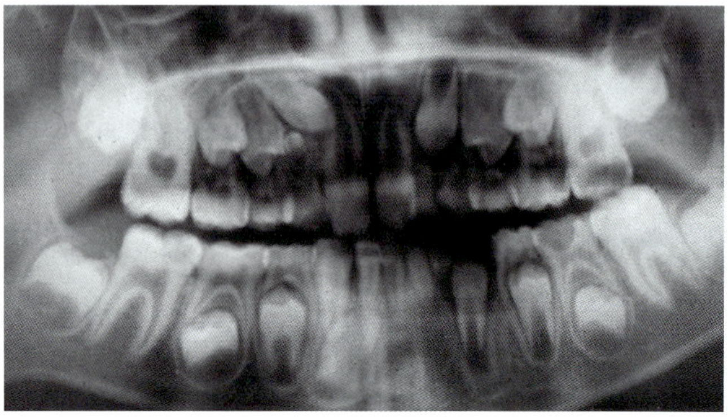

Figure 7.12 OPT showing simple anomalies of the root of 53 (bifid root with the presence of a supernumerary tooth at furcation).

Some authors have characterized fusion by a double crown and a single root, with double root canals; on the contrary, gemination is characterized by a double crown and a single root, but with a single root canal.
A criterion often used by authors relies on the analysis the number of dental elements within the arch: the absence of dental elements adjacent to the anomalous one guides the diagnosis toward fusion, whereas the presence of all dental elements of the normal set suggests gemination.
The complex anomaly (fusion) in the deciduous dentition shows a high risk of being followed by agenesis in the permanent dentition (88.7%) (Tab. 7.5 and Fig. 7.13).

Table 7.5 Presence of fusion in deciduous teeth and permanent dentition agenesis in the experimental and control groups*

	Agenesis in the permanent dentition	Absence of agenesis in the permanent dentition	Total
Fusion in the deciduous dentition	30	4	34
Absence of fusion in the deciduous dentition	12	259	271
Total	42	263	305

* Numbers refer to dental elements.

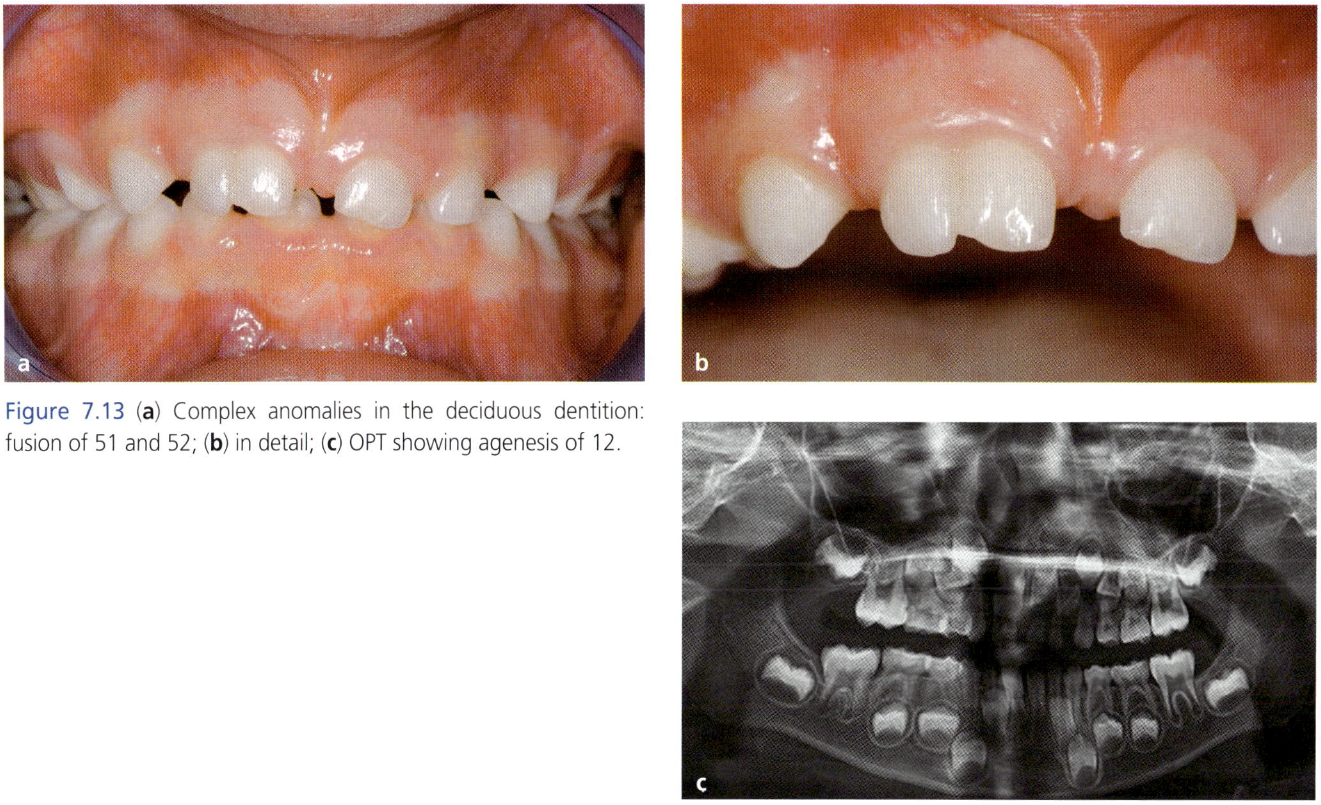

Figure 7.13 (**a**) Complex anomalies in the deciduous dentition: fusion of 51 and 52; (**b**) in detail; (**c**) OPT showing agenesis of 12.

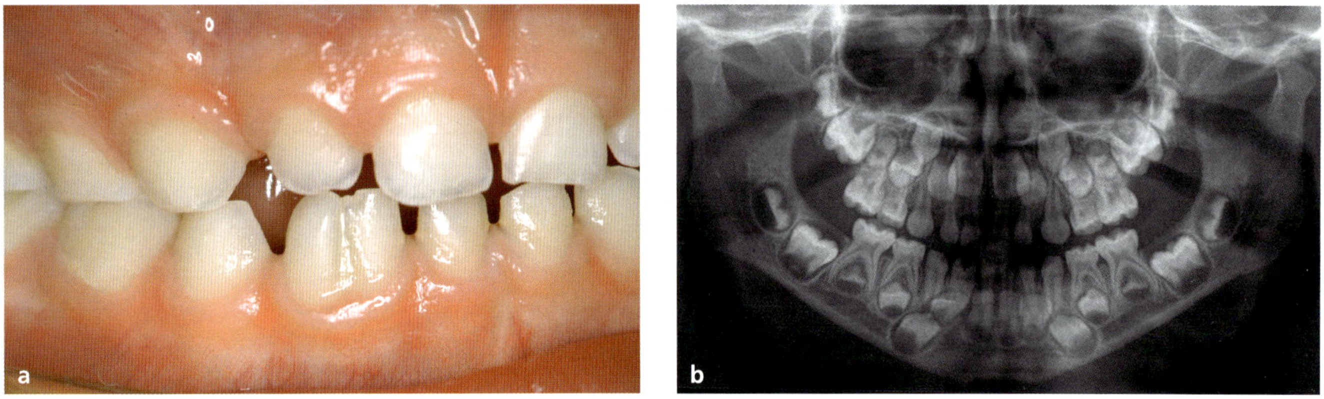

Figure 7.14 (**a**) Gemination of the deciduous dentition. (**b**) OPT.

This prevalence is similar to that reported by Hagman (1988) (75%). The fusion of the upper central incisor with the lateral one is followed by the agenesis of the permanent lateral incisor in six out of seven cases (Marinelli et al, 2012).

Gemination in the deciduous dentition is repeated in the permanent dentition in 45% of cases (Fig. 7.14 and Tab. 7.6). This prevalence rate is similar to that reported by Nik-Hussein and Abdul Majid (59%) (1996) and Skrinjarić and Barac-Furtinović (61%) (1991).

In conclusion, it is important to highlight the existence of linearity and repetitiveness of the several anomalies characterizing the deciduous and permanent dentition. In most cases, a radiographic examination will be sufficient for providing useful details to perform a diagnostic and prognostic assessment of the permanent dentition.

In clinical practice, although the detection of dental anomalies in the deciduous dentition can occur at approximately 2.5–3 years of age, a knowledge of the dental elements listed in this chapter allows postponing the radiographic examination tuntil approximately 5–6 years of age to obtain a better clinical picture and better patient cooperation.

Table 7.6 Presence of gemination in the deciduous dentition and supernumeraries in the permanent dentition in the experimental and control groups*

	Supernumerary teeth in the permanent dentition	Absence of supernumerary teeth in the permanent dentition	Total
Gemination in the deciduous dentition	9	11	20
Absence of gemination in the deciduous dentition	15	256	271
Total	24	267	291

* Numbers refer to teeth.

References

Avery JK. Essentials of oral histology and embryology: a clinical approach. St. Louis: Mosby Year Book; 1992. p. 51-69.

Bolender C. Les anomalies de nombre et de éruption de la denture temporaire. Orthod Fr 1964;39:373.

Boyne PJ. Gemination; report two cases. J Am Dent Assoc 1955;50:194.

Broadbent BH, Broadbent BH Jr, Golden WH. Bolton standards of dentofacial development growth. St. Louis: CV Mosby Co; 1975.

Castaldi CR, Bondarchuk A, MacRae PD, Zacherl WA. Incidence of congenital anomalies in permanent teeth of group of Canadian children aged 6-9. J Can Dent Ass 1966;32:154-9.

Cildir SK, Sencift K, Olgac V, Sandalli N. Delayed eruption of a mandibular primary cuspid associated with compound odontoma. J Contemp Dent Pract 2005;4:152-9.

Clayton J. Congential dental anomalies occurring in 3557 children. J Dent Child 1956;23:206-18.

Enlow DH, Hans MG. Essentials of facial growth. 2nd ed. Philadelphia: W.B. Saunders; 2008.

Grahnen H, Granath L. Numerical variations in primary dentition and their correlation with the permanent dentition. Odont Revy 1961;12:348.

Hagman FT. Anomalies of form and number, fused primary teeth, a correlation of the dentitions. J Dent Child 1988;55:359-61.

Magnusson BO. Tandovertal i den primara dentitionen. Swensk Tandlak T 1959;52:357.

Magnusson BO, Kock G, Poulsen S. Pedodonzia: un approccio sistematico. Milano: Edi-Ermes; 1985.

Magnusson TE. Hypodontia, hyperodontia, and double formation of primary teeth in Iceland. An epidemiological study. Acta Odontol Scand 1984;42:137-9.

Marinelli A, Giuntini V, Franchi L et al. Dental anomalies in the primary dentition and their repetition in the permanent dentition: a diagnostic performance study. Odontology 2012;100:22-7.

Menczer LF. Anomalies of the primary dentition. J Dent Child 1955;22:57-62.

Nik-Hussein NN, Abdul Majid Z. Dental anomalies in the primary dentition: distribution and correlation with the permanent dentition. J Clin Pediatr Dent 1996;21:15-9.

Plaetschke J. Okklusionsanomalien in milchgebiss. Dtsch Zahn-Mund-Kierfereilk 1938;5:435.

Ranta R. Premature mineralization of permanent canines associated with aplasia of their primary predecessor: report of four cases. J Dent Child 1983;50:274-7.

Ravn JJ. Aplasia, supernumerary teeth and fused teeth in the primary dentition. An epidemiologic study. Scand J Dent Res 1971;79:1-6.

Sheehy EC, Odell EW, Al-Jaddir G. Odontomas in the primary dentition: literature review and case report. J Dent Child 2004;71:73-6.

Škrinjarić, I, Barac-Furtinović, V. Anomalies of deciduous teeth and findings in permanent dentition. Acta Stomatol Croat 1991;25:151-6.

Tollaro I, Antonini A, Bassarelli V et al. La fase della dentatura decidua. Milano: Masson; 1990. p. 33-47.

Yassin OM. Delayed eruption of maxillary primary cuspid associated with compound odontoma. J Clin Pediatr Dent 1999;23:147-9.

Yonezu T, Hayashi Y, Sasaki J, Machida Y. Prevalence of congenital dental anomalies of the deciduous dentition in Japanese children. Bull Tokyo Dent Coll 1997;38:27-32.

Chapter 8

Pathologies of the oral mucosa in pediatric dentistry

A. Majorana, E. Bardellini

Physical examination of the oral cavity, at least during the initial visit, should always include assessment of the health status of the oral mucosa. This gains even more importance in the case of children. In fact, it is difficult to obtain the correct pathological medical history in children with mucosal abnormalities, both because of the difficulties children may face in describing and localizing the pain symptoms and the inability to put these into temporal context and link them to previous events, for example traumatic events, and the difficulties in highlighting any modification of the lesions over time. This considerably reduces the opportunities to add additional information to the medical history and makes clinical data interpretation very challenging. Furthermore, partial knowledge of the various pathological manifestations affecting the oral mucosa in children often results in the provision of nonspecific treatment based on the use of inadequate or irritating drugs that alter the initial clinical condition. Add to this the fact that the clinical condition can present with existing abnormalities due to bacterial superinfections or with minor traumas due to children's habit of putting objects in their mouths, and the clinician's difficulty in analyzing a mucosal lesion is understandable. Lastly, the immunological immaturity in children and the reduced mucosal trophism often favor the local extension of the concerned lesion and increase the risk of systemic impairment (Rioboo-Crespo et al, 2005; Mathew et al, 2008).

However, the diagnosis of oral lesions in children is made easier by the limited spectrum of pathologies that affect the oral mucosa compared with the wide variety of abnormalities noted in adults, remembering that, by definition, some abnormalities are typical of the developmental age. From an etiological perspective, abnormalities of the oral mucosa in children can generally be attributed to reactive, infective, and immune-mediated forms or may belong to the so-called nonpathological conditions (Rioboo-Crespo et al, 2005; Mathew et al, 2008).

The clinical aspect of a lesion and the associated signs and symptoms are the starting points to guide the correct process of differential diagnosis. Oral lesions in children essentially present three main clinical aspects: white lesions, ulcerative lesions, and neoformations. In particular, ulcerative lesions include both those, *in the strict sense* of the word, characterized by an onset with an immediate loss of superficial (erosions) or deep (ulcers) tissue and *secondary* lesions, which are caused by the rupture of previous vesicles or blisters, containing an organic fluid at the intra- or subepithelial level, which are generally the consequence of infective or autoimmune pathologies. In fact, it is very difficult to observe vesicles or blisters in the oral cavity because the mechanical action of the tongue and masticatory muscles, together with the macerating action of saliva, cause them to break down after formation (Rioboo-Crespo et al, 2005; Mathew et al, 2008; Scully and Welbury, 1994; Majorana et al, 2010a; Majorana et al, 2010b). The guided diagnostic pathways related to the oral white and ulcerative lesions in children are shown in Figures 8.1 and 8.2.

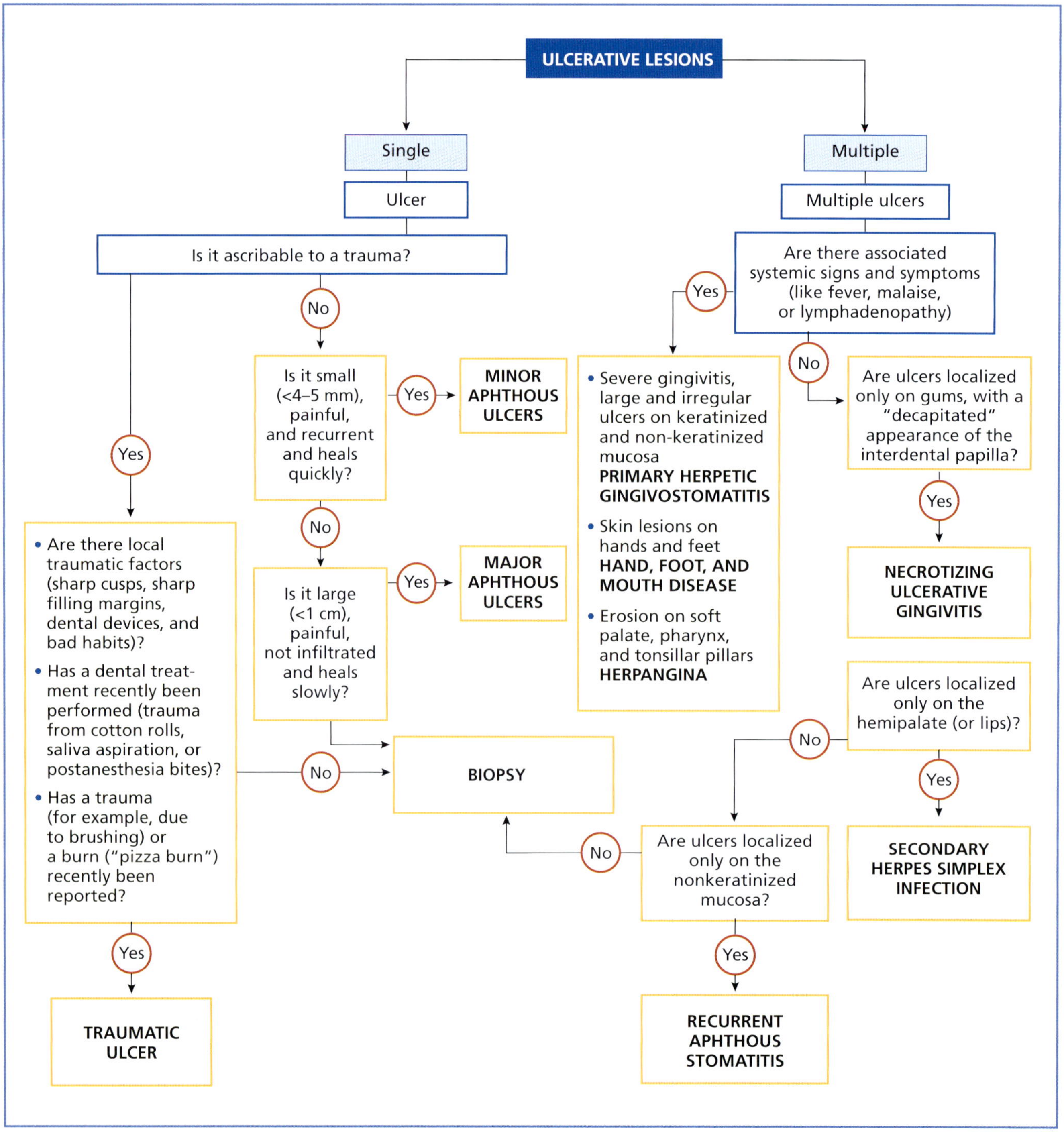

Figure 8.1 Guided approach for the diagnosis of the main ulcerative mucosa lesions in children.

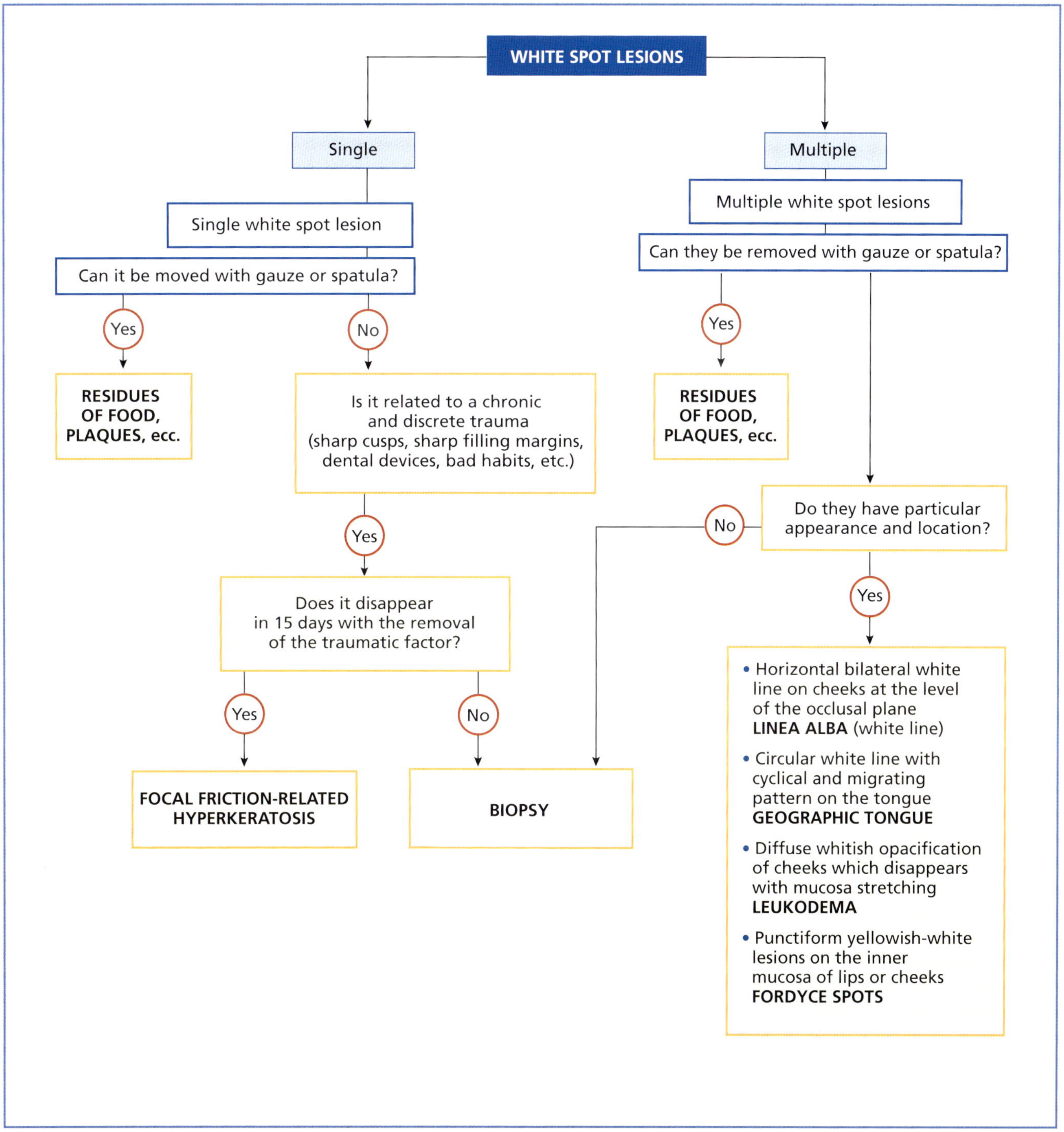

Figure 8.2 Guided approach for the diagnosis of the main white mucosa lesions in children.

Main white lesions

Pseudomembranous candidiasis

Pseudomembranous candidiasis (Fig. 8.3), commonly known as "thrush," is one of the most frequent white lesions found in children. It is an infectious pathology caused by the fungus *Candida albicans*, and its development depends on the establishment of favorable conditions for the growth of this organism, which is a result of the complex interaction between its pathogenicity and the host immune status. The predisposing factors in children include immunological immaturity; antibiotics; inhaled corticosteroid therapy; diabetes and various conditions inducing psychophysical stress, such as viral influenza, malnutrition, and anxiety states, which can act as an optimal substrate for the subsequent development of the fungus. The lesions clinically manifest as detachable whitish plaques spread all over the oral cavity, and their removal leaves an eroded and reddened surface. The plaques comprise colonies of this fungus, keratin debris, inflammatory cells, fibrin, bacteria, and desquamated epithelial cells. The symptoms are generally mild, although they can compromise nutrition in the most severe cases, with the ensuing deterioration of the child's health status. Diagnosis is based on the clinical examination of the lesions and demonstration of the presence of the fungus using the periodic acid–Schiff staining or culture testing. The treatment of immunocompetent patients is based on the administration of topical antifungals (Mathew et al, 2008; Appleton, 2000; Jabra-Rizk et al, 2007; Rozkiewicz et al, 2006).

Focal hyperkeratosis caused by friction

Reactive forms such as focal hyperkeratosis caused by friction are frequently found in children. Focal hyperkeratosis manifests clinically as a single nondetachable white lesion caused by a traumatic mechanical event; in fact, it can frequently be found in the proximity of a local irritating factor, such as the sharp edge of a fractured filling or an orthodontic bracket. The tissue response can be considered a protective mechanism

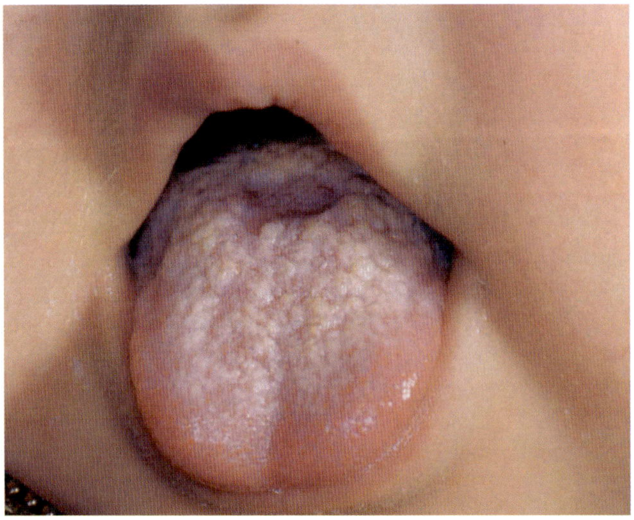

Figure 8.3 Candidiasis.

initiated by the epithelium. From a histological perspective, it is possible to observe hyperkeratosis and variable inflammatory infiltrate in the stroma. Removal of local irritating factors allows the lesion to regress within 2 weeks. The clinical condition of hyperkeratosis also includes more widespread conditions such as the thickening of the linea alba, i.e., the whitish streak on the buccal mucosa running from the labial commissure to the chewing plane in the backward direction, or morsicatio buccarum, i.e., areas of traumatic abrasion of the superficial epithelium of the buccal mucosa with whitish thickenings caused by the habit of cheek biting in children and young people with anxious personalities or nervous conditions. Rarely, this can also be observed in children with psychiatric pathologies or certain disabilities. Both these bilateral conditions can be reduced by stopping the habit of voluntarily chewing the mucosa, which can also be done using protective occlusal plates (Mathew et al, 2008; Sewerin, 1971).

Leukoedema

Leukoedema, considered an anatomical variant of the oral mucosa, involves bilateral opacification of the buccal mucosa, which appears whitish and edematous. As the buccal mucosa stretches, the lesion disappears and subsequently reappears after release. No treatment is necessary (Mathew et al, 2008; Martin, 1992).

Fordyce spots

Fordyce spots are ectopic sebaceous glands that are usually located on the buccal mucosa or the inner lip mucosa in the form of small isolated or confluent yellowish papules. They require no therapy (Mathew et al, 2008).

Hairy tongue (Lingua villosa)

Hairy tongue is an innocuous condition characterized by hypertrophy and lengthening of the filiform papillae due to a delayed desquamation of the stratum corneum or an increased rate of keratinization. It manifests as the formation of a yellowish patina on the tongue, comprising elongated filiform papillae, food residues, cellular debris, and microorganisms. It appears to be associated with insufficient self-cleaning of the tongue due to various factors, such as excessive consumption of soft foods or poor oral hygiene, but might also be related to the alteration of the composition of oral microbial flora caused by thermoregulation disorders (fever) or prolonged antibiotic therapies. Diagnosis is clinically performed, and the lesion tends to spontaneously regress, improving the general condition of patients (after influenza, fever, or prolonged antibiotic therapies) and their oral hygiene condition (Mathew et al, 2008; Majorana et al, 2010).

Geographic tongue

Geographic tongue (Fig. 8.4) (migratory glossitis) is a benign chronic inflammatory condition characterized by a dystrophic desquamative process affecting the filiform papillae; it occurs in children, particularly in those aged less than 10 years. Subsequently, its appearance reduces with age. From a clinical perspective, it is possible to observe multiple smooth and erythematous regions on the dorsum of the tongue, with rounded or irregular shapes surrounded by slightly raised, thin, white/yellowish

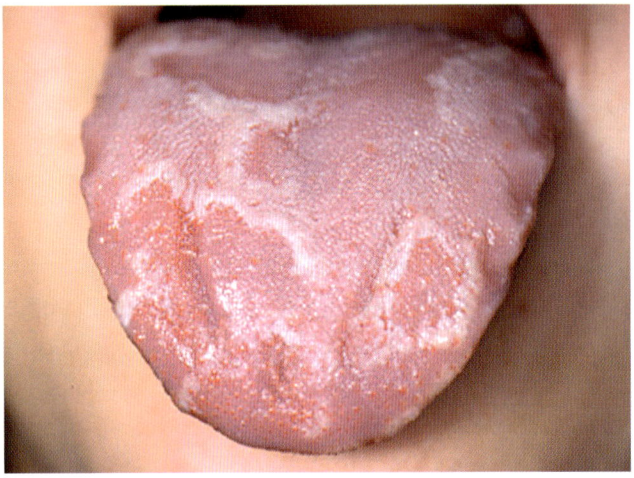

Figure 8.4 Geographic tongue.

margins. Thus, various shapes resembling a geographical map appear on the tongue. These lesions tend to regress spontaneously within a few days or weeks only to reappear later in other parts of the tongue. Thus, they seem to "migrate" over the tongue surface; while there is healing at one margin, there is simultaneous extension of the process at the opposite margin. For this reason, this condition is also called migratory erythema. It is usually asymptomatic, although some patients might feel discomfort eating some foods. From a histological perspective, the central erythematous portion shows lymphocyte and neutrophil infiltration in the epithelium, whereas the white peripheral portion shows hyperkeratosis and acanthosis. The diagnosis is exclusively clinical, and no treatment is required because the pathology is self-limiting (Ray et al, 2007; Miloğlu et al, 2009). Hairy tongue and geographic tongue are frequently related to fissured tongue, a developmental anomaly that is asymptomatic and characterized by the presence of furrows on the tongue surface. The association of fissured tongue with the unilateral paralysis of the facial nerve and facial edema leads to Melkersson–Rosenthal syndrome, which is rare during infancy (Dodi et al, 2006).

Main ulcerative lesions

Real ulcerative lesions

Ulcerative lesions are those occurring because of the loss of tissue (erosive or ulcerative), in the absence of previous vesicles or blisters. These include recurrent aphthous stomatitis, PFAPA syndrome, traumatic ulcer, necrotizing ulcerative gingivitis, and erythema multiforme.

Recurrent aphthous stomatitis

Aphthous stomatitis (Fig. 8.5) is an ulcerative pathology that is most commonly found in the oral mucosa, with an incidence rate of 20%–66%. The etiology is unknown,

although several favoring or triggering factors have been considered, such as vitamin B12 deficiency, folic acid deficiency; iron deficiency; intolerance of certain foods, such as chocolate, nuts, and cheese; drug intolerance; emotional or physical stress; hormonal modifications; local trauma; genetic predisposition, such as HLA-B12, A2, and AW29 antigens in affected subjects; and systemic diseases, such as gluten-induced enteropathy or celiac disease, ulcerative colitis, agranulocytosis, or cyclic neutropenia. The pathogenic mechanism involves the destruction of the oral mucosa, which is mediated by CD8+ T lymphocytes following an altered immunoregulatory mechanism in response to an endogenous or exogenous antigen. It is believed that the basis of this pathology is immune complex vasculitis, i.e., the circulating immune complexes react with the neutrophils present in vessel walls, with the subsequent release of cytoplasmic enzymes, resulting in the destruction of the overlying epithelium (Campisi et al, 2008; Malahias et al, 2009; Albanidou-Farmaki et al, 2008).
Aphthous stomatitis manifests as ulcers within the oral cavity and affects only the nonkeratinized mucosa. The clinical course can be subdivided into four phases:

- *prodromal* phase: burning or itching sensation in the absence of oral lesions (this phase may occasionally be absent and usually does not last more than 24 hours)
- *preulcerative* or *erythematous* phase: emergence of macular or papular erythematous lesions (this phase lasts no more than 24 hours)
- *ulcerative* phase: formation of roundish and painful ulcers with yellow bottoms and erythematous halos
- *reparative* phase: re-epithelialization with *restitutio ad integrum* and withdrawal of pain.

Clinically, there are two forms of aphthous ulcers: minor and major. The minor aphthous ulcers include three types: vulvar, recurrent, and herpetiform aphthae.
Vulvar aphthae are oval ulcers that are usually single (from 2 to 6 at most), ungrouped, and painful and have a diameter smaller than 1 cm; they are covered with a whitish-yellow fibrinous membrane and are surrounded by an erythematous halo. They are frequently located in the fornices, particularly at the level of frenula. They appear 2–4 times annually and heal in approximately 1 week. *Recurrent* aphthae, clinically

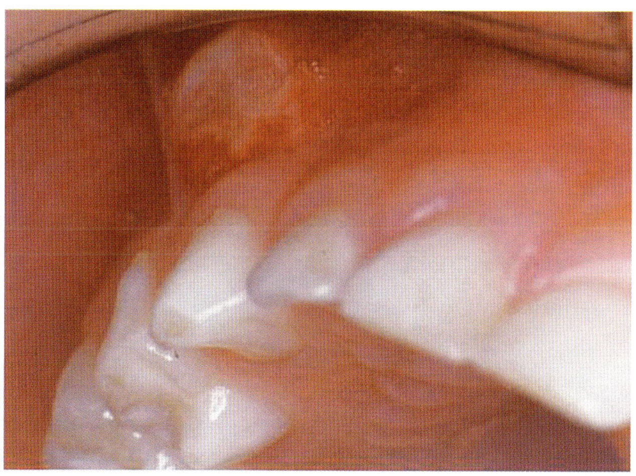

Figure 8.5 Aphthous stomatitis.

similar to the previous ones, evolve suddenly and last for 1 to 2 weeks depending on several factors (psychological, dietary, and systemic) that are able to support incoming injuries. *Miliary* aphthae are small, numerous, and grouped ulcers that are frequently confluent and distributed on both the keratinized and nonkeratinized mucosa. They are also defined as "herpetiform" because of their similarity to herpetic lesions, although they are not preceded by the appearance of vesicles. They can coexist with vulvar aphthae, facilitating, in this case, the diagnosis. They rarely occur in children.

Numerous authors have highlighted a close correlation between recurrent aphthous stomatitis and celiac disease, with a frequency of 20%–60% depending on the records available. It is believed that the pathogeneses of recurrent aphthous stomatitis and celiac disease are similar because aphthous manifestations and intestinal lesions in patients with celiac disease undergo remission following a gluten-free diet and recur in the *challenge* period. Despite the fact that celiac disease in its typical form manifests in the third/fourth trimester of life with a characteristic clinical picture of malabsorption, atypical forms are frequent as well: they appear in late infancy and are accompanied by sideropenic anemia (iron deficiency), short stature, abdominal pain, or occasional diarrhea. The related frequency of these atypical cases underlies important clinical implications, among which there is a possibility to identify the celiac form (otherwise unknown) controlling the clinical course of recurrent aphthous episodes, particularly if the patient has a relevant personal and/or family history (Campisi et al, 2008; Malahias et al, 2009).

Giant aphthae and syndromic forms should be added to the group of major aphthosis. Giant aphthae are large-sized ulcers (1–5 cm), usually with irregular margins that are not hard and surrounded by an erythematous halo; the bottom is covered by a yellowish exudate with a soft base. Healing takes weeks or months with frequent recurrences. The scarring leaves fibrous areas; therefore, the recurrence of necrotizing aphthae at the same site might cause deformations and mutilations. *Syndromic* forms are characterized by an association between classic oral aphthae and lesions in other regions of the body. In particular, they are associated with genital and cutaneous aphthae in Neumann's bipolar aphthosis; with genital and ocular aphthae in the tripolar aphthosis of Behcet's disease; and aphthae at other sites, such as ocular, articular, cutaneous, or vascular sites, in the multipolar aphthosis of Touraine. However, these are typical clinical conditions in adult patients (Tunes et al, 2009; Sun et al, 2009; Alli et al, 2009).

The diagnosis is generally clinical based on the location (non-keratinized mucosa) and clinical aspect (round ulcers) of lesions as well as the medical history of recurrent episodes. The treatment is usually symptomatic. In children, it is especially based on filling substances containing hyaluronic acid that attenuate pain and speed up reparative and disinfectant processes, whose purpose is to prevent bacterial superinfections that might influence the duration and severity of ulcers. As aphthae are caused by an immunological defect, the related treatment also includes drugs that regulate the immune response, i.e., topical cortisones. These reduce the duration and severity of ulcers but do not influence the frequency of aphthous episodes. Topical therapy can be initiated very early, even before the development of the ulcer, and subsequently continued until the final recovery.

PFAFA or Marchall's syndrome

PFAFA syndrome (periodic fever, aphthous stomatitis, pharyngitis, and adenopathy), which has only recently been established from a diagnostic perspective, is characterized by episodes of recurrent high fever, recurrent aphthous stomatitis, pharyngitis, and satellite adenopathy and is frequently accompanied by headache and abdominal and articular pain. PFAFA syndrome usually manifests before 5 years of age and is normally benign and self-limiting. To date, the related etiology remains unknown (Valenzuela et al, 2009; Femiano et al, 2008).

Traumatic ulcers

Among ulcerative lesions in children, those of a reactive nature, i.e., traumatic ulcers, are particularly frequent (Fig. 8.6). Traumatic ulcerative lesions can have various origins such as "mechanical" trauma similar to that from neonatal teeth, leading to Riga–Fede ulcers in the anterior lingual area in infants (Fig. 8.7) (Choi et al, 2009; Ceyhan, 2009); foreign bodies, such as toys or dental equipment; bad habits or iatrogenic maneuvers, such as tongue suction and dehydration caused by rolls or cottons; or self-harm, such as accidental bites during chewing and postanesthesia bites after dental treatment or, more specifically, "physical" (burns from hot foods) or "chemical" (generally of intragenic nature: caused by the use of hydrogen peroxide, hypochlorite, or eugenol during dental visits) self-harm. Traumatic ulcers are single and painful ulcerative lesions with surfaces that may be red or covered by a yellowish-white exudate and with thin erythematous edges that are located at sites easily subject to traumas, such as arches or cheeks. These ulcers, which appear to lack substance upon palpation, heal after the removal of the associated cause or spontaneously within 6–10 days. The reparative process can frequently be slowed down by the onset of bacterial superinfections, which tend to make the lesions larger and deeper. The diagnosis is clinical: it is important to find the correlation between ulcers and current or previous traumatic factors that might have caused the mucosal tissue to lacerate (Rioboo-Crespo et al, 2005; Majorana et al, 2010).

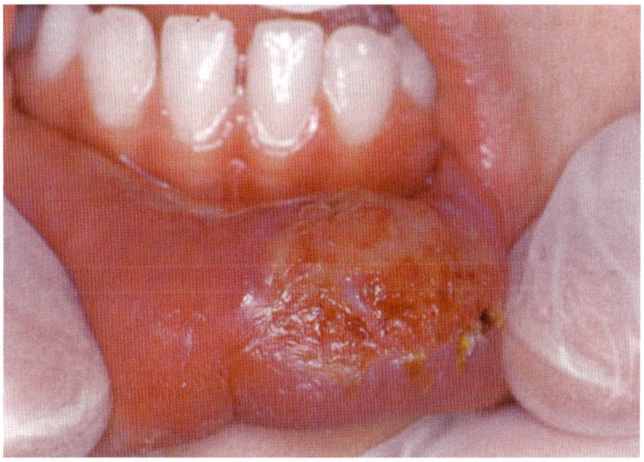
Figure 8.6 Traumatic ulcer.

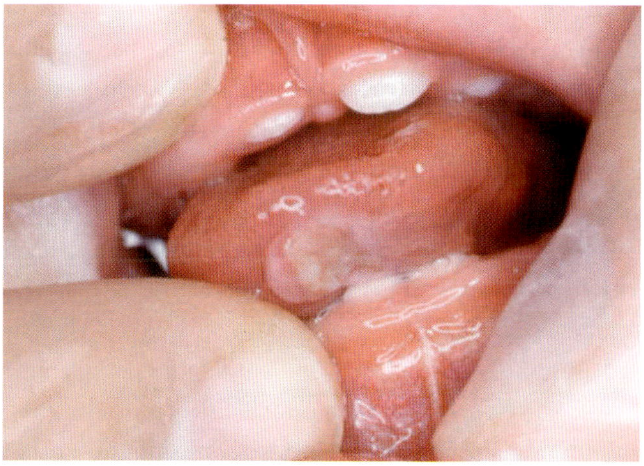
Figure 8.7 Riga–Fede syndrome.

Necrotizing ulcerative gingivitis

This is caused by fusiform bacilli and spirochetes; it rarely appears in preschool age and occasionally manifests between 6 and 12 years of age. It clinically manifests as severe gingival inflammation characterized by edema, redness, spontaneous bleeding, pain, and necrosis of interdental papillae, which appear "decapitated." Additionally, it is accompanied by hyperthermia, poor appetite, general malaise, and halitosis. In addition to a targeted antibiotic approach, the related treatment is based on careful professional and home hygiene measures (Oh et al, 2002; Perdikogianni et al, 2009; Rai et al, 2009).

Erythema multiforme

This is a mucocutaneous pathology with an immune-mediated pathogenesis caused by several factors, such as viruses, drugs, or *Mycoplasma pneumoniae* infections, and it can manifest particularly during adolescence. In particular, erythema multiforme is frequently associated with recurrent infections caused by *Herpes simplex* virus (HSV). It involves typical cutaneous lesions with a rosette-like structure associated with mucosal lesions frequently involving more than two areas. At the oral level, it shows large erosive/ulcerative lesions on the buccal mucosa, tongue, and palate, in addition to erosive lesions that progress to form crust-like structures on the lips (Fig. 8.8). In some cases, the clinical condition can be so severe as to constitute Steven–Johnson syndrome (Lam and Ulloa-Gutiérrez, 2008; Koh and Tay, 2009; Levi et al, 2009).

Secondary ulcerative lesions

Among secondary ulcerative lesions, i.e., those caused by the rupture of vesicles or blisters, it is possible to identify infectious lesions, i.e., primary or secondary herpetic stomatitis; herpangina; and hand, foot, and mouth disease.

Primary herpetic gingivostomatitis

In most people, the first contact with HSV-1, which usually occurs during childhood or early adolescence through saliva or direct contact with labial lesions, is followed by no clinical manifestation, and the virus remains in a latent state at the level of trigeminal neurons. In contrast, in some subjects (approximately 10% of cases), it is possible to identify primary herpetic stomatitis (Fig. 8.9), i.e., vesiculobullous eruptions extending throughout the oral cavity, which rapidly results in an erosive/ulcerative condition that is frequently coupled by superinfections and accompanied by severe gingivitis, as well as systemic signs and symptoms such as fever, loss of appetite, malaise, and cervical lymphadenopathy. The diagnosis is generally clinical, and the treatment is supportive; i.e., a diet comprising soft foods and adequate hydration, together with local antipyretics/analgesics and antiseptics. Additional diagnostic examinations include cytology and the use of monoclonal or immunofluorescent antibodies. The level of circulating antibodies only provides information related to the exposure to viruses and cannot be used to exclude or confirm current infection (Tovaru et al, 2009).

Herpes labialis

After infection, HSV-1 remains latent in the sensitive trigeminal ganglion cells. Its periodic reactivation, caused by factors such as sunlight, stress, fever, diet, or traumas, results in recurrent unilateral lesions on the lips or hard palate. Early signs include paresthesia and irritation at the site of origin, followed by redness and formation of vesiculobullous lesions, which rapidly evolve into the related erosive/ulcerative form. Healing occurs spontaneously in approximately 7–10 days (Chayavichitsilp et al, 2009).

Herpangina

Caused by coxsackievirus infections herpangina clinically manifests as aphtha-like erosions/ulcers of the oropharynx, absence of gingivitis, cervical lymphadenitis, fever, malaise, irritability, loss of appetite, and nausea. Pain during swallowing leads to loss of appetite for a few days. Therefore, it is important to alleviate pain symptoms using supportive treatment such as use of local antiseptics, analgesics, and antipyretics, with the possible addition of antibiotics. Small epidemics are possible but rare. Diagnosis is clinical, and treatment is symptomatic (Yamashita et al, 2005).

Hand, foot, and mouth disease

This disease too is caused by coxsackievirus infection and manifests as a clinical condition comparable to that of herpangina. The disease is characterized by cutaneous eruption of red papules, which evolve into superficial vesicles within a few days, typically located on the palms of the hands and soles of the feet (Suzuki et al, 2009). Both herpangina and hand, foot, and mouth disease can occur following infection with human enterovirus 71, the main organism responsible for the development of epidemic encephalitis (Chen et al, 2007; Wang and Liu, 2009).

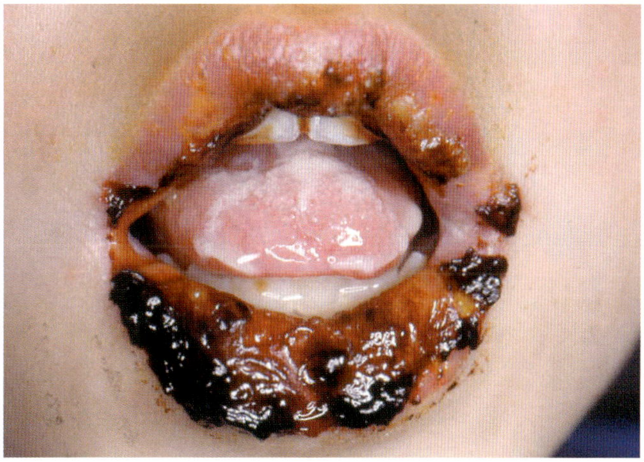

Figure 8.8 Erythema multiforme.

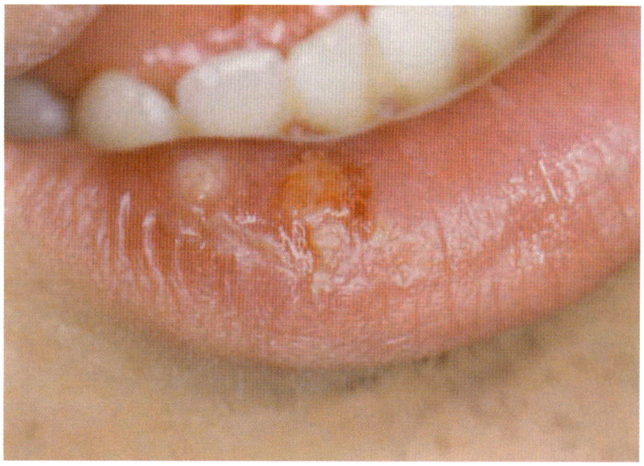

Figure 8.9 Primary herpetic gingivostomatitis.

Neoformations

Mucoceles

Mucoceles occur rather frequently in children (Fig. 8.10). They manifest as a translucent, cupuliform, painless growth that is usually caused by mucous extravasation following the traumatic rupture of a salivary gland duct. They are especially common on the lower lip and are rarely found on the floor of the mouth, where they are called *ranulae*. They rupture easily, leading to the secretion of saliva. Apparent healing occurs, which is usually followed by relapse. Diagnosis is simple, but in case of doubt or an excessive increase in volume, surgical removal is advisable (Shah et al, 2009; Boj et al, 2009; Sousa et al, 2002).

Fibrous hyperplasia

It is a reactive, exophytic, pedunculated, or broadly sessile growth that is pinkish in color and has a soft texture; it is located at the level of the buccal mucosa or tongue and is caused by chronic irritating factors such as bad habits, dental equipment, or uneven fillings. It is surgically removed after histological confirmation (Sousa et al, 2002; Tamarit-Borrás et al, 2005).

Papillomas

These have a viral origin, e.g., human papilloma virus, and can appear as a pedunculated lesion with a verrucous surface, white or pink in color, and can be located on the palate, tongue, or other sites such as gums and lips. They are treated by surgical removal (Sousa et al, 2002).

Traumatic fibroma

These are rare lesions occurring in children. They appear as sessile growths that are pink and variable in size and are caused by chronic trauma resulting in reactive fibrous hyperplasia of the connective tissue. They are treated by surgical removal (Mathew et al, 2008; Tamarit-Borrás et al, 2005).

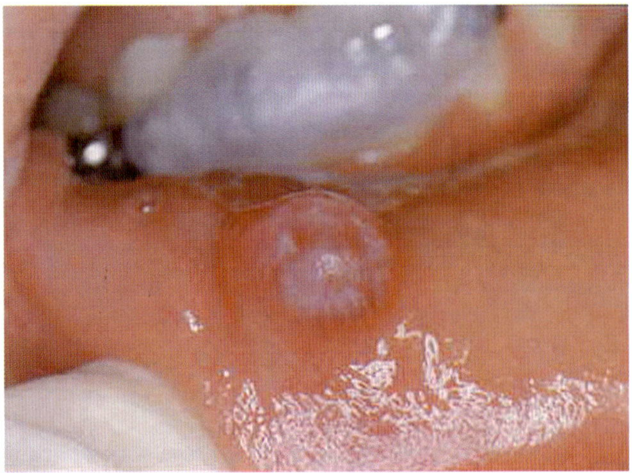

Figure 8.10 Mucocele.

Conclusions

In light of the most common clinical conditions of oral mucosa pathologies in immunocompetent children, assessing the clinical characteristics of a lesion during diagnosis assumes importance considering the possible modifications caused by bacterial superinfections and the improper use of swabs and mouthwashes. Reactive lesions are very frequent in children; therefore, it is important to identify previous or current traumatic factors that might have favored their onset. Furthermore, the single or multiple nature of the lesions, associated with the presence or absence of systemic symptoms, helps guide the management of diagnosis and treatment. In conclusion, it is necessary to note the relative frequency of neoplastic pathologies in children, particularly lymphomas, and the related necessity of never overlooking lesions and sending specimens for biopsy in case they do not regress.

References

Albanidou-Farmaki E, Deligiannidis A, Markopoulos AK et al. HLA haplotypes in recurrent aphthous stomatitis: a mode of inheritance? Int J Immunogenet 2008;35(6):427-32.

Alli N, Gur G, Yalcin B, Hayran M. Patient characteristics in Behçet disease: A retrospective analysis of 213 Turkish patients during 2001-4. Am J Clin Dermatol 2009;10(6):411-8.

Appleton SS. Candidiasis: pathogenesis, clinical characteristics and treatment. J Calif Dent Ass 2000;28:942-8.

Boj JR, Poirier C, Espasa E et al. Lower lip mucocele treated with an erbium laser. Pediatr Dent 2009;31(3):249-52.

Campisi G, Di Liberto C, Carroccio A et al. Coeliac disease: oral ulcer prevalence, assessment of risk and association with gluten-free diet in children. Dig Liver Dis 2008;40(2):104-7.

Ceyhan AM, Yildirim M, Basak PY et al. Traumatic lingual ulcer in a child: Riga-Fede disease. Clin Exp Dermatol 2009;34(2):186-8.

Chayavichitsilp P, Buckwalter JV, Krakowski AC, Friedlander SF. Herpes simplex. Pediatr Rev 2009;30(4):119-29; quiz 130. Review.

Chen KT, Chang HL, Wang ST, Cheng YT, Yang JY. Epidemiologic features of hand-foot-mouth disease and herpangina caused by enterovirus 71 in Taiwan, 1998-2005. Pediatrics 2007;120(2):e244-52.

Choi SC, Park JH, Choi YC, Kim GT. Sublingual traumatic ulceration (a Riga-Fede disease): report of two cases. Dent Traumatol 2009;25(3):e48-50.

Dodi I, Verri R, Brevi B et al. A monosymptomatic Melkersson-Rosenthal syndrome in an 8-year old boy. Acta Biomed 2006;77(1):20-3.

Femiano F, Lanza A, Buonaiuto C et al. Oral aphthous-like lesions, PFAPA syndrome: a review. J Oral Pathol Med 2008;37(6):319-23. Review.

Koh MJ, Tay YK. An update on Stevens-Johnson syndrome and toxic epidermal necrolysis in children. Curr Opin Pediatr 2009;21(4):505-10. Review.

Jabra-Rizk MA, Torres SR, Rambob I et al. Prevalence of oral *Candida* species in a North American pediatric population. J Clin Pediatr Dent 2007;31(4):260-3.

Lam J, Ulloa-Gutiérrez R. Erythema multiforme associated with varicella. An Pediatr (Barc) 2008;69(3):281-2.

Levi N, Bastuji-Garin S, Mockenhaupt M et al. Medications as risk factors of Stevens-Johnson syndrome and toxic epidermal necrolysis in children: a poole analysis. Pediatrics 2009;123(2):e297-304.

Malahias T, Cheng J, Brar P et al. The association between celiac disease, dental enamel defects, and aphthous ulcers in a United States cohort. J Clin Gastroenterol 2010; 44(3):191-4.

Majorana A, Bardellini E, Flocchini P. Principali manifestazioni patologiche non neoplastiche nelle mucose orali del bambino (dossier). Dental Cadmos 2010;78(5).

Majorana A, Bardellini E, Flocchini P et al.Oral mucosal lesions in children from 0 to 12 years old: ten years experience. Oral Surg Oral Med Oral Pathol Oral Radiol Endod 2010;110(1).

Martin JL. Leukoedema: a review of the literature. J Natl Med Assoc 1992;84(11):938-40. Review.

Mathew AL, Pai KM, Sholapurkar AA, Vengal M. The prevalence of oral mucosal lesions in patients visiting a dental school in Southern India. Indian J Dent Res 2008;19(2):99-103.

Miloğlu O, Göregen M, Akgül HM, Acemoğlu H. The prevalence and risk factors associated with benign migratory glossitis lesions in 7619 Turkish dental outpatients. Oral Surg Oral Med Oral Pathol Oral Radiol Endod 2009;107(2):e29-33.

Oh TJ, Eber R, Wang HL. Periodontal diseases in the child and adolescent. J Clin Periodontol 2002;29(5):400-10.

Perdikogianni H, Papaioannou W, Nakou M et al. Periodontal and microbiological parameters in children and adolescents with cleft lip and/or palate. Int J Paediatr Dent 2009;19(6):455-67.

Rai K, Supriya S, Hegde AM. Oral health status of children with congenital heart disease and the awareness, attitude and knowledge of their parents. J Clin Pediatr Dent 2009;33(4):315-8.

Ray R, Pyle MA, Sawyer DR et al. Prevalence and etiology of erythema migrans among children in northeast Ohio. Quintessence Int 2007;38(5):409-16.

Rioboo-Crespo MdelR, Planells- del Pozo P, Rioboo-Garcia R. Epidemiology of the most common oral mucosal diseases in children. Med Oral Patol Oral Cir Bucal 2005;10(5):376-87.

Rozkiewicz D, Daniluk T, Zaremba ML et al. Oral *Candida albicans* carriage in healthy preschool and school children. Adv Med Sci 2006;51(Suppl 1):187-90.

Scully C, Welbury R. Color atlas of oral diseases in children and adolescents. London: Wolfe; 1994.

Sewerin IA. Clinical and epidemiologic study morsicatio buccarum-labiorum. Scand J Dent Res 1971;79(2):73-80.

Shah SK, Le MC, Carpenter WM. Retrospective review of pediatric oral lesions from a dental school biopsy service. Pediatr Dent 2009 Jan-Feb;31(1):14-9.

Sousa FB, Etges A, Corrêa L, Mesquita RA, de Araújo NS. Pediatric oral lesions: a 15-year review from São Paulo, Brazil. J Clin Pediatr Dent 2002;26(4):413-8.

Sun A, Wang YP, Chia JS, Liu BY, Chiang CP. Treatment with levamisole and colchicine can result in a significant reduction of IL-6, IL-8 or TNF-alpha level in patients with mucocutaneous type of Behcet's disease. J Oral Pathol Med 2009;38(5):401-5.

Suzuki Y, Taya K, Nakashima K et al. Study on risk factors for severe hand-foot-and-mouth disease. Pediatr Int 2010;52(2):203-7.

Tamarit-Borrás M, Delgado-Molina E, Berini-Aytés L, Gay-Escoda C. Removal of hyperplastic lesions of the oral cavity. A retrospective study of 128 cases. Med Oral Patol Oral Cir Bucal 2005;10(2):151-62.

Tovaru S, Parlatescu I, Tovaru M, Cionca L. Primary herpetic gingivostomatitis in children and adults. Quintessence Int 2009;40(2):119-24.

Tunes RS, Anjos TC, Martins GB et al. Prevalence of Behcet's syndrome in patients with recurrent aphthous ulcerations in Brazil. Rheumatol Int 2009;29(8):875-8.

Valenzuela PM, Majerson D, Tapia JL, Talesnik E. Syndrome of periodic fever, aphthous stomatitis, pharyngitis, and adenitis (PFAPA) in siblings. Clin Rheumatol 2009;28(10):1235-7.

Wang SM, Liu CC. Enterovirus 71: epidemiology, pathogenesis and management. Expert Rev Anti Infect Ther 2009;7(6):735-42.

Yamashita T, Ito M, Taniguchi A, Sakae K. Prevalence of coxsackievirus A5, A6, and A10 in patients with herpangina in Aichi Prefecture, 2005. Jpn J Infect Dis 2005;58(6):390-1.

Chapter 9

Dentoalveolar traumatology in pediatric dentistry

E. Spinas

Among the vast range of dental pathologies affecting children, traumatic lesions affecting the deciduous and permanent dentition (hereinafter referred to as TDI) have a remarkable incidence rate, affecting 25%–30% of the population, with a certain variability depending on the regional location, race, and statistical parameters considered.

Such a high incidence rate is the result of the obvious multifactorial nature of these lesions. Not all traumatic events affecting the oral cavity can be considered predictable and preventable, considering that the most frequent causes of traumatism are, at all latitudes, *falls* and *playing*, but it is not conceivable to stop children from playing and socializing. At the same time, however, there are precise anatomical markers that characterize children and adolescents who will be more easily and more severely affected by such traumatic events: among these, Angle's class II and especially increased dental *overjet* (OVJ; particularly beyond 5–6 mm) are prevalent, and children who present with such abnormalities should be identified and treated at an early stage.

Therefore, we need to increase the awareness of associations of professionals, practitioners, and pediatric and orthodontic experts in order to draw greater attention to interceptive and preventive issues related to such pathologies while anticipating radical reforms of the national preventive health system. For example, Italy is known to be one of the countries with a large ratio of people who participate in sports activities; however, it is also one of the countries least involved in establishing adequate campaigns to raise awareness about and prevent the actual risk of orofacial trauma associated with both amateur and professional sports.

Epidemiology

Dental trauma affects between 15% and 30% of the population, with several age-associated peaks of incidence. The first peak occurs in the deciduous dentition phase between 1 and 3 years of age; in this age group, individuals have low motor coordination even if they are starting their first movement-related experiences, such as crawling, walking, running, and ascending and descending stairs, and first socialization experiences, such as attending kindergartens and visiting playgrounds, which are often the first recreational activities.

During the period of permanent teething, there are two characteristic peaks of incidence of dentoalveolar trauma: the first occurs between 8 and 12 years of age (the beginning of adolescent socialization, also linked to the practice of the first individual and group sports and games activities); the second occurs between 15 and 21 years, an age group characterized by competitive sport activities or those with greater risk of traumatism, the first autonomous road movements with motorcycles and other means of motor transport, and by injuries resulting from youth socialization-related conflicts.

Epidemiological variables

The epidemiological variables used to characterize dental traumatic lesions are as follows:

- sex
- location
- predisposing factors.

Sex. Males suffer from dentoalveolar trauma more frequently than their female peers (incidence ratio of males:females = 3:2).

This difference tends to diminish gradually after the age of 10 years and decreases to zero in adulthood. This pattern is characteristic of the evolution of habits and customs of our society, in which girls tend to emulate the activities practiced by their male peers, such as smoking and alcohol abuse, leading to increased participation in life and sport habits usually associated with males, such as football, violent and/or acrobatic sports, and extreme sports.

Location. Dentoalveolar injuries most commonly affect the upper arch, especially in the anterior region, and in particular the upper central incisors (80%–90% of cases, depending on statistics). The upper lateral teeth are affected in 10%–18% of individuals. In the remaining 2%–4% of cases, the lower incisor or the lateroposterior groups are involved (the latter usually at a more advanced age). We should not forget the superior premolar trauma— characteristic of falls or certain sports—as a consequence of indirect trauma transmitted through the jaw, such as in football, boxing, and martial arts.

Dentoalveolar injuries are frequently limited to a single tooth but may simultaneously affect several dental elements (two, three, or more teeth) depending on the etiological agent; traumas affecting multiple regions are more frequent in sports and road traffic accidents than in other circumstances. Their severity and degree of expression depend on the object causing the harm, as described in the following sections.

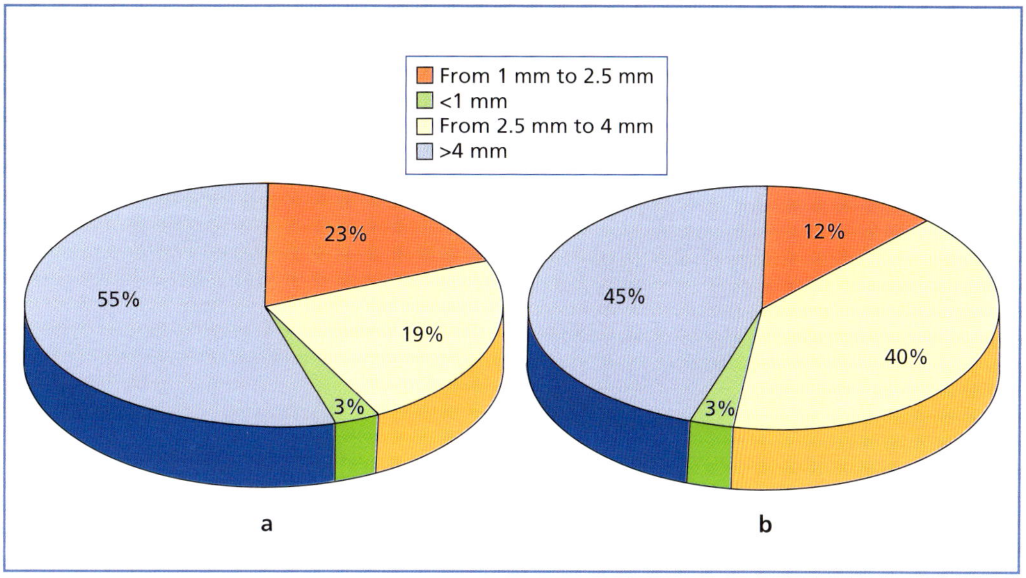

Figure 9.1 Traumatism percentage considering the different overjet (**a**) and overbite (**b**) values.

Predisposing factors. Anatomical factors play an important role in determining dental trauma. Anomalies of the intermaxillary joints and dental arch occlusion, particularly Angle's class II, are of great importance.

The role of an increased OVJ is equally important (Fig. 9.1a). It has been shown that individuals with an OVJ greater than 4–6 mm report traumatic lesions more frequently than those with a normal OVJ. The increase in OVJ leads to a proportionate increase in risk (Fig. 9.2).

Bauss et al (2004) confirmed that 10.3% of their study sample (1,367 orthodontic patients) had experienced dental trauma during treatment, with a maximum incidence in the age range of 11–15 years, predominantly in the upper central incisors (79.6%) and more frequently in patients with increased OVJ and upper lip incompetence.

Shulman and Peterson (2004) also reported an increase in the *odds ratio* of traumatic injuries in a sample of 13,057 patients in the NHANES III study, which was directly proportional to the increase in OVJ.

The dental overbite (OVB), if increased, can also be a predisposing factor (see Fig. 9.1b), although it is less relevant than increased OVJ, especially if the OVB has a value greater than 5–6 mm. Again, a greater OVB considerably increases the risk. In older age, it also contributes to the occurrence of distinctive coronal-radicular fractures of the incisors and premolars with an indirect mechanism (traumatism transmitted through the jaw).

Additionally, open anterior bite, upper lip incompetence, and macrodontia in the upper central incisors (Fig. 9.3) also favor the occurrence of dental traumatic lesions. These conditions are often associated with syndromic forms, typically in mouth breathers who also show a tendency to higher prognathism.

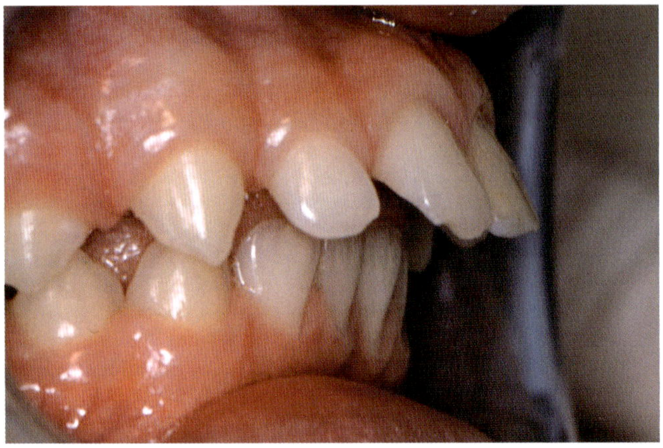

Figure 9.2 Adolescent patient with increased dental overjet.

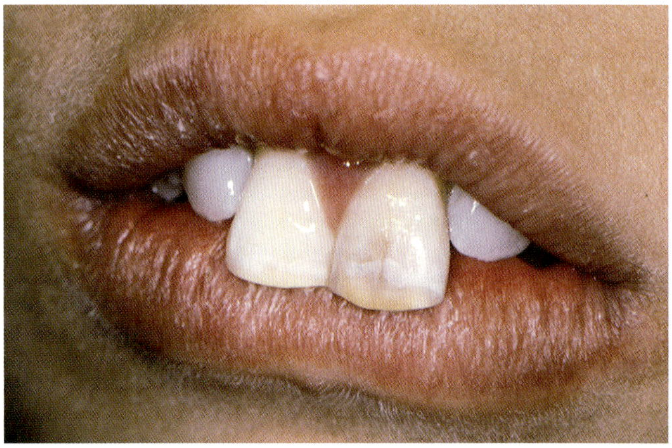

Figure 9.3 Patient with labial incompetence and macrodontia of the upper central incisors.

Among the causes that lead to the occurrence of TDI that are reported in the literature (Glendor, 2009), environmental factors (Tab. 9.1) are particularly important; they can be interpreted as facilitating factors and are always particularly relevant during adolescence. Among these factors, the inadequacy of a child's area of residence, especially if situated in suburban areas, and the presence of small-scale crime and bullying are increasingly important in the occurrence of these pathologies.
The failure to meet safety standards of the environments in which the recreational and sport activities take place, e.g., school gyms, kindergartens, swimming pools, and playgrounds, and the state of conservation and maintenance of the equipment used are equally important.

Table 9.1 Etiopathogenetic factors of traumatic lesions of the anterior teeth

Dental	Caries, devitalized teeth, amelogenesis imperfecta, fluorosis, ankylosis, macrodontia
Dentofacial	Labial incompetence, open bite, prognathism, increased overjet and overbite, crowding
General	Age, sex, sports, social context, epilepsy, disability
Contributing factors	Mechanism of action (direct or indirect); characteristics of the blunt object; angle, speed, and force of impact

Frequency of possible causes of dentoalveolar injuries

Within the designation of domestic accidents, we include several events with playful causes, falls, and contact between individuals and/or objects, irrespective of whether they are involuntary (accidental) or voluntary (pushes and violent games). These events are the most frequent causes of dentoalveolar injuries in preschool age and are strongly influenced by environmental factors (regional), customs, level of control, and quality of the facilities and area of residence of the individual.
Road traffic injuries refer to pedestrian, bicycle, and motor vehicle accidents; depending on the age of the persons involved, they may be caused by neglecting the use of protective equipment, e.g., failure to use special car seats or safety belts, distraction, carelessness, and lack of cycling or road crossing proficiency, especially in individuals aged between 6 and 12 years.
This group of TDIs mainly includes complex and multiple lesions and lesions simultaneously involving hard and soft tissues (wounds, abrasions, and lacerations), basal bone (maxillary fractures), and supporting tissues (alveolar fractures) (Tab 9.2).

Sports-related trauma

As shown in Table 9.2, injuries occurring during sports activities vary between 20% and 25%. Their frequency, which is low during childhood, increases between the ages of 8 and 16 years and diminishes again as age increases.
It is undeniable that there are some sports activities that predispose participants to dental trauma and other activities that can be considered only potentially at risk (Tab. 9.3).

Table 9.2 Frequency of possible causes of dentoalveolar trauma

40%	Domestic accidents (accidental trauma)
25%–30%	Road accidents
20%–25%	Sports accidents
5%–10%	Injury, aggression, accidents at work and other less conceivable causes

Table 9.3 Classification of different types of sports with risk of trauma

Statistically dangerous	Skateboarding, skiing, basketball, field hockey, ice hockey, soccer, rugby, martial arts, handball
Potentially dangerous	Ice skating, mountain biking, weight throwing, volleyball, water polo, surfing, weight-lifting, acrobatic gymnastics, tennis, golf, football, gymnastics, lacrosse, baseball, racquetball, inline skates, boxing
Potentially and statistically dangerous	Squash, wrestling, equestrian sports, rugby, handball

It is necessary to compare the incidence of dental trauma in different sports with the number of individuals who actually participate in these sports to obtain the real *incidence* of trauma related to each discipline.

It is apparent that different types of sports are associated with a different risk of suffering injuries of variable severity, depending on whether the use of blunt objects (sticks, clubs, balls, and disks or pucks in hockey, baseball, or handball), the achievement of high speeds (skating, surfing, motorcycle racing, and cycling), the need for physical contact between players (water polo, basketball, martial arts, and rugby) or the association of some of these factors, for example, in ice and field hockey, horse-riding, or polo, are envisaged.

In addition, players' inexperience, primarily when practicing risky sports during childhood or adolescence, or the aggressive nature of the sport (particularly inherent in certain sports) contribute to an increase in the likelihood of facial and, therefore, dentoalveolar trauma.

Hence, in some sports (sometimes just for lower age groups and/or female players), it is obligatory to use special extraoral protection (for example, full-protection helmets in ice hockey for women and players aged under 16 years) or intraoral protection (*mouthguards*), such as in all specialized combat sports.

However, it should be noted that in many violent competitive activities, including at the professional level, the use of intraoral protection is not so frequent and is often left to the discretion of the player.

In all disciplines in which these protective standards have been made mandatory, the percentage of events with dental trauma has been drastically reduced; in American football, for instance, the rates of oral trauma have been reduced to below 2% and brain concussion episodes have also been significantly reduced.

Main features of dental trauma

The main factors that influence the type, severity, or expressiveness of the lesions are as follows:

- intensity of the traumatic force, i.e., the force of the impact between the blunt object and the individual
- direction of application of the force
- resilience of the blunt object
- form of the blunt object.

Intensity. The faster the impact on the dentoalveolar structures, the greater is the likelihood of damage to the hard tissues (crown fractures). If the speed is lower, however, soft tissue damage and periodontal lesions (dislocations) will be relatively more likely to occur.

Direction. Direction of the force can determine the extent of the fracture lines, both at the level of the dental crowns and the roots (horizontal and/or vertical fractures).

Impact force and resilience. With regard to fractures, the severity of the lesion appears to be directly proportional to the elasticity of the blunt object; if this is rather elastic, less severe fractures or dislocations are more likely to occur.

Form of the blunt object. The smaller the object, the less the area of application of the force will be, and, therefore, the greater its extent per unit of surface. Therefore, there will be an increased likelihood of fracture at the expense of dislocation. This factor is relevant, for example, in some sport disciplines in which it is possible to precisely predict the outcome of any dental trauma and, consequently, to provide adequate means of protection.

Classification of traumatic lesions

The following tables (Tab. 9.4-9.7) present some of the most commonly used classifications of traumatic dental lesions.

Table 9.4 WHO Classification, 1992

Class	Features
1	Enamel fractures, including infractions
2	Crown fracture without pulpal involvement
3	Crown fracture with pulpal involvement
4	Root fracture
5	Crown–root fracture
6	Unspecified dental fracture
7	Dental luxation
8	Dental intrusion or extrusion
9	Avulsion
10	Other traumatic injuries (including soft tissue lacerations)

Table 9.5 Ellis and Davey classification, 1945

Class	Type of trauma
I	Simple crown fracture involving only enamel
II	Extensive crown fracture involving enamel and dentin without pulp exposure
III	Extensive crown fracture involving enamel and dentin with pulp exposure
IV	Loss of pulp vitality with or without loss of crown structure
V	Avulsion
VI	Root fracture with or without crown fracture
VII	Traumatic tooth dislocation with or without crown or root fracture
VIII	Total cervical crown fracture
IX	Trauma of deciduous teeth

Table 9.6 Classification by Andreasen and Andreasen, 1990

- Enamel infraction
- Enamel fracture
- Enamel and dentin fracture
- Crown fracture with pulp exposure
- Crown–root fracture
- Root fracture

Table 9.7 Classification by Spinas, 2002

Class	Type of trauma
A	Simple crown fractures (enamel) involving a coronal angle (mesial or distal) or exclusively the incisal margin
B	Complex fractures involving mesial or distal angles and the incisal surface
B1	Pulp involvement is also present
C	Complex fractures involving the incisal surface and at least one-third of the crown surface
C1	Pulp involvement is also present
D	Complex fractures involving the root (crown–root fractures)
D1	Pulp involvement is also present
H	All fractures with a silent or necrotic pulp, even if the fractures are not complicated

Prevention of dentoalveolar trauma

Although caries, a disease strongly linked to lifestyle, is preventable, the same principle does not apply to trauma affecting the orodental structures; because a trauma is an accidental event that is beyond the individual's control, the chances of preventing it are low. In public health, the crucial question is whether there are effective preventive actions, i.e., whether it is possible to reduce the incidence of dental trauma and its complications within the population.

Indeed, in today's health culture, we exceedingly use the term "*prevention*" as preventive practices are not only always applicable but also and above all are a safe way to achieve living a life without disease. The slogan "prevention is better than cure" is grounded on an ethical foundation by which it is intended to justify the primacy of preventive medicine over curative medicine regardless of its limitations (all diseases cannot always be prevented), costs (the cost-benefit ratio is often negative), and real benefits (often more assumed than ascertained).

Prevention activities should focus on four levels:

- informing individuals and equipping the environment
- correcting predisposing factors
- protecting parts exposed to possible injuries
- preventing post-traumatic relapses.

Informing individuals and equipping the environment

Informing individuals involved in social activities and risky sports about attitudes and precautions to be taken to prevent face-to-face trauma is of paramount importance. Information dissemination activities should extensively be conducted at all schools (from primary to high school) where daily fun, recreational, and sports activities are conducted (teachers and directors of education should be motivated and educated in this field) and should involve clear and simple teaching materials, such as posters on the walls and leaflets distributed individually that could summarize the preventive and more immediate treatment procedures.

The information will be mainly aimed at the youngest players as well as at their parents and the sports team/club they belong to, including managers, trainers, coaches, sports and corporate physicians, and physiotherapists, and above all those who should know the technical and health problems associated with sport trauma; moreover, information dissemination meetings should be arranged regularly (every 6–12 months).

Information dissemination should also be conducted institutionally by the relevant ministries and national institutions to encourage the organization to implement national plans for the prevention of orofacial trauma.

Correcting predisposing factors

The correction of predisposing factors involves the early identification and treatment of pathologies or anatomical conditions that promote trauma and that can be included in the occlusal and/or gnathological group of anomalies.

The anomalies that should be first recognized by family pediatricians and submitted to pediatric dentists for treatment are as follows:

- pathological forms that increase superior prognathism, favoring the impact between the upper arch and the external bodies
- skeletal and dental class II
- increase of OVJ and/or OVB
- bad habits that increase OVJ
- presence of retained and/or impacted teeth that cause a *point of least resistance* of the maxillary bones.

Individuals with such predisposing factors should be identified before their participation in sports activities that are considered among the most frequent causes of orofacial trauma.
The treatment of these conditions is clearly of the conventional orthodontic or interceptive type, is mobile or fixed, and is aimed at the attenuation and correction of any discrepancies. To the greatest extent possible, the treatment should not hinder or delay the start of socialization activities.

Protecting parts exposed to possible injuries

Protection must be ensured by the use of equipment such as helmets and protective masks and intra- and extraoral devices such as mouthguards as well as by the adoption of rules and regulations to facilitate proper and supervised practice of activities that involve a high risk of falls, clashes, and/or contact between participants, such as at kindergartens, playgrounds, and facilities adapted to the type of activity envisaged and by complying with the safety standards of the environment and facilities.
Sports that do not require extraoral facial protection should include at least intraoral protection; i.e., a *mouthguard* appropriate for the person's age and discipline.

Preventing post-traumatic relapses

If a trauma with the abovementioned levels of prevention has occurred because of noncompliance, the outcomes of the lesions should be mitigated. The implementation of appropriate and early therapies limits the personal consequences (in terms of disability) and the social costs of trauma, thereby reducing the costs of rehabilitation. For this, information and refresher courses must be implemented and regularly proposed among the professionals involved in the reception and treatment of head pathologies.
These obviously affect not only general healthcare professionals (emergency services, pediatricians, and nurses) and specialists (pediatric dentists, orthodontists, and oral hygienists) but also staff employed in public facilities (janitors, caretakers, instructors, and teachers), who must at least know the general rules of first aid (recovery and maintenance of detached dental elements).
As highlighted above, it is very difficult to implement real and effective strategies to prevent the occurrence of traumatic events at a young age because of the randomness and quickness at which such events occur.

There is, however, a possibility to eliminate or at least mitigate the devastating effects of these pathologies in at least the 25% of cases that can be traced with certainty to individual and group sports activities with high traumatic risk that are usually started at a fairly young age, e.g., basketball, handball, hockey, martial arts, and mountain biking. To this end, *mouthguards* should be made more widely available and should be used.

Mouthguards

These devices allow direct prevention. They protect the upper incisors from direct frontal impact; provide protection against soft tissue tears by distancing them from the teeth (very important in athletes with fixed orthodontic devices); protect all dental elements from indirect trauma resulting from a violent impact that acts with the arches in occlusion; reduce the risk of fractures of the jaw resulting from blows coming from below; and reduce the force with which trauma on the jaw can be indirectly transmitted to the teeth, skull, neck, and temporomandibular joint (prevention also in the context of cerebral concussion).

It is important to stress that the use of mouthguards should be encouraged in children who engage in contact sports particularly for two reasons: the greater severity of some traumas when they occur in growing children (8–12 years) and an easier acceptance of mouthguards if applied at an early age.

It has been shown that younger athletes show greater compliance with all types of mouthguards compared with older athletes who have previously practiced sports without wearing them. In addition, if mouthguards are worn during training, they are better tolerated and used in competitions or in high-level competition, in which the risk of trauma is greater.

Çetinbas and Sönmez (2006) reported the results of a survey of 22 coaches from 15 high schools in Ankara (Turkey) to assess their knowledge of the use of *mouthguards* and the frequency of mouthguard use among students aged between 11 and 18 years. None of the adolescents included in this age group used mouthguards during sport activities; hence, there is the need to encourage the use of mouthguards, especially among coaches, who are ideal vehicles of information transmission.

At the request of the Italian Society of Dentistry of Sport, the Center for the Study of Dental Facial Trauma of the University of Cagliari conducted an epidemiological survey of 4,000 athletes, 1,000 of whom were middle-school students from the provinces of Cagliari and Nuoro (Ranalli et al, 1999). The survey results showed that 30% of the sample population had experienced trauma during sport activities and 60% of the trauma incidences affected the dental area.

The students' level of knowledge and application of general rules for the prevention of dental traumatic events was also assessed. Only 2% said that they knew how to use a mouthguard and used one, and approximately 35% said that they would use one if it was provided for free.

Spinas (2007) conducted a survey of 300 young basketball players and highlighted the very poor knowledge regarding *mouthguard* use (10% of the sample population) and the even less frequent usage (only three subjects), which was usually motivated by having already experienced an orodental trauma.
Mouthguards are conventionally classified into three categories:

1. **Stock mouthguards**, or ready-to-use mouthguards, which are available in various standard sizes, are currently in disuse because they are not easily adaptable and have *absolutely insufficient* retention power (Fig. 9.4).
2. **Semi-individual mouthguards (self-made)**, which are preformed and are intra-orally modeled, are usually considered not very efficient. They include the classic *Boil and Bite* mouthguard and those of the new generation, including the ProGuard and similar models (*Boil and Bite* N.G.) (Fig. 9.5 and 9.6).
3. **Custom-made mouthguards**, known as *individual* mouthguards, are built in a laboratory using a model of the user's dental arches. This type is subdivided into *monolaminar* and *multilaminar* mouth protectors depending on the type and number of protective layers of material and on the construction technique, with the application of low or high pressure on the materials (Fig. 9.7).

Considering the data in the literature and the numerous clinical screenings, it is clear that choosing an *individual mouthguard* fully meets an athlete's anatomical–functional and safety requirements. However, mouthguards should be applied for individuals who have *completed tooth eruption and alignment* (not younger than 12 years of age) (Fig. 9.8).
The explanations provided by athletes to explain why they do not use oral protection include poor grip, bulk, hard oronasal breathing, dry mouth, and difficult phonation.
Many of these are in fact reasons associated with the poor quality of the mouthguards used, and for this reason, it would be advisable that a mouthguard, to be defined as such, should meet some precise requirements (Tab. 9.8).
The preformed *Boil and Bite mouthguards* seem to be particularly suitable for use *in adolescent sportspersons*. They have an optimal structure, are made of quality materials, and offer the undeniable advantages of being adaptable to individuals during the mixed dentition phase (7–11 years), *being able to be customized several times* (Spinas, 2009), and being able to follow the evolution of dental transition and alveolar growth. The reduced construction time and competitive cost make it the mouthguard of choice for pediatric patients and/or in orthodontic treatment (Fig. 9.9).

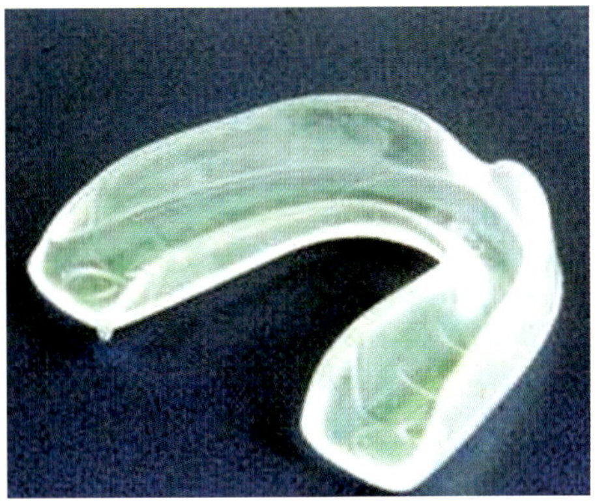

Figure 9.4 Standard *mouthguard*; it is considered ineffective and its use should be discouraged.

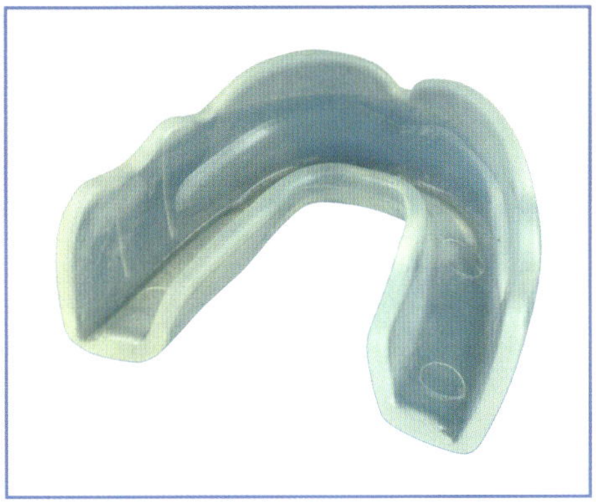

Figure 9.5 Conventional *Boil and Bite mouthguard*; its oral adjustment is complicated.

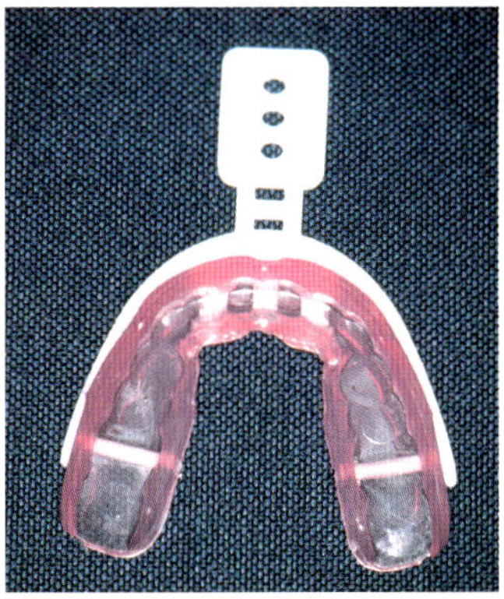

Figure 9.6 *New-generation Boil and Bite mouthguard*; it is easily customisable, and it has a good intra-oral grip.

Figure 9.7 (**a**) Multi-layered individual *mouthguard*; it is the most effective from the anatomical-functional point of view. (**b**) The scheme shows the number of possible layers.

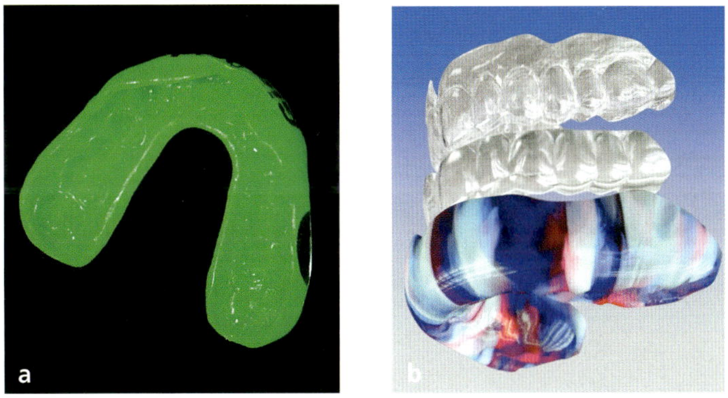

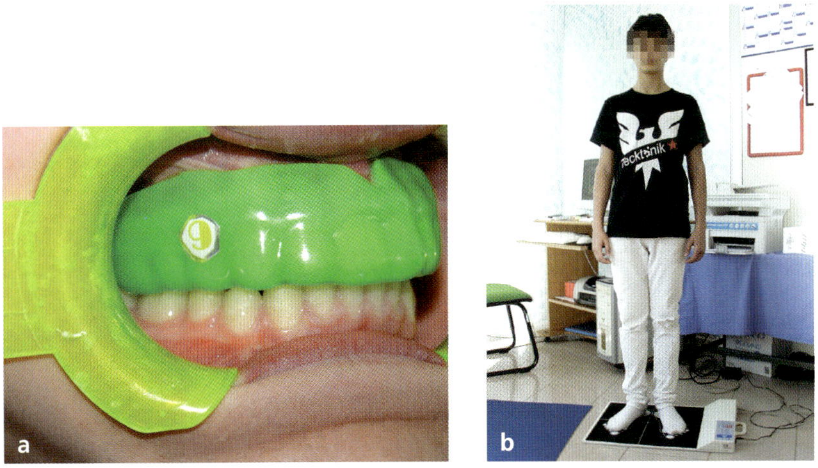

Figure 9.8 (**a**) Individual *mouthguard* placed in the oral cavity; the functional and aesthetic features are considered. (**b**) The postural-balance analysis is often used to achieve the proper mouthguard operability.

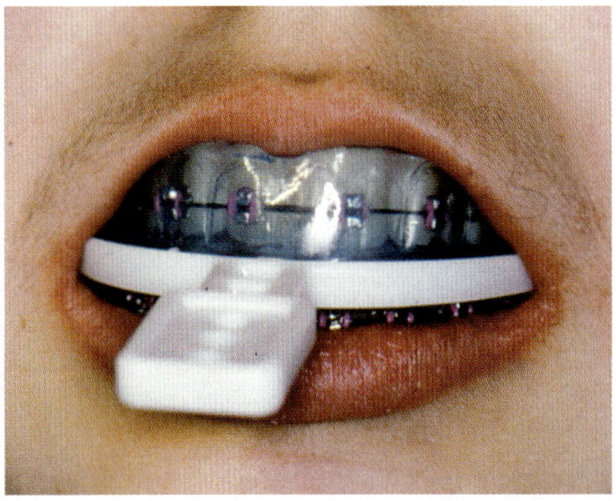

Figure 9.9 *New-generation Boil and Bite mouthguards* are the best type of mouthguards in young patients undergoing dentistry treatment: they can be customized several times in order to adjust to the therapeutic progress.

Table 9.8 Suitability features of mouthguards

• Should be made of a resilient material as a material that is too rigid could cause soft tissue lacerations while not providing any shock-absorbing effect
• Should have rounded edges
• Should be odorless, tasteless, nonporous, and easily washable
• Should not have unwanted orthodontic effects or should not put the jaw in a forced position
• Should be adherent and retentive: in order to obtain retention, the athlete should not have to keep the arches in occlusion; otherwise, the **mouthguard** interposing itself would prevent open mouth breathing
• Should be resistant to the effect of salivary fluids and should not undergo delamination
• Should not be bulky and should not reduce breathing spaces or prevent the athlete from speaking
• Should have a vestibular shield extending approximately 5–6 mm above the gingival margin to provide maximum protection while extending palatally for approximately 1–2 mm; Yamada et al. (2006) have shown that the ability to defend against traumatic forces does not vary with the position of the **mouthguard's** palatal edge relative to the cervical margin of the teeth, provided the palatal surface of the teeth is completely covered.
• Should have a thickness of at least 3–4 mm on vestibular surfaces and 3 mm on the occlusal surface. Recently, Takeda et al. (2004) confirmed that the effectiveness of the mouth guard in dispersing traumatic forces decreases with occlusal thicknesses below 3 mm.
• Should allow contact between the arches with the interposition of an occlusal thickness of 2–3 mm so that if the jaw undergoes a trauma that results in forced closure, the energy is distributed across the entire maxillary arch. Occlusally, it is essential that the impressions of the mandibular and maxillary dental elements are recorded and reproduced, although not excessively accentuated (the necessary thickness of the mouth guard and its shock-absorbing effect would be reduced). However, especially in dynamic sports, it is not crucial to have locking of the antagonist arch in occlusion, but a certain degree of "occlusion leeway" in which the athlete can enter and exit easily is essential.
• Should have a Vickers hardness of at least 78 shore A
• Should be modifiable as needed
• Should be affordable

Treatment of dental trauma

If prevention has not been implemented or has not been successful, rational treatment of traumatic injury should be administered.
The relevant clinical implications—sometimes dramatic for young patients and their families and associated with the possible, and sometimes serious, sequelae of traumatic injuries—require the immediate intervention of experienced clinicians. From this perspective, it is necessary to establish a proper clinical diagnostic plan, starting from the objective examination of the injured party and the lesions.

First examination

The first examination of the injured individual is always a particularly important therapeutic event, especially when it is conducted as an emergency, i.e., immediately or soon after the traumatic event.
The first examination must be conducted calmly but with the utmost care and following well-tested protocols; its specific features will depend on the age of the patient and the circumstances in which the trauma occurred.
Moreover, the increasing number of forensic problems related to medical professional activity has led to increased attention in the collection of data regarding the first objective examination of the injured individual.
The importance of a prompt and effective clinical diagnosis is of considerable psychological, functional, and esthetic importance, which a healthcare professional cannot deliberately ignore.

The first examination consists of the following steps:
1. establishment of the pathology
2. psychological approach
3. history, including current illness and past medical/clinical history
4. collection of preexisting documentation if available
5. objective clinical examination
6. instrumental examinations, such as sensitivity tests, x-rays, and photographs
7. verification and evaluation of the collected data
8. implementation of the treatment plan
9. certification of clinical diagnostic activity.

Disease identification

This initial point has already been discussed: accurate identification allows the clinician to save considerable time and energy. It must first be made clear that the clinician and staff consider the treatment of dental trauma as a code red event, i.e., an event that in most cases takes precedence over any other pathology and/or scheduled treatment and therefore motivates a change in the diary and appointments for the day.

First and foremost, in such pathologies, four-handed procedures are always necessary for the correct and seamless treatment progress; moreover, prompt diagnosis and surgery are obviously essential for the success of the procedure or at least for the attenuation of future issues. It is also possible to establish a ranking of the interventions that need priority: first, the treatment of exarticulations and dislocations needs immediate intervention, especially if the patient is very young (7–11 years of age).

Coronal-radicular fractures, root fractures, and pulp exposures also need to be treated promptly, whereas concussions, subluxations, and uncomplicated crown fractures can be treated with a delay of a few hours.

The role of individuals who receive the message or the phone call that anticipates the arrival of a trauma patient is also crucial because they have to understand the gravity of the situation and organize and prepare the appropriate dental team interventions within a few minutes. Below we propose a procedure that unifies the various events in which therapeutic action can be expressed in these complex pathologies (Tab. 9.9).

Table 9.9 Treatment options for various categories of crown trauma (according to Spinas classification)

Class	Treatment
Class A	• Reattachment of the fragment • Reconstruction using composite material • Fracture margin remodeling with simulation of physiological abrasion (only for minimal substance losses)
Classes B and C	• Reconstruction using composite material • Reattachment of the fragment
Classes B1 and C1	• In deciduous teeth: pulpotomy, followed by the application of pure calcium hydroxide and composite reconstruction • In immature permanent teeth: two-stroke pulpotomy with calcium hydroxide and composite reconstruction • In teeth with apex formed: direct encapsulation and subsequent composite reconstruction. Follow-up to monitor pulp vitality • In teeth with compromised pulp: root canal therapy and composite reconstruction (possible use of fiber intracanal pins)
Classes D and D1	• Surgical extrusion • Gingivectomy with apical repositioning and bone surgery • Orthodontic extrusion • Orthodontic extrusion with orthodontic reintroduction

Psychological approach

This follows the standards and well-known procedures in pediatric dentistry and should be adapted to the age of the child; it should be implemented by properly qualified staff and should be addressed not only to the trauma patient (child or adolescent) but also to those present at the time of the examination (parents, relatives, and friends). It should be possibly implemented by trained personnel with previous experience in such pathological situations. In case the trauma has affected a very young individual, the objective examination and clinical emergency is always conducted in the presence of a parent (generally the mother), who also physically supports the young patient.

Anamnesis

History of the current disease. The subjective symptomatology and the patient's impressions regarding the trauma, including the intensity, extension, and irradiation, are recorded. This report is easy in the presence of alert and oriented patients aged more than 5–6 years, but it becomes more difficult and less precise with patients aged less than 4 years.
An initial general evaluation of the patient's neurological status is also conducted to ensure that uncertain situations are referred to the responsible departments and that strictly stomatognathic surgery is delayed.

Recent medical history. The modalities of the occurrence of the trauma are reconstructed, and the time, place, causes, and dynamics (sport, accidental, domestic, road, and aggression) of the incident are reported; in particular, the blunt object that caused the injury is described. In some cases, it is possible to detect conflicting versions in the child's and/or his or her caregivers' reports; in this case, further investigation is needed, especially in the case of very young subjects with perioral skin tissue lesions that are not clearly associated with the trauma itself or if they have recurrent traumatic situations, including abuse of means of correction in families or kindergartens.

Family, pharmacological, and past pathological history. Document collection may be delayed in cases of urgency, except for the more strictly medicopharmacological section (drug intolerance/allergy, epilepsy, diabetes, hepatic crisis, etc.). Moreover, given the particularly high incidence of many infectious diseases, it is advisable to complete this documentation as soon as possible. All data should be collected in a special folder.

Collection of preexisting documentation

Whenever a patient who has suffered a trauma is examined by a physician, it is essential to ascertain whether he/she has already been assessed by other healthcare professionals, such as dentists, doctors, or emergency department physicians, for the same trauma, which examinations have been performed, particularly x-rays, and which treatments have been administered. It is very important to verify the correctness of information reported in such documents (certifications and consultations) and, in the event that errors or omissions are detected (as soon as therapeutically possible), to refer the patient to these facilities to correct the errors in the medical records, particularly if they result from emergency room examinations, because these certificates play a significant role in the possible subsequent (frequent) forensic activities consequential to the stabilization of the traumatic outcomes.

Clinical objective examination

A careful objective examination is indispensable to make a correct diagnosis and therefore to establish a valid treatment plan.

The examination of the traumatized patient begins with the clinician's observation of the lateral, anterior, and upper profiles of the face to evaluate the possible presence of asymmetry and/or depressed areas caused by fractures, edema, and contusions.

The inspection of the extraoral tissues allows the clinician to search for wounds or scarring results that can predict the site and the type of a concurrent injury; the lips, tongue, and fornix should be investigated first.

The palpation of the mandibular edge and the maxillary process is also particularly important considering the high frequency of fractures. These examinations should ideally be performed by doctors in maxillofacial hospital departments, but it is good practice not to overlook them, especially if the subject is first examined by a dentist.

The intraoral examination is conducted by checking the integrity of the gum, alveolar mucosa, and in the absence of such evidence, the buccal mucosa. Tearing, swelling, and hemorrhagic processes may be observed in these tissues, which may be the telltale sign of underlying maxillary fractures.

With regard to hard tissues, the integrity of the coronal surface of the teeth is analyzed, and their axial position and the possible presence of horizontal and axial mobility are then assessed; for this maneuver, the handles of the mirror and the mirror itself are used. The palpation of the alveolar process can detect the presence of possible underlying bone fractures.

Instrumental examinations

The following examinations generally complete the clinical objective examination.

Pulp sensitivity test. The main tests used to evaluate pulp sensitivity are the cold test (ethyl chloride) and the electrical test. It should be noted that after the traumatic event, the tooth is in a state of shock that can last for a few days; therefore, it is recommended to repeat the test during the subsequent checks. Response reliability is very limited in subjects aged less than 5 years and in the deciduous teeth. It is advisable to extend the test not only to teeth objectively affected by the trauma but also to the adjacent dental elements and those in an antagonistic relation.

Photographs. Photographic documentation is fundamental in both pre- and post-trauma situations. It consists of at least five photographs: a photo of the face (1/8x), a frontal photo of the area where the trauma is located, a photo of the clinical sequelae (fistulae, tissue laceration, etc.), a frontal photo of the occlusion arches (1/2x), and a photo of the lingual area where the trauma occurred. Photography must always be performed and must be stored responsibly as it is an incontrovertible attestation of the initial lesions.

X-rays. It is essential to perform intraoral x-ray examination for traumatized teeth as well as for adjacent and antagonist teeth. The x-rays must be taken using a centering device to obtain optimal images, which are easily repeatable and, therefore, comparable to evaluate the result in time.
Orthopantomography provides the first image of the oral and articulotemporal areas; indeed, fractures of the jaw, particularly condylar fractures, which are very frequent in juvenile traumatism, are initially identified using this modality.

Verification and evaluation of the collected data

This step involves analysis and synthesis of all the information collected and is considered useful for the preparation of a correct and timely therapeutic plan; examinations that are poorly defined or open to interpretation must be repeated if possible.

Implementation of the treatment plan

This last stage first requires the approval of the treatment plan and the informed consent of the patient (or caregivers in case the patient is a minor). Using safety measures and experience gained over the years, the clinician should perform the interventions necessary for the correct treatment of the highlighted lesions with the aim of promoting the healing or attenuation of the disabling effects of the trauma.
It is known that dental trauma in both deciduous and permanent dentition can often lead to disabling consequences; these can be avoided both with early and correct treatment interventions, both with the prompt management, control, and maintenance of the treatment in the subsequent months (follow-up).
Of course, the type of procedure varies depending on the type of trauma and the urgency code assigned to it.
In some types of trauma, such as dislocations and exarticulations, that occur in school or during sport activities, an initial intervention should be immediately performed at the place where the traumatic event occurred, but this is possible in very few situations. Obviously, because of such limitations, the timeliness and validity of some procedures lose much of their significance and, consequently, the possibility of *complete recovery* of the anatomical injury is reduced.

Certification of the clinical diagnostic activity

A written statement of the procedures performed and above all a description of the patient's health status before and after the specialist intervention are ethical and legal obligations that should not be neglected and should normally be performed by every clinician. With this statement and with the support of the other diagnostic investigations, a complete picture of the post-traumatic conditions can be obtained; this is of extreme importance to the injured patient in the medical and legal processes that frequently result from such harmful events.

Trauma in the deciduous dentition

With regard to traumas that can affect very young patients and consequently the deciduous teeth, we must mainly refer to subjects aged between 1 and 3 years. As mentioned previously, falls and clashes during recreational activities are the main causes of such traumatic events; the places at greatest risk are homes (falls from stairs and fixed structures resulting in direct trauma to the face or teeth), nurseries or kindergartens (clashes between children), and playgrounds (falls from slides, rides, tricycles, and bicycles).
Traumas in this age group are difficult to control and prevent; in the first place, all activities should be monitored at kindergartens, where children are often involved in recreational and gymnastic activities, and, in particular, the environments in which such games are played (closed or open spaces) should be controlled to check compliance with safety standards, especially related to the presence of pavements or fixed obstacles, such as steps and curbs.
In such environments and in the presence of children aged less than 4 years, hyperkinesis, incoordination, and absence of inhibitory restraints lead to frequent falls and clashes between children; these should be adequately prevented with greater vigilance and participation of control personnel.
Additionally, some sports are taken up at a very early age, e.g., skiing, swimming, and gymnastics, and children often start practicing such activities at 3–4 years of age and need appropriate protective equipment and trained personnel for the control and proper conduct of the exercises, for example, by creating small groups under close supervision.
We should not underestimate the use of skateboards, skates, and bicycles, which, at such ages—with the attempt to switch from training wheels to proper wheels—represent a difficult phase, during which falls are particularly frequent.
For the present discussion, it is clear that the most interesting age range is that between 1 and 3 years because children are more involved in such activities and because the deciduous dentition is in the phase of completion and motor incoordination is still remarkably present.
Facial trauma in such children mainly affects the upper anterior elements; the occlusal alterations, e.g., increased OVJ, are important predisposing factors. In 70% of cases, these traumas are dislocations, with a very high frequency of intrusions and exarticulations. Coronal and coronal-radicular fractures are less frequent because of the crown–root relationship (always close to the 1:1 ratio) and because of the remarkable elasticity of the alveolar processes that favors the mobilization of the dental elements.
With regard to lacerated and contused wounds and/or ecchymosis and extensive chin hematomas with altered occlusal function (note that at this age, children hardly use their hands to protect themselves in frontal falls), the presence of possible condylar fractures (head and branch) should not be overlooked and should always be investigated using x-ray, orthopantomography, and submental vertex radiography.
In most cases, however, a *gentle* approach is needed in such children, who are most likely to be at their first dental examination, and they should have a nontraumatizing memory of this experience and the following examinations.

Crown fracture

Uncomplicated traumas of the deciduous teeth, which only affect the dental crown without pulp involvement, are reported infrequently, first because they are often underestimated by parents and second because of their low functional influence; these type of lesions are examined by physicians only when they occur along with pulp lesions (concomitant subluxation phenomena) with the onset of abscess and draining fistula or for a silent hyperpigmentation of the dental crown. Such phenomena can often occur long after the traumatic event (Figs. 9.10 and 9.11).

In case of simple crown fractures involving the loss of enamel and/or dentin, the therapy of choice involves the use of composite resin in reconstruction procedures. In case of pulp involvement (pulp necrosis), the treatment of choice is pulpectomy with intracanal absorbent material in order to not hinder the progress of the physiological root exfoliative process; in such cases, periodic clinical and intraoral x-ray examinations are necessary to evaluate the normal evolution of the process (Fig. 9.12).

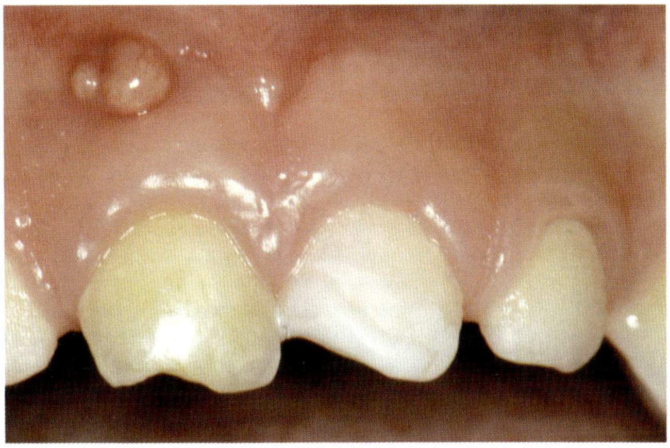

Figure 9.10 5.1 Necrosis in a deciduous tooth with abscess, subsequent to a concussion; 6.1 deciduous tooth treated for a simple crown fracture.

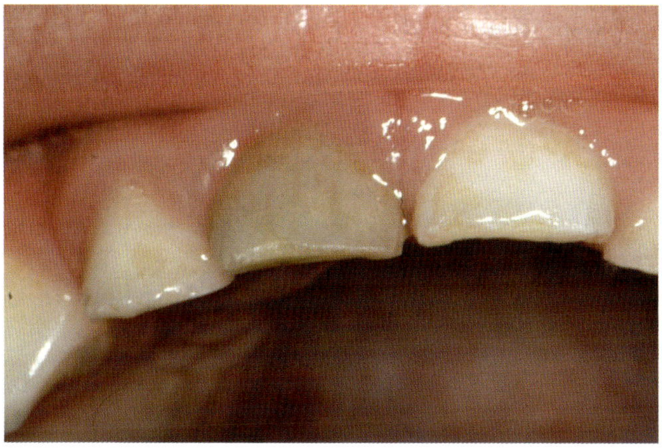

Figure 9.11 5.1 Late and asymptomatic emergence of necrosis in a deciduous tooth.

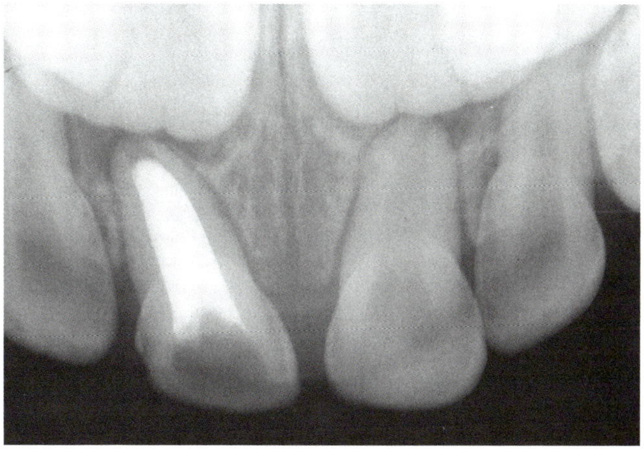

Figure 9.12 X-ray of the root-canal treatment of 5.1 tooth using absorbable materials.

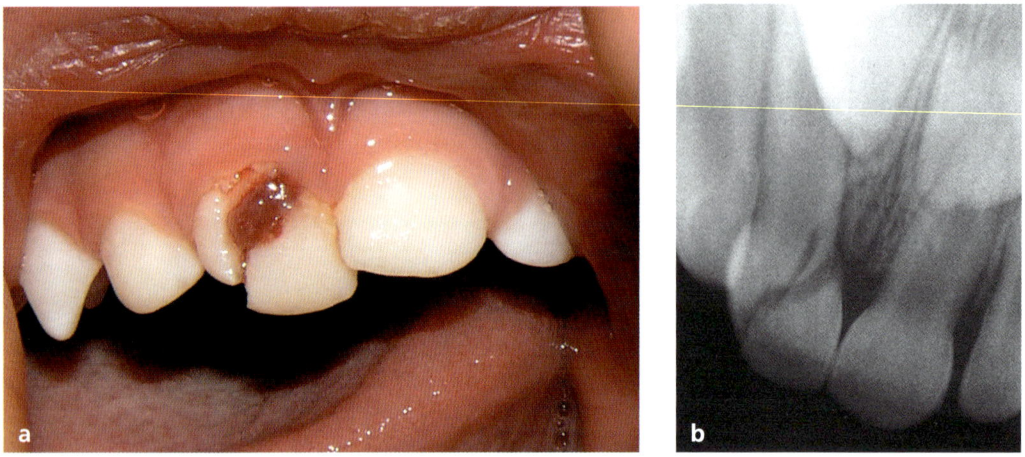

Figure 9.13 Coronal-radicular fracture of 5.1 tooth with pulp exposure (**a**) and related X-ray (**b**).

Coronal-radicular fractures

In case of extensive crown fractures that also affect the dental root, the direct involvement of the dental pulp is very frequent (Fig. 9.13). The prognosis of such traumas is usually poor as it is difficult to apply the range of interventions that are available for permanent dental elements to the deciduous ones.

Thus, preservation of the traumatized element involves the removal of the fractured coronal fragment (Fig. 9.14) and the preservation of the remaining radicular fragment after proper treatment of the pulp stump. The success of this intervention also depends on the cooperation of the child and the experience of the operating team. In cases in which the root stump cannot be saved, its removal and the subsequent design and application of a "space maintainer" should be conducted.

Radicular fractures

Traumas that affect only the root are infrequent (3%–5% of deciduous traumatisms) but must be correctly diagnosed because they are often confused with extrusive luxation (Fig. 9.15). If the fracture fissure is horizontal and is located between the middle and apical third, treatment can be performed by splinting (solidarization) of the affected teeth to the adjacent healthy teeth to heal periodontal tissues (Fig. 9.16a-c). In contrast, fracture of the apical third does not require particular attention as it evolves into a spontaneous resorption of the distal fragment.

Orthodontic *bracket* splints and wire or simple braided wire and *composite resin* can be used; the former are preferred as they also allow axial repositioning of the coronal fracture fragment (if extruded), although they require more investigative interventions and are less tolerated by children.

In the absence of clear signs of pulp involvement, it is not necessary to proceed with the devitalization of the concerned element; with regard to the fate of the radicular fragment—distal to the fracture fissure—it usually develops against a phenomenon of physiological rhizolysis that can be only partially more rapid (Fig. 9.16d). The described treatment requires frequent follow-up, especially in the first 6 months after the trauma, and regular x-ray verification of the evolution of the normal phenomena of dental transition. The result may be positive (Fig. 9.16e).

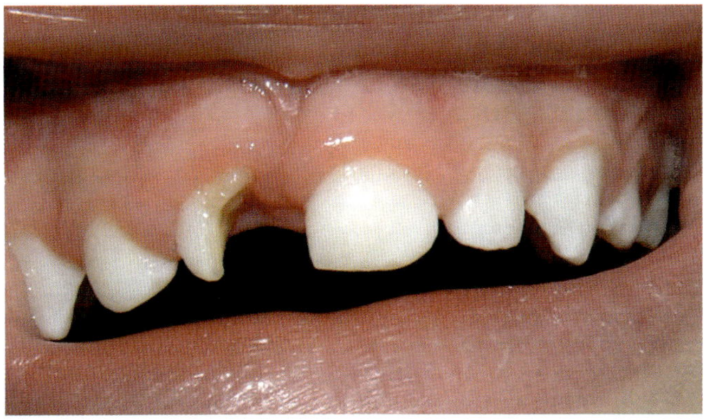

Figure 9.14 Debridement of the fractured crown fragment of 5.1 tooth.

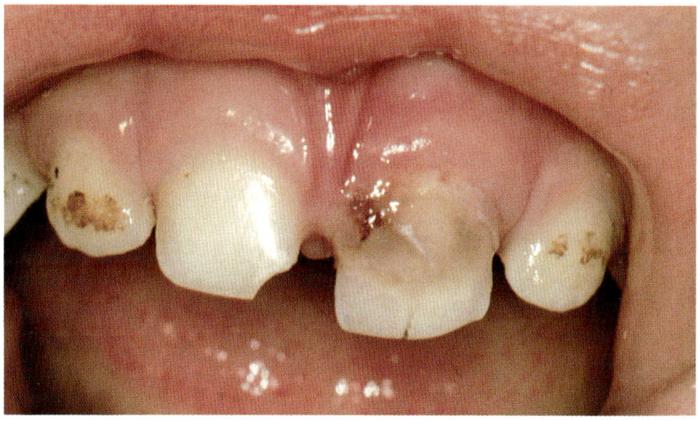

Figure 9.15 Extruded 6.1 deciduous tooth; a differential diagnosis with root fractures is needed.

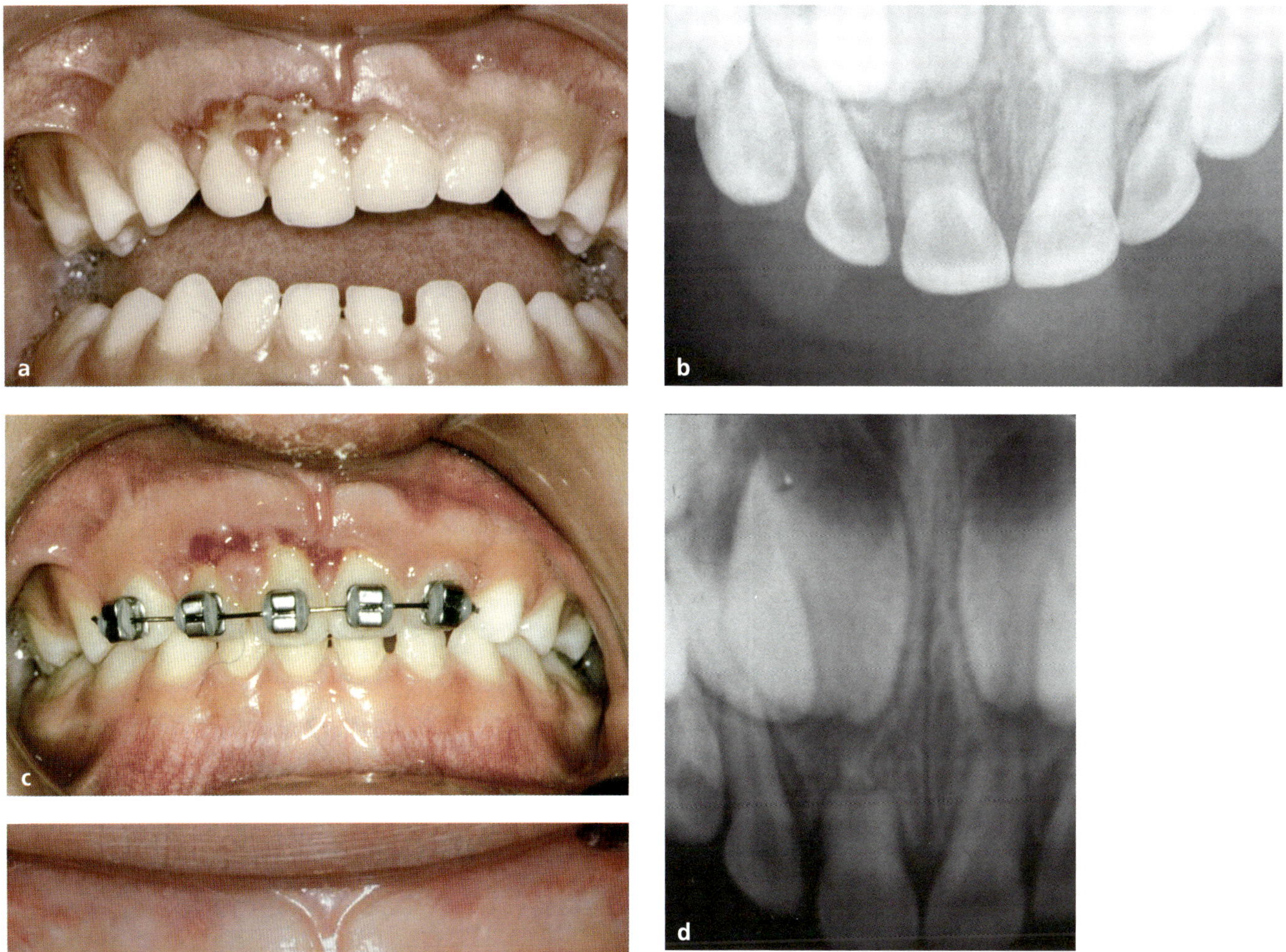

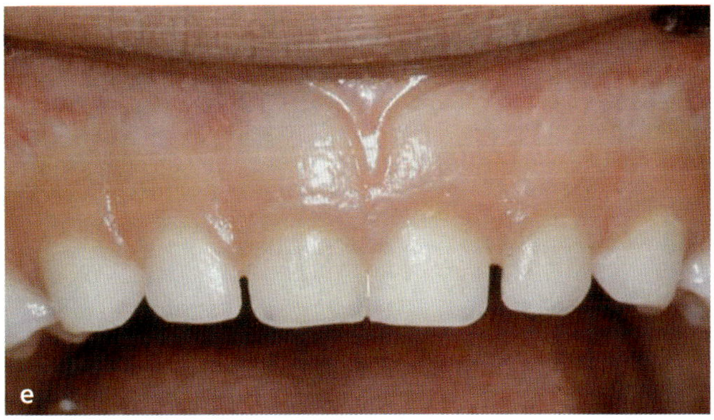

Figure 9.16 (**a**) Oral image of a suspect fracture of 5.1 tooth root that needs X-ray verification. (**b**) Occlusal X-ray image of 5.1 tooth: root horizontal fracture is observed. (**c**) Replacement of the crown fracture and splinting of 5.1. (**d**) Control X-ray 12 months after the trauma: normal rizalysis of the root apical fragment is observed. (**e**) Clinical check 18 months after the trauma: no sign of pathology is observed.

Tooth luxation

As already anticipated, deciduous tooth luxations are the most frequent events needing dental attention. These include concussions, subluxations, and extrusive, intrusive, and lateral luxations and exarticulations.

With regard to concussions and subluxations (Fig. 9.17), these types of traumas can often be ignored because the child is unlikely to report intense pain; soft tissue bleeding and dental mobility may be lacking or reduced, and, for this reason, it is easier to identify outcomes related to such events rather than the event itself.

The yellowing of the dental crown is a very frequent outcome in case of a subluxation; this optical phenomenon that is visible in x-ray examinations is caused by the *obliteration of the pulp canal* of the affected tooth. In this situation and in the absence of pulp symptoms such as abscess and fistula, no treatment should be provided, and only the normal development of the dental transition should be monitored with regular biannual visits.

Extrusive luxations are characterized by visible axial displacement of the crown and with accentuated mobility and interference in occlusion (displacement is often in a palatal direction). They require early treatment intervention shortly after the trauma. The treatment involves an attempt to manually replace the tooth or teeth involved in

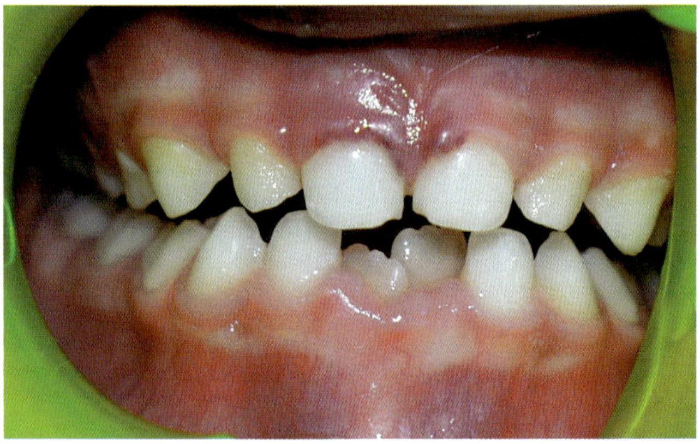

Figure 9.17 Concussion and sub-dislocation of 5.1 tooth.

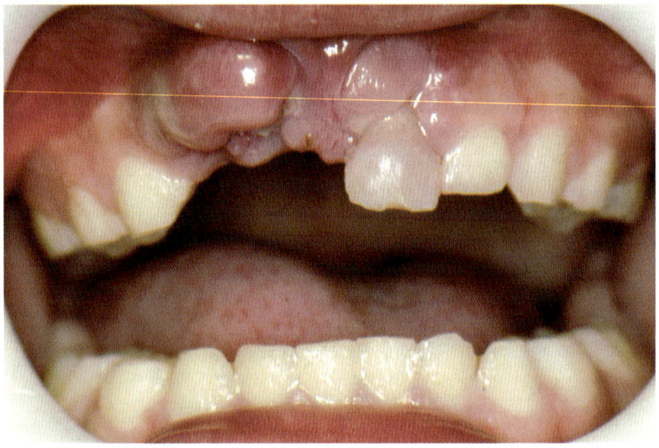

Figure 9.18 Complete intrusive dislocation of 5.1 tooth concomitant with 6.1 tooth necrosis.

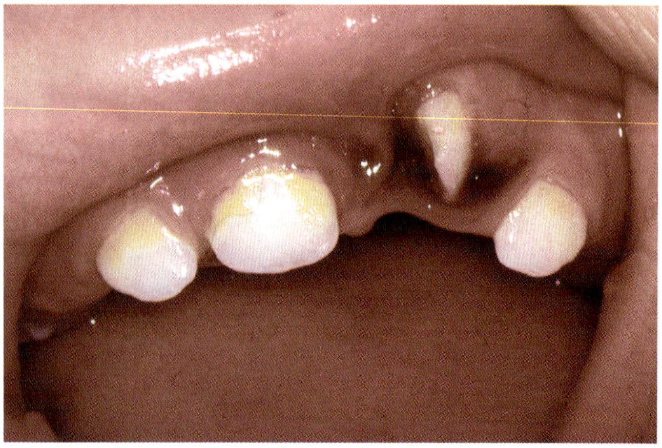

Figure 9.19 Intrusive dislocation of 6.1 with vestibular bone fracture.

addition to soft tissue treatment (medication and sutures) to stem the often-present bleeding. A differential diagnosis should also be made with root fractures via an intraoral x-ray examination.

In the case of an intrusive luxation, total or partial disappearance of the affected tooth inside the alveolar process can be observed (Fig. 9.18); this usually occurs *with vestibular displacement of the root and palatal displacement of the crown*, which, depending on the degree of maturation of the root apex, may involve perforation of the soft vestibular bone plate (Fig. 9.19).

In the intrusive movement, the root apex often comes into contact with the bud of the homologous developing permanent tooth; this contact, depending on the age of the child and the stage of maturation of the forming tooth, can result in permanent outcomes, which are only visible at the time of eruption of the permanent tooth in the arch (hypoplasia of enamel and dentin, Fig. 9.20); in the most serious cases, it may result in the cessation of the development of the permanent dental bud or its morphological—coronal and/or radicular—variation (dilaceration), with difficult eruption or, in more limited cases, the need for extraction of the tooth due to the impossibility of recovering the arch (Fig. 9.21).

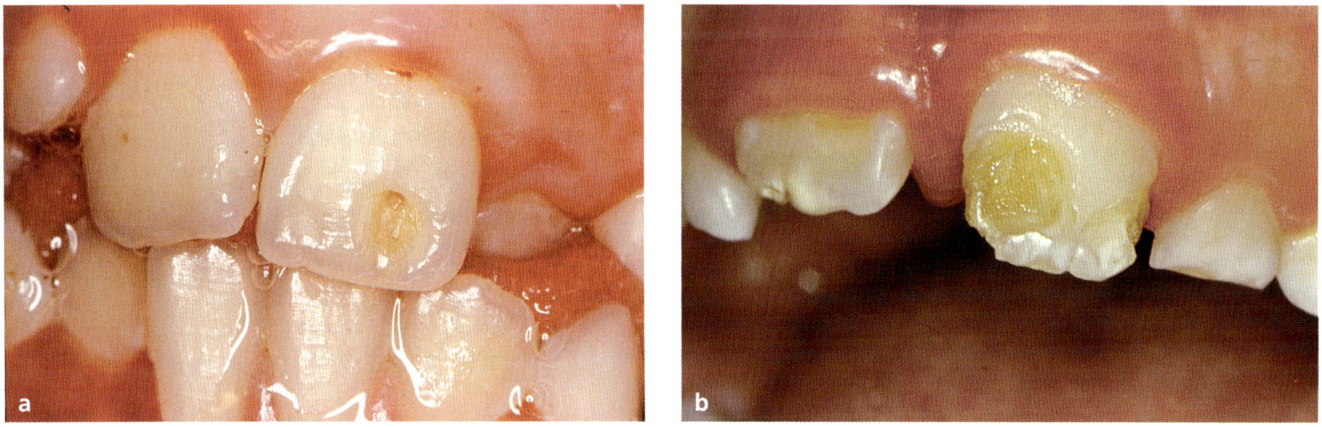

Figure 9.20 (**a**) 2.1 tooth crown local hypoplastic outcome, subsequent to 6.1 intrusive dislocation. (**b**) Severe enamel-dentin outcome of 2.1 tooth crown, subsequent to 6.1 intrusive dislocation.

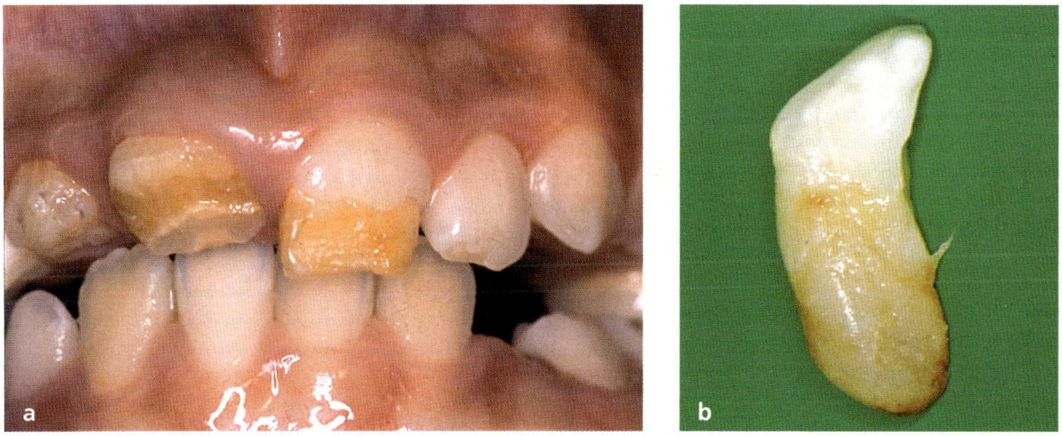

Figure 9.21 (**a**) Laceration of 1.1 crown and severe 2.1 hypoplasia, subsequent to a severe 5.1 and 6.1 dislocation. (**b**) Extracted lacerated tooth due to the impossibility of recovering the arch.

Therefore, it is always necessary to reassess the injured young patient shortly after the trauma in order to perform an evaluation of the severity of the event, arrange any immediate interventions, and decide whether recovering the intrusive deciduous teeth is useful or possible.
In the case of delayed examination, it is always necessary to conduct simple examinations, such as occlusal x-ray, to ascertain the position of the luxated teeth and/or the presence of exarticulations (always look for the avulsed tooth).
For intrusive teeth that do not interfere with the growing buds of permanent teeth, waiting 60–90 days is a possible treatment option. During this period—if there are no infraocclusion events—the tooth will spontaneously regain an appropriate position in the arch (Fig. 9.22). This method requires frequent checks and parental cooperation at home but can often be followed by necrosis of the intrusive tooth and/or obliteration of the canal with yellowing of the crown.
If the tooth does not spontaneously re-erupt, infraocclusion of the intrusive tooth, also known as pseudoankylosis (Fig. 9.23a), will occur; this will require avulsion of the tooth at the appropriate time, which is motivated by the potential obstruction to the normal eruption of the homologous permanent tooth that this element can create (Fig. 9.23b); regular x-ray evaluation and the commitment of the young patient are necessary.
Traumatic avulsions or exarticulations are no less frequent in deciduous teeth (Fig. 9.24); in these cases, it is important to first look for the detached element; if it is not identified, a differential diagnosis with full intrusive luxations should be conducted by performing an x-ray examination, or the rare but not to be overlooked hypothesis of inhalation or ingestion of the dental element should be considered. In such situations, it is evident that the general symptoms guide the medical staff to the correct location of the phantom tooth.
If the child has a detached tooth, some considerations must be made:

- what is the age of the child?
- what are the general and local conditions of the alveolus?
- what are the conditions of preservation of the avulsed dental element?
- where and how was the avulsed dental element stored?

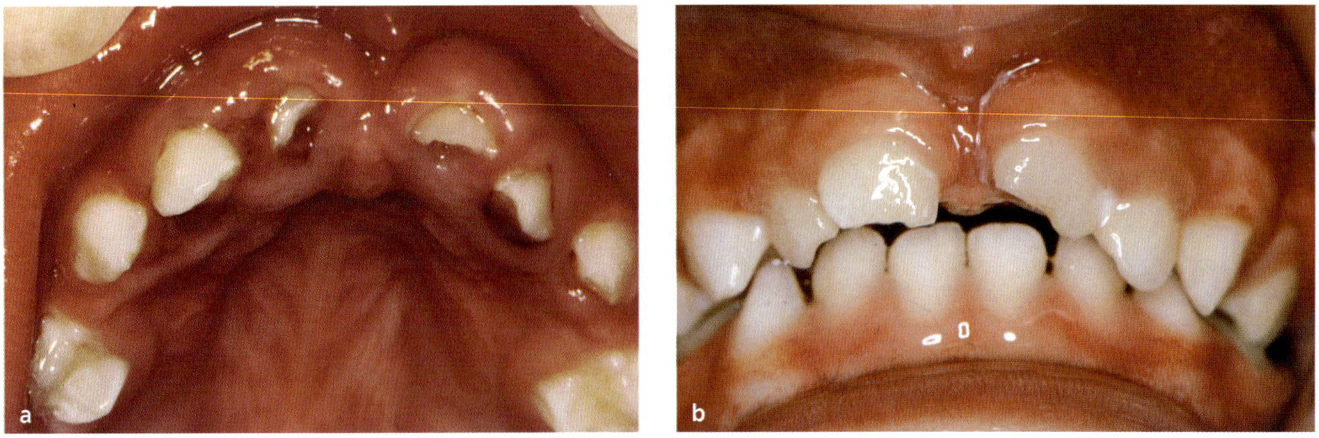

Figure 9.22 (**a**) 5.1, 6.1, and 6.2 intrusive dislocation (concomitant with crown fractures). (**b**) Spontaneous re-eruption of the intruding teeth 30 days after the trauma.

In principle, protocols suggest not to re-implant a deciduous tooth because children offer little cooperation and have a disadvantageous apical anatomy of the young deciduous tooth (children aged up to 2 years); in addition, the objective difficulty in providing adequate stabilization of the replanted tooth, the need for extensive pharmacological cover, and the risk of loss of the splint when the child eats should be considered. In the literature, re-implantation of avulsed deciduous incisors have been described, although usually in patients aged more than 3 years (rhizolysis improves the apical conformation of the root) and are usually performed soon after the traumatic event (Fig. 9.25). However, *substantial negative opinion on this therapeutic approach remains*. In such cases, there is an evident need for the functional maintenance of the child's arches, and therefore, when dental losses occur in children aged between 2–4 years, we should evaluate the need for maintenance or reopening of the eruptive space for future permanent teeth (Fig. 9.26) and the preservation of correct respiratory, phonetic and, if possible, esthetic parameters (Fig. 9.27) with the use of small removable plates equipped with mini expansion screws and active nickel–titanium arms if required.

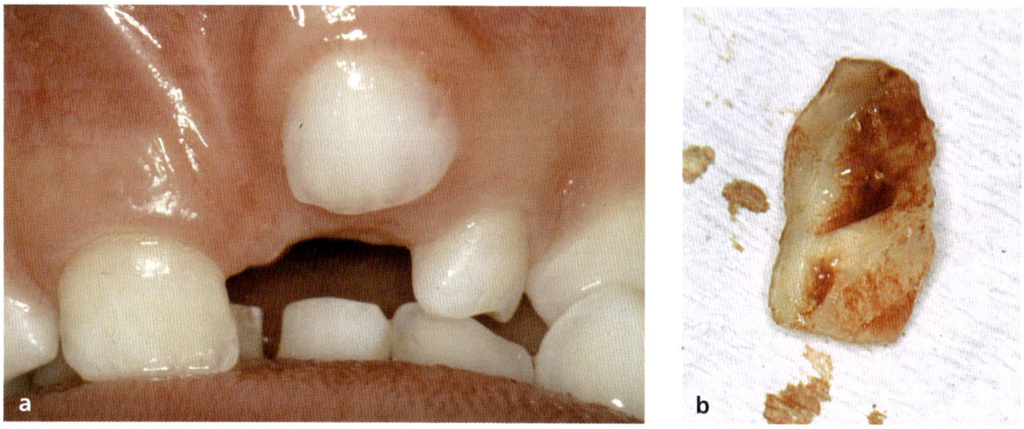

Figure 9.23 (**a**) Infra-occlusion subsequent to a 6.1 intrusive trauma. (**b**) Extracted infra-occluded tooth.

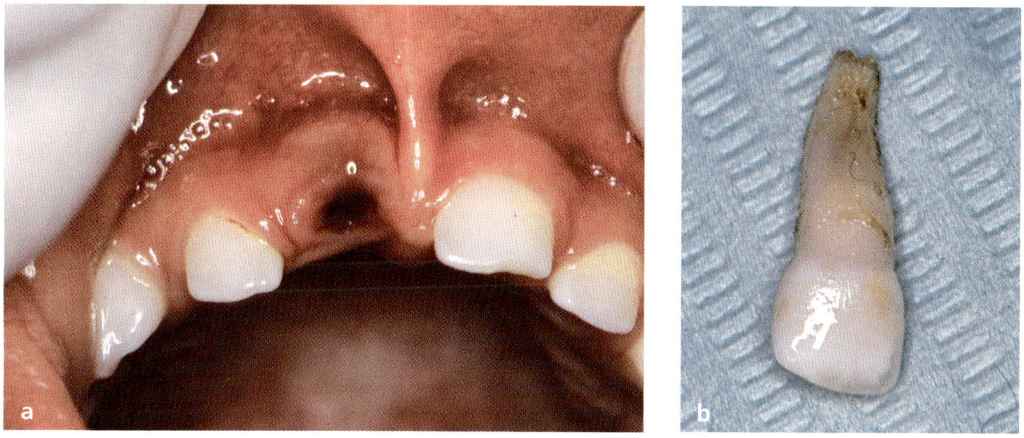

Figure 9.24 (**a**) Intra-oral image of 5.1 deciduous incisor detachment. (**b**) Detached 5.1 tooth; notice the complex root morphology.

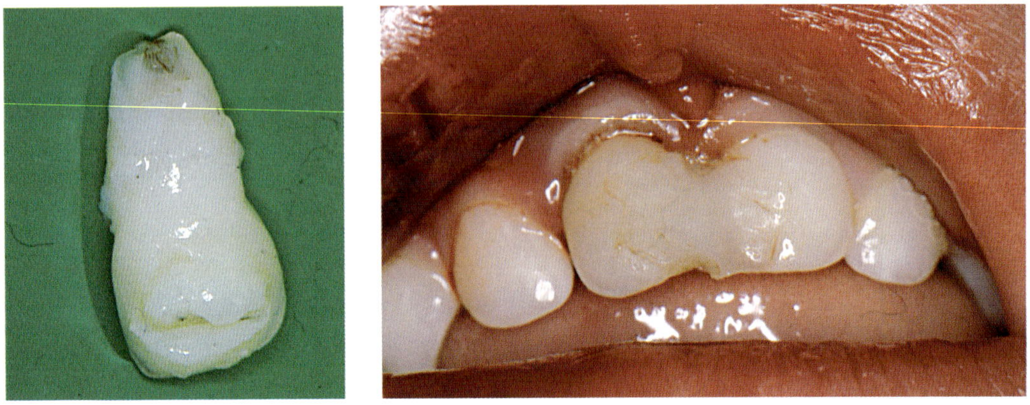

Figure 9.25 (**a**) Detached 5.1 deciduous tooth; notice the root reduced length: in this case, repositioning the alveolus is easier. (**b**) Post-replant image of 5.1 tooth splinted to 6.1.

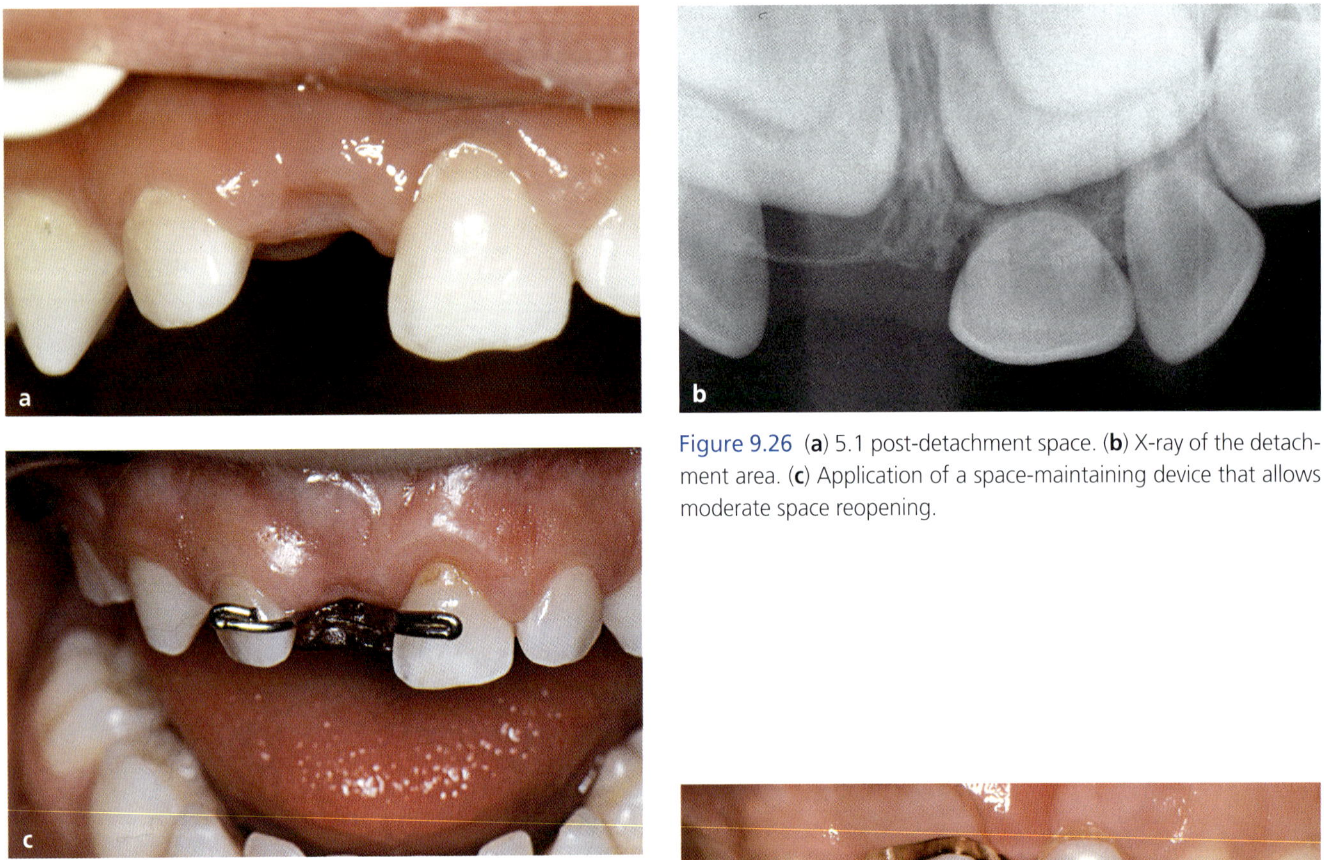

Figure 9.26 (**a**) 5.1 post-detachment space. (**b**) X-ray of the detachment area. (**c**) Application of a space-maintaining device that allows moderate space reopening.

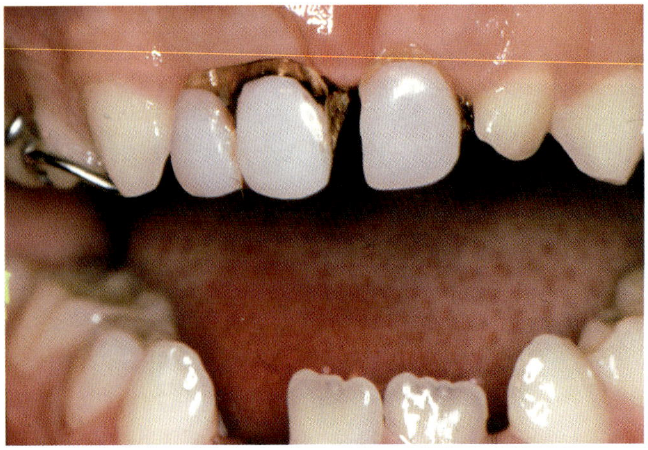

Figure 9.27 Aesthetic space-maintaining device, which is useful in case of multiple detachments or prolonged eruption periods.

Table 9.10 Treatment approach to deciduous dental lesions

Type of trauma	Immediate therapy	Follow-up
Avulsion	Local treatment, occlusal x-ray, tooth recovery, no re-implantation.	Need for mobile space maintainer and verification of permanent tooth eruption
Intrusive luxation	Local treatment, occlusal x-ray, manual repositioning, expected re-eruption of the deciduous tooth (if the visit is delayed)	Occlusal x-ray, permanent eruption and deciduous exfoliation examination, check for tooth color and vitality (necrosis); in case of infra-occlusion. consider extracting the intruding tooth
Extrusive luxation	Local treatment, occlusal x-ray, manual repositioning, check differential diagnosis with root fracture	Orthodontic reintrusion (if the visit is delayed), color vitality (necrosis)
Subluxation	Local treatment, occlusal x-ray, increased mobility, orthodontic splint	Follow-up x-ray, check for tooth color and vitality (necrosis), check for mobility and physiological exfoliation
Crown fracture	Considering the extent of the fracture and vitality, pulp treatment if it is exposed	Composite reconstruction, pulpotomy using absorbable material, intraoral x-ray, check for exfoliation
Root fracture	Check differential diagnosis with extrusive luxation, orthodontic splint (30–60 days)	Intraoral x-ray; check for necrosis, mobility, and physiological exfoliation
Coronal-radicular fractures	The tooth is usually extracted; it is advisable to proceed in two stages, starting with the mobile fragment	Space maintainer, periodic check-ups

To complete the brief discussion on such traumatic events, Table 9.10 summarizes the methodology of therapeutic approaches for the most frequent deciduous dental lesions and the general rules of immediate intervention and follow-up. We highlight the importance of periodic follow-ups. Moreover, the correct skeletal growth and physiological dental transition should be monitored.

Trauma in the permanent dentition

Regarding permanent teeth, in accordance with the aims of this study, we will deal with traumatic events that most frequently affect adolescents. For traumatic events, the intervention protocols to be implemented—in case of pulp and exarticulation exposure (complete dislocation of the dental element)—are of particular importance.

Crown fractures involving the enamel and dentin

Crown fractures are the most frequently examined lesions. Uncomplicated tooth enamel fractures are the most common types. These substance losses always require rehabilitative dental treatment, while simple fractures of the enamel (Fig. 9.28) are often considered by first aid providers or by the patients themselves as not deserving of examination and treatment by the dentist and, therefore, easily acceptable (considering their limited extent), especially if they do not result in complications (subsequent necrosis due to concussion); thus, they are often undiagnosed or underestimated.

Crown fractures with fragment recovery are events that can lead to the best reconstructive results. The fragment, usually enamel and dentin, must be kept in milk or saline solution if possible to prevent dehydration (Fig. 9.29), so that the professional may use it for the reconstruction of the dental element if needed. The operational features of this technique are described later in this chapter.

When the fragment is unavailable, the standard rehabilitation treatment for coronal fractures (both enamel and enamel-dentin) (Fig. 9.30) involves the use of composite resins at least up to the age of 18–20 years, when the size and morphology of the fracture are limited; in all other cases, and especially in later ages, it is necessary and advisable to provide a prosthetic gold–porcelain or ceramic crown or alternatively, a ceramic veneer.

Complicated crown fractures involving the enamel and dentin

These types of lesions always require urgent dental treatment because of pulp exposure. They require special attention and proper diagnosis, especially when they involve patients aged between 9 and 11 years or in cases involving the presence of an obvious immaturity of the root system, both in terms of wall thickness and root apex width.

Permanent teeth with immature apex

If clinical and radiographic signs as well as thermal and electrical sensitivity tests do not indicate that the pulp is extensively compromised, pulp vitality should be maintained by direct capping or partial pulpotomy (Fig. 9.31). In contrast, if the pulp is widely and visibly involved, it is more appropriate to perform pulpotomy extending to the whole visible pulp (Fig. 9.32).

Pulpotomy techniques have the greatest success; they consist of the removal of the exposed pulp tissue (often exposure of a single pulp cornet can occur), followed by the application of powdered calcium hydroxide to the pulp wound and self-hardening calcium hydroxide overload for the mechanical protection of the site.

Pulpotomy is a two-stage technique, i.e., it involves reopening of the exposed pulp area previously treated with calcium hydroxide to detect the formation of a dentinal barrier (dentin bridge) below the previous pulp wound.

Clinical evaluation should be supported by the preserved response to the sensitivity tests and by the absence of pathological images in the periapical radiographic examination (Fig. 9.32c).

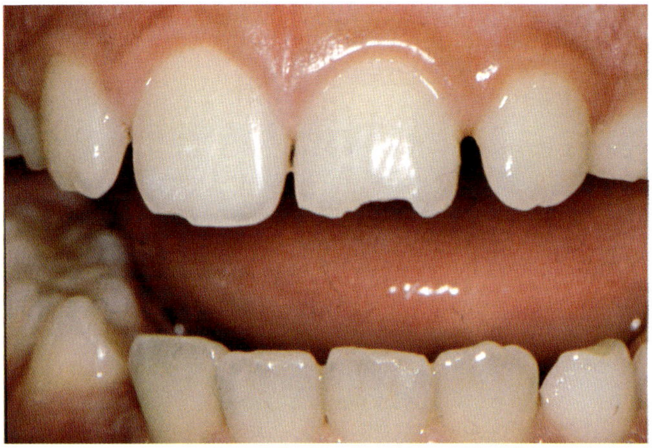

Figure 9.28 2.1 permanent tooth involved in a simple enamel crown fracture.

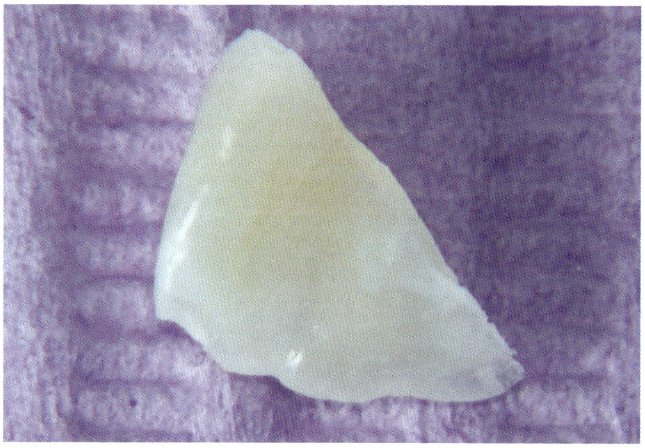

Figure 9.29 Crown fracture of an incisor; to maintain good aesthetics, the fragment should be stored in saline solution.

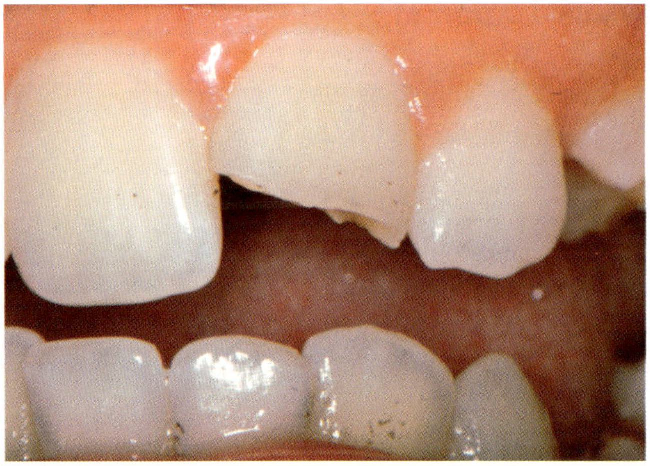

Figure 9.30 2.1 tooth involved in a wide enamel-dentin fracture.

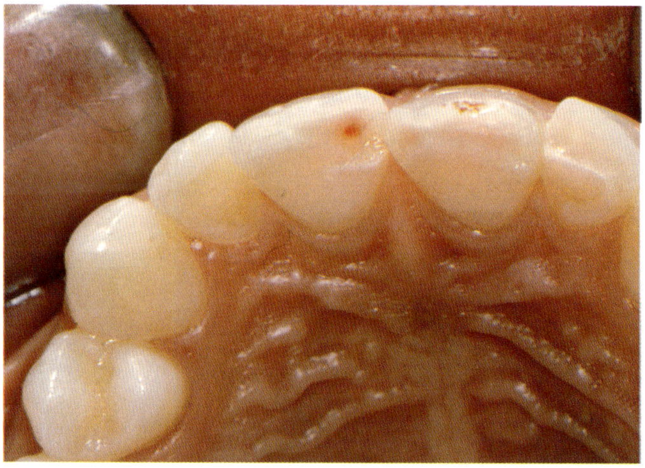

Figure 9.31 1.1 palatal image which shows a crown fracture with pulp exposure; 2.1 tooth also shows a wide crown fracture with significant pulp exposure.

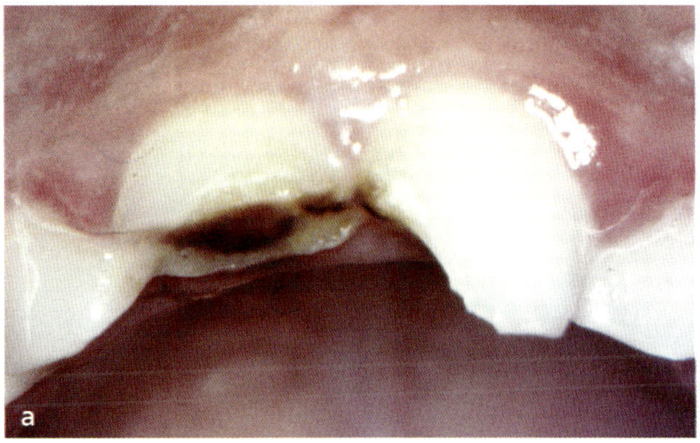

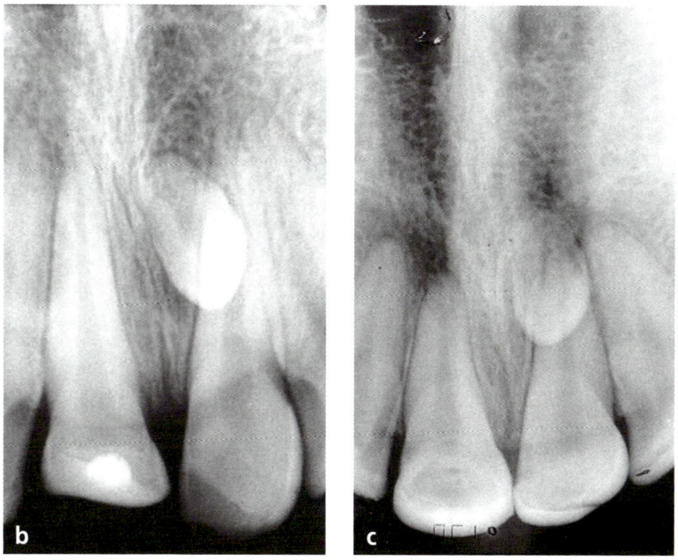

Figure 9.32 (**a**) 1.1 palatal image which shows a crown fracture with pulp exposure; in these cases, a wide pulpotomy is necessary. (**b**) X-ray 60 days after the pulpotomy (notice the presence of a mesiodens). (**c**) The same tooth 1 year after the trauma and after the reconstruction with compound resins.

In case of a positive result, it will be possible to complete the final reconstruction of the fractured crown with the use of composite resins or the correctly stored original fragment.
In the event of the onset of irreversible pulpitis or pulp necrosis, a pulpectomy should be performed, followed by apexification with calcium hydroxide or alternative materials, such as MTA.
In case of pulp necrosis of a dental element with an immature apex, the impossibility of spontaneous radicular maturation and therefore the need for induced radicular maturation, with increased risk of failure and/or subsequent possible fractures of the root walls, may occur.
The purpose of specialized pulpotomy treatment should be the maintenance of pulp viability and consequently normal root apex formation.

Permanent teeth with formed apex

The procedure of choice is direct capping using calcium hydroxide paste in case of mild and recent pulp exposure, followed by crown reconstruction, usually in the same session or subsequently. In case the pulp is compromised, pulpectomy should be performed and, once endodontic treatment is completed, reconstruction of the crown can be conducted immediately using the abovementioned techniques.
In case of extensive coronal mutilation, it is advisable to place a carbon fiber or glass pin inside the canal lumen (Fig. 9.33). In some cases, the reconstructive phase may be combined or preceded by *bleaching* therapy of the dental tubules. Rehabilitation using indirect gold stump pins should be postponed to a later age.
After treatment, the patient should be instructed to use the reconstructed teeth, and caution should be recommended, especially when chewing hard food.
Teeth with coronal fracture without pulp impairment should be controlled over time to prevent complications; follow-up should be repeated for at least 12–24 months. It is always advisable for young sportspersons who have suffered a coronal fracture with conservative reconstruction to get accustomed to wearing a *mouthguard*.

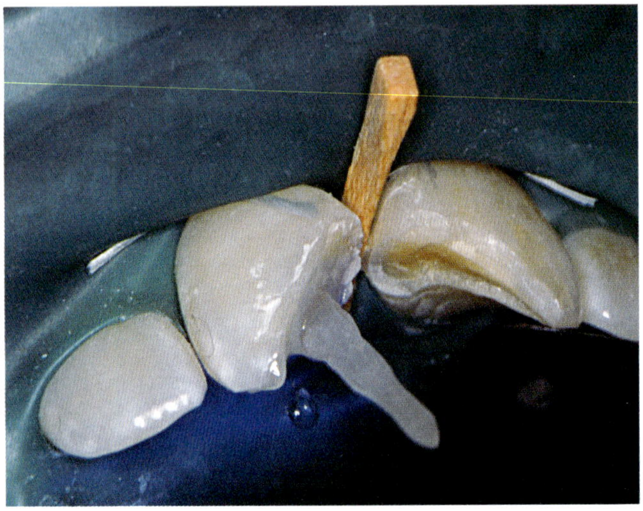

Figure 9.33 1.1 tooth after pulpotomy; it was necessary to place an aesthetic pin to achieve the optimal conservative finalisation.

Coronal frame reattachment technique

Coronal fragment reattachment is a suitable alternative to composite resin reconstruction, especially if there is a single fragment that is perfectly coincident with the residual crown, and also in case of mutilations of both the enamel and dentin.

The prognosis depends on the proper storage of the fragment (in saline solution in a refrigerator) in order to prevent unesthetic chromatic alterations and dehydration, which could facilitate subsequent enamel lesions.

After isolating the field using a rubber dam, the fracture fissure must be cleaned with pure pumice. At this stage, the perfect match between the edges of the stump and the fragment is verified and the enamel and dentin are smoothed, washed with water, and dried. Next, adhesive is applied, and it should be polymerized according to the manufacturer's instructions. This method must always be conducted *four-handed* in order to adhere to the indicated times and obtain the desired results.

A photopolymerizable composite of suitable color is then inserted between the two surfaces of the fracture and possibly inside the pins specially constructed on the two portions of the crown (where the residual stump and fragment have sufficient thickness).

The material is then polymerized, holding the appropriate lamp on the entire fracture fissure so as to ensure adequate and deep polymerization of the compound (60 seconds is sufficient).

If the fracture involves the point of contact, it is more appropriate to reconstruct it entirely in composite resin to increase its durability.

If the esthetic result is not considered satisfactory, for example, because of excessive visibility of the fracture fissure or too jagged a margin, a *circumferential or delayed vestibular bevel* may be constructed so as to allow better integration of the fragment and therefore a more natural appearance (Fig. 9.34).

In a study evaluating 20 elements treated using the fragment reattachment technique in adolescents after 7 years, Spinas (2004) found that only 25% of the restorations carried out with this technique after 5 years were functionally and esthetically still in good condition, while all the other teeth had already undergone renewal (25%) or needed cosmetic re-intervention at the attachment area (50%). This study confirmed that the method, although very valid, is dependent on proper oral hygiene and requires frequent controls and timely adjustments.

However, fragment reattachment is a treatment that does not always have to be performed urgently but can be postponed to when it is associated with pulpotomy.

Coronal-radicular fractures

Coronal-radicular fractures are lesions involving the crown, root, and frequently, the pulp apparatus. They are traumatic events that require extensive efforts by the clinician from the perspective of rehabilitation owing to their extreme complexity.

Temporary reconstructive techniques can be applied *in adolescents*, with definitive finalization in adulthood with the application of a complete crown.

Low (cervical) coronal-radicular fractures are always complicated; in such cases, it will be usually necessary to perform root canal therapy (Fig. 9.35), which, in case of radicular immaturity, will need an intermediate phase of root treatment (apexogenesis/apexification); thereafter, it may be necessary to place a pin in the root canal (fiberglass or quartz pins), following which it will be possible to proceed with orthodontic extrusion of the root with or without resection of periodontal fibers, with subsequent reattachment of the coronal fragment, if available, or composite resin reconstruction.

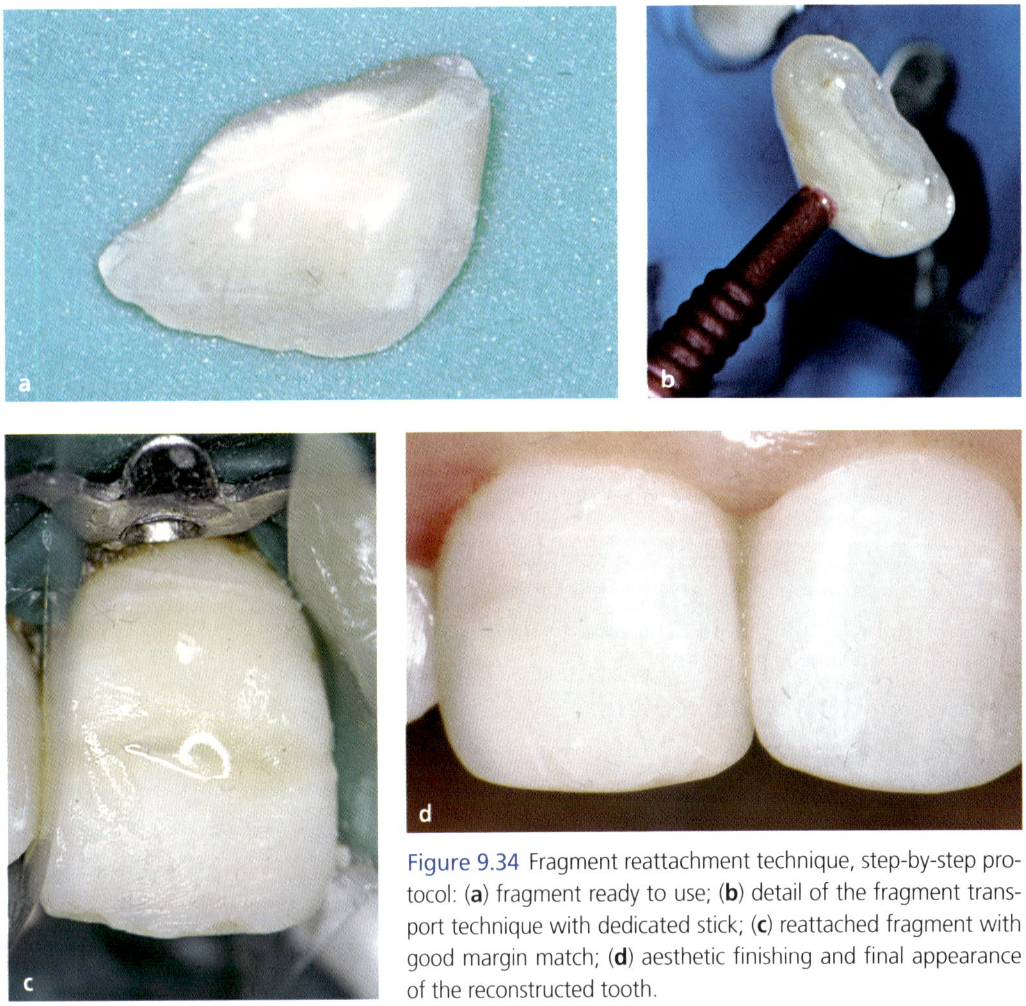

Figure 9.34 Fragment reattachment technique, step-by-step protocol: (**a**) fragment ready to use; (**b**) detail of the fragment transport technique with dedicated stick; (**c**) reattached fragment with good margin match; (**d**) aesthetic finishing and final appearance of the reconstructed tooth.

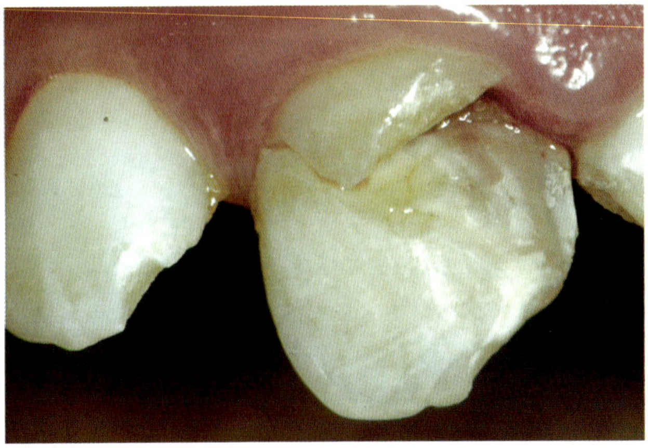

Figure 9.35 Complicated 1.1 coronal-radicular fracture.

For the limited extension fractures with the shape of a flute beak, it is possible to proceed with gingivectomy and immediate reconstruction of the fractured zone.
The other techniques described in the literature, such as apically repositioned flap, intra-alveolar transplant, and extrusive surgical luxation, have little application in the juvenile age range. In contrast, the technique described in 2005 by Spinas, which involves orthodontic extrusion in rehabilitative treatment followed by radicular-coronal intrusion of the injured tooth, is interesting (Fig. 9.36). However, it requires good orthodontic dexterity.

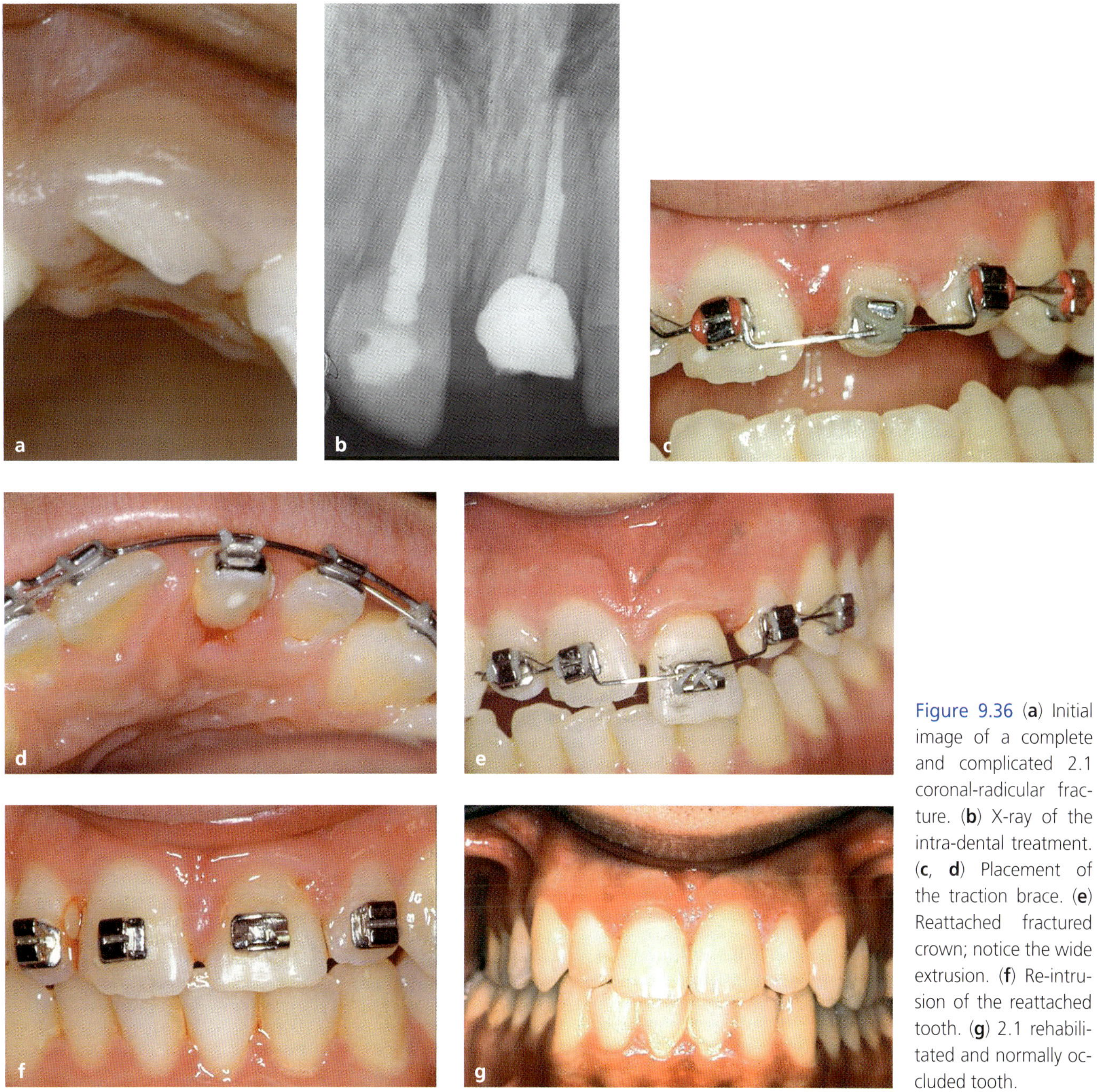

Figure 9.36 (**a**) Initial image of a complete and complicated 2.1 coronal-radicular fracture. (**b**) X-ray of the intra-dental treatment. (**c**, **d**) Placement of the traction brace. (**e**) Reattached fractured crown; notice the wide extrusion. (**f**) Re-intrusion of the reattached tooth. (**g**) 2.1 rehabilitated and normally occluded tooth.

Root fractures

Root fractures are often associated with very violent traumatic events, such as road accidents, falls, abuse, and contact sports, and account for approximately 4% of complicated trauma cases.

Oblique or horizontal radicular fracture

First, x-ray must be performed for accurate diagnosis, and the exact location of the fracture line must be established (apical, middle or cervical third); the localizations at the middle and cervical third are the most difficult in terms of treatment: indeed, in apical fractures (2–3 mm from the apex), the application of a rigid splint for 30 days is sufficient to achieve a very high likelihood of success.

The horizontal fractures of the middle third (Fig. 9.37) may involve mobility of the coronal fragment and its possible extrusion or alternatively may be silent; however, such fractures must be suspected in the presence of coronal-radicular fractures of the adjacent teeth or those resulting from trauma caused by fast-moving and rigid blunt objects, such as sports or road accidents. Intraoral x-ray examination (repeated after 24 hours) can help in differentiation because it provides specific images (fracture line diastasis), even if the cone images are currently considerably more precise and recommended compared with any other conventional technique.

In the presence of pulp vitality, only rigid splinting (for 30–45 days) should be performed; regular checks should then be performed in order to verify vitality and promote healing by applying cement to the radicular surface at the fracture fissure (modeled on the bone callus).

In few cases, root canal treatment may be necessary (Fig. 9.38): it must be limited to the coronal tract. If complications occur, it should involve the distal tract to the fracture fissure. Finally, preventive root canal therapy with radicularly immature teeth should be avoided.

The *evolution of horizontal root fractures* should follow the following pattern:

- healing with calcified tissue (dentin and cement)
- healing with fibrous connective tissue
- healing with interposition of bone tissue
- no healing by interposition of granulation tissue.

Vertical root fracture

In the case of a vertical root fracture, the element cannot be maintained, and an appropriate treatment for the replacement of the affected tooth must be implemented because of the age of the patient. In select cases, intentional self-transplantation (premolars to be extracted for orthodontic purposes are used) or closing of the orthodontic space or conservation of space with mobile or fixed maintainers can be considered; the Maryland bridge in Fiber-reinforced composite (FRC) is the most suitable esthetic and functional solution in adolescents.

In individuals at the end of their skeletal growth period, proceeding with root extraction and placement of a bone-integrated implant using a conventional technique or a post-extraction technique should be considered.

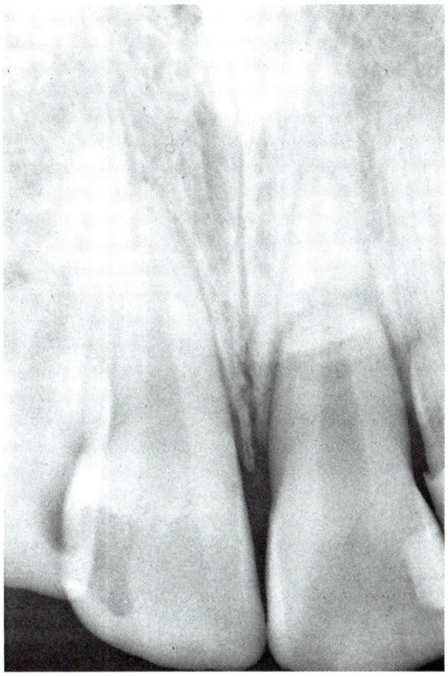

Figure 9.37 2.1 horizontal root fracture (medial third).

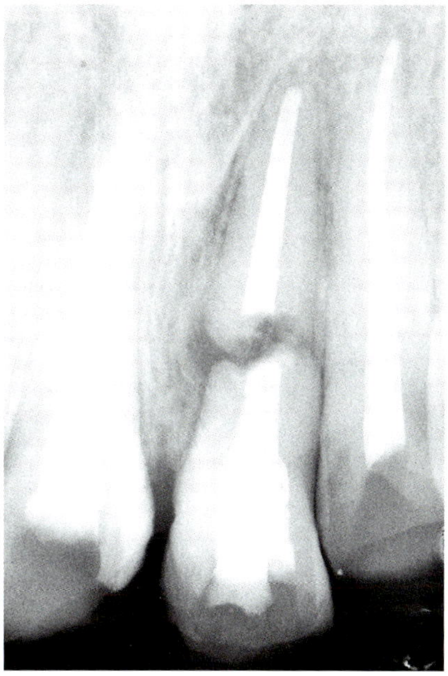

Figure 9.38 Root canal treatment of 2.1 root fracture, extended to the distal fragment due to an infection; notice the healing with interposition of fibrous connective tissue.

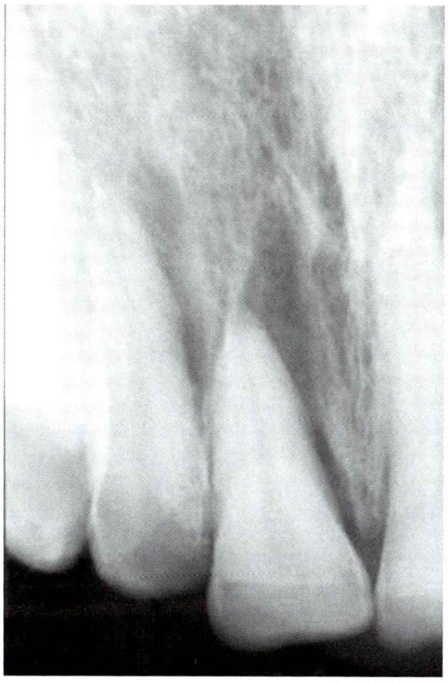

Figure 9.39 Double lateral dislocation X-ray (1.1 and 1.2 teeth).

Dental luxations

Dental luxations are more frequent in cases of trauma with reduced impact speed or those resulting from objects with a low modulus of elasticity; they manifest with visible displacement of the dental element inside its alveolus with possible fracture of its walls.

However, luxations may be associated with coronal fractures of the same or adjacent elements, thereby requiring combined treatment.

They are classified as intrusive, extrusive, and lateral depending on the direction of displacement. They require immediate and accurate diagnosis, possibly immediately after the trauma or as early as possible, by clinical examination and appropriate x-ray examinations (periapical intraoral x-ray with a centering device).

In case of a luxation, it is necessary to relocate the dental element to its correct position inside the alveolus as early as possible. If this maneuver is not conducted within a reasonable timeframe (30–60 days), it is very likely that the condition will evolve into ankylosis and/or substitute external radicular resorption (usually in intrusive and lateral luxations).

From a prognostic perspective, the most serious luxations are the intrusive and lateral ones because these are often associated with pulp lesions (interruption of the vascular-nervous beam) and/or fractures of the alveolar, palatal or vestibular cortex (Fig. 9.39).

Extrusive lesions may simulate or be associated with radicular fractures. Radiographic diagnosis is therefore essential to define the nature of the lesion (periapical x-ray or cone-beam x-ray examination).

Immediate repositioning should be performed manually if the luxation is not associated with root incarceration in the cortex, which strongly affects the possibility of immediate manual repositioning.
The repositioned luxated element must be splinted, i.e., joined, to the adjacent elements and followed-up for at least 30–60 days. This follow-up also applies to cases of extrusive luxations.
If the luxation is not examined within 24 hours, manual repositioning becomes impossible; *surgical repositioning or, alternatively, an orthodontic procedure* is needed.
Surgical repositioning is indicated only in case of incarceration of the intruding element in the bone cortex because it is the only way to reposition the element. In all other cases, surgical repositioning is not recommended owing to the possibility of loss of vitality outcomes and *external root resorption*, which often follows such a procedure. Thus, slow orthodontic repositioning (with fixed equipment) with the initial correct relocation of the traumatized tooth and alignment to the adjacent teeth is preferable in cases of dislocation with a delayed examination (Fig. 9.40). This results in a semi-rigid orthodontic splintering that is further usable for the next restraining and stabilizing period; the total length of restraining is approximately 60 days.

The following types of splinting can be used:
- rigid splinting with composite resin or braided wire and composite resin
- semi-rigid splinting with a titanium splint (titanium trauma splint) that can be used only in the phase of retention of luxations.

Luxations are not free from negative outcomes; *obliteration of the canal lumen* is one of the most frequent and characteristic complications, particularly in teeth with open apex, and may remain asymptomatic for a long time (Fig. 9.41), with a late slight yellowing of the crown and poor response to sensitivity tests.
This reactive pulp evolution should not be interpreted as a pathological event; therefore, intervening with endodontic treatments is *definitely contraindicated* if there are no further signs of pulp disease, including periapical radiotransparency, mobility, or percussive pain.

Traumatic exacerbation or avulsion

Luxations also include exarticulations (complete extrusive dislocations), the most dreaded and unfortunate dental lesion, especially among 8–12-year-olds, as they may cause, if not properly treated, permanent outcomes that are difficult to be rehabilitated using prosthetics. It follows that such events must be dealt with swiftly, adequately, and completely.
Immediate dental replanting is the ideal treatment for traumatic avulsions in adolescents. There is also a possibility of *late replanting*; however, the prognosis is less favorable using this method.
As mentioned before, the prognosis of such treatment depends on the timeliness of replanting and is particularly *positive if treatment is performed within 30–60 minutes* after the trauma. In addition, the prognosis strongly depends on the proper preservation of the detached element by the first rescuers.

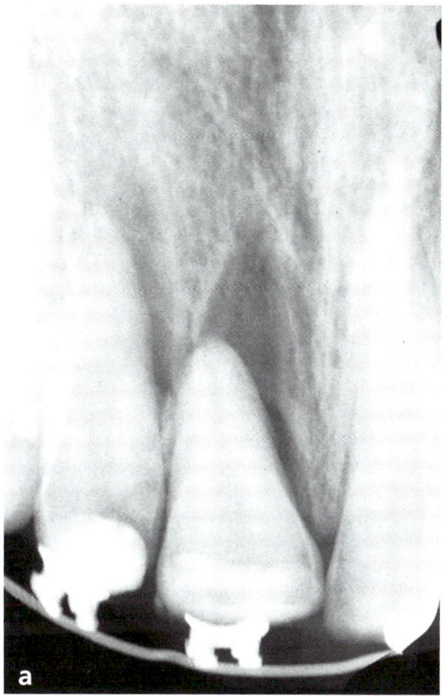

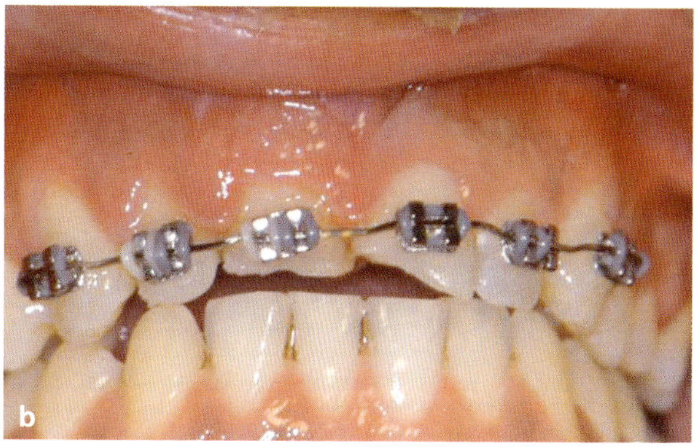

Figure 9.40 (**a**) X-ray of the dislocated tooth repositioning. (**b**) Clinical image of dental repositioning braces.

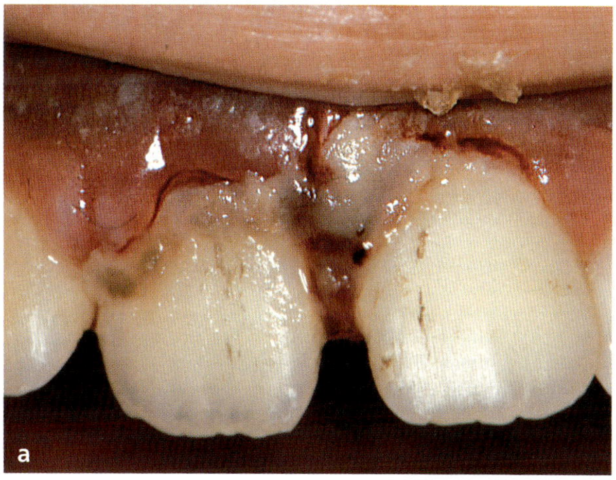

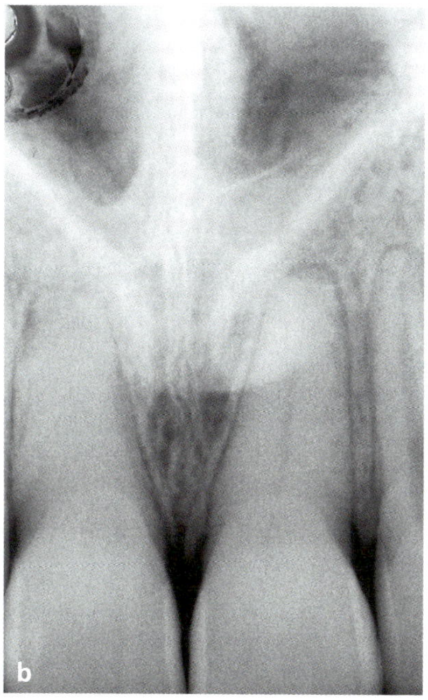

Figure 9.41 (**a**) Severe 1.1 and 2.1 dislocation and gingival soft tissue traumatism. (**b**) X-ray 18 months after the trauma: complete obliteration of 1.1 canal and partial obliteration of 2.1 is clearly observed.

The humid environment ideal for the preservation of the detached tooth is Hank's balanced salt solution (HBSS), followed by fresh milk, saline solution, saliva, and water in descending order of adequacy (Tab. 9.11).
The rescuers must therefore ensure that the detached element is constantly hydrated by one of these means during transport to the nearest dental clinic. The prognosis is completely dependent on the competence and information of the first-aid providers on the treatment protocols for dental luxations.

Table 9.11 Suitable preservation solutions for detached dental elements

Solution	Validity	Preservation time
Water	x	
Saliva	xx	1–2 h
Saline solution	xxx	2–3 h
Milk	xxxxx	Up to 8 h
HBSS	xxxxxx	24 h
Viaspan	xxxxxxxxx	Up to 48 h

x: least recommended; xxxxxxxxx: most recommended.

Some studies show that adolescents, their relatives, paramedical staff, and a large proportion of staff working in schools and sports facilities have insufficient knowledge of the subject; as a result, they are totally incapable of providing correct and timely therapy.

In a survey of 211 Kuwaiti students, Andersson et al (2006) found that the vast majority of respondents had little knowledge about avulsions and re-implantation and the stages of emergency treatment.

Even in dentistry classes, the level of knowledge of dental trauma management procedures is not high.

Hu et al (2006) reported the results of a survey of 230 generic dentists and 70 Brazilian endodontists. The study found a low level of knowledge on emergency treatment of traumatic injuries, especially among general dental practitioners. Thus, while 93.4% of dentists understood the need to perform replanting of the detached teeth within 30 minutes, only 59.1% knew that semi-rigid splinting is the most suitable splinting and that it should be maintained for up to 2 weeks.

Immediate dental replanting is an emergency therapeutic procedure; it provides a very good prognosis and requires not less than 8–10 years of residence of the tooth in the arch. The prognosis becomes less favorable in cases of late replanting because the survival of the root of the replanted tooth is considerably reduced because of certain phenomena, which are described below.

Immediate replanting

Replanting should be quickly performed to maintain the viability of the periodontal ligament (PDL), whose cells and fibers begin to degenerate within 60 minutes after trauma. If replanting is performed within 60 minutes after the detachment, it is very likely that the PDL will heal, with no root ankylosis.

Maintenance of the tooth in a humid environment and timely replanting is therefore essential for the preservation of the PDL. Ideally, the tooth should be replanted immediately after the trauma by nonmedical personnel, such as parents, teachers or coaches, who are present at the time of the detachment; they should be properly informed about the correct procedures to be performed in order to minimize the time the detached tooth is in an extraoral environment. If this does not happen, as often occurs, the patient must be promptly sent to the nearest dental care facility while keeping the tooth detached in a suitable humid environment (Fig. 9.42).

The replanting must be performed after verifying the adequacy of the element, confirming of the patency and structural adequacy of the alveolus, and cleaning the tooth and alveolus with saline solution (Fig. 9.43).

The tooth should be placed back in its normal position, correctly splinted to the adjacent elements (or to the nearest ones able to hold the restraint). The *health status of the pulp* should be assessed subsequently (within 7 days after the trauma).

After a week, in approximately 80% of cases of teeth with mature apex, pulpectomy of the re-inserted element and closing of the endodontic space must be performed, first provisionally using Ledermix paste and after approximately 15–30 days with the application of a calcium hydroxide dressing. Subsequently, in the absence of signs of external inflammatory resorption, the canal space should be closed definitively with gutta-percha and cement.

In *immature* (open apex) *elements*, endodontic treatment should be conducted using the same calcium hydroxide dressing as that used when initiating an apexification procedure; after 6–12 months, it usually leads to the closing of the apex, which must be followed by definitive closing of the endodontic space with cement and gutta-percha.

In *very immature elements that are re-implanted* under optimal conditions, pulp viability is often maintained and should be assessed every 2 weeks for at least 1 year using appropriate sensitivity tests and control x-rays; this phenomenon occurs because of the regenerative recovery of totipotent cells in the periapical spaces (Hertwig's epithelial sheath) and because of vessel proliferation. This regenerative and distributive process often involves an evolution toward the obliteration of the pulp canal, which can be accompanied by complete root development.

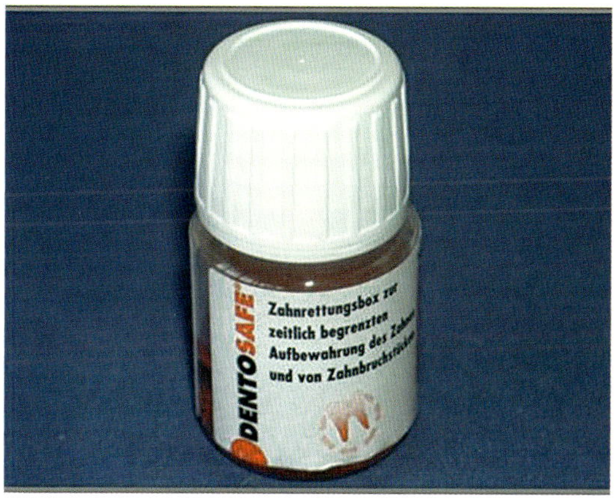

Figure 9.42 Ideal storing solution for detached teeth containing HBSS (trade preparation).

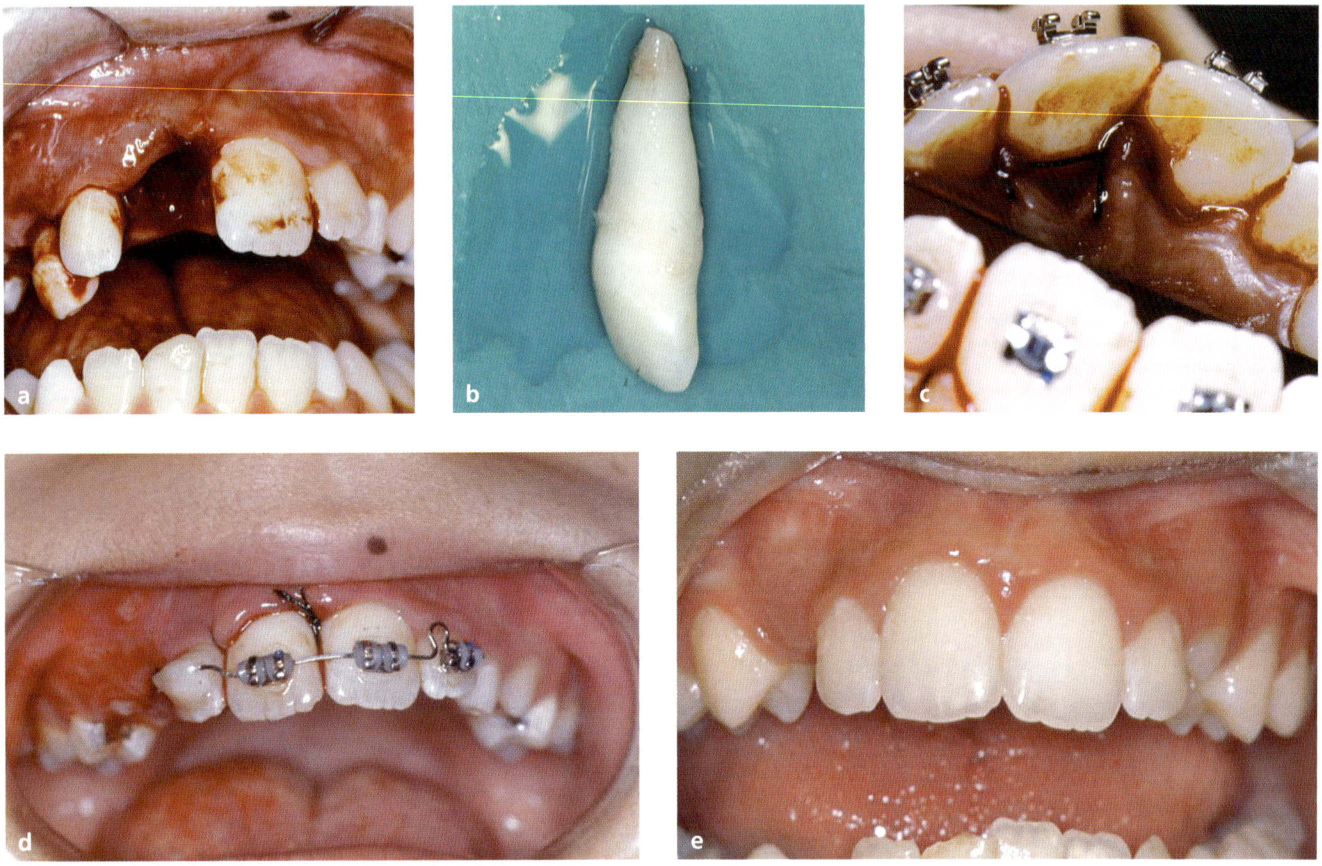

Figure 9.43 (**a**) Traumatic detachment approx. 2 hours after the accident. (**b**) 1.1 detached and stored in a wet environment; replantation is possible. (**c**) Replanted tooth, palatal image. (**d**) Replanted 1.1 tooth, splinted to the adjacent teeth. (**e**) Clinical check 30 months after the replant: the clinical conditions are optimal.

Delayed replanting

If the detached tooth is not appropriately stored i.e., it is not hydrated, or if the time after detachment is long (more than 1 hour), late replanting should be performed.
This treatment is advisable in adolescence because even if the element has a safe *replacement resorption of the root* (with ankylosis), it guarantees, at least temporarily, the preservation of esthetics and function, as well as the maintenance of the arch space and bone volume necessary for future prosthetic rehabilitation.
In adults, if replanting is not indicated, post-extraction rehabilitation or deferred technique can be selected; in any case, resorption phenomena in adults are less striking than in adolescents.
The *limitation* of late replanting, as already mentioned, is linked to the decay of the cells of the PDL, whose function cannot be restored. Therefore, the practice is to remove the PDL of the detached element before replanting. The tooth is kept in a 2% fluorine solution and antibiotic for 60 minutes and is then cleaned and inserted into the alveolus, which is also properly cleaned (elimination of the clot). Finally, the tooth is splinted according to the techniques described above.

In this case, endodontic treatment can be performed extraorally using a retrograde technique. It is essential to avoid bacterial contamination of the root.
If there are doubtful cases from the diagnostic perspective, i.e., the opportunity to perform an immediate or delayed replanting, immediate replanting should be indicated, thereby preserving the PDL if it is not particularly contaminated (some authors recommend the use of amelogenin-like substances to promote the healing of the PDL); otherwise, we should proceed as recommended for delayed replanting by performing root canal therapy within 2 weeks to reduce the risk of external inflammatory resorption.
Frequent x-ray examinations are recommended during the first 3 months after replantation to follow the patient's progress and to evaluate the presence of initial signals of radicular resorption (surface resorption), which can be completely transient. General supportive drug therapies (7–10 days) and anti-tetanus serum prophylaxis should not be neglected.

Prevention and treatment of post-replantation complications

Septic complications can be avoided by administering general antibiotics, e.g., tetracyclines; antibiotic solutions may also be used to dip the tooth (30 minutes) before replanting.
Anti-inflammatory, tetanus serum prophylaxis, and strict rules of oral hygiene should also be adhered to and recommended, such as application of chlorhexidine gel to the trauma site.
Complications associated with radicular resorption vary and are partly predictable.
Transient and reversible external radicular resorptions are usually favorable consequences of immediate replanting and recede as a result of antibiotic therapy (if the preset splinting is correct and maintained for approximately 14 days).
If the endodontic treatment of the replanted tooth is not conducted within the time specified in the protocol, *inflammatory external radicular resorption* is likely to occur in adolescents; it rapidly evolves and is completed within 30–60 days, leading to the early loss of the replanted tooth (Fig. 9.44).
A frequent outcome of delayed replantation is *root resorption with bone replacement*, which is more or less rapid depending on the patient's age and the timing of replanting. The greater the permanence of the tooth in an extraoral environment, the greater the rate of root resorption. The prevention of ankylosis also depends on the proper treatment of the tooth outside the alveolus (alveolar conditions, endodontic treatment, and radicular surface with 2% fluorine).
The most favorable prognosis allows a permanence of the replanted tooth in the arch for 5 to 10 years. The *most unfortunate outcome* in adolescents is *ankylosis of the replanted tooth*, which appears as an infraocclusion (Malmgren et al, 2002). Such infraocclusion manifests itself beginning at 11–13 years and becomes more marked with the progress of the skeletal growth of the individual; at the end of the growth period, it can manifest itself with bony gaps of approximately 7–10 mm (Fig. 9.45).
Thus, there is a need to reduce the impact of such infraocclusions in both functional and esthetic terms considering that it is not advisable and acceptable to refuse performing late replantation in a young injured person (8–11 years), although it is clear

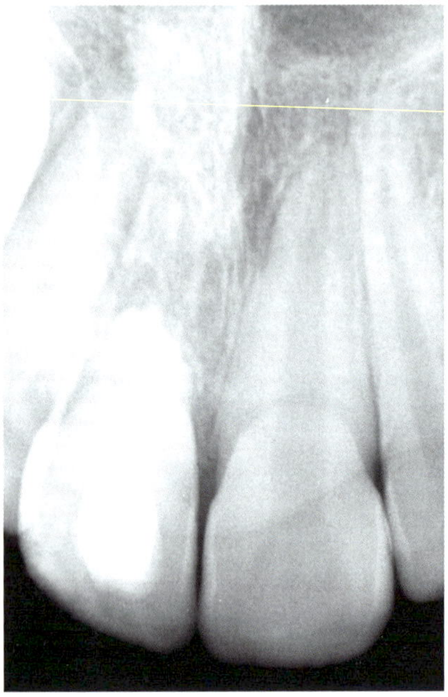

Figure 9.44 The tooth has been treated with a tardive replant (3 hours after the detachment), and root-canal therapy started 40 days after the replant. As seen in the X-ray images, a year after the accident, there is a significant radicular reabsorption with bone replacement. The treatment with calcium hydroxide can slow down complete root reabsorption.

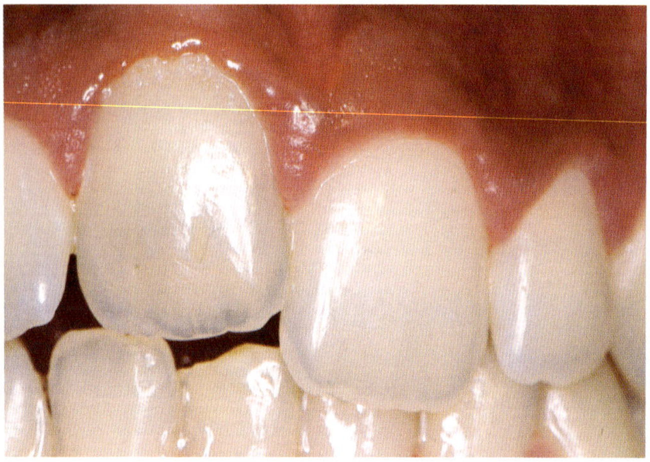

Figure 9.45 The image shows 1.1 infra-occlusion (subsequent to ankylosis); the tooth had been tardively replanted when the patient was 10 years and now, at 15 years, it shows a vertical bone gap of about 6 mm.

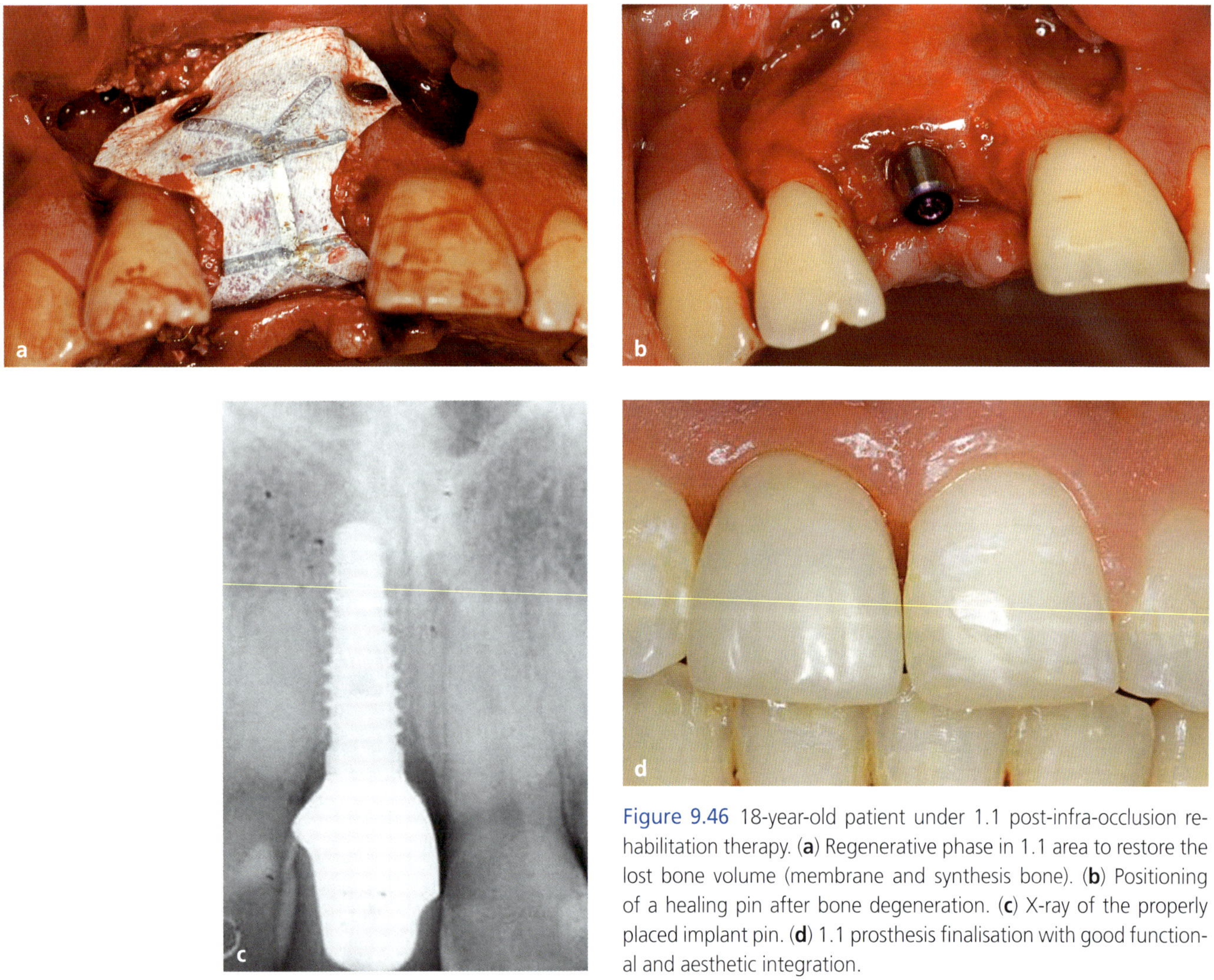

Figure 9.46 18-year-old patient under 1.1 post-infra-occlusion rehabilitation therapy. (**a**) Regenerative phase in 1.1 area to restore the lost bone volume (membrane and synthesis bone). (**b**) Positioning of a healing pin after bone degeneration. (**c**) X-ray of the properly placed implant pin. (**d**) 1.1 prosthesis finalisation with good functional and aesthetic integration.

that this late replanted tooth will certainly evolve into ankylosis and consequent infra-occlusion.

As explained before, infraocclusion will begin to manifest at the age of 11–13 years; this is the perfect time to make reasonable choices to avoid further bone loss. The alternatives proposed are as follows:

- ankylosed tooth extraction and orthodontic space closure
- tooth extraction and self-transplantation of premolar extracted for orthodontic purposes
- tooth decoronization of the ankylosed tooth and subsequent application of temporary prosthesis
- intentional replanting of the ankylosed tooth
- deciduous canine self-transplantation, only in younger patients (Pohl et al, 2008).

If the first two solutions are feasible in selected patients, all the reported solutions are practicable by very experienced clinicians and require, in any case, very intense cooperation from the child and his or her family members.

If none of the procedures described are performed, at 18–20 years of age, we will need to intervene at the site of ankylosis using regenerative methods, such as bone grafting, which is important for the restoration of the lost bone tissue, followed by appropriate implant-prosthesic rehabilitation techniques that guarantee adequate results to the esthetic area in question (Fig. 9.46).

In conclusion, the authors believe that the best treatment in case of traumatic detachment is the correct and rapid reintegration of the tooth into the alveolus in the shortest possible period and the proper preservation of the tooth. Hence, there is a need to provide appropriate dental storage ("Save a tooth® kit" containing HBSS, with long-term storage and at an affordable price) to sports and school facilities, especially in primary and secondary schools, where such traumas occur most frequently, and to trauma patients who are at a critical age. The distribution of such kits should be widespread in areas that are rural and far from dental care facilities that are equipped to receive traumatized patients. These kits, currently with a long shelf life (3 years), also have reasonable costs for large-scale use. Below we propose a scheme of the procedures to be undertaken in traumatic events that occur in adolescents and in permanent teeth (Tab. 9.12).

Table 9.12 Summary of the types and times of intervention and recovery with regard to trauma in permanent teeth

Lesion	Treatment	Recovery
Crown fracture without pulp exposure	• May be delayed (24–48 h) • Should be performed by a pediatric dentist	• Does not entail consequences if no other concomitant lesions (luxations) are present
Crown fracture with pulp exposure	• Can be immediate in specialist facilities • Pulpotomy/capping treatment	• Treatment duration is short (30 min) and should allow function to be resumed immediately • Outcomes of mild/medium-severity are possible
Crown–root fracture	• Can be delayed • Requires evaluation of the extent of fracture and pulp exposure (if any)	• Results in significant functional and esthetic impairments • Recovery is delayed and requires complex rehabilitation recovery interventions
Root fracture	• Should be immediate (splinting) and should be performed in specialist facilities • Requires diagnostic tests within 48 h	• Results in significant functional and partially esthetic impairments. • Recovery is delayed and requires follow-up for 30–60 days • Possible outcomes.
Dislocation	• Must be immediate with repositioning and splinting • Requires a delayed phase of check-ups and follow-ups	• Recovery can be immediate if injury is of limited severity • If treatment is postponed, recovery may require a long time and may involve possible consequences.
Avulsion	• Must be immediate and always continued in specialized facilities	• Functional recovery is delayed (48–72 h) and may be complicated by responses to therapies and patient age (resorption). • There are always outcomes of considerable severity.

References

Andersson L, Al-Asfour A, Al-Jame Q. Knowledge of first-aid measures for avulsion and replantation of teeth: an interview of 221 Kuwaiti schoolchildren. Dent Traumatol 2006; 22:57-65.

Andreasen JO, Andreasen FM. Essential of traumatic injuries to the teeth. Copenhagen: Ed. Munskgaard; 1990.

Andreasen JO, Bakland LK, Matras RC, Andreasen FM. Traumatic intrusion of permanent teeth. Part 2. A clinical study of the effect of preinjury and injury factors, such as sex, age, stage of root development, tooth location and extent of injury including number of intruded teeth on 140 intruded permanent teeth. Dent Traumatol 2006;22:90-8.

Andreasen JO, Bakland LK, Matras RC, Andreasen FM. Traumatic intrusion of permanent teeth. Part 3. A clinical study of the effect of treatment variables such as treatment delay, method of repositioning, type of splint, length of splinting and antibiotics on 140 teeth. Dent Traumatol 2006;22:99-111.

Barrett EJ, Kenny DJ. Survival of avulsed permanent maxillary incisors in children following delayed renplantation. Endod Dent Traumatol 1997;13: 269-75.

Bauss O, Röhling J, Schwestka-Polly R. Prevalence of traumatic injuries to the permanent incisors in candidates for orthodontic treatment. Dent Traumatol 2004;20(2):61-6.

Bornstein MM, Wolner-Hanssen AB, Sendi P, von Arx T. Comparison of intraoral radiography and limited cone beam computed tomography for the assessment of root-fractured permanent teeth. Dent Traumatol 2009;25:571-7.

Borum MK, Andreasen JO. Sequelae of trauma to primary maxillary incisors. I. Complications in the primary dentition. Endod Dent Traumatol 1998;14:31-44.

Burden DJ. An investigation of the association between overjet size, lip coverage, and traumatic injury to maxillary incisors. Eur J Orthod 1995;17(6):513-7.

Caprioglio C, Caprioglio A, Caprioglio D. La traumatologia nei denti decidui. Quaderni di traumatologia Dentaria. Bologna: Edizioni Martina; 2007.

Caprioglio D, Manna A, Paglia L. Manuale di traumatologia dento-alveolare. Milano: Ed. Ciba; 1996.

Çetinbas¸ T, Sönmez H. Mouthguard utilization rates during sport activities in Ankara, Turkey. Dent Traumatol 2006;22:127-9.

Cvek M. A clinical report on partial pulpotomy and capping with calcium hydroxide in permanent incisors with complicated crown fracture. J Endod 1978;4:232-7.

Cvek M, Andreasen JO, Borum MK. Healing of 208 intralveolar root fractures in patients aged 7-17 years. Dent Traumatol 2001;17:53-62.

Doyle DL, Dumsha TC, Sydiskis RJ. Effect of soaking in Hank's balanced salt solution or milk on PDL cell viability of dry stored human teeth. Endod Dent Traumatol 1998;14:221-4.

Ellis RG, Davey KW. The classification and treatment of injuries to the teeth of children. Chicago: Year Book Mediacal Publisher Inc.; 1945.

Feliciano KM, de Franca Caldas A Jr. A systematic review of the diagnostic classifications of traumatic dental injuries. Dental Traumatol 2006;22:71-6.

Gargiulo AW et al. Dimensions and relations of the dentogingival junction in humans. J Periodontol 1961;32:261.

Glendor U. On dental trauma in children and adolescents. Incidence risk, treatment, time and costs. Swed Dent J Suppl 2000;14:1-52.

Glendor U. Aetiology and risk factors related to traumatic dental injuries: a review of the literature. Dent Traumatol 2009;25:19-31.

Heithersay GS. Combined endodontic-orthodontic treatment of transverse root fractures in the region of the alveolar crest. Oral Surg 1973;36:404-15.

Holan G. Long-term effect of different treatment modalities for traumatized primary incisors presenting dark coronal discoloration with no other signs of injury. Dent Traumatol 2006;22:14-7.

Hu LW, Prisco CDR, Bombana AC. Knowledge of Brazilian general dentists and endodontists about the emergency management of dento-alveolear trauma. Dent Traumatol 2006;22:113-7.

Kahnberg KE. Surgical extrusion of root-fractured teeth. A follow-up study of two surgical methods. Endod Dent Traumatol 1988;4:85-9.

Lieger O, von Arx T. Orofacial/cerebral injuries and the use of mouthguards by professional athletes in Switzerland. Dent Traumatol 2006;22:1-6.

Loh T, Sae Lim V, Yian TB, Liang S. Dental therapist' experience in the immediate managment of traumatized teeth. Dent Traumatol 2006;22:66-70.

Maeda Y, Kumamoto D, Kumamoto Y, Kazunori I. Effectiveness and fabrication of mouthguards. Dent Traumatol 2009;25:556-64.

Malmgren B, Malmgren O. Rate of infraposition of reimplanted ankylosed incisors related to age and growth in children and adolescent. Dent Traumatol 2002;18:28-36.

Malmgren O, Malmgren B, Frykholm A. Rapid orthodontic extrusion of crown root and cervical root fractured teeth. Endod Dent Traumatol 1991;7:49-54.

Marushima M. Pulpal healing using calcium hydroxide preparation [in Japanese]. J Oral Med 1958;25:149.

Matalon V, Brin I, Moskovitz M, Ram D. Compliance of children and youngsters in the use of mouthguard. Dent Traumatol 2008;24:462-7.

Nakabayashi N, Kojima K, Masuhara E. The promotion of adhesion by the infiltration of monomers into tooth substrates. J Biomed Mater Res 1982;16:265-73.

Nakabayashi N, Nakamura M, Yasuda N. Hybrid layer as a dentin-bonding mechanism. J Esthet Dent 1991;3:133-8.

Oginni AO, Adekoya-Sofowora CA, Kolawole KA. Evalutation of radiographs, clinical signs and symptoms associated with pulp canal obliteration: an aid to treatment decision. Dent Traumatol 2009;25:620-5.

Öz IA, Haytaç MC, Toroğlu MS. Multidisciplinary approach to the rehabilitation of a crown-root fracture with original fragment for immediate esthetics: a case report with 4-year follow-up. Dent Traumatol 2006;22:48-52.

Pohl Y, Filippi A, Kirschner H. Results after replantation of avulsed permanent teeth. II. Periodontal healing and the role of physiologic storage and antiresorptive- regenerative therapy. Dent Traumatol 2005;21:93-101.

Pohl Y, Geist P, Filippi A. Tranplantation of primary canines after loss or ankylosis of upper permanent incisors. A prospective case series study on healing and survival. Dent Traumatol 2008;24:388-403.

Ranalli DN, Spinas E, Altana M. Metodiche innovative di prevenzione dei traumi dento-facciali nello sport. Dent Mod 1999;5:77-92.

Shulman JD, Peterson J. The association between incisor trauma and occlusal characteristics in individual 8-50 years of age. Dent Traumatol 2004;20:67-74.

Simonsen RJ. Restoration of the fractured central incisor using original tooth fragment. J Am Dent Assoc 1982;105:646-50.

Spinas E, Altana M. A new classification for crown fractures of teeth. J Clin Pediatr Dent 2002;26(3):225-31.

Spinas E, Melis A, Savasta A. Therapeutic approach to intrusive luxation injuries in primary dentition. A clinical follow up study. Eur J Paediatric Dent 2006 Dec;7(4):179-86.

Spinas E, Melis A. Approccio conservativo al trattamento delle fratture traumatiche corono-radicolari. In: Progressi in Odontoiatria. Torino: UTET; 2005. p. 231-73.

Spinas E, Savasta A. Prenvention of traumatic dental lesions: cognitive research on the role of mouthguards during sport activities in paediatric age. Eur J Paediatric Dent 2007 Dec;8(4):187-92.

Spinas E. Odontoiatria e sport. Milano: Edizioni Edi ermes; 2009.

Spinas E. A biological conservative approach to complex traumatic dento-alveolar lesions. J Clin Pediatric Dent 2003 Fall;28(1):1-10.

Spinas E. Longevity of composite restorations of traumatically injured teeth. Am J Dent 2004;17(6): 407-11.

Takeda T, Ishigami K, Ogawa T et al. Are all mouthguards the same and safe to use? The influence of occlusal supporting mouthguards in decreasing bone distortion and fractures. Dent Traumatol 2004;20:150-6.

Tenca JI, Tsamtsouris A. Continued root end development: apexogenesis and apexification. J Pedod 1978;2:144-57.

Trope M. Root resorption of dental and traumatic origin: classification based on etiology. Pract Periodont Aesthet Dent 1998;10:515-22.

Tsukiboshi M. Il trattamento dei traumi dentali. Milano: Scienza e tecnica dentistica Edizioni Internazionali; 2000.

Wilson RD, Maynard JG. Intracrevicular restorative dentistry. Int J Periodontics Restorative Dent 1981;4:34.

Zachrinsson BU, Jacobsen I. Long term prognosis of 66 permanent anterior teeth with root fractures. Scand J Dent Res 1975;83:345-54.

Chapter 10

Dental materials in pediatric dentistry

L. Breschi, E. De Stefano Dorigo, M. Ferrari

Prevention materials

Fluoride agents for professional topical treatment

The safety and effectiveness of fluoride for the prevention and control of caries have been previously documented (Adair, 2006). There are various mechanisms of action of fluoride for protection from caries, including remineralization of enamel and alteration of bacterial metabolism (Featherstone, 2000) (Table 10.1). Topical application of fluoride should be based on the assessment of the carioreceptivity risk while considering the daily dose that patients are exposed to (Adair, 2006).

Professional treatments have been shown to significantly reduce the incidence of caries in children at moderate or high risk (American Dental Association Council on Scientific Affairs, 2006; Bader et al, 2001). Over time, a series of methods and technologies have been developed for the application of various fluoride compounds on tooth surfaces; the pharmaceutical forms most commonly used in clinical practice are gels and varnishes.

Fluoride gels

Fluoride gel has the advantage of being easy to use, especially if applied using special trays, and is particularly indicated for the simultaneous treatment of multiple teeth. Various fluoride agents are available in gel form for topical application; the most stud-

Table 10.1 Mechanisms of action of fluoride

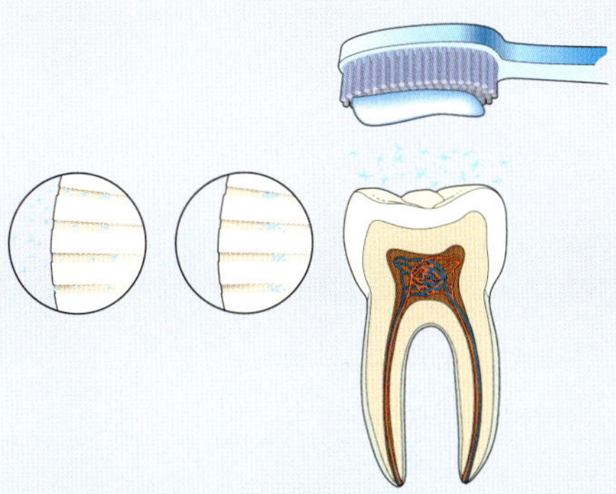

- Incorporation of fluoride into enamel microstructure with the production of fluorapatite $Ca_{10}(PO_4)_6(OH)_2+2F^- \; Ca_{10}(PO_4)6F_2+2OH^-$
- (Hydroxyapatite) (fluorapatite)
- Fluoride promotes remineralization
- It is an inhibitor of some bacterial enzymes
- The F^- ion influences the absorption of acquired film and bacterial aggregation because of its affinity for Ca^{2+} ion

ied and recommended fluoride agents are 2% sodium fluoride (NaF; 9,000 ppm) and 1.23% acidulated fluorophosphate (APF; 12,300 ppm) (Adair, 2006).
APF products are composed of a mixture of NaF, hydrogen fluoride (HF), and orthophosphoric acid, with the addition of coupling agents, coloring agents, and flavoring agents in an aqueous gel. They have low pH values, which favor fluoride absorption at the enamel level, and phosphate ions, which help contain fluoride dissolution.
Among fluoride agents, 2% neutral NaF gels are chemically very stable, do not irritate the gingival mucous membranes, and do not present a risk of discoloration of dental elements or restorative materials. They are also indicated in the use of glass ionomer cement and composite or ceramic restorations because they do not cause the unintentional etching effect caused by compounds with low pH.
New thixotropic gels introduced in the market have the capability to become fluid under pressure in order to facilitate penetration into interproximal areas and then return to their original consistency once removed, thereby ensuring better adherence to the tooth surface.
Prophylaxis with pumice is not an essential prerequisite (Johnston and Lewis, 1995); instead, appropriate precautionary measures should be taken to prevent children from ingesting the gel.

Fluoride varnishes

Fluoride varnishes have the advantages of achieving good adherence to the tooth surface, increasing contact time, and decreasing fluoride ingestion risk. Hence, these varnishes are particularly indicated for the treatment of single dental elements. The most commonly used varnishes are those with 5% NaF (225,000 ppm) (Adair, 2006; Petersson et al, 2004). Although further quality clinical studies are needed, the effectiveness of varnishes is comparable to that of gels.
A recent literature review of the Cochrane Database of Systematic Reviews reported a caries reduction rate of 33% in deciduous teeth and 46% in permanent teeth (Marinho et al, 2005). Some of these products are marketed with recommended application times of less than 4 minutes, although some studies suggest that increasing the application time leads to a greater efficacy (Adair, 2006).
The frequency of professional treatments should be 6 monthly for patients at moderate risk of caries and quarterly for those at high risk (American Dental Association Council on Scientific Affairs, 2006; Kallestal, 2005).

Sealants

Pit and fissure sealants are materials that, because of micromechanical adhesion to the enamel, create a barrier against the bacteria responsible for caries in the areas most prone to this pathology. Pit and fissure caries are in fact the most rapid and prevalent type of caries, representing more than 80% of all caries in the permanent dentition of young individuals (Brown et al, 1996). The effectiveness of sealants in caries prevention is related to their durability. Retention of the sealant should be assessed via regular checks to allow early intervention for restoring the sealant in case of total loss or leakage.

Chemically, sealants are similar to composite resins that are used as restorative materials, mainly differing in their viscosity, which is lower and allows their deep penetration in to pits and fissures. Basically, sealants are single-component photopolymerizable resin systems that comprise diluted methacrylate monomers such as bisphenol A-glycidyl methacrylate (bis-GMA or Bowen resin) or urethane dimethacrylate (UDMA) and are used in association with the etching techniques proposed by Buonocore to increase enamel retention (Buonocore, 1955).

The acid most commonly used for etching is 37% orthophosphoric acid. The recommended application time of 15 seconds is considered sufficient to etch the enamel at an appropriate depth to ensure good sealant retention (Duggal et al, 1997). The acid should be carefully rinsed to stop the demineralization reaction and remove any etch residue (Fig. 10.1).

Resins with inorganic fillers whose content can reach 75% are available in the market. Clinicians should be aware of the quantity of filler in the sealant used by them to ensure adequate application. Indeed, high percentages of filler improve mechanical properties; however, they require greater caution with regard to polymerization and careful occlusion control at the end of the procedure.

Color-changing sealants such as Clinpro™ (3M ESPE) are also available; it changes color from pink to white during polymerization, owing to the addition of titanium

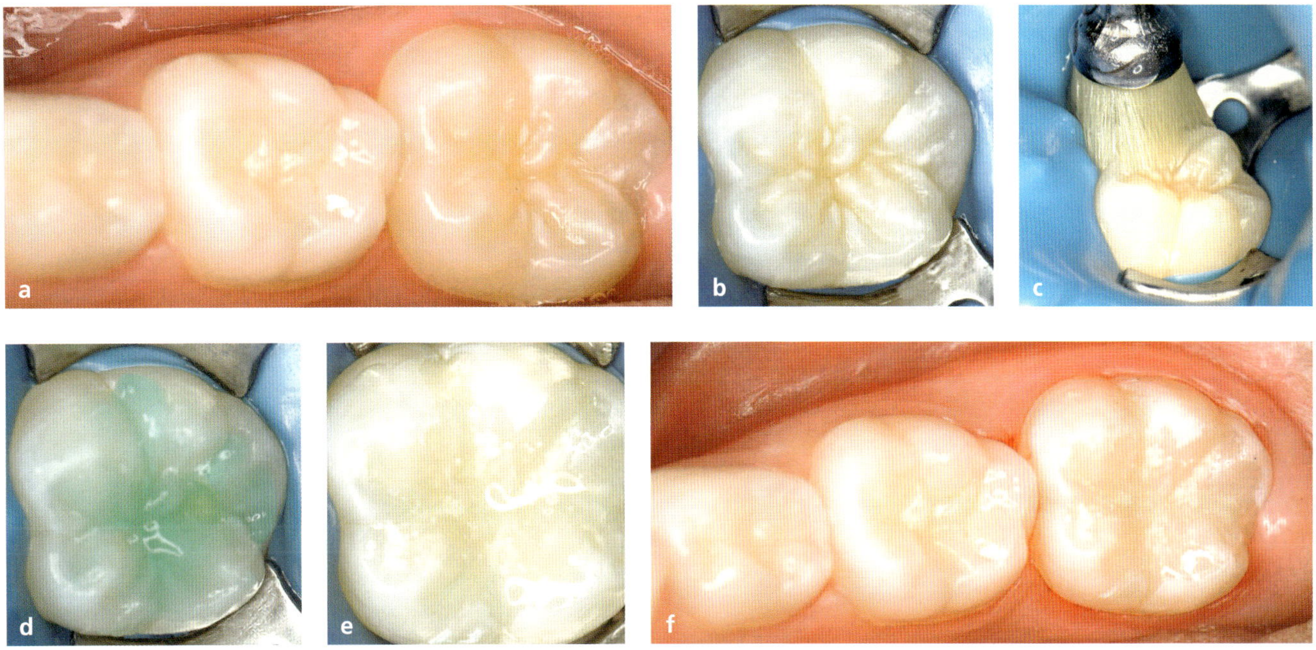

Figure 10.1 Step-by-step sealing procedure. (**a**) Initial clinical presentation. (**b**) Proper operative field isolation using a rubber dam. (**c**) Appropriate cleansing of fissures and pits to remove the salivary pellicle, plaque, and any other contaminant. (**d**) Etching with orthophosphoric acid gel for 15–30 seconds. (**e**) After polymerization, the sealant appears properly spread on the tooth surface. (**f**) Final image of the sealing after clamp and rubber dam removal.

dioxide, thereby allowing correct adaptation in the fluid phase and a quick evaluation of the integrity of the sealant at subsequent checks. Another sealant available is Helioseal Clear Chroma (Ivoclar-Vivadent), a clear and translucent sealant that changes color to olive green when exposed to curing light. However, the preferred products are those containing opacifying agents. This is because the presence of the sealant should be easily verifiable during placement and at subsequent follow-ups.

Previously, to reduce the caries risk at sealant edges, products containing fluoride were also available, but there are no clinical studies demonstrating their effectiveness (Vrbic, 1999). The fluoride present in the sealant resin has extremely low availability and release values compared with other dental materials such as glass ionomer cements (García-Godoy et al, 1997). More recent fluoride inclusion methods have increased the availability of fluoride by decreasing its association with resin chemistry. Nevertheless, some authors claim that the use of fluoride sealants is appropriate and state that although there is no evidence regarding the clinical benefit provided by these sealants, no negative effect on their retention has been identified (Morphis et al, 2000).

Glass ionomer cements have also been evaluated as sealants for their hydrophilicity and their distinctive fluoride-releasing feature. However, because of their fragility and susceptibility to break under high masticatory loads, their use as sealants is historically contraindicated.

To draft guidelines on the use of pit and fissure sealants, the American Dental Association conducted a literature review that revealed limited and contradictory evidence on a significant reduction in the incidence of caries using glass ionomer cements compared with resin-based sealants (Beauchamp et al, 2008; Pardi et al, 2003; Pardi et al, 2005; Pereira et al, 2003; Taifour et al, 2003; Songpaisan et al, 1995). In particular, a very low retention rate was observed (Ahovuo-Saloranta et al, 2004). Therefore, glass ionomer cements are currently recommended as a transitional sealant material for tooth surfaces considered at high risk for caries development that do not allow good insulation, such as partially erupted elements. Further studies on resin-modified glass ionomer cements compared with resin-based sealants should be conducted to provide scientific evidence of their effectiveness.

Restoration materials

Glass ionomer cements

Traditional

Glass ionomer cements are materials comprising a base powder [calcium fluoroaluminosilicate (SiO_2-Al_2O_3-CaF_2-Na_3AlF_6-$AlPO_4$), barium glass, and zinc oxide] and an acidic liquid (aqueous solutions of 47.5% polyacrylic acid and itaconic or maleic acid copolymer and 5% tartaric acid), which react as a result of an acid–base reaction between the two components (Fig. 10.2).

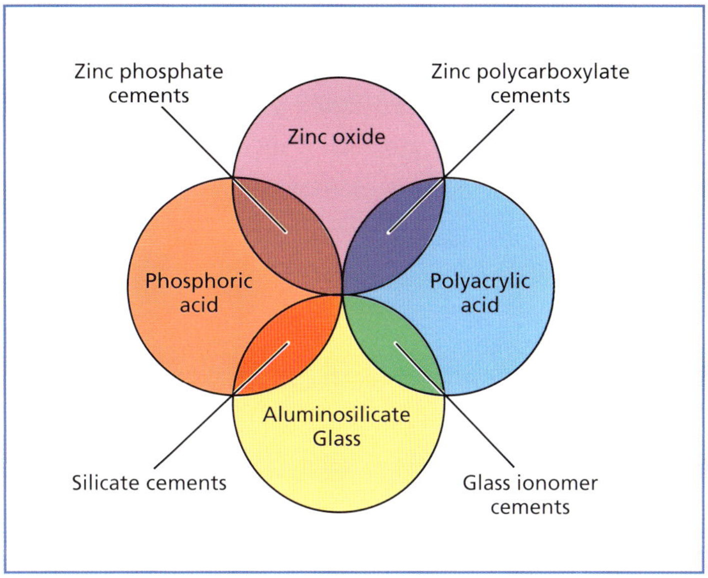

Figure 10.2 Composition of cements used in dentistry.

The activation process occurs in three phases (Fig. 10.3):

- acid dissolution of polyacrylic acid
- gelation: release of Ca^{2+} ions, which react with COO^- groups (the reaction takes place within the first 3 hours)
- hardening: release of Al^{3+} ions, which react with COO^- groups (the reaction takes more than 24 hours).

Tartaric acid binds to Al^{3+} ions, thereby removing them from polyacrylic acid.
Several formulations that can be used as a restoration or cement material and as a cavity base or *liner* are available in the market.
Their distinguishing feature is the ability to release fluoride after setting (F^- ions not involved in the bonds), thereby creating a variation in the mineralization of tooth surfaces in contact with them and preventing the potential formation of secondary caries (Tam et al, 1997). The fluoride release increases in the first week, reduces in the following 6 months, and remains constant for at least 3 years. Some studies have shown that fluoride release continues for at least 5 years (Swartz et al, 1984). Glass ionomer cements also play the role of fluoride *reservoirs*; they can absorb fluoride from toothpastes, mouthwashes, gels, and varnishes (Donly and Nelson, 1997). Because of their preventive action due to fluoride, these cements have been especially indicated for the cementation of preformed steel crowns, space maintainers, and orthodontic bands in patients with high carioreceptivity (Donly et al, 1995).
During the setting reaction, the cement ions interact with calcium and phosphate ions present in enamel and dentin. Improved adhesion can be achieved if the dentin surface is first treated with a mild acid, such as polyacrylic acid, which allows the removal of the *smear layer* (Powis et al, 1982). The strength of the bond with dentin, however, is quite low compared with those of composite materials and modified glass ionomer cements. Solubility in aqueous environments is high in the early stages, whereas it is good once setting has been achieved (Crisp et al, 1980). Therefore, it is necessary to be very care-

ful in avoiding contact with oral fluids in the initial stages of the acid–base reaction (Negm et al, 1982).

Their fragility and poor resistance to wear have led to the development of materials with better mechanical properties, such as modified glass ionomer cements.

Cermets

Cermets are glass ionomer cements reinforced with metal powders. Silver is the most commonly used metal, although other metals such as tin, gold, titanium, and palladium have been used.

The reaction type is acid–base, similar to that occurring in other glass ionomer cements. The silver present in these cements confers a grayish color to the restorations, which negatively affects their esthetic features, and a degree of radiopacity that is not achievable using traditional glass ionomer cements.

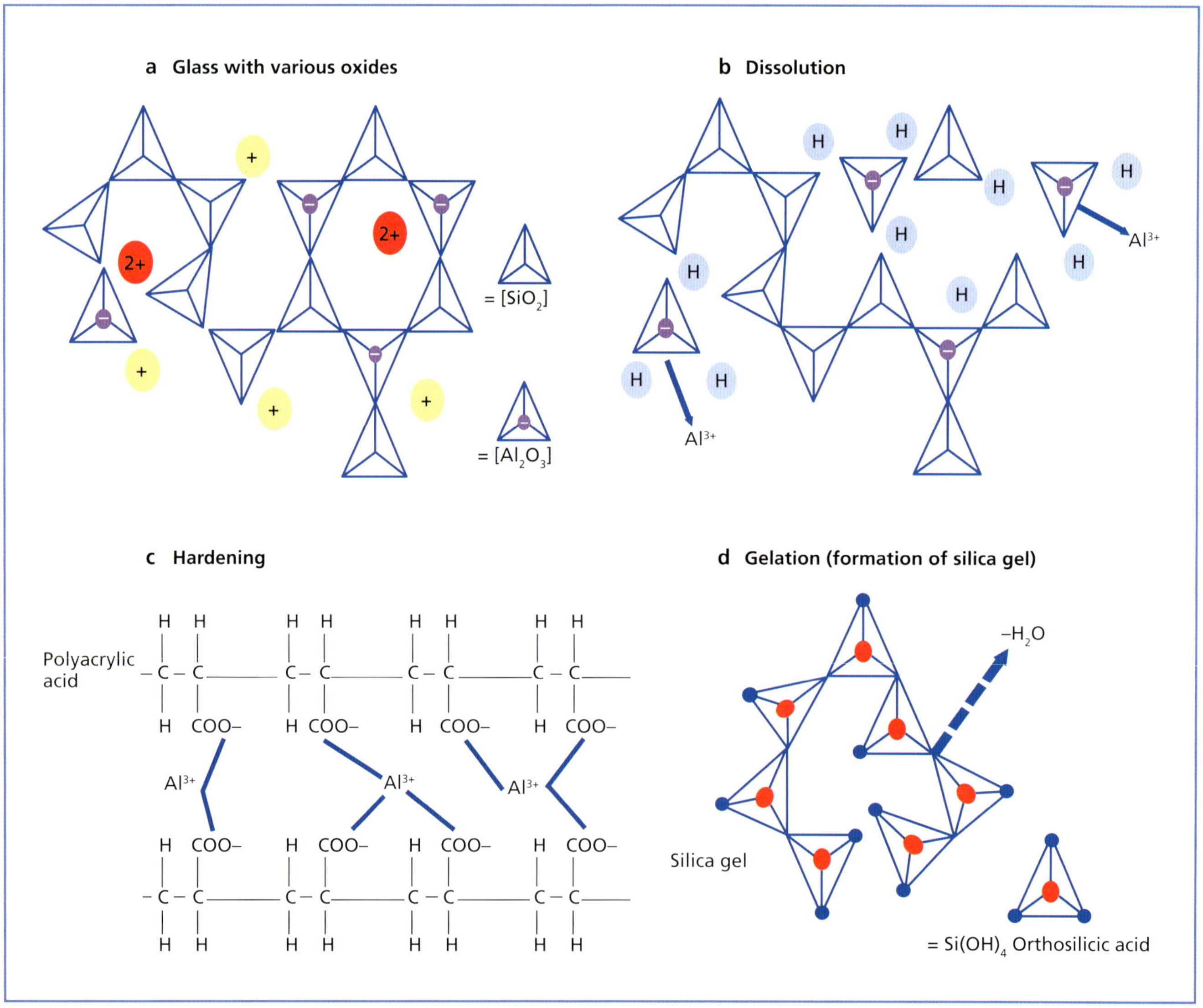

Figure 10.3 (**a**) Glass with various oxides. (**b**) Acid dissolution. (**c**) Hardening. (**d**) Gelation.

The mechanical characteristics of cermets such as compression and fatigue resistance are improved, whereas their *flexural strength* and abrasive wear resistance test results are similar to those of traditional glass ionomer cements. Finally, the fluoride release from these restorations is significantly lower than that from conventional glass ionomer cements (Craig, 1998).

Resin-modified glass ionomer cements

These are direct derivatives of the traditional glass ionomers with the addition of a resin component. The need for a modified glass ionomer material fundamentally arises from the need to improve some mechanical properties and reduce moisture susceptibility after mixing, with advantages such as fluoride release remaining unchanged (Yoshii et al, 1992).

The setting reaction is caused by an acid–base interaction, typical of traditional glass ionomers, with an associated polymerization reaction (auto- or photo-activated) of the resin's methacrylic component.

For surface conditioning, a mild acid can be used, such as citric or polyacrylic acid (Kato et al, 1995), for 15 seconds.

Analyses performed using a scanning electron microscope have highlighted that resin-modified glass ionomers create a hybrid layer, which is not present in conventional glass ionomer cements (Forsten et al, 1998). Usually, these materials have a lower solubility in aqueous environments (Cho et al, 1995; Quackenbush et al, 1998) and greater compression and wear resistance than traditional glass ionomer cements (Kerby et al, 1992). The better mechanical and esthetic properties make these materials preferable to conventional glass ionomer cements for deciduous tooth restoration (Vilkinis et al, 2000; Rutar et al, 2002; Donly et al, 1999; Croll et al, 2001).

Composites

Composite materials, which are based on the principles of dentin/enamel adhesion, represented a decisive and substantial turning point in restorative dentistry as a universal material for direct restoration. Composite resins are materials that comprise a polymer combined with inorganic vitreous particles.

The polymer constitutes the composite matrix in which the inorganic particles serving as fillers are dispersed and are chemically bound to the polymer through a binding agent (Ferracane, 2011). This three-dimensional combination of chemically different materials, with a distinct interface separating the components, results in the formation of a new material with mechanical properties that are generally superior to those of the separate individual components.

Essentially, the physical–mechanical properties of composites are determined by the matrix to filler quantitative ratio, filler type, resin matrix chemical structure, and polymerization type.

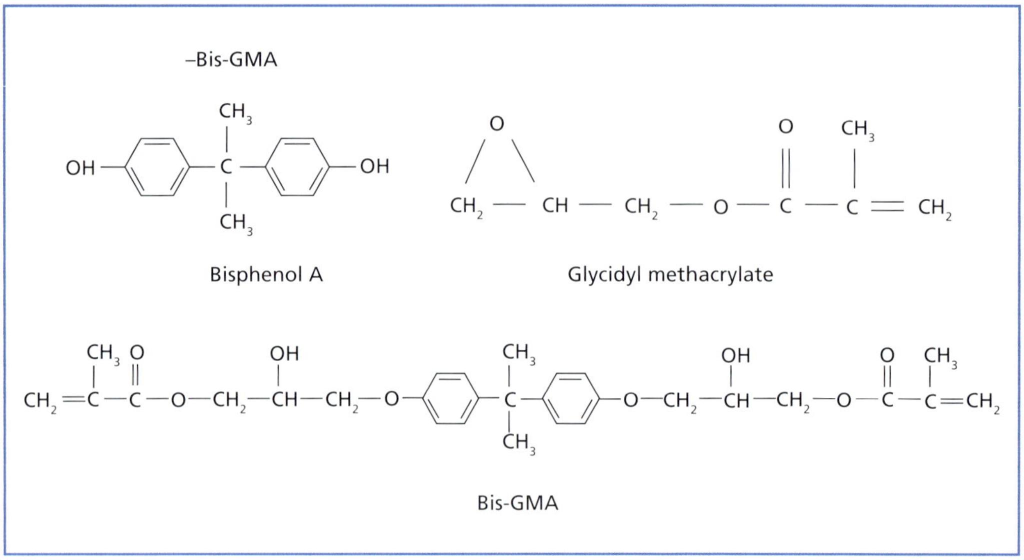

Figure 10.4 Bis-GMA formation.

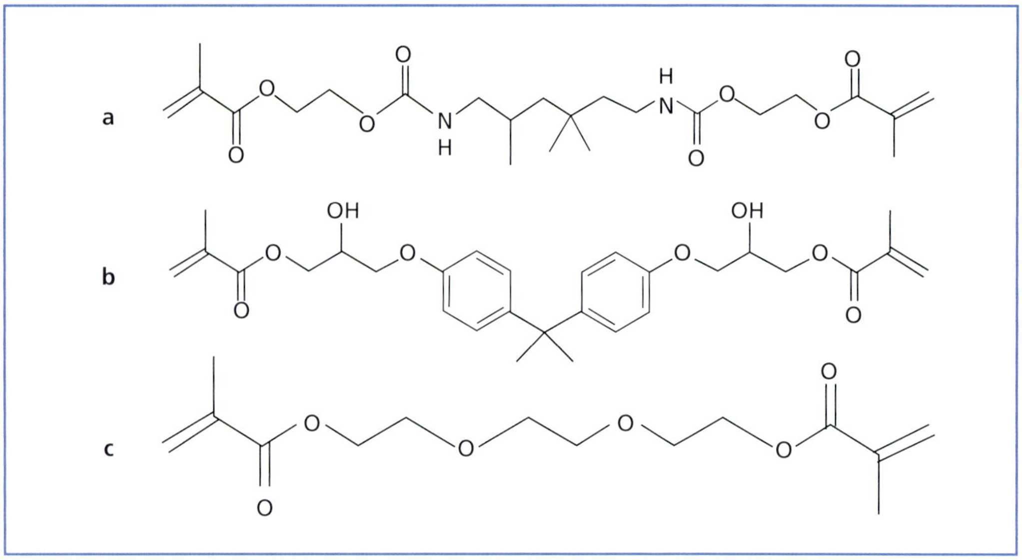

Figure 10.5 Monomers frequently present in the organic matrix of composites and their chemical formula: (**a**) bis-GMA, (**b**) TEGMA, and (**c**) UDMA.

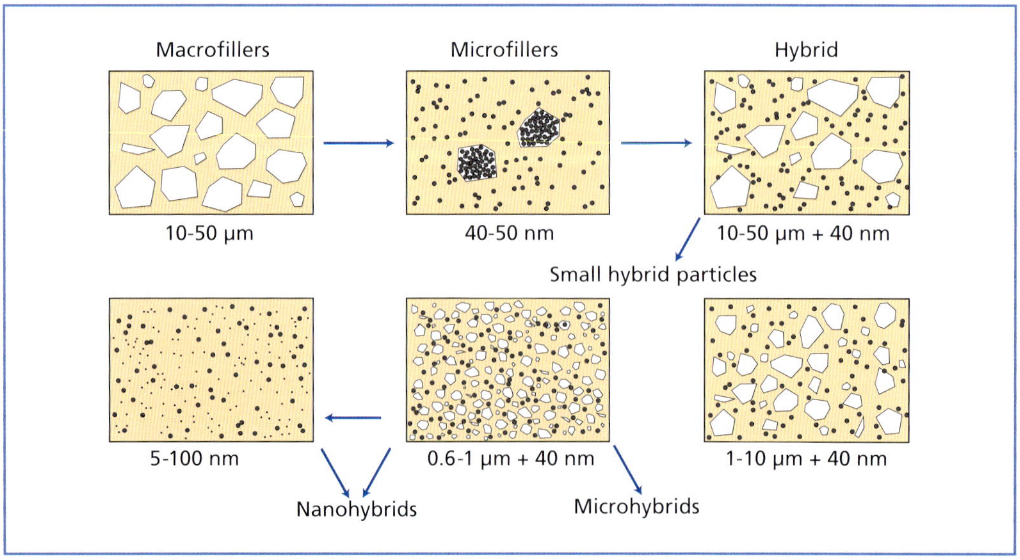

Figure 10.6 Size of fillers used in most common composites (Ferracane, 2011).

Composites used for direct restoration are light-cured. Thus, the setting reaction is induced following exposure to a light of suitable intensity and wavelength to induce the formation of a polymer, i.e., a molecule consisting of elementary units repeated n number of times within the same molecule. The number of elementary units (monomers) varies from a few thousand to millions. The length of the molecules or their molecular weight has considerable influence on the polymer properties: usually, melting temperature, rigidity, and viscosity increase with increasing molecular weight. The most widely used polymers available on the market are methacrylate resins such as bis-GMA, or Bowen resin, which is the reaction product of one bisphenol A molecule and two dicidyl-methacrylate molecules, or UDMA (Fig. 10.4).
Bis-GMA is a highly viscous liquid and is mixed with diacrylate monomers of lower molecular weight, such as EGDMA or triethylene glycol dimethacrylate (TEDDMA). An inhibitor, such as hydroquinone, is often added in trace amounts (Fig. 10.5).
The inorganic matrix is the substance added to a composite material as a filler to counteract the lack of resistance of the organic matrix itself. Thus, the composite mechanical properties are enhanced, the hardness and compression resistance are increased, and the thermal expansion coefficient is decreased, and at the same time, the esthetic characteristics are improved (Ferracane, 2011).
The filler may vary according to chemical composition, size, and quantity. Based on composition, there are silica-based particles and particles with a complex chemical composition, such as barium, zinc, strontium, lithium, aluminum, borosilicate, zirconium, and ceramic glasses.

According to the particle size, there are six types of fillers (Fig. 10.6):

- mega fillers, from 2 to 0.5 mm
- macro fillers, from 100 to 10 µm
- medium fillers, from 10 to 1 µm
- mini fillers, from 1 to 0.1 µm
- micro fillers, from 0.1 to 0.01 µm
- nano fillers, from 0.01 to 0.005 µm (Bayne et al, 1994).

The function of coupling agents is to improve the bond between the organic matrix and filler; hence, they contribute to increase the material's biomechanical properties. Coupling agents are mainly silanes, which are deposited on the filler particles. Methoxy silane groups are partially hydrolyzed with the OH groups present on the filler, thereby binding to it. During polymerization, the double bonds of the molecule react with the oligomer, leading to continuity in the final structure, which improves the mechanical properties (Fig. 10.7).
Composites allow a more conservative approach in dental element preparation, outdating Black's old concept of "*extension for prevention*," which prevailed for more than a century. In fact, using these materials, small carious lesions can be restored without removing healthy tissue and sealing the remaining dental element. This technique has been described as preventive resin restoration. The minimally invasive conservative approach becomes especially relevant in the conservative treatment of deciduous

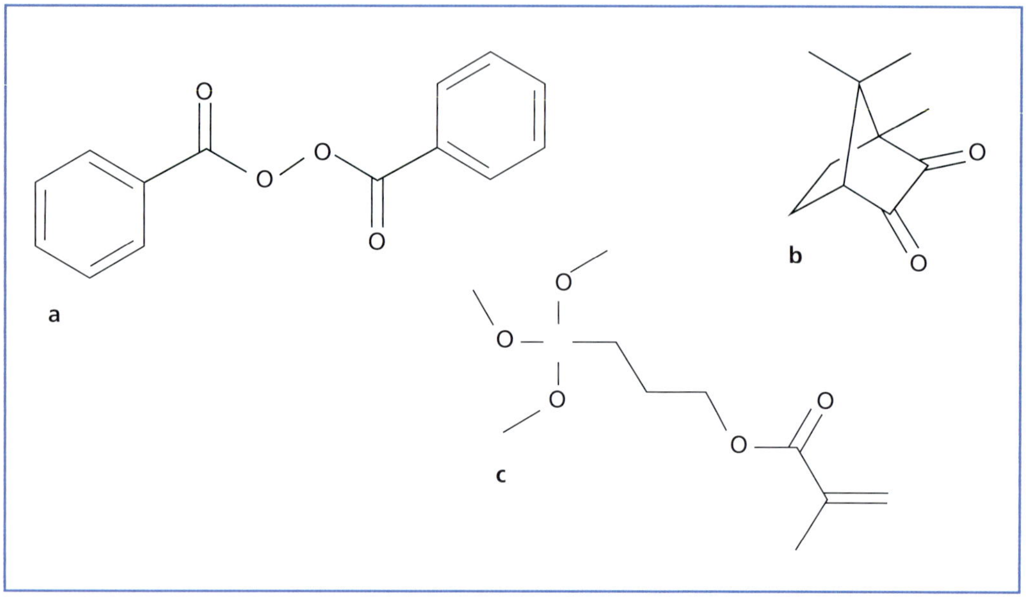

Figure 10.7 Polymerization starters and chemical formula of silanes: (**a**) benzoyl peroxide, (**b**) camphorquinone, and (**c**) silane.

teeth, which have a particularly less enamel and dentin thickness compared with the permanent teeth.

Universal composites have a consistency that allows them to be applied and modeled, whereas *flowable* composites are directly applied into cavities through a syringe as they have a low viscosity due to reduced filler content or the presence of surfactants. *Packable* composites, which are more viscous and compact, have lower workability but high resistance not because of an increase in filler content but because of modifications in the distribution of the size of the fillers or usage of other filler types, such as fibers. Recently, ormocers (*organically modified ceramics*) have also been introduced; these are silicon-based hybrid organic–inorganic polymers.

In pediatric dentistry, these materials are indicated for any class of restorations on both deciduous and permanent teeth (Donly and García-Godoy, 2002). However, there are situations in which composite restorations in children and adolescents may be contraindicated: operative technique and patient cooperation strongly influence the usage of these materials, and adequate moisture control of the operative field can be difficult to achieve in younger patients.

Table 10.2 summarizes the features of composite material components.

Amalgam

Dental amalgam is a multi-phase alloy derived from the reaction between liquid mercury and a powder containing several metals, such as silver, tin, and copper. Through the mechanical process of "trituration," the various components are mixed together; this gives rise to a product with plastic consistency, allowing it to be molded into previously prepared dental cavities. Once condensed and adapted to the cavity shape, the alloy hardens, forming a stable metal restoration.

Table 10.2 Features of composite materials components

	Components	Function
Organic resin	Bis-GMA, UDMA	Resin monomers responsible for the fluid component of the material
	EGDMA, TEGDMA	Viscosity determinants to promote correct handling
	Activator – Photoactivator: camphor quinone – Dual activator: tertiary amines + benzoyl peroxide	Polymerization reaction inhibitors–activators
Inorganic filling	Silica (glass of barium, zinc, strontium, lithium, aluminum, borosilicate, zirconium, and ceramic)	Responsible for esthetic biomechanical features and the radio-opacity of the composite material
Coupling agent	Silane	Responsible for the coupling between the inorganic filler and organic resinous matrix

Dental amalgam has been used as a restorative material since 1880 and until adhesive dentistry gained popularity. Many studies have demonstrated the longevity of amalgam restorations. In deciduous teeth, the patient's age plays a fundamental role in the lifespan of these restorations.

The choice to use amalgam should be considered for individual patients. These restorations often require the removal of a large amount of healthy tissue to ensure adequate retention. Hence, as far as possible, more conservative restorations are indicated, such as those with composite resins or glass ionomer cements. On the other hand, in cases of severe impairment of the dental element with potential pulp involvement, the most appropriate choice is restoration with preformed metal crowns.

Preformed metal crowns

Reconstruction of deciduous molars using preformed metal crowns was introduced in 1950 with the aid of stainless steel crowns; soon, the metal used for fabricating the crowns was changed to nickel–chromium-based alloys. The use of preformed metal crowns is indicated in cases in which other conservative techniques do not allow satisfactory rehabilitation given the high degree of dental element impairment. Preformed crowns allow the masticatory function to be restored and can function as space maintainers for several years. If restoration is properly performed using these crowns, intervention using other prosthetic measures until is usually not required exfoliation (Seale, 2002).

Clinical studies have shown that in children aged less than 4 years, preformed metal crowns have twice the clinical success compared with amalgam restorations (Levering et al, 1988; Hunter, 1985).

Enamel/dentin adhesive systems

With the use of orthophosphoric acid, proposed by Buonocore "*to make the tooth more receptive to resin monomers*," a new approach was established in restorative dentistry, i.e., adhesive dentistry (Buonocore, 1955). This differs from the previous restorative dentistry in the possibility of using materials that, due to adhesion, guarantee an optimal adaptation to dental elements, thereby modifying the principles of cavity preparation and eliminating the need for retention.

In adhesive dentistry, the various properties of dental tissues should be taken into account.

Adhesion to enamel

Enamel consists of 96%–97% inorganic material, comprising hydroxyapatite crystals, and low amounts of organic material (1%–2%) and water (4%–12%).

Through etching with a strong acid (37% orthophosphoric acid) for 15–30 seconds, a partial demineralization of the enamel can be obtained, with the formation of a porous surface, allowing the resin adhesive to wet and penetrate it (Pashley et al, 2011); this enables micromechanical adhesion (Buonocore, 1955). For deciduous tooth enamel, it is advisable to extend the etching time to up to 60 seconds.

It is very important that no contaminant is present on the enamel at the time of application of the adhesive system; if this occurs, the bond would indeed be very weak in the presence of the primary organic film covering the surface (Brännström et al, 1989).

Adhesion to dentin

Dentin comprises 70% hydroxyapatite, 18% organic material (type 1 collagen), and 12% water (Breschi et al, 2008).

Dentin is a moist tissue crossed by numerous canaliculi, the dentinal tubules, whose number and diameter vary according to the coronal distance (Breschi et al, 2008). Another characteristic is the presence of a layer, called dentinal mud or *smear layer*, that forms following mechanical instrumentation and is characterized by a thickness varying between 0.5–5 μm and 3–10 μm (Pashley et al, 1984; 2011); this layer is weakly bound to dentin. The reduction in dentinal permeability induced by the smear layer constitutes an obstacle to the penetration of adhesive resins and therefore to dentin adhesion.

Smear layer removal is performed through acid etching (Breschi et al, 2008). This allows dissolution of the inorganic component, leading to exposure of the organic component, which mainly comprises collagen fibers. The treatment, if excessively long at the dentinal level, leads to denaturation of collagen proteins. It is therefore advisable not to exceed dentin etching beyond 15 seconds. After inactivation of the acid by adequate rinsing, it is also important to avoid the collapse of the demineralized collagen fibers due to an overly vigorous drying phase (Breschi et al, 2008; Pashley et al, 2011). To address this issue, *primers* have been introduced; these are molecules that are able to function as spacers of collagen fibers and favor the penetration of the adhesive agent into the surface micropores (Pashley et al, 2011; Liu et al, 2011).

The adhesive leakage process peaks with the formation of a layer called a *hybrid layer* or resin–dentin interdiffusion zone (Nakabayashi et al, 1982).

Classification of adhesive systems and methods of clinical application

Each adhesive system contains an acid *etching* agent (etchant) to increase the surface free energy, a *primer* agent to increase the wettability of the adhesive system, and a resin (*bonding*) agent to infiltrate the surface and form the bond. These chemical compounds can be combined to determine the adhesive system.

Adhesive systems can be classified into two categories: *etch-and-rinse* and *self-etch* (or *etch-and-dry*) (Tab. 10.3) (Breschi et al, 2008).

The *etch-and-rinse* system involves the application of an etching agent to the enamel and dentin and subsequent rinsing to remove the acid and salts formed during the demineralization process (Pashley et al, 2011). The simultaneous application of *etchant* to the enamel and dentin is called the *total-etching* technique. The acid (generally 35%–37% orthophosphoric acid in gel form) exposes enamel prisms and completely removes the *smear layer* from the dentin surface. Furthermore, it demineralizes collagen fibers in the intact dentin below the smear layer, thereby leaving a substrate that is porous and more easily impregnated by *primers* and *bonding* agents, which can be distinct (3-step) or combined in a single solution (2-step) (Breschi et al, 2008).

Etch-and-rinse 3-step adhesives involve three consecutive steps: etching, *priming*, and *bonding*. They are the most studied among all adhesives and allow high adhesion values to be obtained (Breschi et al, 2008; Pashley et al, 2011); they are considered reference adhesive systems and have very stable adhesion values over time (Liu et al, 2011) (Fig. 10.8).

Etch-and-rinse 2-step adhesives conform to the same principle of etching, but priming and bonding are combined in a single step. Therefore, these adhesives ensure a simplified clinical procedure but often require the application of *multiple layers*; otherwise,

Table 10.3 Classification and application of adhesive systems and brand names of some adhesive systems currently available

Etch-and-rinse		**Self-etch (or etch-and-dry)**	
3-step	2-step	2-step	1-step
Generation IV	Generation V	Generation VI	Generation VII and VIII
Etching 1. Apply for 15 seconds 2. Rinse thoroughly for 15 seconds 3. Dry gently without overdrying the dentin **Primer** 4. Apply 1–5 layers of primer and bonding agent with gentle blowing to encourage evaporation of the solvent **Bonding** 5. Apply one layer; blow gently to obtain a uniform layer 6. Polymerize	**Etching** 1. Apply for 15 seconds 2. Rinse the water abundantly for 15 seconds 3. Dry gently without overdrying the dentin **Primer and bonding** 1. Apply 1–5 layers of primer and bonding agent; blow gently to encourage evaporation of the solvent 2. Polymerize	**Etching and primer** 1. Apply for the time specified by the manufacturer and dry gently without rinsing **Bonding** 1. Apply one layer; blow gently to obtain a uniform layer 2. Polymerize	**Etching and primer and bonding** 1. Apply 1–5 layers of *etchant* and *primer* and *bonding* agent; blow gently at the end to promote evaporation of the solvent 2. Polymerize
• Adper Scotchbond Multi-Purpose (3M ESPE) • Gluma Solid Bond (Heraeus Kulzer) • Optibond FL (Kerr) • PermaQuick (Ultradent) • Syntac (Ivoclar Vivadent)	• Adper Scotchbond 1XT (3M ESPE) • Excite (Vivadent) • Gluma Comfort Bond (Heraeus Kulzer) • One-Step Plus (Bisco) • PQ1 – PEAK LC (Ultradent) • Prime & Bond NT, XP-Bond (Dentsply)	• AdheSE (Ivoclar Vivadent) • Clearfil Protect Bond (Kuraray) • One-Step Plus (Bisco) • Peak SE (Ultradent)	• AdheSE One (Ivoclar Vivadent) • Adper Prompt L-Pop (3M ESPE) • All-Bond SE (Bisco) • Clearfil S3Bond (Kuraray) • I-Bond (Heraeus Kulzer) • XENO V (Dentsply)

the adhesive layer is so thin that it does not function as a *shock absorber*. The adhesive interface created by these systems tends to degrade over time because of the hydrolysis phenomena of monomers and the instability of dentinal collagen (Breschi et al, 2008; Liu et al, 2011).

The *self-etch* system, unlike the *etch-and-rinse* system, involves the application of an acid system, followed by drying (hence, it is also called *etch-and-dry*; Breschi et al, 1998). In fact, instead of the acid being rinsed off the surface, it is neutralized by the salts produced during demineralization (Van Meerbeek et al, 2011). Because the acid is already mixed with the primer, any washing would be a clinical error because it would also remove the *primer*, which is indeed necessary to properly permeate the substrate. After the etching phase, the *bonding* agent is applied, which can be performed separately (2-step) or combined with the *etchant/primer* application (1-step); they can also be in a single container or in separate containers and mixed at the time of use. In this respect, the application of a self-etch adhesive provides a lower-grade demineralization than that obtained with orthophosphoric acid and simultaneous infiltration because it does not remove the smear layer and forms the so-called *modified smear layer* (Van Meerbeek et al, 2011). The most prominent morphological difference between the *self-etch* system and the *etch-and-rinse* system is the formation of a hybrid layer less than 1-μm thick, with few prominent *resin tags* (considering that tubules are not opened via separate etching).

Self-etch 2-step systems involve the application of a *self-etching primer* with acidic features that treats the substrate by modifying the *smear layer* and increasing the wettability of the surface, followed by the application of a *bonding* agent (Van Meerbeek et al, 2011). These adhesive systems have demonstrated excellent adhesive capabilities, comparable to those of the *etch-and-rinse 3-step* systems, and their stability over time appears to be ensured by the formation of a chemical bond with the dentin mineral component that adds to micromechanical adhesion (Van Meerbeek et al, 2011).

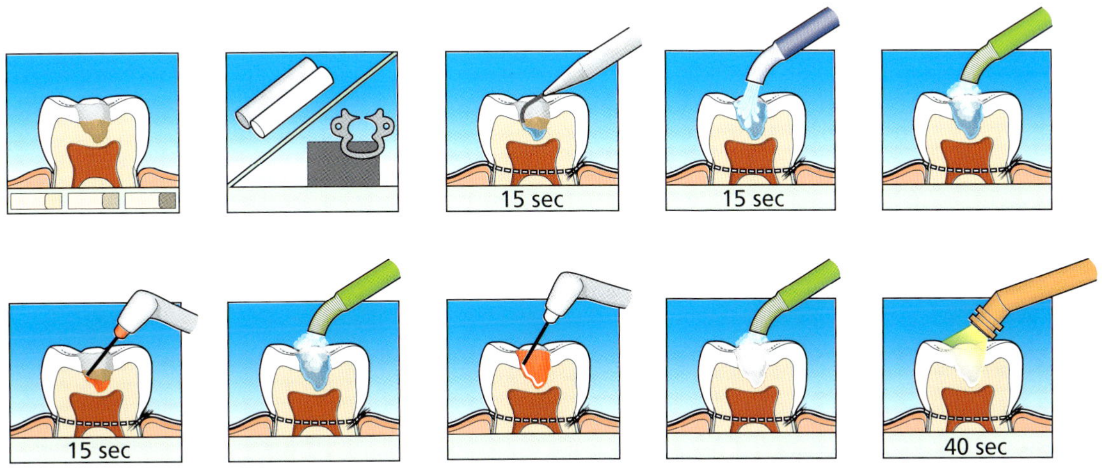

Figure 10.8 Application method of an *etch-and-rinse 3-step* adhesive system.

However, there are still doubts about the interface stability at the enamel level; thus, some manufacturers suggest enamel pretreatment using a selective etching technique (Pashley, 1984; Breschi et al, 2008; Van Meerbeek et al, 2011).
Self-etch 1-step systems include the three fundamental components of adhesive systems in a single step. They can be packaged in separate containers to be mixed at the time of use (VII generation) or be packaged as a single solution (VIII generation). These super-simplified systems were introduced with the aim of reducing operating times, combining substances that were supplied separately in previous systems. While ensuring an undoubted simplification compared with the multistep systems, their stability over time is lower than that of other classes of adhesive systems (Breschi et al, 2008; Liu et al, 2011).
In vitro studies have demonstrated that adhesion values in the deciduous and permanent teeth are comparable (Greenwell et al, 1990; Garcia de Araujo et al, 1997); therefore, apart from the extension of etching times, especially on enamel (up to 60 seconds), there are no differences in the application of an adhesive system on a deciduous or permanent dental element.

Materials for endodontics

Indications for the different endodontic treatments and, consequently, for materials to be used in the different clinical situations depend on the pulp status: whether it is vital, and in this case if inflammation is reversible or irreversible, or necrotic (American Association of Endodontics, 2003). Materials used in pediatric endodontics differ from those used in adult patients because the clinical situations to be addressed are different. It is necessary to have materials that are biocompatible and do not irritate any residual pulp tissue; ensure dental pulp seal; and, in case of deciduous elements, are reabsorbed simultaneously with root resorption.

Zinc oxide and eugenol

Zinc oxide and eugenol (ZOE) has long been considered the material of choice for filling the root canals of deciduous elements because of its easy workability and good sealing capabilities. However, it has low antibacterial activity, and its reabsorption is slower than that of deciduous roots compared with iodoform paste (Özalp et al, 2005); it can also produce black mucosal pigmentation. Therefore, currently, it is no longer possible to consider ZOE the gold standard of root canal filling materials. In endodontics, ZOE finds more use as a temporary filling material that is used between sessions considering its excellent marginal sealing capacity.

Calcium hydroxide

Calcium hydroxide was introduced in dentistry in 1921 and, together with mineral trioxide aggregate (MTA), is considered the gold standard for direct pulp capping and apexification (see Chapter 12). Calcium hydroxide has excellent antibacterial properties. In fact, a study showed 100% reduction in the microorganisms associated with pulp infections 1 hour after contact with calcium hydroxide (Stuart et al, 1991). Owing to its alkaline pH, it favors biological healing and the formation of a mineralized tissue barrier.

As shown by some studies, calcium hydroxide has a history of long-term clinical success, even up to 10 years after treatment (Matsuo et al, 1996; Accorinte et al, 2006). It has high solubility, low compression resistance, and is not able to provide a good marginal seal; therefore, it should not be used for temporary restorations. To ensure successful treatment, it is necessary to combine calcium hydroxide with a material capable of providing a good seal to dental restoration, such as glass ionomer cement, ZOE, or an adhesive material.

Iodoform paste

Since 2009, the American Academy of Pediatric Dentistry has considered iodoform paste (KRI paste) to be the best filling material for deciduous canals (AAPD, 2009). It has good bactericidal action, and its rate of resorption is comparable to that of root resorption of deciduous elements. Iodoform paste is biocompatible and easily transportable inside the canals; the only contraindication is esthetics: over time, it can cause a brownish-yellow pigmentation of the crown (Barja-Fidalgo et al, 2011).

Mineral trioxide aggregate

MTA consists of calcium oxide in the form of tricalcium silicate, dicalcium silicate, or tricalcium aluminate, with the addition of bismuth oxide for radiopacity; it is commercially available as a powder to be mixed with water. It has been used for endodontic therapy in adult patients since the 1990s, but indications for its use in the treatment of permanent elements in pediatric patients have been increasing.

MTA is biocompatible; has high antibacterial potential because of the strongly alkaline pH of 12; and can stimulate cytokine release by pulp fibroblasts, which in turn stimulate the formation of mineralized tissue (Rodd et al, 2006). Hence, it is beginning to be considered the material of choice, instead of calcium hydroxide, for both apexification and direct pulp capping of permanent elements; it can be said that 1 g of MTA is equivalent to 24 g of calcium hydroxide. Additionally, it has a good compression resistance and offers an excellent marginal seal compared with calcium hydroxide (Srinivasan et al, 2009). Moreover, recent studies have suggested that it can be used to seal the pulp chamber of deciduous elements that are not fully formed in order to facilitate apexogenesis (Felippe et al, 2006).

The disadvantages of this material are related to its hardening requirements and time. In fact, complete hardening of MTA requires a damp environment and 140 minutes (Islam et al, 2006). Consequently, when using it as a capping material, two sessions will be required before proceeding to final restoration.

It is necessary to bear in mind that although MTA shows excellent results in clinical practice, it is not an easily workable material for inexperienced clinicians.

Ferrous sulfate

Ferrous sulfate (15.5%) promotes pulpal hemostasis through a chemical reaction with blood. It has been proposed as a pulpotomy agent because it can control pulpal hemorrhage and form a metal–protein clot protection over the vital radicular pulp. Its use is limited to achieving hemostasis after pulpotomy in deciduous elements, following which a dressing with calcium hydroxide should be applied on root canal openings; an adhesive restoration is then placed to ensure the seal (Rodd et al, 2006).

Formocresol

Formocresol consists of 35% formaldehyde and tricresol. This substance is used as a dressing to achieve hemostasis after pulpotomy in deciduous elements. It maintains its effect even with a 1:5 dilution in water. In 2004, the International Agency for Research on Cancer issued a press release stating that there is sufficient evidence that formaldehyde is involved in the pathogenesis of nasopharyngeal carcinoma (IARC, 2004). Clearly, a single exposure does not entail risk for the patient; however, in general, formaldehyde is a cytotoxic, mutagenic, and carcinogenic substance, and its usage is considered to be outdated, especially when treating pediatric patients.

Root canal irrigation materials

For irrigating the canals of deciduous elements, both saline solution and 2% sodium hypochlorite solution can be used. One needs to be careful to irrigate gently, especially when using 2% sodium hypochlorite, to avoid damaging the permanent element bud.

Alginates

This impression material falls within the class of irreversible hydrocolloids. It mainly comprises alginic acid (extracted from marine algae), which acts as a reagent; a calcium salt soluble in water, such as calcium sulfate dihydrate, which in aqueous solution can react with soluble alginate; a retarder that regulates the hardening time, such as trisodium phosphate; a gypsum setting accelerator, such as potassium sulfate; a filler (diatomaceous earth); and flavoring and coloring agents (Cook, 1986). It is available as a powder. The mixing time is approximately 1 minute, and the ideal temperature at which the reaction should take place is approximately 21°C.
The alginate powder is mixed with water. Sodium phosphate reacts with calcium sulfate to allow adequate processing time; subsequently, the remaining calcium sulfate reacts with the insoluble sodium alginate, which forms a gel with water. The reaction time can be shortened by increasing the temperature or powder to water ratio. Alginates are the most widely used impression materials as they are easy to handle, low cost, elastic, and highly hydrophilic. However, they have some disadvantages including low tear resistance and inability to reproduce the minutest surface details like, for example, elastomers. Additionally, they are dimensionally unstable as they contain

a large amount of water. Therefore, it is necessary to pour the impression as quickly as possible or, alternatively, store it in a moist environment. In orthodontics, alginate is still widely used for the preparation of study models at the beginning and end of treatment as well as for fabricating appliances that do not require a high reproduction of detail, such as thermoformed fixing aligners, Hawley retainers, space maintainers, and indirect splinting.

Waxes

Waxes are thermoplastic materials that easily soften and warp under the action of heat and become stiff again upon cooling. They are widely used in dentistry because their properties allow easy processing by shaping them into desired forms (Millstein, 1985). According to their use and properties, which depend on chemical composition, different types of waxes are used. They can be classified as natural waxes, comprising hydrocarbons and esters (with the addition of alcohols and organic acids in some types), and synthetic waxes (comprising various complex organic compounds), which are used to a limited extent and are often mixed with natural waxes. To obtain the desired properties, suitable additives are added such as stearic acid, mineral oils, and natural resins. In orthodontics, wax is primarily used for bite registration to examine the occlusion and determine the relationship between the bone bases and dental arches.

While taking impressions, it is necessary to use the wax in habitual occlusion and occasionally in centric relation to identify the manner in which the two arches are related. The wax is softened in a hot water bath, and the patient is then asked to bite it; following this, the wax is left in place for a few seconds and cooled with a cold air jet to start the solidification process.

It is also used in the fabrication of some appliances, such as during construction bite registration for the Fränkel or Andresen appliance and many other functional appliances.

References

Accorinte M, Reis A, Loguercio A et al. Influence of rubber dam isolation on human pulp responses after capping with calcium hydroxide and an adhesive system. Quintessence Int 2006;37(3):205-12.

Adair SM. Evidence-base use of fluoride in contemporary pediatric dental practice. Pediatr Dent 2006:28(2):133-42.

Ahovuo-Saloranta A, Hiiri A, Nordblad A et al. Pit and fissure sealants for preventing dental decay in the permanent teeth of children and adolescents. Cochrane Database Syst Rev 2004;(3):CD001830.

American Academy of Pediatric Dentistry. Guideline on pulp therapy for primary and young permanent teeth. Pediatr Dent 2009;(31)6:179-86.

American Association of Endodontists. Glossary of Endodontic Terms. 7th ed. Chicago: American Association of Endodontists; 2003.

American Dental Association Council on Scientific Affairs. Professionally-applied topical fluoride: Evidence-based clinical recommendations. J Am Dent Assoc 2006;137(8):1151-9.

Bader JD, Shugars DA, Bonito AJ. A systematic review of selected caries prevention and management methods. Community Dent Oral Epidemiol 2001;29(6):399-411.

Barja-Fidalgo F, Moutinho-Ribeiro M, Amorim Oliveira MA, Heloìsa de Oliveira B. A systematic review of root canal filling materials for deciduous teeth: is there an alternative for zinc oxide-eugenol. ISRN Dent 2011;367318.

Bayne SC, Heymann HO, Swift EJ Jr. Update on dental composite restorations. J Am Dent Assoc 1994;125(6):687-701.

Beauchamp J, Caufield PW, Crall JJ et al. American Dental Association Council on Scientific Affairs. Evidence-based clinical recommendations for the use of pit and fissure sealants. J Am Dent Assoc 2008;139(3):257-68.

Brännström M, Mattson B, Torstenson B. Critical review of lining materials and technics for fillings. Dent Cadmos 1989;57(1):13.

Brännström M. Communication between the oral cavity and the dental pulp associated with restorative treatment. Oper Dent 1984;9(2):57-68.

Breschi L, Mazzoni A, Ruggeri A Jr et al. Dental adhesion review: aging and stability of the bonded interface. Dent Mater 2008;24:90-101.

Brown LJ, Kaste L, Selwitz R, Furman L. Dental caries and sealant usage in U.S. children, 1988-1991: selected findings from the Third National Health and Nutrition Examination Survey. J Am Dent Assoc 1996;127:335-43.

Buonocore MG. A simple method of increasing the adhesion of acrylic filling materials to enamel surfaces. J Dent Res 1955;34:849-53.

Cho E, Kopel H, White SN. Moisture susceptibility of resin modified glass ionomer materials. Quintessence Int 1995;26:351-8.

Cook W. Alginate dental impressions material: chemistry, structure, properties. J Biomed Mater Res 1986;20(1):1-24.

Craig R. Materiali per l'odontoiatria restaurativa. Milano: Masson; 1998.

Crisp S, Kent BE, Lewis BG et al. Glass ionomer cement formulations. II. The synthesis of novel polycarboxylic acids. J Dent Res 1980;59:1055.

Croll TP, Bar-Xion Y, Segura A, Donly KJ. Clinical performance of resin-modified glass ionomer cement restorations in primary teeth. A retrospective evaluation. J Am Dent Assoc 2001;132(8):1110-6.

Donly KJ, García-Godoy F. The use of resin-based composite in children. Pediatr Dent 2002;24(5):480-8.

Donly KJ, Istre S, Istre T. In vitro enamel remineralization at orthodontic band margins cemented with glass ionomer cement. Am J Orthod Dentofacial Orthop 1995;107(5):461-4.

Donly KJ, Nelson JJ. Fluoride release of restorative mate-rials exposed to a fluoridated dentifrice. ASDC J Dent Child 1997;64(4):249-50.

Donly KJ, Segura A, Kanellis M, Erickson RL. Clinical performance and caries inhibition of resin-modified glass ionomer cement and amalgam restorations. J Am Dent Assoc 1999;130(10):1459-66.

Duggal MS, Tahmassebi JF, Toumba KJ, Mavromati C. The effect of different etching times on the retention of fissure sealants in second primary and first permanent molars. Int J Paediatr Dent 1997;7:81-6.

Featherstone JD. The science and practice of caries pre-vention. J Am Dent Assoc 2000;131(7):877-99.

Felippe WT, Felippe CS, Rocha MJC. The effect of mineral trioxide aggregate on the apexification and periapical healing of teeth with incomplete root formation. Int Endod J 2006;39:2-9.

Ferracane JL. Resin composite state of the art. Dent Mater 2011;27:29-38.

Forsten L. Fluoride release and uptake by glass ionomers and related materials and its clinical effect. Biomaterials 1998;19(6):503-8.

García de Araujo FB, García-Godoy F, Issao M. A comparison of 3 resin bonding agents to primary tooth dentin. Pediatr Dent 1997;19(4):253-7.

Garcia-Godoy F, Abarzua I, De Goes MF, Chan DC. Fluoride release from fissure sealants. J Clin Pediatr Dent 1997;22:45-9.

Greenwell AL, Johnsen D, DiSantis TA et al. Longitudinal evaluation of caries patterns from the primary to the mixed dentition. Pediatr Dent 1990;12(5):278-82.

Hunter B. Survival of dental restorations in young patients. Community Dent Oral Epidemiol 1985;18(5):285-7.

International Agency for Research on Cancer. IARC classifies formaldehyde as carcinogenic to humans. IARC 2004 Press release n. 153.

Islam I, Chang HK, Yap AUJ. X-ray diffraction analysis of mineral trioxide aggregate and Portland cement. Int Endod J 2006;39:220-5.

Johnston DW, Lewis DW. Three-year randomized trial of professionally applied topical fluoride gel comparing annual and biannual applications with/without prior prophylaxis. Caries Res 1995;29(5):331-6.

Kallestal C. The effect of five years' implementation of caries-preventive methods in Swedish high-risk adolescents. Caries Res 2005;39(1):20-6.

Kato S, Tosaki S, Hirota K. Effect of tooth surface conditioning materials on glass ionomer bonding. J Dent Res 1995;74:206.

Kerby RE, Mc Glumpny EA, Holloway JA. Some physical properties of implant abutment luting cements. Int J Prosthod 1992;5:321-9.

Kielbassa AM, Uchtmann H, Wrbas KT, Bitter K. In vitro study assessing apical leakage of sealer-only backfills in root canals of primary teeth. J Dent 2007;35:607-13.

Levering NJ, Messer LB. The durability of primary molar restorations: I. Observations and predictions of success of amalgams. Pediatr Dent 1988;10(2):74-80.

Liu Y, Tjäderhane L, Breschi L et al. Limitations in bonding to dentin and experimental strategies to prevent bond degradation. J Dent Res 2011;90:953-68.

Marinho VCC, Higgins JPT, Logan S, Sheiham A. Fluoride varnishes for preventing dental caries in children and adolescents. Cochrane Database Syst Rev 2005;3.

Matsuo T, Nakanishi T, Shuimizu H, Ebisu S. A clinical study of direct pulp capping applied to carious-exposed pulps. J Endod 1996;22(10):551-6.

Millstein PL. An evaluation of occlusal indicator wax. J Prosthet Dent 1985;53:570-2.

Morphis TL, Toumba KJ, Lygidakis NA. Fluoride pit and fissure sealants: a review. Int J Paediatr Dent 2000;10:90-8.

Nakabayashi N, Kojima K, Mashuara E. The promotion of adhesion by the infiltration of monomers into tooth substrates. J Biomed Mater Res 1982;16:265-73.

Negm MM, Beech DR, Grant AA. An evaluation of mechanical and adhesive properties of polycarboxylate and glass ionomer cements. J Oral Rehabil 1982;9:161.

Osborne JW, Summitt JB. Extension for prevention: is it relevant today? Am J Dent 1998;11(4):189-96.

Özalp N, Saroglu I, Sönmez H. Evaluation of various root canal filling materials in primary molar pulpectomies: an in vivo study. Am J Dent 2005;(18)6:347-50.

Pardi V, Pereira AC, Ambrosano GM, Meneghim Mde C. Clinical evaluation of three different materials use as pit and fissure sealant: 24-months results. J Clin Pediatr Dent 2005;29(2):133-7.

Pardi V, Pereira AC, Mialhe FL et al. A 5-year evaluation of two glass-ionomer cements use as fissure sealants. Community Dent Oral Epidemiol 2003;31(5):386-91.

Pashley DH. Smear layer: physiological considerations. Oper Dent 1984;3:13-29

Pashley DH, Tay FR, Breschi L et al. State of the art etch-and-rinse adhesives. Dent Mater 2011; 27:1-16.

Pereira AC, Pardi V, Mialhe FL et al. A 3-year clinical evaluation of glass-ionomer cements use as fissure sealants. Am J Dent 2003;16(1):23-7.

Petersson LG, Twetman S, Dahlgren H et al. Professional fluoride varnish treatment for caries control: A systematic review of clinical trials. Acta Odontol Scand 2004;62(3):170-6.

Powis DR, Folleras T, Merson SA, Wilson AD. Improve adhesion of a glass ionomer cement to dentin and enamel. J Dent Res 1982;61:1416-22.

Quackenbush BM, Donly KJ, Croll TP. Solubility of a resin-modified glass ionomer cement. ASDC J Dent Child 1998;65(5):310-2, 354.

Rodd HD, Waterhouse PJ, Fuks AB et al. Pulp therapy for primary molars. Int J Paediatr Dent 2006;16(Suppl 1):15-23.

Rutar J, McAllan L, Tyas MJ. Three-year clinical performance of glass ionomer cement in primary molars. Int J Paediatr Dent 2002;12(2):146-7.

Seale NS. The use of stainless steel crowns. Pediatr Dent 2002;24(5):501-5.

Songpaisan Y, Bratthall D, Phantumvanit P, Somridhivej Y. Effects of glass ionomer cement, resin-based pit and fissure sealant and HF applications on occlusal caries in a developing country field trial. Community Dent Oral Epidemiol 1995;23(1):25-9.

Srinivasan V, Waterhouse P, Whitworth J. Mineral trioxide aggregate in paediatric dentistry. Int J Paediatr Dent 2009;19:34-47.

Stuart K, Miller C, Brown C Jr, Newton C. The comparative antimicrobial effect of calcium hydroxide. Oral Surg Oral Med Oral Path 1991;72:101-4.

Swartz ML, Phillips RW, Clark HE. Long-term fluoride release from glass ionomer cements. J Dent Res 1984;63(2):158-60.

Taifour D, Frencken JE, van't Hof MA et al. Effects of glass ionomer sealants in newly erupted first molars after 5 years: a pilot study. Community Dent Oral Epidemiol 2003;31(4):314-9.

Tam LE, Chan GP, Yim D. In vitro caries inhibition effects by conventional and resin-modified glass ionomer restorations. Oper Dent 1997;22(1):4-14.

Tjan AHL, Castelnuovo J, Liu P. Bond strength of multi-step and simplified-step systems. Am J Dent 1996;9(6):269-72.

Van Meerbeek B, Yoshihara K, Yoshida Y et al. State of the art of self-etch adhesives. Dent Mater 2011;27:17-28.

Vilkinis V, Hörsted-Bindslev P, Baelum V. Two-year evaluation of Class II resin-modified glass ionomer cement/composite open sandwich and composite restorations. Clin Oral Investig 2000;4(3):133-9.

Vrbic V. Retention of a fluoride-containing sealant on primary and permanent teeth three years after placement. Quintessence Int 1999;30:825-8.

Yoshii E, Kanaoka T, Hirota K. Biological evaluation of a new light cured glass ionomer cement for restorative filling. Fourth World Biomaterials Congress 1992; p. 53.

Chapter 11

Conservative treatment of carious lesions in pediatric dentistry

M. Bossù, L. Ottolenghi, A. Polimeni

Introduction and etiology of carious lesions

Carious pathology is a chronic degenerative process of multifactorial etiology defined as a transmissible disease. It affects the dental hard tissues and is initially characterized by infection and thereafter by demineralization of the affected tissues, resulting in cavity formation.
The process of the development of carious lesions requires the coexistence of three components that are temporally interrelated:

- presence of cariogenic bacteria with acidifying characteristics in the plaque
- substances promoting bacterial growth and adhesion that act as a metabolic substrate for acid formation (carbohydrates)
- host-related factors.

At the oral cavity level, the presence of saliva causes the enamel surface to be covered with acquired salivary pellicle, which is characterized by the presence of some glycoproteins and mucus. In addition, there are numerous microorganisms that form a mucobacterial plaque, which in turn can adhere to the salivary pellicle. The presence of this substrate is considered to be physiological, and its shift toward disease depends on the duration for which it has been present on the tooth surfaces, which can favor the accumulation of pathogenic bacterial colonies (Fig. 11.1).
The bacteria most commonly found in pathogenic plaque are *Streptococcus mutans* and *Lactobacillus*, which have acid-producing and acid-tolerant features, respectively. Two components are evident within the bacterial plaque: the corpuscular fraction, i.e., bacteria, leukocytes, and epithelial cells, and the amorphous fraction, i.e., salivary glycoproteins and dietary carbohydrates. As can be seen, the crucial factor in the process of caries development is diet and, therefore, the consumption of rapidly fermentable substances such as carbohydrates.
Because carious lesions are the result of enamel demineralization, it is important to consider the pH of the tooth surface itself. The critical pH value is 5.5, and the presence of glucose-6-phosphate hydrolase, a bacterial enzyme, may decrease the pH, initiating the decalcification of the hydroxyapatite in the enamel.

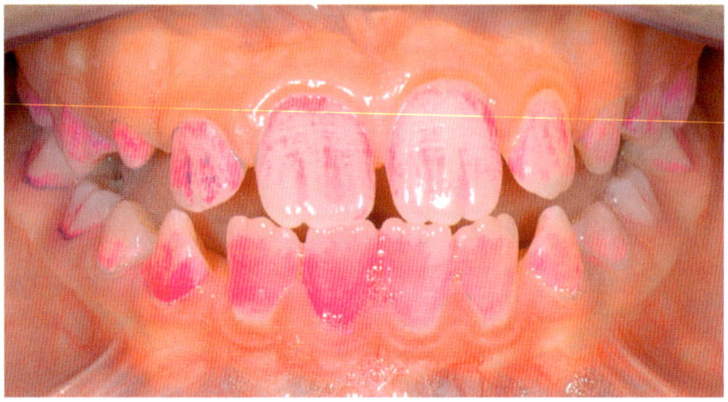

Figure 11.1 Evaluation of plaque on dental surfaces.

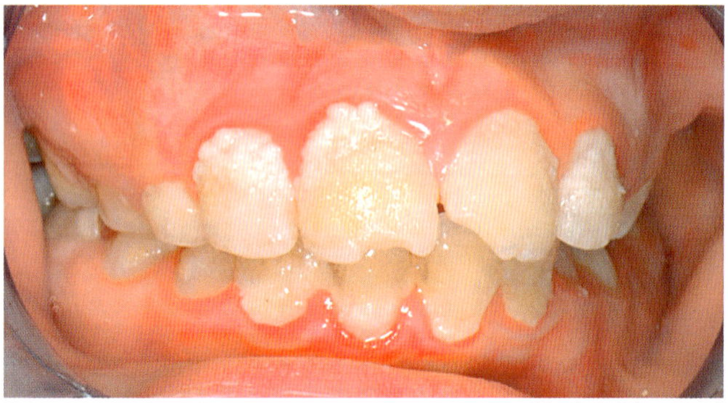

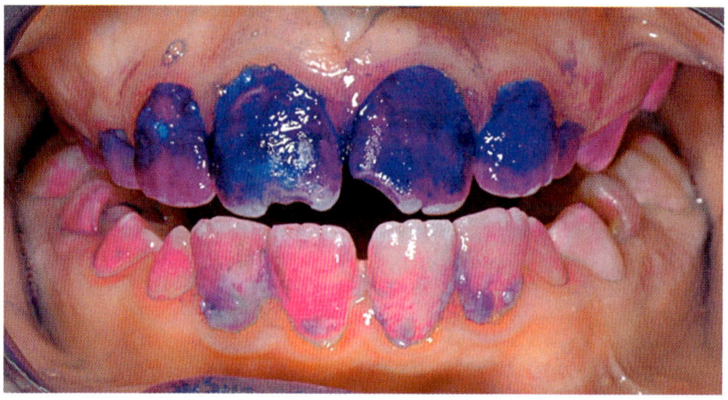

Diagnosis

International Caries Detection and Assessment System (ICDAS) method

The diagnosis of caries is based on the history of the lesion present on the tooth surface at the time of clinical examination and does not provide indications on the future course of the disease.

To prepare an adequate treatment plan for dental caries, it is necessary to implement an appropriate diagnostic system because different intervention criteria are set based on the severity of the lesion.

The diagnostic means most widely used to record carious lesions are as follows:

- direct observation
- delicate probing of the tooth surface (WHO-CPI-PSR probe) (Fig. 11.2)
- bitewing radiographs.

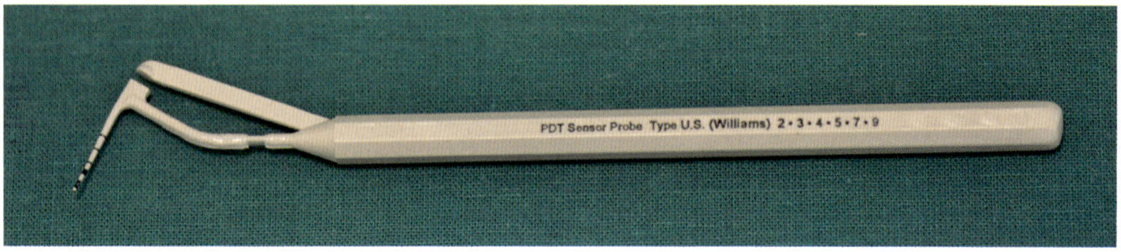

Figure 11.2 WHO-CPI-PSR probe.

The use of low-magnification optical systems and alternative techniques such as fiber-optic transillumination and fluorescence laser is useful and desirable.
Physical examination of the hard tissues should be performed under suitable lighting, and the tooth surface should be observed after thorough cleaning, first wet and then after air-drying, because the refraction difference between a portion of healthy and demineralized enamel is greater when saliva is removed from the porous enamel.
In case of uncertainty or to confirm the visual inspection findings, a WHO-CPI-PSR probe should be used gently along the tooth surface to evaluate its roughness (demineralization) or the presence of a minimal cavity limited to the enamel. The spherical end of the probe is slid along the suspect surface; a limited discontinuity is detected if the probe tip "drops" into the enamel surface lesion. The use of a sharp probe (sickle probe) is not advisable: if "pressed" on a sub-surface lesion, it can cause irreversible damage, favoring cavitation.

ICDAS codes

- 0: sound tooth surface (Fig. 11.3)
- 1: initial enamel lesion visible on the tooth surface after drying (Fig. 11.4)
- 2: enamel change visible even when the surface is wet (Fig. 11.5)
- 3: cavitated enamel lesion without dentinal involvement visible through the enamel (Fig. 11.6)
- 4: underlying dentinal shadow visible through the enamel with or without localized enamel damage (undermining caries) (Fig. 11.7)
- 5: frank cavitation with dentin exposure (Fig. 11.8)
- 6: cavity with extensive dentin exposure (Fig. 11.9).

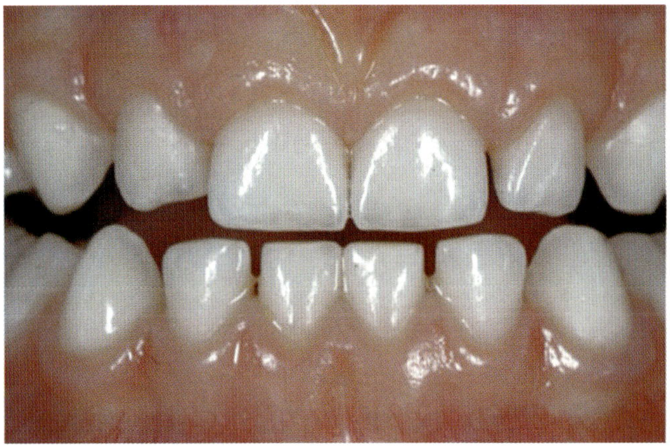

Figure 11.3 ICDAS index 0: sound surface.

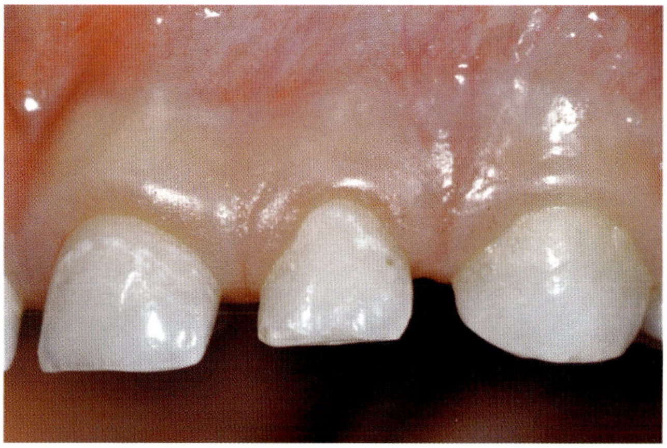

Figure 11.4 ICDAS index 1: initial enamel lesion (visible only after prolonged drying of the tooth and confined to furrows and fissures).

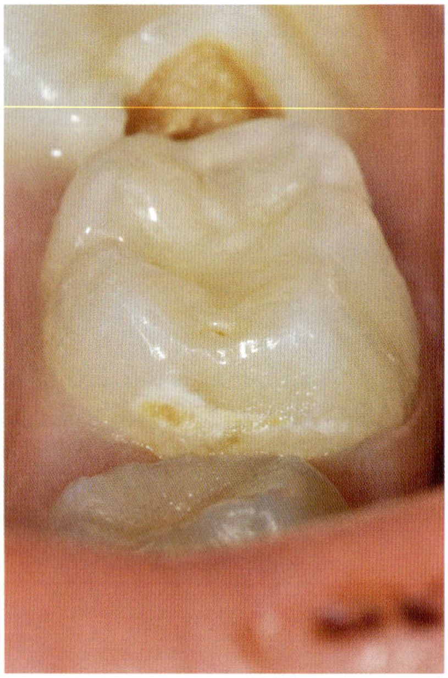

Figure 11.5 ICDAS index 2: clear and clearly visible enamel change.

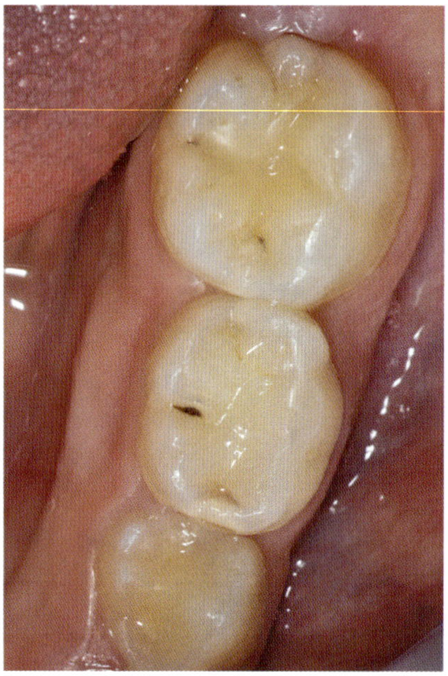

Figure 11.6 ICDAS index 3: localized cavitated enamel lesion without visible signs of dentinal damage.

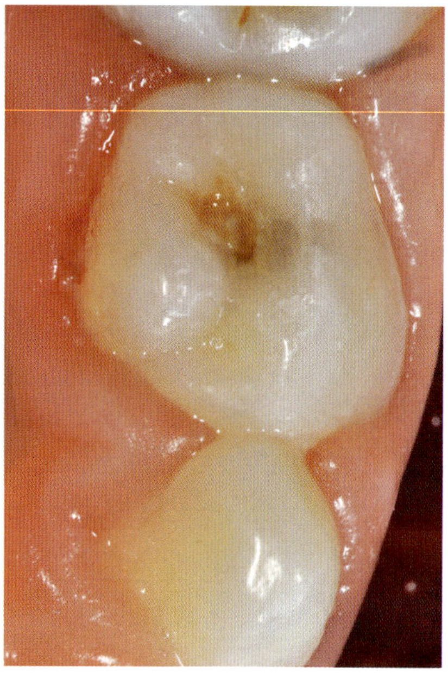

Figure 11.7 ICDAS index 4: area of underlying dentinal shadow visible through the enamel.

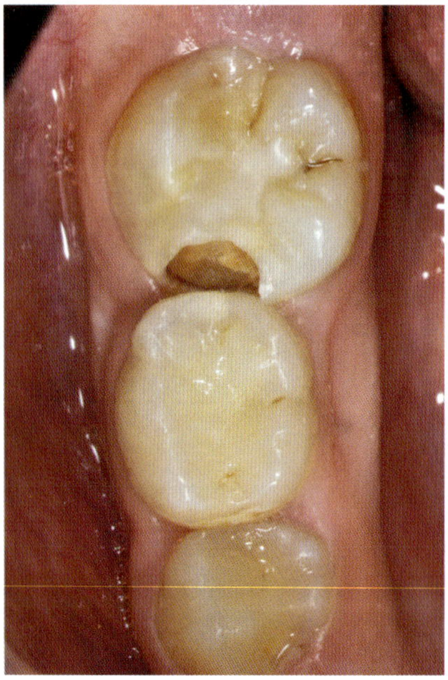

Figure 11.8 ICDAS index 5: frank cavitation with dentin exposure.

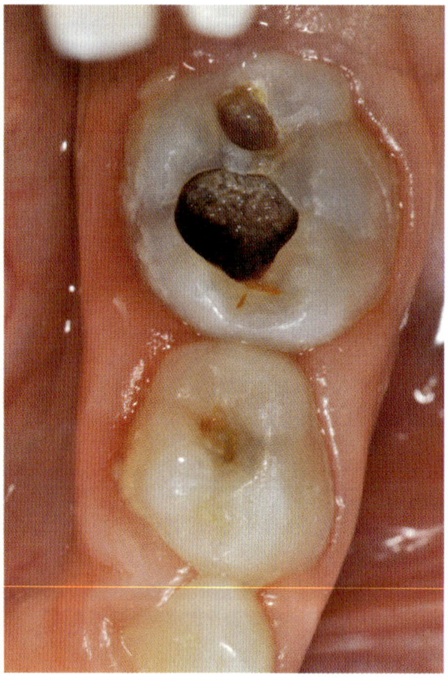

Figure 11.9 ICDAS index 6: destructive lesion with dentin exposure.

Sound tooth surface: code 0. Absence of obvious signs of caries and/or altered enamel translucency after prolonged drying (5 seconds). If tooth surfaces exhibit developmental defects, such as enamel hypoplasia, fluorosis, tooth wear (attrition, abrasion, and erosion), or intrinsic or extrinsic stains, they are coded as sound (Fig. 11.3).

Initial enamel lesion visible on the surface after tooth drying: code 1. On wet tooth surfaces, discoloration attributable to carious activity is not evident; however, after prolonged drying, an opacity (white or brown lesion) that is not consistent with the clinical appearance of sound enamel is visible (Fig. 11.4).

Enamel change visible even when the surface is wet: code 2. An opacity (carious lesion) or discoloration (white or brown lesion) not consistent with the clinical appearance of sound enamel is visible on both wet and dry tooth surfaces. When the lesion affects the mesial or distal smooth surfaces, it can be seen directly via either buccal/labial or palatal/lingual observation. In addition, via occlusal observation, this opacity or discoloration may appear as a shadow confined to the enamel seen through the marginal ridge (Fig. 11.5).

Cavitated enamel lesion without dentinal involvement visible through the enamel: code 3. Presence of an intense opacity on wet tooth surfaces caused by the carious lesion (white spot) and/or brown discoloration wider than natural fissures or pits.
After drying, a lack of continuity is seen on the smooth enamel surface, indicating demineralization. Fissures and pits may appear wider than normal, but there is neither dentin exposure on smooth surfaces or at the base of the cavity nor discontinuity.
In case of uncertainty or to confirm the visual inspection findings, a WHO-CPI-PSR probe should be gently slid along the tooth surface to confirm the presence of a cavity apparently confined to the enamel. The spherical end of the probe slides along the junction; a limited discontinuity is detected if the probe tip "drops" into the lesion present on the enamel surface (Fig. 11.6).

Underlying dentinal shadow visible through the enamel with or without localized enamel damage (undermining caries): code 4. A dentinal shadow is present on the wet tooth and is visible through the apparently sound enamel (loss of continuity but without exposure of the underlying dentin). This shadow, which is more visible when the tooth is wet, presents itself as an intrinsic bluish, grayish, or brownish stain that must be clearly associated with a carious lesion of the tooth tissue. If the examiner believes that the carious lesion initially developed on an adjacent surface and no evidence of lesions on the smooth surface of the tooth being examined is found, code "0" will be assigned to this surface (Fig. 11.7).

Frank cavitation with dentin exposure: code 5. Cavitation of the opaque enamel and/or discoloration (white or brown) of the exposed dentin visible at clinical examination. In case of uncertainty, the WHO-CPI-PSR probe is used to confirm the presence of a cavity in the dentin. This is achieved by sliding the round tip of the probe along the surface: any cavity in the dentin is detected when the ball tip of the probe enters into the lesion gap (Fig. 11.8).

Cavity with extensive dentin exposure: code 6. Obvious loss of tooth structure, with a large and deep cavity in which the dentin is clearly visible both on the walls and the bottom. The marginal ridge may not be present. The cavity involves at least half the tooth surface and can possibly reach the pulp (Fig. 11.9).

Isolation of the operative field

In the field of dentistry, many treatment procedures require isolation of the operative field for various reasons (Fig. 11.10). In pediatric dentistry, the importance of isolation is related not only to the use of specific materials but also to the less capacity of children to control swallowing, thereby preventing accidental ingestion of foreign bodies (burs, endodontic instruments, etc.). A well-positioned dam also protects soft tissues from contact with irritating and unpleasant substances (etchants). In addition to protecting the young patient, the use of rubber dams has some advantages for the clinician as well: good visibility of the operative field, absence of saliva and therefore of bacterial contamination during the procedures, and better outcomes.

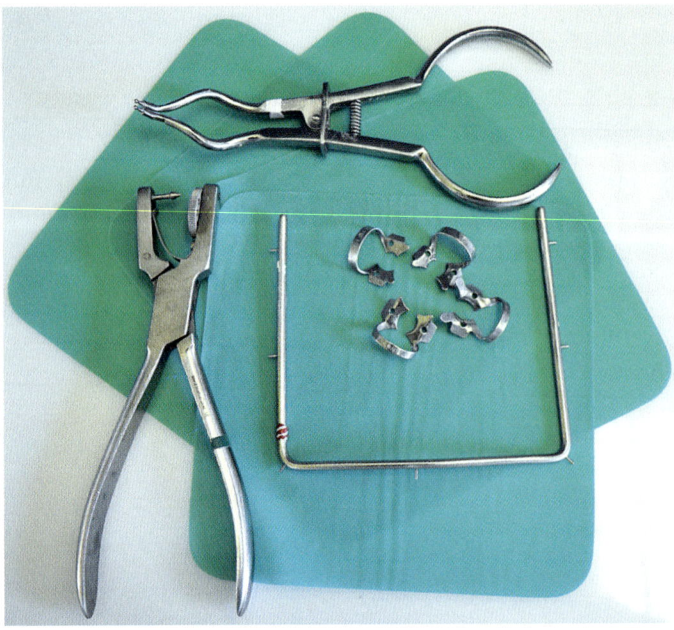

Figure 11.10 Instruments for operative field isolation.

Unfortunately, the use of rubber dam is sometimes not possible in pediatric dentistry because of incompletely erupted or badly positioned dental elements or the lack of cooperation of the child. In such cases, clinicians should implement all available procedures to make the operative field as suitable as possible for treatment, such as using suction, dental cotton rolls, and liquid dams.
Rubber dam sheets are made of latex and are available in various thicknesses, giving them different elasticity and isolating ability. The most commonly used thicknesses are medium (0.2 mm) and heavy (0.25 mm) depending on whether the procedure involves anterior or posterior regions of the dental arches. Dam positioning entails the use of devices such as the rubber dam punch, which has a tip that makes clear and precise holes when inserted into the holes in a rotating disc on the opposite handle. The holes on the disc have different diameters, allowing the most appropriate adaptation to the dental anatomy. After positioning, a Young frame keeps the sheet stretched. To place clamps on dental elements, clamp forceps are required, and finally, the use of a waxed dental floss is essential for both the insertion of the dam into the interdental spaces and ligation of the dental elements. Clamps or hooks have the essential role of keeping the dam fixed on dental elements; they are selected in accordance with the position of the dental element in the arch and its anatomy and the type of isolation required. Clamps feature different shapes that allow an optimal positioning on all dental elements (molars, premolars, and anterior teeth). When testing the selected clamp on the dental element, especially in the case of a pediatric patient, it is advisable to secure the clamp to a piece of dental floss tied to the buccal hole to allow quick recovery if it were to fall into the oral cavity. It is possible to isolate multiple dental elements by ligating the elements adjacent to the clamped one using dental floss. There are various operative techniques for rubber dam positioning; however, in pediatric dentistry, the use of winged clamps is preferred as it is possible to assemble the clamp and dam outside the oral cavity and apply them simultaneously on the dental element to be treated. When removing the dam after completing the restoration, care should be taken to remove any residue from the interdental spaces.

Operative procedures

Noninvasive dentistry

The treatment of noncavitated carious lesions in both permanent and deciduous dentition involves a noninvasive approach and aims to arrest or reverse the pathological process of caries to avoid the application of conservative restorations with varying degrees of complexity. This result is achieved via methods that can be used in both a professional setting and at home:

- daily brushing (at least twice a day) with a toothpaste promoting enamel remineralization/repair (containing fluoride, hydroxyapatite, or similar substances)

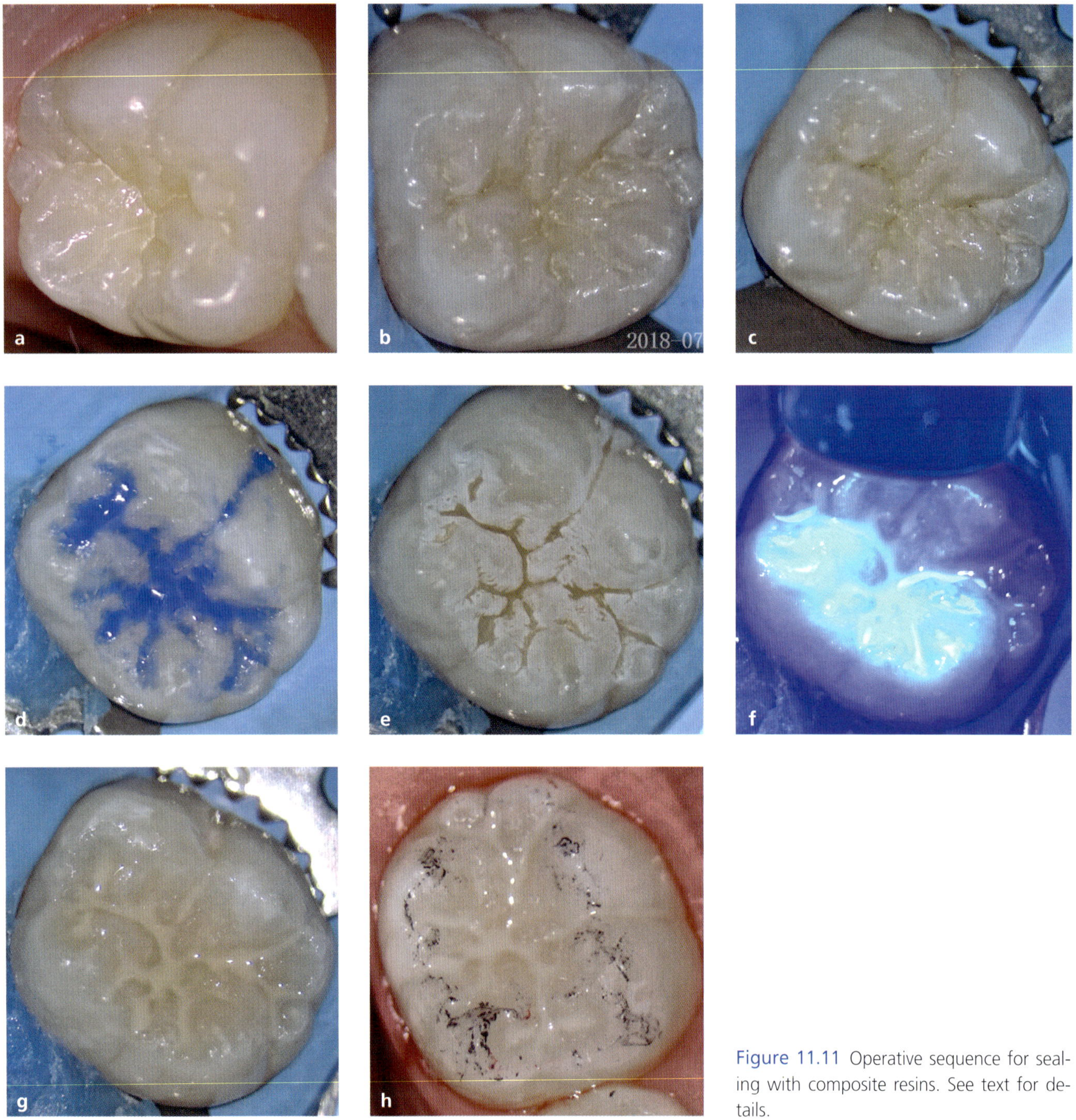

Figure 11.11 Operative sequence for sealing with composite resins. See text for details.

- use of a gel or mousse containing fluoride and/or casein products (casein phosphopeptide–amorphous calcium phosphate [CPP–ACP])
- professional topical application of varnishes and lacquers or gels with high fluoride concentration (see Chapter 6)
- pit and fissure sealing.

Pit and fissure sealing (ICDAS codes 0-1 and 2). Clinical diagnosis of caries is based on the absence of obvious signs or the presence of demineralized enamel (white spots or brown discoloration) at the bottom of occlusal or buccolingual pits, fissures, or fossae, with a clear change in enamel translucency after prolonged drying (5 seconds). Molar pits or fissures, particularly in permanent dentition, are the sites where carious lesions are most frequently found. Caries prevention in these sites is one of the fundamental objectives of pediatric dentistry. A 15-year longitudinal study showed that pit and fissure sealant treatment reduces the onset of caries by 62% (Simonsen, 1991). The Italian national guidelines for the promotion of oral health and the prevention of oral diseases in children and adolescents (Recommendation No. 3 - Update November 2013) state that "sealants are indicated for all children and adolescents, although the greatest benefits are achieved in subjects and dental elements at high risk of caries," and recommend clinical assessment every 6–12 months to verify tooth integrity.
Currently, two types of *sealant* materials are used: composite resins and glass ionomer cements (low- or high-viscosity). Resin *sealants* have a greater retention than low-viscosity glass ionomer cements, but their ability to prevent tooth decay depends on moisture control in the operative field. Therefore, in cases of barely erupted teeth (in patients at high risk of caries) or badly positioned teeth, which are therefore difficult to isolate, the use of low-viscosity glass ionomer cements is recommended.

Sealing with composite resins: operational sequence

- Isolate the operative field using a rubber dam (Fig. 11.11a, b)
- Cleanse the tooth surface thoroughly, avoiding fluoridated and/or oily products.
- Rinse with air and water sprays to remove any material residue (Fig. 11.11c)
- Etch the tooth with 37% orthophosphoric acid for 30 seconds and then rinse the treated surface thoroughly (for at least 30 seconds) (Fig. 11.11d)
- Dry the surgical field and the treated enamel thoroughly to obtain optimal drying of pits and fissures (Fig. 11.11e)
- Apply a thin layer of sealant on the pits and fissures
- Cure and evaluate resin hardening and integrity (Fig. 11.11f)
- Verify that the sealant extends over all pits and fissures, and evaluate its degree of retention (Fig. 11.11g)
- Remove the dam and check the occlusion (Fig. 11.11h).

Clinical case

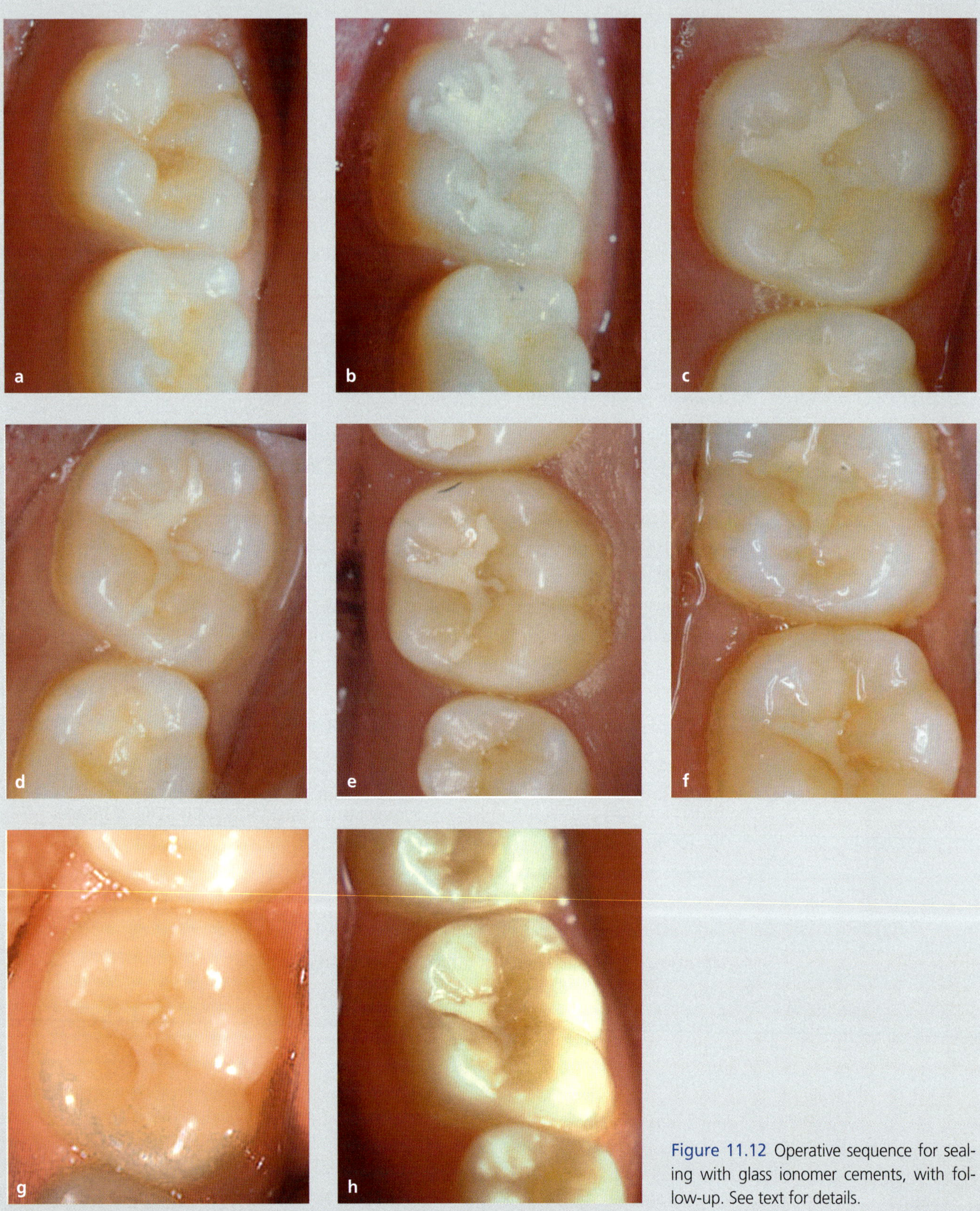

Figure 11.12 Operative sequence for sealing with glass ionomer cements, with follow-up. See text for details.

Sealing with glass ionomer cements: operational sequence

- Isolate the operative field using cotton rolls and surgical suction
- Cleanse the tooth surface thoroughly, avoiding fluoridated and/or oily products
- If required, use a conditioner
- Rinse with air and water sprays to remove any material residue
- Dry the surface without drying it out completely (because cement adhesion is better on moist enamel)
- Apply the cement and cure for the time specified by the manufacturer (approximately 30 seconds)
- Verify that the cement extends over all pits and fissures, and evaluate its degree of retention
- Evaluate the occlusal relationship with the antagonist.

See the clinical case described in Figure 11.12.

Minimally invasive dentistry

Minimally invasive dentistry comprises all treatment protocols involving the removal of carious tissue with the utmost respect for and preservation of healthy dental tissues. When proceeding with the esthetic functional rehabilitation of dental elements affected by the caries process, it is necessary to account for the extension of the carious lesion because operative techniques may vary depending on the anatomical part to be reconstructed. However, there are significant differences regarding the materials used in deciduous dentition compared to permanent dentition. Notably, despite considering glass ionomer cements and compomers to be useful in some restorative situations, many authors use composite resins for restorations in the posterior regions.

Selective enameloplasty plus sealing (PRR-1 by Simonsen, 1977–1980) (ICDAS code 3)

The treatment of small carious lesions on the occlusal surface through selective enameloplasty and fissure sealants (Fig. 11.13) is indicated when there is an intense opacity on the wet tooth, such as white spots, and/or a brownish discoloration wider than natural pits and fissures.

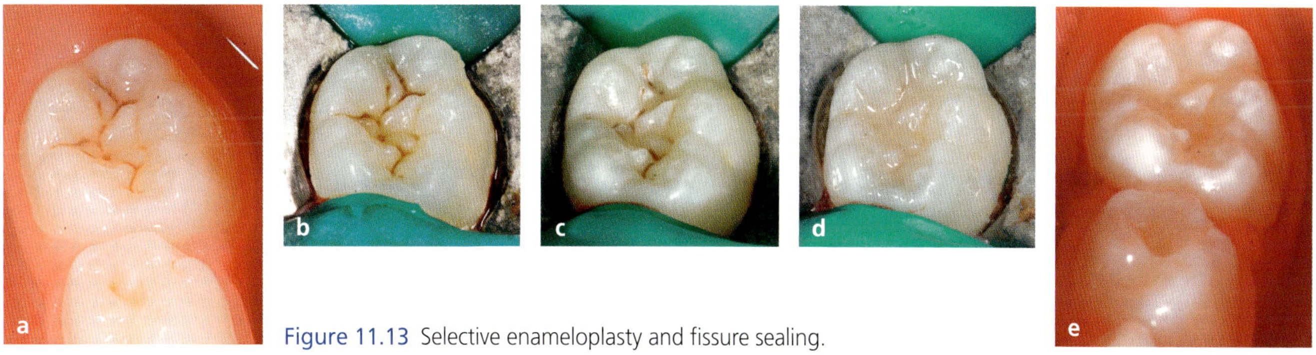

Figure 11.13 Selective enameloplasty and fissure sealing.

After drying, a lack of continuity is seen on the smooth enamel surface, indicating the presence of significant demineralization. Pits and fissures may appear wider and more open than normal, but there is no discontinuity or dentin exposure on the smooth surfaces or at the base of the cavity.

Operative sequence

- Isolation of the operative field using a rubber dam
- Thorough cleansing of the tooth surface using nonoily pumice and a bicarbonate jet
- Rinsing of tooth surfaces with air and water sprays to remove porous residues
- Opening of small cavities on the affected fissures
- Etching with 37% orthophosphoric acid for 30 seconds, followed by copious rinsing of the treated surface for at least 30 seconds
- Drying, followed by the application and polymerization of an appropriate adhesive system
- Application of a thin layer of sealant on pits and fissures
- Polymerization for 20 seconds (evaluation of the complete setting of the resin and its retention)
- Dam removal and occlusal check.

Preventive Resin Restorations (PRR-2 by Simonsen, 1977-1980) (ICDAS code 4)

Preventive resin restoration (PRR) is indicated when the wet tooth shows a dentinal shadow that is visible through the apparently sound enamel, which can appear without signs of localized enamel cavitation (Fig. 11.14).
The first operative step is selection of the color to be used for the restoration (Fig. 11.14a), followed by the isolation of the operative field using a rubber dam, which is always necessary when using composite resins (see Fig. 11.14b). The next step is a thorough cleansing of the tooth using a brush, water and pumice, or a bicarbonate jet. Access to the carious lesion involves the use of coarse-grained (100 µm) diamond-coated micro burs under copious irrigation, and care should be taken not to engage enamel tissue that is not affected by the caries process. Selectivity is also necessary when removing the underlying demineralized dentin, and a rosette burr should be used, preferably a tungsten carbide one. Once the complete removal of the decayed tissues has been achieved, the finishing of the resulting cavity is carried out using a fine-grained (40 µm) diamond-coated burr, preferably mounted on a multiplier handpiece, always with copious irrigation (Fig. 11.14c). The following steps describe the preparation of the substrate that will receive the adhesive system and filling material. The conditioning of the surface varies according to the tissue to be treated. Enamel consists of a mineral phase that contains large hexagonal crystals of hydroxyapatite comprising calcium phosphate salts. These crystals form enamel prisms; in 1955, Buonocore understood the need to treat this surface with acids (etching) to transform a smooth and polished surface into an irregular one, increasing its free energy and facilitating capillary infiltration of liquid acrylic resins. The material of choice for enamel etching is 37% orthophosphoric acid, applied for 30

seconds (Fig. 11.14d). The second tissue to be conditioned is the dentin, the preparation of which, performed using rotating instruments, leads to the formation of a *smear layer* on the surface and *smear plugs* at a deeper level (organic and inorganic debris). The presence of debris reduces the permeability of the dentin; etching with 37% orthophosphoric acid for 15 seconds allows its demineralization as well as debris removal (Fig. 11.14e). After 30 seconds, etched surfaces are rinsed, taking care to remove the acid completely, using air and water sprays for at least 30 seconds (Fig. 11.14f). Following cavity cleansing, any excess liquid in the operative field should be removed and the tooth should be dried using suction to avoid the complete dehydration of the dentinal substrate and the collapse of collagen fibers within the tubules (Fig. 11.14g). Such cavity treatment allows the subsequent adhesive procedures to be performed using the *wet technique*, involving application of the primer for 30 seconds (Fig. 11.14h). Once the tissue is primed, the primer is spread with light air blow (see Fig. 11.14i) and then polymerized using halogen light for 40 seconds at

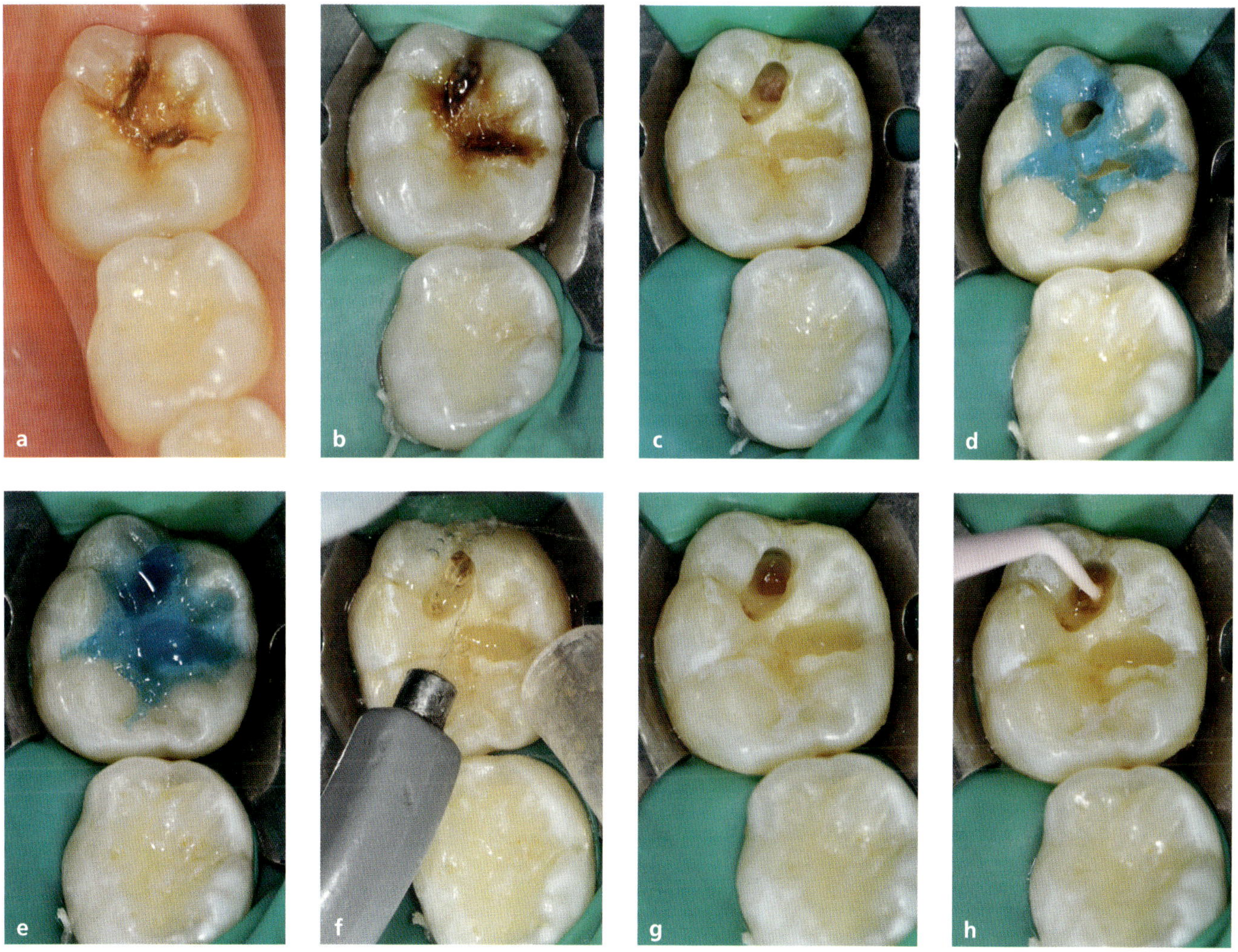

Figure 11.14 (**a–u**) Preventive resin restoration. See text for details.

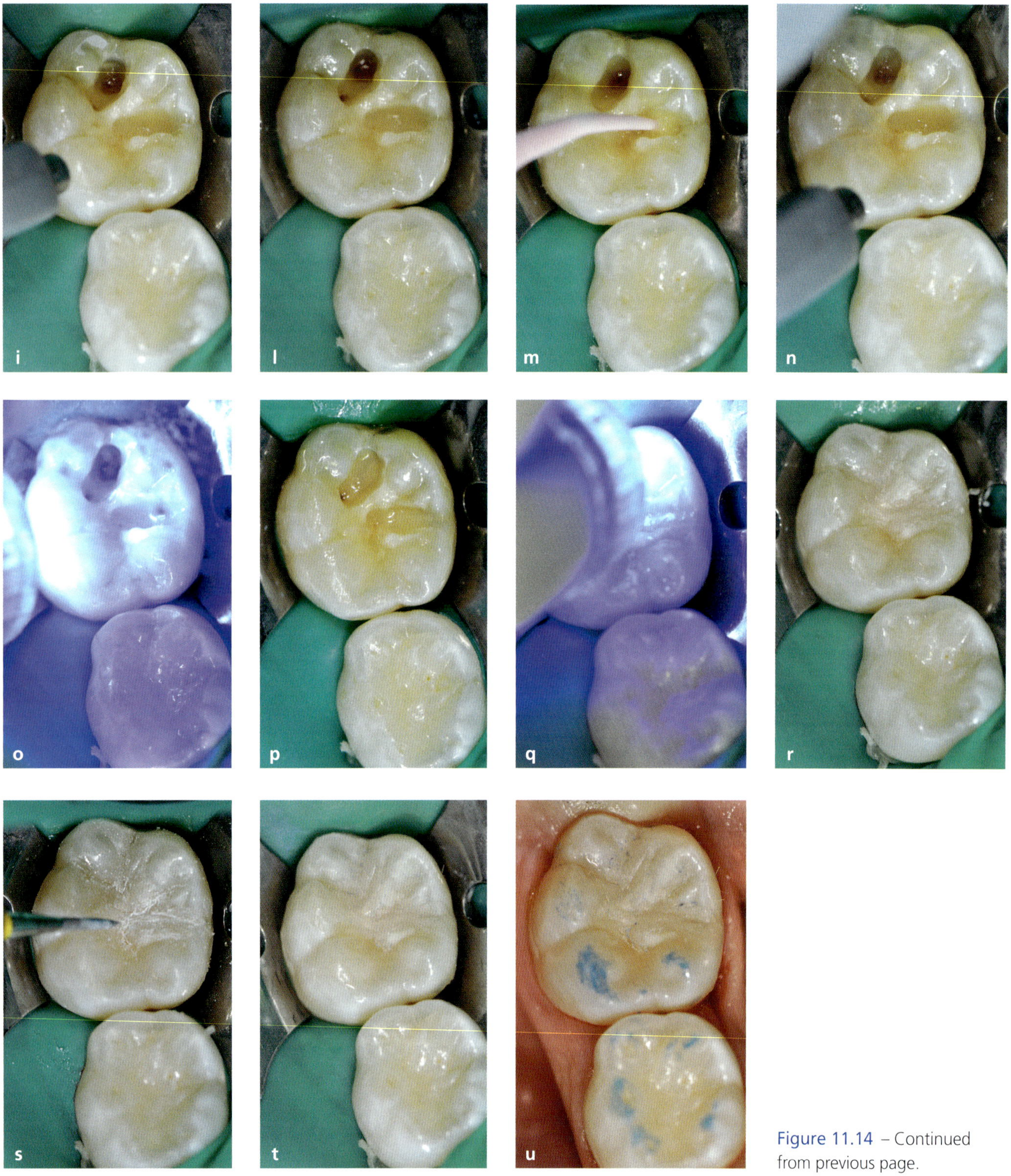

Figure 11.14 – Continued from previous page.

standard power (Fig. 11.14l). The steps for application of a bonding agent are the same (Fig. 11.14m–o). Occlusal anatomy restoration requires anatomical stratification (Fig. 11.14p). The application should be incremental, with each increment polymerized for 40 seconds (Fig. 11.14q). Once the restorative phase is completed (Fig. 11.14r), any excess material can be removed using a fine-grained (20 μm) diamond-coated burr (Fig. 11.14s). After removal of the rubber dam and evaluation of the occlusal contact (Fig. 11.14t), the last steps are smoothening with the silicone rubber, polishing with the brush and diamond paste, and final finishing with the felt pad and aluminum oxide paste.

Atraumatic restorative treatment (ICDAS codes 5-6)

Atraumatic restorative treatment (ART) is an interim therapy preceding definitive restoration (Fig. 11.15). The fundamental principle of this type of intervention is identification of an "affected" dentin layer below the "infected" and discolored dentin, which is often soft and pigmented but not infected (Fusayama, 1979). This technique allows the stabilization of active carious lesions using manual tools to remove the severely weakened enamel and infected dentin.

The "affected" dentin can be remineralized using fluoride-releasing glass ionomer cements (indirect pulp capping), thereby allowing a minimal amount of tissue to be removed (owing to limited enamel and dentin thickness of deciduous molars) and reducing intervention times (in noncooperative patients). This method is widely used in developing countries, where it is even performed by dental auxiliary personnel or in situations with poor availability of dental equipment.

It is important to remember that the child should be checked regularly to prevent any occurrence of complications and to schedule the placement of final restoration as soon as possible.

Indications:

- caries extended to dentin
- no pulp involvement
- access to the lesion possible using manual instruments.

Contraindications:

- carious lesion with pulp exposure
- access difficult using manual instruments.

Operative sequence

- Plexus or nerve block anesthesia (Fig. 11.15a)
- Isolation of operative field using cotton rolls and suction or using a rubber dam if possible (Fig. 11.15b)
- Tooth surface cleansing using sterile cotton pellets
- Removal of infected dentin using manual instruments, starting from the cavity walls and taking care to remove all the caries from the enamel–dentin junction to prevent the progression of the lesion and ensure a good marginal seal (Fig. 11.15c)

- Subsequent removal of dentin from the cavity floor to reduce the patient's sensitivity and discomfort during excavation
- Cleansing of the residual dentin surface and occlusal and lateral cavity surfaces following completion of the excavation phase by rubbing a brush soaked in a weak acid (conditioner) for 10–15 seconds (Fig. 11.15d)
- Rinsing with saline solution and drying of all treated surfaces using a sterile cotton pellet

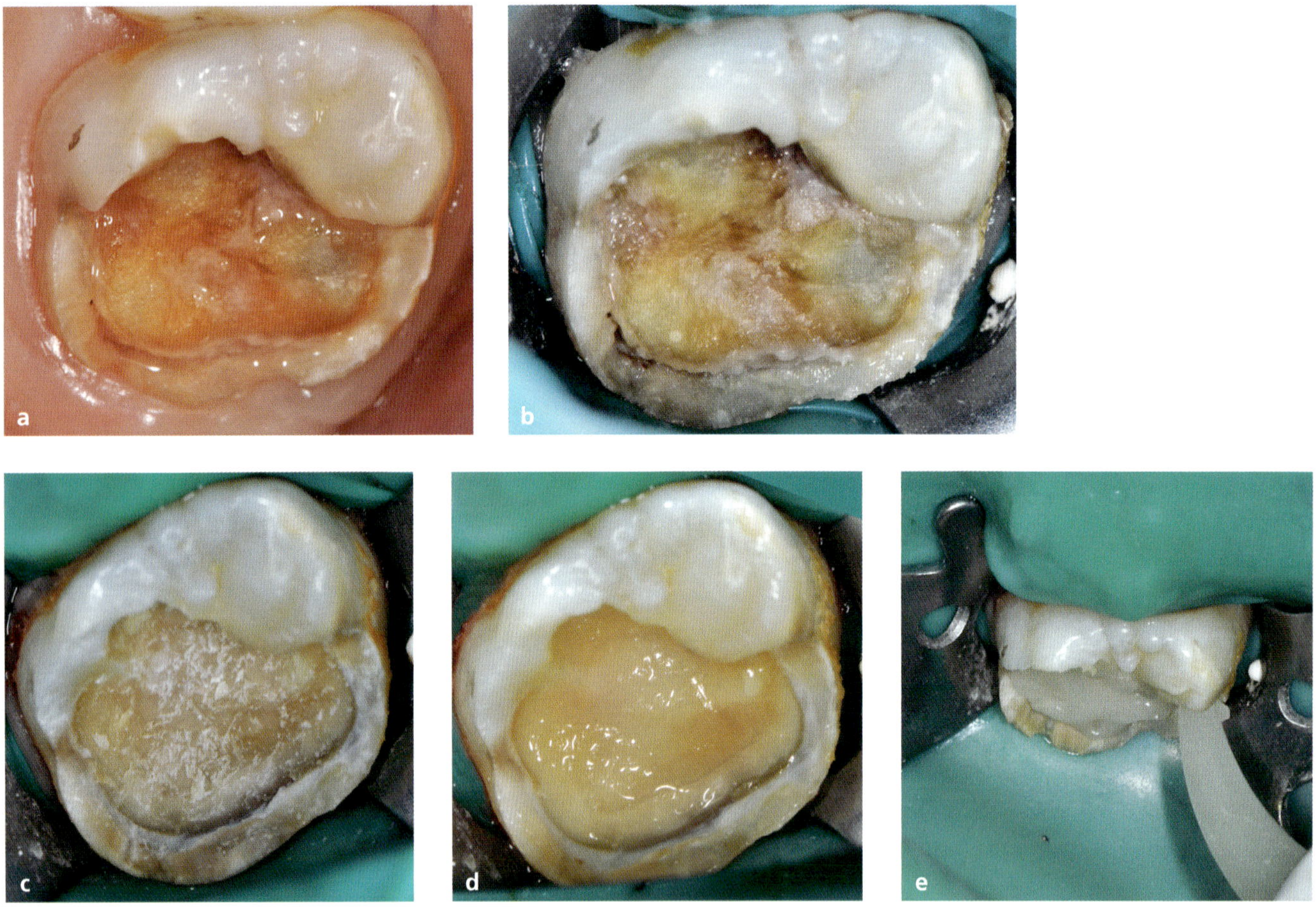

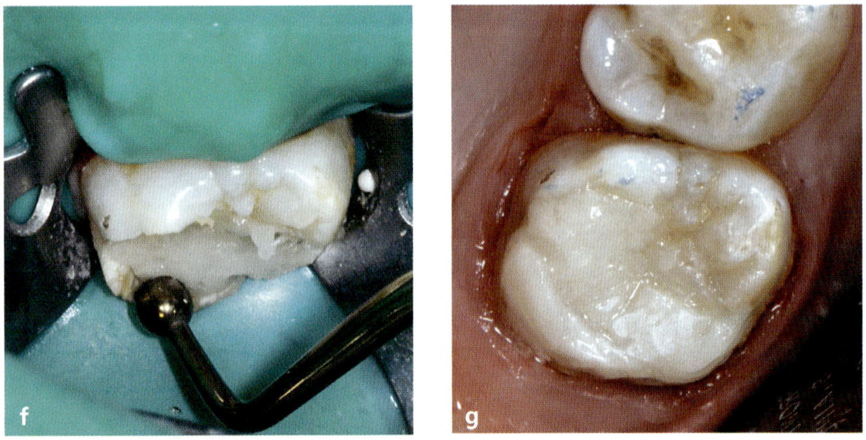

Figure 11.15 (**a–g**) Atraumatic restorative treatment.

- Preparation of glass ionomer cement and application in the cavity in large amounts, exerting slight pressure to allow the best possible adaptation to cavity walls (Fig. 11.15e, f)
- Removal of any excess cement, evaluation of occlusal contact, and application of a varnish on the surface to prevent water uptake or loss (Fig. 11.15g).

Restorative dentistry

Restorative treatment aims to restore the anatomical features of teeth that are altered by caries or trauma. Dental tissue restoration must reproduce the original shape and size of the tooth while maintaining the healthy tissues and reducing the risk of secondary caries. With regard to materials currently used in pediatric dentistry, the authors' choice tends toward the use of composite resins, whereas glass ionomer cements or compomers are used in certain situations only. Amalgam usage, because of the controversy concerning the presence of mercury, is contraindicated in patients aged less than 6 years (Italian Ministry of Health Decree of October 10, 2001) and is not recommended by the authors in light of the principle of "bioeconomy" of healthy tissue, which is the basis of modern adhesive dental techniques.

Direct restorations

In pediatric dentistry, the direct restoration technique is definitely the most commonly used dental restoration method. It is used in the conservation of deciduous and permanent elements as it proves to be the most simple and least invasive, allowing minimal cavity preparation and requiring shorter intervention times (single session).

Direct or semi-direct restoration technique in anterior regions

The selection of the technique and materials to be used in anterior restorations is not always easy and cannot be based solely on technical considerations. The selection criteria available to the clinician are the child's age and ability to cooperate, the extent of injury, the number of teeth involved, and the possibility of a morphological and functional restoration of the damaged tooth. Usage of glass ionomer cements in the management of caries in an anterior deciduous tooth can be an excellent method to rehabilitate a 2-year-old child esthetically and functionally, whose behavior does not allow the placement of a composite resin restoration, because it does not require rubber dam placement and local anesthesia administration. At a subsequent age, from the esthetic and functional perspectives, the child will be able to undergo a more suitable treatment using composite resins.
Semi-direct restoration of a permanent central incisor fractured following a trauma requires impression taking and preparation of a diagnostic wax-up that is used to make a rigid silicone matrix to be used as a guide for composite layering. After selecting the color and isolating the field with a rubber dam and cervical ligations, the next step is the preparation and finishing of the margins.

After tooth cleansing, the enamel and dentin undergo etching, followed by treatment with traditional adhesive systems. The first application of composite material involves the positioning of a thin layer of enamel (0.5 mm) on the matrix to recreate the entire palatal and interproximal portions of the restoration, slightly increasing the thickness at the contact point between the restoration and the tooth.
Once the material has been adapted using a thin spatula, it is polymerized using halogen light for 40 seconds at standard power.
Before removing the matrix, a mass of dentin is applied in the cervical and central areas that consolidates the fragment. The modeling subsequently proceeds without the silicone support to improve visibility and range of movement.
The application of masses of dentin continues until the enamel–dentin junction is reached, polymerizing each material increment for 40 seconds and taking care to recreate the anatomical and chromatic features of the adjacent dental element. The final increment of enamel composite is applied on the entire dentin mass surface as a single layer to avoid the formation of seams and microporosities. Polymerization occurs as described above, and any excess is removed using very fine-grained diamond burs. After removing the rubber dam, it is necessary to pay careful attention to the finishing and polishing phases of the restoration (Fig. 11.16).

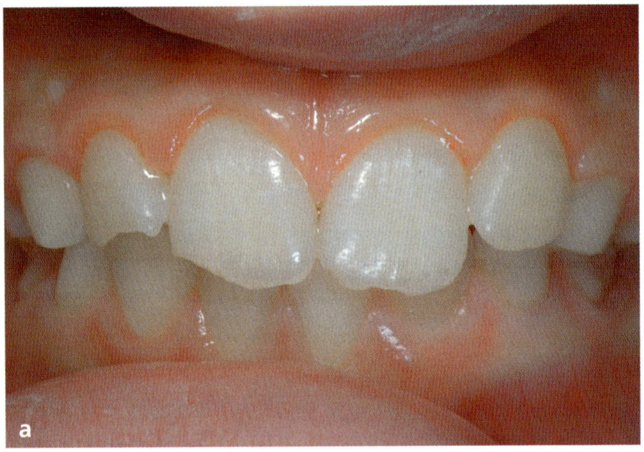
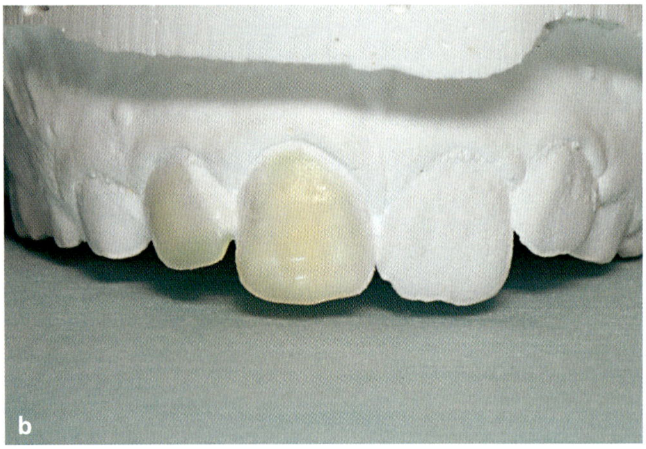
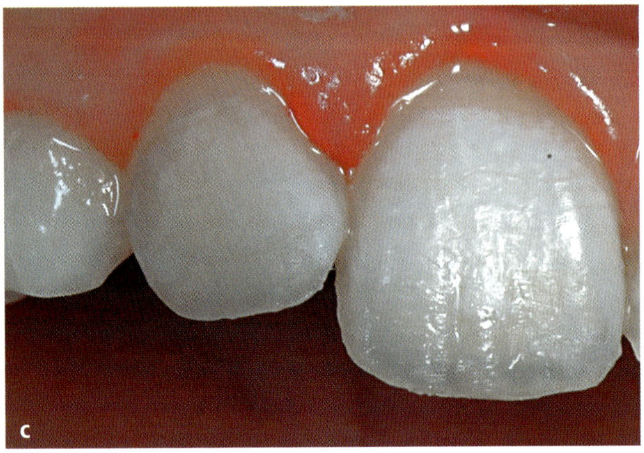

Figure 11.16 (**a–c**) Direct or semi-direct reconstruction technique in anterior regions. See text for details.

Direct reconstruction technique in posterior regions

Black's class I restoration. To perform a Black's class I composite resin direct restoration in a deciduous or permanent tooth, the first step of conservative treatment involves the administration of anesthesia, if needed; selection of the material and its color; and isolation of the field (Fig. 11.17a, b).

The operative sequence is as follows:

- Cavity design follows the carious lesion extent; access through the enamel requires the use of a cylindrical or truncated-cone coarse-grained (100 μm) diamond bur with a flat tip and rounded corners
- For a more selective intervention, the soft dentin should be removed using a tungsten carbide rosette bur mounted on a low-speed handpiece and/or manual instruments (Fig. 11.17c)
- The cavity walls are finished using fine-grain (40 μm) diamond burs, and the edges are subsequently smoothened using an abrasive rubber
- It is recommended to disinfect the exposed dentin by applying sterile cotton pellets soaked in 0.2% chlorhexidine for 1 minute
- Currently, it is believed appropriate to apply a thin layer of glass ionomer cement at the bottom of deep cavities to increase restoration elasticity and reduce dental pulp shock injury. The material should be spread uniformly in the deepest part of the cavity; this is followed by polymerization for 40 seconds or, in the case of self-curing materials, the setting time (sandwich technique) (Fig. 11.17d, s)
- Hard tissue etching requires 37% phosphoric acid, which should act on enamel for 30 seconds and on dentin for 15 seconds (Fig. 11.17f)
- After copious rinsing with air and water sprays to completely remove the gel, the cavity is dried via suction to avoid excessive dehydration of the exposed dentin.
- Application of the adhesive system for enamel and dentin conditioning is performed. The authors recommend using small brushes that, when rubbed on dentin, allow the fluids to penetrate perfectly into dentinal tubules. In such cases, the primer is applied first (Fig. 11.17g), followed by the bonding agent (Fig. 11.17h), which is spread with a light air blow and then polymerized using halogen light for 40 seconds at standard power (Fig. 11.17i)
- When the adhesive seal photopolymerization is completed, the authors perform tooth restoration using an anatomical multilayering technique with single composite increments of 2 mm, followed by polymerization for 40 seconds (Fig. 11.17l). Once the reconstruction of the triangular cusp ridges with masses of dentin is completed, tooth modeling is performed via the application of masses of enamel on marginal ridges and the more superficial occlusal layers (Fig. 11.17m)
- Any excess is removed with very fine-grained (20 μm) diamond burs, and the complete restoration should be finished and polished using a silicone or impregnated brush
- After removing the rubber dam, occlusal check is performed (Fig. 11.17n).

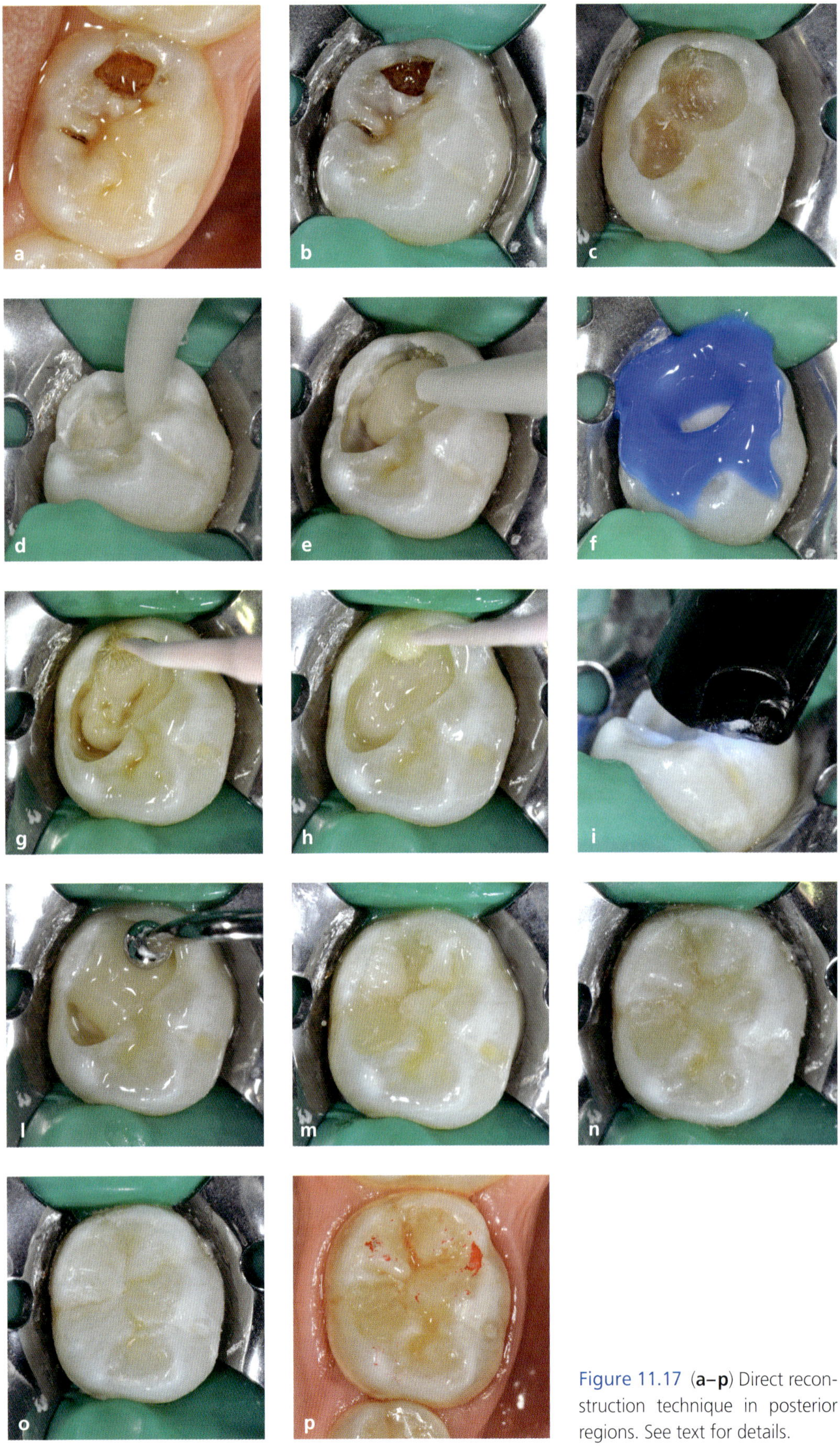

Figure 11.17 (**a–p**) Direct reconstruction technique in posterior regions. See text for details.

Black's class II restoration. Direct restorative treatment of interproximal cavities should be limited to small- or medium-sized carious lesions with a suitable amount of cervical enamel (Fig. 11.18). The principle of maximum conservation of healthy hard tissues entails preserving the proximal ridges, enamel bridges, and occlusal surfaces, even if not completely supported by dentin, when possible. In the presence of interproximal caries, which require the placement of a direct restoration with adhesive technique, cavity preparation should respect the topography of the carious lesion and comprise a round-shaped interproximal box with the smoothening of enamel margins without creating an actual chamfer finish line. The marginal ridge is accessed using a coarse-grained (100 µm) cylindrical diamond bur with rounded head angles. After removing the carious lesion using a tungsten carbide rosette bur mounted on a contra-angle handpiece with a 1:1 ratio, the axial edges are finished with diamond burs of the same design as that of the previous one but with a finer grain (40 µm) or using a long or short flame burr. The smoothing of the cervical step is performed using a dental chisel. After careful cavity preparation, the matrix and wooden wedge are positioned. Next, "adhesive restoration" is performed: etching of hard tooth tissues using 37% orthophosphoric acid (15 seconds for the dentin and 30 seconds for the enamel); rinsing with air and water sprays to remove the acid; and cavity drying via suction, followed by the application of primer and bonding agent. The first step in the morphological and functional restoration of a dental element involves restoration of the proximal wall. Application of a thin vertical layer of enamel material that recreates the interproximal wall contours and transforms the class II cavity into a class I cavity. After removal of the matrix, the marginal ridge undergoes further polymerization and evaluation for the presence of an adequate contact surface using dental floss. At this point, a thin layer of *flowable* composite is placed at the bottom of the cavity, and the composite masses are stratified using the technique described for class I restorations. The technique

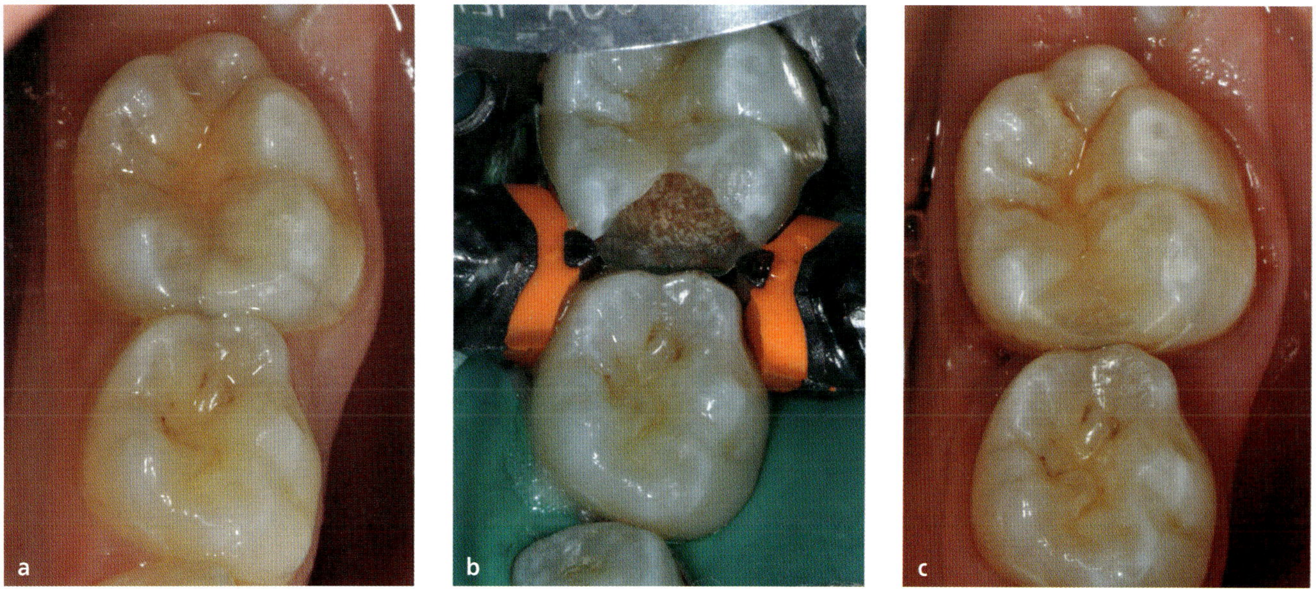

Figure 11.18 Direct reconstruction technique in posterior regions in the permanent dentition.

used by the authors for occlusal surface restoration involves anatomical multilayering, with the application, modeling, and polymerization of various layers of composite resin for dentin and enamel. When reconstruction is completed, the entire restoration is polymerized for 60 seconds, and after dam removal, the occlusal check is performed, along with the finishing and polishing of the definitive tooth surfaces.

Suggested readings

Gutmann JL, Solomon E. Evidenced-based review of clinical studies on indirect pulp capping. J Endod 2009;35(8):1147-51.

Buonocore MG. A simple method of increasing the adhesion of acrylic filling materials to enamel surfaces. J Dent Res 1955;34(6):849-53.

Burke FJ, Crisp RJ, James A et al. Two year clinical evaluation of a low-shrink resin composite material in UK general dental practices. Dent Mater 2011;27(7):622-30. Epub 2011 Apr 22.

Daly D, Waldron JM. Molar incisor hypomineralisation: clinical management of the young patient. J Ir Dent Assoc 2009;55(2):83-6.

Fusayama T. Two layers of carious dentin; diagnosis and treatment. Oper Dent. 1979; 4(2):63-70.

Gotler M, Ratson T. Molar incisor hypomineralization (MIH): a literature review. Refuat Hapeh Vehashinayim 2010;27(2):10-8,60.

Hill EE. Decision-making for treatment planning a cantilevered fixed partial denture. Compend Contin Educ Dent 2009;30(9):580-5; quiz 586, 606.

Kemoli AM, van Amerongen WE. The dilemma of selecting suitable proximal carious lesions in primary molars for restoration using ART technique. Community Dent Health 2011;28(1):12-6.

Killian CM, Croll TP. Nano-ionomer tooth repair in pediatric dentistry. Pediatr Dent 2010;32(7): 530-5.

Leinfelder KF. Posterior composites. State-of-the-art clinical applications. Dent Clin North Am 1993;37(3):411-8.

Marks LA, Faict N, Welbury RR. Literature review: restorations of class II cavities in the primary dentition with compomers. Eur Arch Paediatr Dent 2010;11(3):109-14.

Mickenautsch S, Yengopal V, Banerjee A. Atraumatic restorative treatment versus amalgam restoration longevity: a systematic review. Clin Oral Investig 2010;14(3):233-40. Epub 2009 Aug 18.

Naasan MA, Watson TF. Conventional glass ionomers as posterior restorations. A status report for the American Journal of Dentistry. Am J Dent 1998;11(1):36-45.

Willmott NS, Bryan RA, Duggal MS. Molar-incisor-hypomineralisation: a literature review. Eur Arch Paediatr Dent 2008;9(4):172-9.

Yengopal V, Harneker SY, Patel N, Siegfried N. Dental fillings for the treatment of caries in the primary dentition. Cochrane Database Syst Rev 2009 Apr 15;(2):CD004483.

Chapter 12

Endodontics in pediatric dentistry

M. Bossù, G. Di Giorgio, A. Polimeni

Pediatric endodontics is the branch of pediatric dentistry involved with the treatment of dental pulp in pediatric patients. Treatment intervention for this group of patients requires the involvement of dental elements from the deciduous and permanent dentition.

Endodontic treatment of deciduous teeth

The diagnosis is based on medical history, particularly that related to recent pathological events, which allows information regarding the cause that led the patient to seek medical attention to be collected. Furthermore, the diagnosis is based on physical and radiographic examination. The necessary examinations include orthopantomography and periapical radiography. The first examination provides a general clinical picture of the stomatognathic apparatus to be obtained for detecting the presence of all permanent elements and the fulfillment of dentition transition times. The second examination facilitates the evaluation of the element to be treated, and in particular, the extension of the disease affecting the pulp, the presence of periapical lesions, the level of resorption, and the possible involvement of the corresponding permanent elements by phlogistic processes (Fig. 12.1 and 12.2).

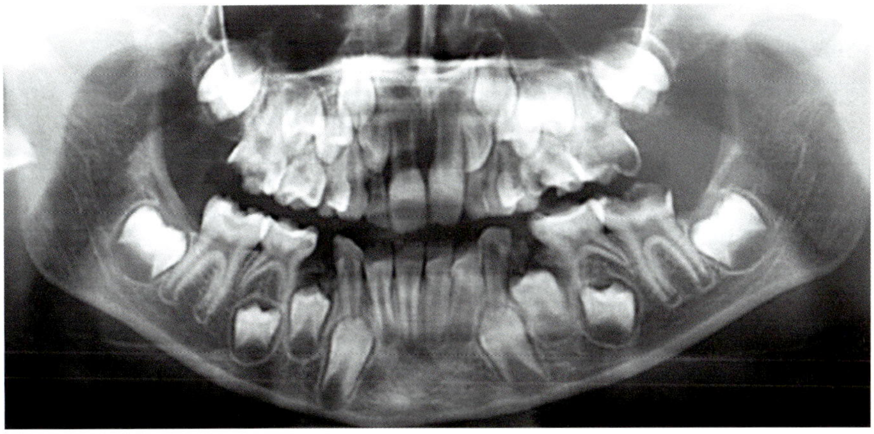

Figure 12.1 From the panoramic radiograph of the dental arches, it is possible to observe the presence of diffuse carious lesions, the level of development of radicular apexes, as well as the phase of dentition exchange and the position of the buds of permanent dental elements.

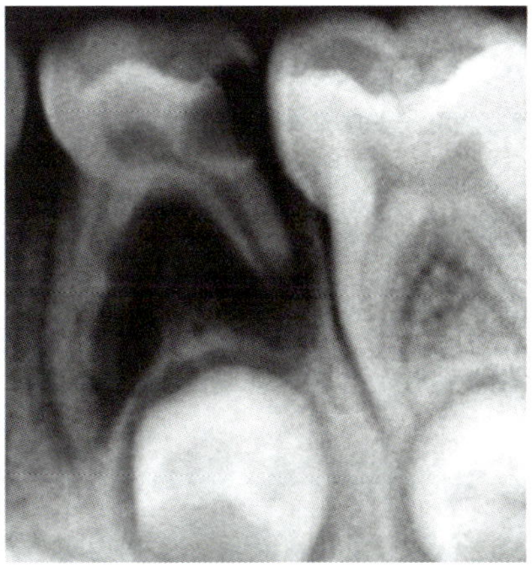

Figure 12.2 Intraoral periapical radiograph, which allows precise evaluation of the extension of the bone lesion and the possibility of treating the affected dental element.

Pediatric dentists should consider the continuous metamorphosis of the patient's dentition that occurs during pediatric age and should know the exact techniques and materials to use in various clinical scenarios. The main goal of pulp treatment is to consider the state of the entire stomatognathic apparatus. The maintenance of the deciduous dentition is essential for the appropriate development of the permanent dentition and for the oral health of children because it contributes to the establishment of a stable, functional, and esthetically harmonious occlusion. In this regard, it is important to remember that the carious and/or traumatic lesion can cause abscesses and early loss of space within the arch, thereby negatively influencing the formation and eruption of the corresponding permanent tooth. Therefore, it is necessary to prevent and treat these pathological events even though endodontic treatment might occasionally be necessary for deciduous teeth, so that they can preserve their anatomical integrity until the transition is completed (Fig. 12.3-12.7). Endodontic treatment of deciduous

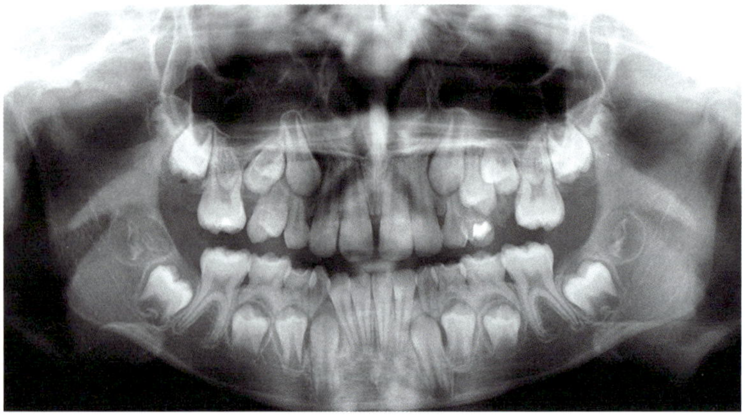

Figure 12.3 From the panoramic radiograph of the dental arches, it is possible to confirm the loss of space at the detriment of the left and right upper second premolar. It is also possible to identify the presence of a supernumerary tooth at the level of 4.8.

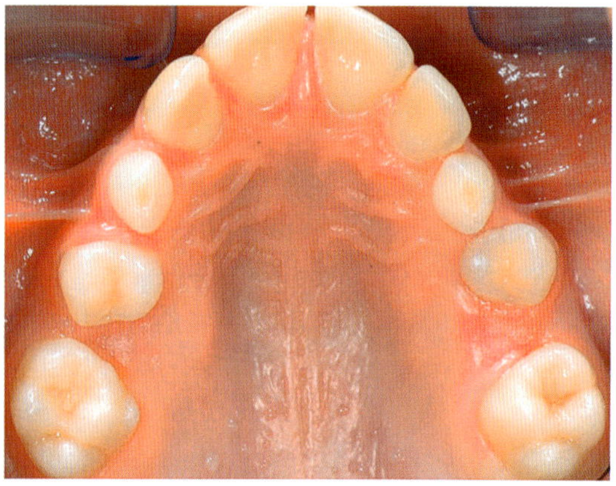

Figure 12.4 Clinical view of the upper arch, from which it is possible to identify the loss of space for the eruption of two second premolars.

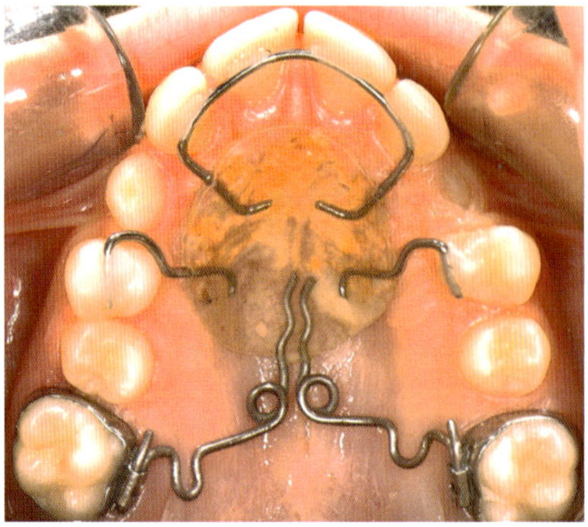

Figure 12.5 Positioning of an orthodontic device of the *pendulum* type, which has created space necessary for the eruption of premolars.

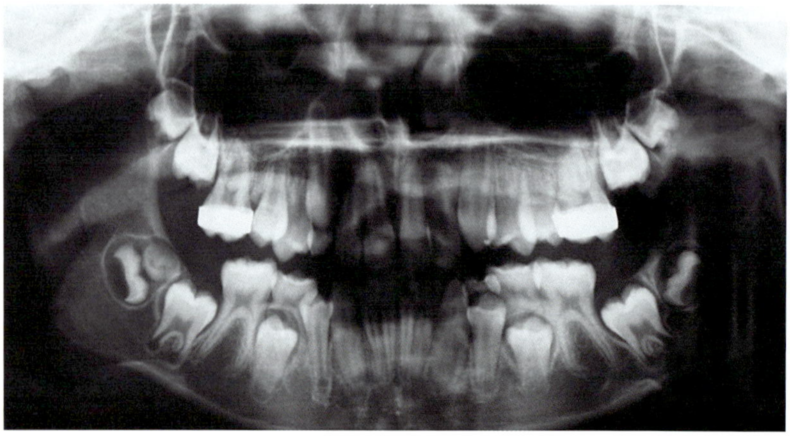

Figure 12.6 Orthopantomographic view after eruption.

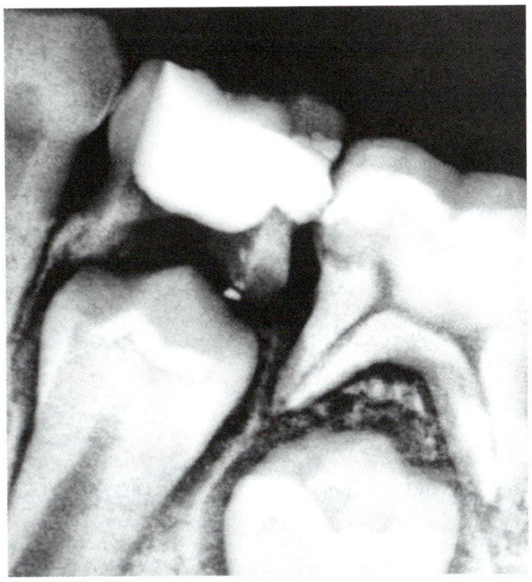

Figure 12.7 From the intraoral periapical radiographic examination, it is possible to note the need for performing extraction of the dental element.

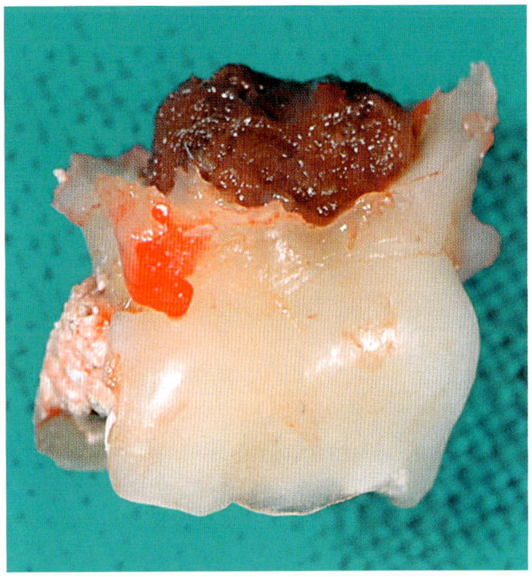

Figure 12.8 Dental element after extraction, which indicates that there has been a previous attempt at therapy.

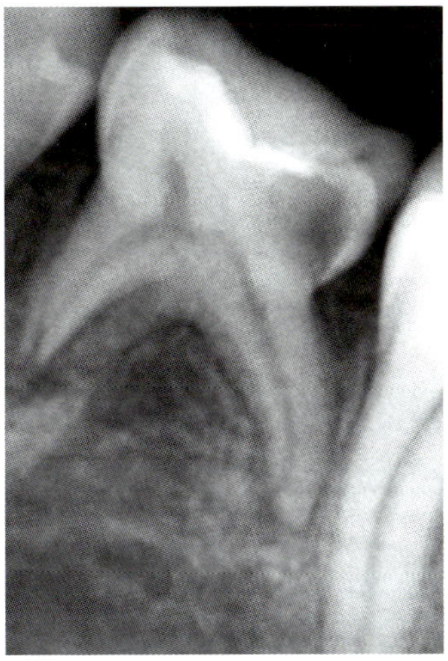

Figure 12.9 From the intraoral periapical radiograph, it is possible to conclude that there is a need for endodontic therapy for 7.5, with agenesis of the corresponding permanent element.

elements can be more or less complex depending on the type of lesion and the extent to which the pulp has been affected by a pathology.

The selected treatment depends on the analysis of several variables:

- extent to which the pulp has been affected
- level of resorption (Fig. 12.8)
- vitality of the dental element
- abscesses of long duration
- agenesis of the corresponding permanent element (Fig. 12.9)
- age of the patient.

After assessing the individual cases and excluding the need for extraction (destroyed or nonrestorable crowns, marked interradicular and periapical osteolysis, advanced resorption, severe systemic pathology, and patient's age), the types of treatment are as follows:

- pulpotomy
- pulpectomy.

Pulpotomy

Pulpotomy is the most widely used endodontic treatment for deciduous elements in cases wherein, after accidental pulp exposure (iatrogenic event) or trauma, only the pulp chamber is affected, provided that there is no symptom and no clinical sign of pulpal pain. The medical history should exclude spontaneous pain, tenderness to percussion or palpation, and previous abscess. Vitality tests must have positive outcomes.

Pulpotomy is contraindicated in the presence of mucosa and periodontium alterations such as swelling, fistulas, pathologic tooth mobility, internal root resorption, pulpal calcification, or excessive bleeding of the radicular pulp during the treatment procedure, with the latter considered a sign of irreversible pulpal inflammation.
The goal of this treatment is to preserve the vitality of the root pulp, favoring the physiological resorption process.
The surgical technique requires a local plexus and nerve block anesthesia with or without adrenaline in the area of intervention. The operative area is isolated using a rubber dam. The hard tissue affected by the carious lesion is eliminated; once the oral cavity is cleansed, the pulp chamber is opened using a diamond bur fitted to a dental turbine, and subsequently, the pulp at the level of the root canals is removed under abundant irrigation to avoid possible lesions or overheating of the residual pulp. The cavity created is then cleansed with abundant irrigation using a physiological solution, and the surface is swabbed with an imbued sterile cotton pellet without exerting pressure on the exposed tissue. When bleeding has ceased spontaneously (no more than 4 minutes), the selected material is applied on the root pulp and a temporary reconstruction is placed. After taking a control x-ray, a visit is scheduled for the following week. At the follow-up, the patient undergoes a physical examination, and, if there are no signs or symptoms of pulp inflammation, definitive reconstruction is performed using composite materials or, alternatively, glass ionomer cements.
The ideal material for pulpotomy should be innocuous for the pulp and protect the root pulp integrity without interfering with the physiological resorption process.
Many materials have been used over the years, such as formocresol, glutaraldehyde, ferric sulfate, calcium hydroxide, and bioactive cements.
Formocresol was introduced in 1904 by Buckley with the following composition: 19% formaldehyde, 35% cresol, 15% glycerin, and 31% water. It has been considered the best material to treat the pulp of deciduous dentition for more than 60 years. Pulpotomies performed with formocresol have a success rate ranging between 55% and 98%. Formocresol is placed at the end of the root canals using a cotton pellet and must be maintained for 5 minutes and then gently removed. The pulp tissue appears brown but does not show bleeding; subsequently, a temporary filling is performed.
Histological studies show that formocresol produces a layer of coagulative necrosis on the pulp adjacent to the lesion, which in time becomes colliquative because of the release of hydrolytic enzymes by neutrophil leukocytes. Nevertheless, formocresol has long been considered the best dressing material; however, concerns regarding its use have recently been raised. Berger and Rolling (1972) and Lambjerg and Hansen (1978) conducted research on pulpotomies performed using formocresol and demonstrated chronic inflammation and necrosis of the radicular pulp. Furthermore, Myers et al (1978) showed the systemic distribution of formocresol used for pulpotomy and some allergenic and mutagenic properties of formaldehyde on animal models. Pruhs et al (1977) highlighted the relationship between pulpotomies performed using formocresol on deciduous elements and enamel defects on the corresponding permanent elements. Many concerns have been raised about the use of formocresol in humans, especially because of its potential toxicity and carcinogenicity. Finally, the Interna-

tional Agency for Research on Cancer determined formaldehyde to be carcinogenic (2004), impelling scientists and technicians to find alternative materials for their operative procedures.

Glutaraldehyde was introduced in 1985 by Gravenmade, who proposed it as a chemical agent that can replace formocresol for the pulpotomy of deciduous elements to eliminate the adverse effects of formaldehyde. Its action on chamber pulp is achieved through the formation of insoluble macromolecular protein bonds, which are followed by lower apical migration and reduced systemic absorption, leading to lower toxicity. Through the action of glutaraldehyde, superficial coagulative necrosis is produced, which causes an instant and more compact fixation at the level of the chamber pulp, leaving a greater quantity of vital tissue. It is used at a concentration of 2%–2.5%, following the same operative procedure used for formocresol.

However, at concentrations higher than 0.5%, this drug is considered a dangerous substance because of its sensitizing properties and because it causes irritation in the eyes, skin, and respiratory tract. Glutaraldehyde can only be used in combination with strict preventive measures, such as the use of suitable rooms, adequate air changes, extractor hoods, and personal protection equipment, as well as compliance with codified usage procedures for the protection of staff and patients and installation of appropriate signs regarding danger and disposal. In light of the above, the use of glutaraldehyde in clinics was discontinued in Italy a long time ago.

Calcium hydroxide is used routinely in endodontics as intracanal medication for dental elements with necrotic pulp, primarily because of its high pH (12.5), which gives it excellent antibacterial activity and a strong capacity to inactivate the bacterial endotoxin lipopolysaccharide. Despite its wide application in dentistry, its use is not highly recommended in the treatment of vital deciduous elements (direct capping and pulpotomy) because of the frequency of failures related to chronic pulp inflammation and/or internal radicular resorptions (Fig. 12.10). It is believed that the high contents of pulp tissue cells in deciduous elements can be responsible for the failures of this treatment because mesenchymal cells can differentiate into odontoclasts in response to either the carious lesion or the treatment itself and produce resorption lesions on dentin and cementum.

Among the drugs that have been tested, only ferric sulfate seems to be a promising alternative to formocresol and glutaraldehyde. It acts by inducing hemostasis through the formation of iron–protein complexes in contact with blood in acidic conditions, thereby sealing cut blood vessels. The use of ferric sulfate is recommended because once the chamber pulp is removed, clot formation prevents problems associated with blood extravasation from occurring, thereby preventing the onset of inflammation or internal resorption, which are important factors for the failure of pulpotomies performed using calcium hydroxide.

Several comparative studies in the literature have focused on ferric sulfate and other materials; the most important aspect highlighted by these studies is that, with the equal rate of clinical and radiographic successes, this material performs an exclusively local action, with no systemic diffusion and no resulting toxicity unlike formocresol and glutaraldehyde.

Recently, satisfactory results have been obtained with bioactive cements such as mineral trioxide aggregate (MTA), which is composed of tricalcium silicate, tricalcium aluminate, tricalcium oxide, and gypsum. Mixing this powder with liquid produces crystals of calcium oxide with amorphous structure. This substance starts solidifying within less than 3 hours and completely hardens within the next 72 hours. MTA has the capacity to form hard tissue in contact with the pulp, as well as the capacity to induce rapid cellular growth in vitro.

The preparation of the cavity to access the pulp requires the same steps that have been previously described (Fig.12.11a, b). Once hemostasis has been achieved (Fig. 12.11c), MTA is directly placed in contact with the radicular pulp (Fig. 12.11d, Video 12.1); subsequently, an imbued cotton pellet is inserted—an important step, as this material sets in a moist environment. This is followed placing a temporary filling and taking a postoperative periapical control x-ray (Fig. 12.11e, f). After approximately 1 week and after having performed a clinical examination to identify the clinical signs of pulpal pain, the temporary filling and cotton pellet are removed, and, if the material has acquired optimal solidity (Fig 12.11g), definitive reconstruction using adhesive systems available in the market can be performed (Fig. 12.11h). Subsequently, it is necessary for the child to undergo periodical clinical and radiographic tests to inspect the integrity of the coronal restoration and ensure that there is no sign of periapical pain (Fig. 12.11l). It is possible to observe, particularly in cases involving patients aged more than 4 years, the formation of a dentin bridge (Fig 12.12). MTA has proved to be an excellent material for the maintenance of pulp tissue integrity, with success rates of 95%–98% in the medium and long term.

The histological analysis of pulp tissues in animals and humans shows lower inflammatory response, lower hyperemia, and fewer cases of pulp necrosis. MTA is extremely effective in reducing the penetration of microorganisms, as well as being biocompat-

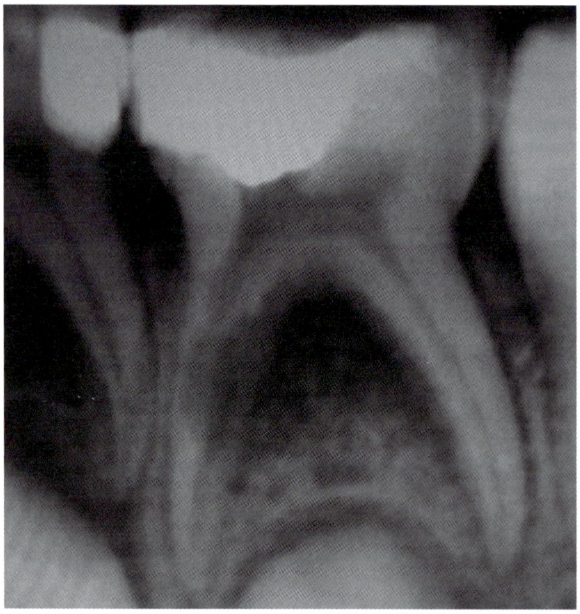

Figure 12.10 Intraoral periapical radiograph, which highlights internal resorption after capping with calcium hydroxide.

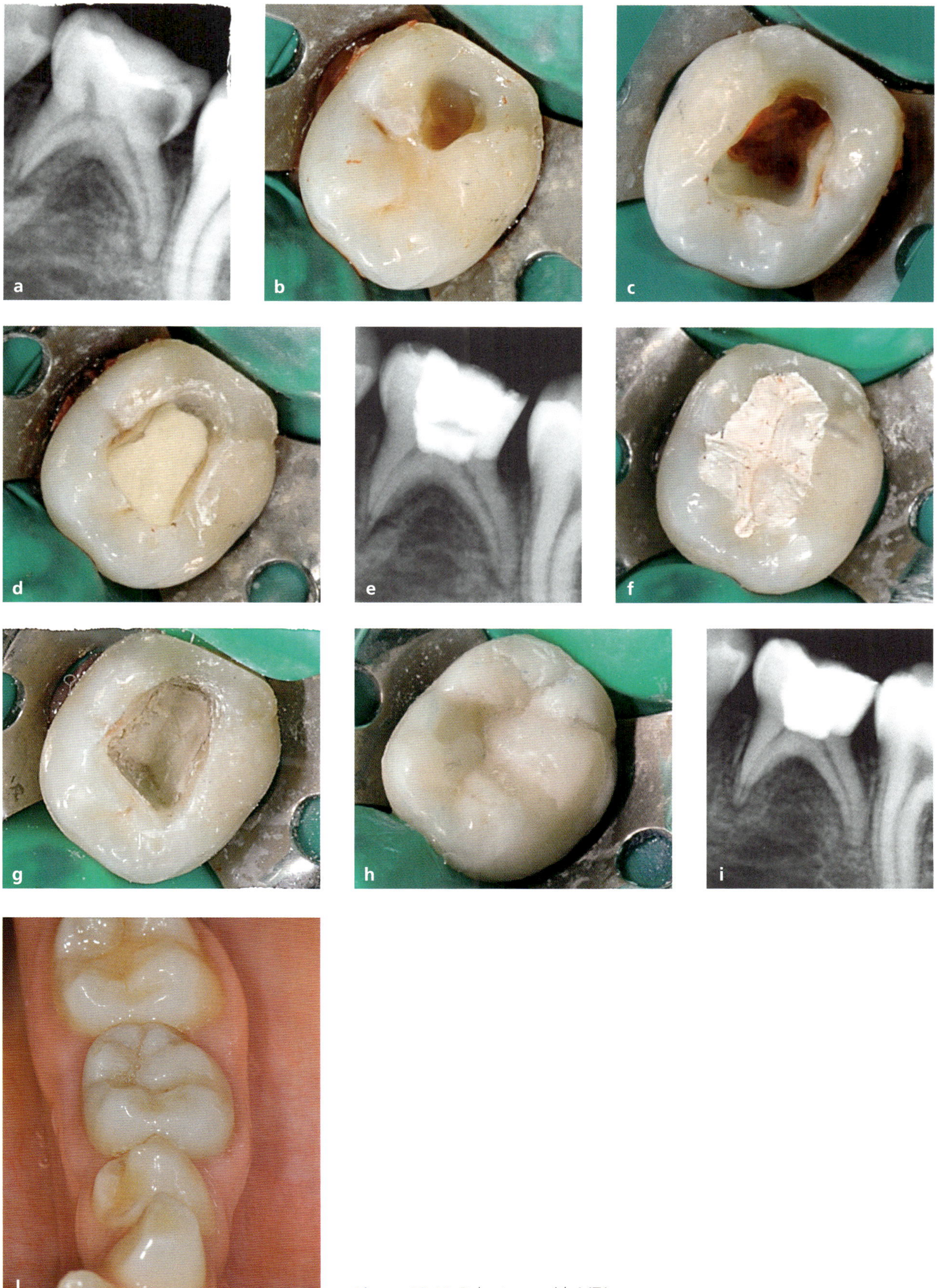

Figure 12.11 Pulpotomy with MTA.

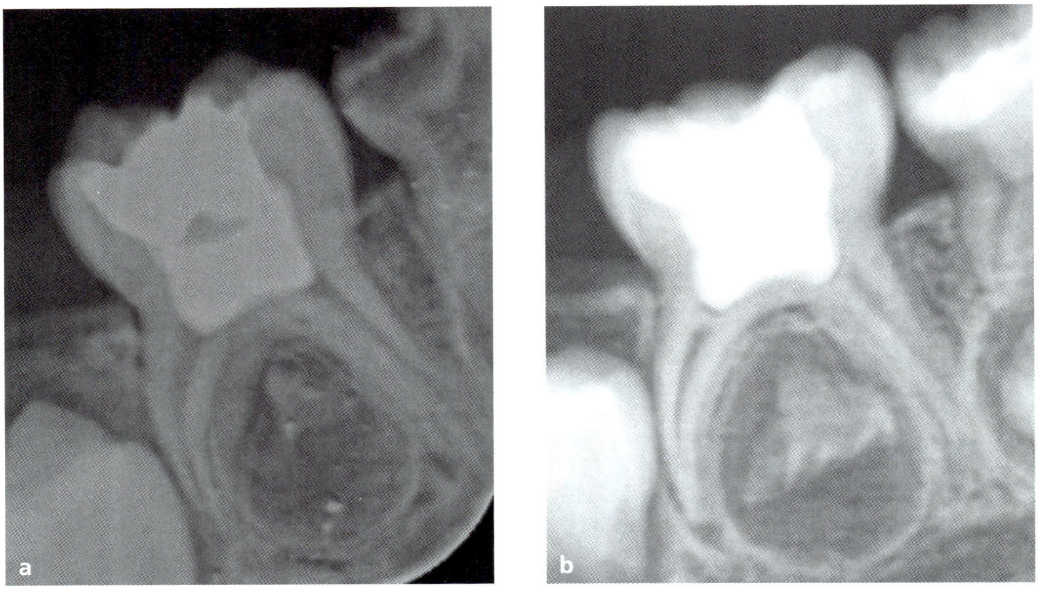

Figure 12.12 Pulpotomy with MTA in a 3-year-old patient. (**a**) Postoperative x-ray; (**b**) control Rx at 6 months, from which it is possible to note the formation of the dentin bridge.

ible and bioinductive and having facultative antibacterial effects, but this is not an effect specific for anaerobic bacteria.

Pulpectomy

Pulpectomy is an endodontic treatment that requires the removal of the entire pulp, both coronal and radicular. It is indicated in cases in which the pulp is vital but irreversibly inflamed or nonvital owing to advanced carious or traumatic lesions.

The indications for pulpectomy include spontaneous or percussion-induced pain, pulp necrosis, abscess processes, or presence of fistulas.

The aim of the endodontic treatment of deciduous elements is to evaluate inflammation and therefore eliminate pathogenic bacteria from the canal system. The bacteria most frequently present are gram-positive anaerobic microorganisms such as *Streptococcus viridians*, *Peptostreptococcus*, and *Actinomyces viscosus*. Gram-positive microorganisms include *Bacteroides melaninogenicus* and *Fusobacterium nucleatum*.

The endodontic treatment of deciduous elements is influenced by several factors, mainly related to the anatomy of the root, the thickness of the pulp chamber floor, and the impossibility to establish the exact position of the apical foramen both from a clinical and radiological perspective, an effect that occurs because of the change that takes place during the physiological resorption process. Owing to the peculiarity of physiological resorption, detecting the radicular length through periapical radiology may be inaccurate. To date, measurement of radicular length using electronic methods appears to be the most reliable method to avoid over-instrumentation, which might cause lesions on the bud of the permanent element located under the root of the deciduous element.

The abundant irrigation of radicular canals is equally important in the endodontics of deciduous teeth. After removing the radicular pulp, cleansing is crucial for creating the most sterile environment possible. For this purpose, the irrigating substance par excellence is undoubtedly 5.25% sodium hypochlorite, which, in addition to dissolving organic substances and cleansing the lateral canals, has a bactericidal action against gram-negative and gram-positive microorganisms, which are associated with reduced toxicity.
To shape the canals, based on their clinical experience, the authors suggest the use of Ni-Ti rotating instruments for the following reasons:

- they are considerably time saving, i.e., the procedure takes 35 minutes using manual instrumentation and just 12 minutes using mechanical instrumentation (in the case of nonexpert practitioners)
- they guarantee safety as the instruments mounted on a contra-angle reduce the risk of accidental ingestion when it is impossible to place the rubber dam
- they ensure adequate access to the apical third and easy penetration of the irrigating agents and medications used.

The need to shape the canal arises from the need to allow the irrigating agent to wet the entire radicular surface, and it should not be considered a fundamental step for the ensuing tridimensional filling of the radicular system, which occurs with the permanent elements.
Among the possible disadvantages of mechanical instrumentation, the risk of compromising the stability of the dental element should not be overlooked because of excessive consumption of healthy dentin tissue. To avoid this complication, it is important to perform an accurate preoperative investigation and, where appropriate, select instruments with lower conicity (02, 04). Many researchers agree that total removal of the pulp tissue in the radicular canals of deciduous elements cannot be achieved because of their complex and variable morphology. For this purpose, Ni-Ti instruments can be directed in the desired direction with active cutting angles because they have an output bore. To this end, endodontic instruments with active cutting angles that allow a more selective bore are available in the market.
The ideal material for root canal filling of deciduous elements should have several properties: it should be innocuous for periapical tissues and the buds of permanent teeth as well as be completely reabsorbed if accidentally pushed beyond the apex; it should have a sterile action and be perfectly reabsorbable complying with the natural resorption times. Furthermore, it should be easy to insert in the canals and adhere to the penetration walls, should not shrink, and should easily be removed, if necessary, without discoloring the tooth. Therefore, it is recommended not to use materials that are difficult to reabsorb, cannot be reabsorbed at all, and can displace the erupting permanent elements (Fig. 12.13 and 12.14).

Zinc oxide eugenol (ZOE) was the first canal filling material recommended for deciduous elements and was described by Sweet et al in 1930. The other materials used for this purpose include iodoform paste and calcium hydroxide. Many studies have been conducted, especially comparative studies, to identify a material that would be as close as possible to the ideal one.

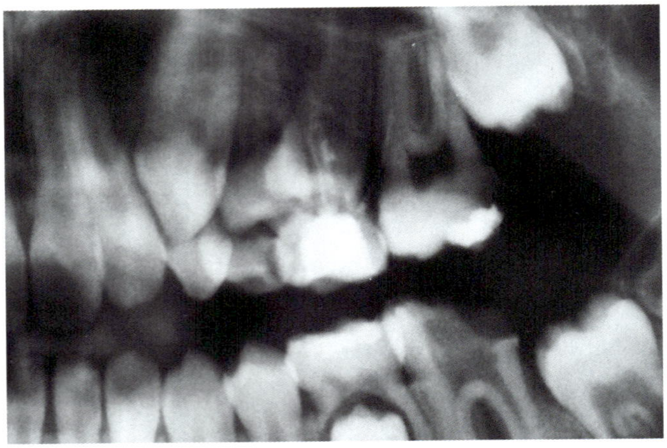

Figure 12.13 Details of panoramic radiograph, which highlights the de-positioning of the bud of 2.5 owing to the presence of nonresorbable material.

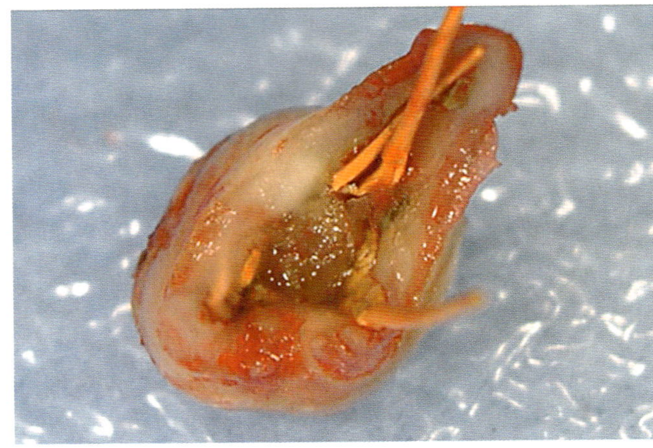

Figure 12.14 Extracted tooth, which shows the use of a nonresorbable material as endodontic filling.

Despite its wide use, ZOE is far from being the ideal material. It has a limited antibacterial activity and, if pushed beyond the apex, can push the corresponding permanent tooth given its solidity; it can cause irritation for the periapical tissues and can cause rearrangement. However, it shows good coronal sealing activity, which is a very important property strictly related to the healing of periapical lesions, as shown by the related scientific literature.
Iodoform paste has found widespread use; its success is linked to its good antibacterial activity, although the studies of Woodhouse and White highlighted a less favorable response on periapical tissues compared with ZOE owing to the presence of chlorophenol. Furthermore, patients show intolerance toward the smell emanated by iodoform paste.
Iodoform paste has recently been reintroduced in combination with calcium hydroxide. This mix is harder than ZOE, more easily removable in case of retreatments, and does not interfere with the eruption of permanent teeth if accidentally pushed out of the apex; furthermore, it is radiopaque and histologically innocuous compared with the buds of permanent teeth.
Calcium hydroxide is widely used in pediatric endodontics for the treatment of necrotic dental elements, which represent an example of a periapical lesion. Its mechanism of action is linked to its alkalinity and the presence of calcium ions. Alkalinity intervenes against the inflammatory process both locally and with the activation of alkaline phosphatases, which are very important enzymes for restructuring hard tissues. Calcium hydroxide has a lower resorption time than ZOE, but this does not constitute a disadvantage for deciduous elements, whose roots must undergo a physiological resorption process: their filling is intended to keep them free from infective processes until the change of dentition.
Our clinical experience, based on the use of calcium hydroxide as a dressing material placed inside the canals and subsequently removed to perform canal refilling with ZOE placed at the coronal third, has achieved appreciable and stable results (Fig. 12.15).

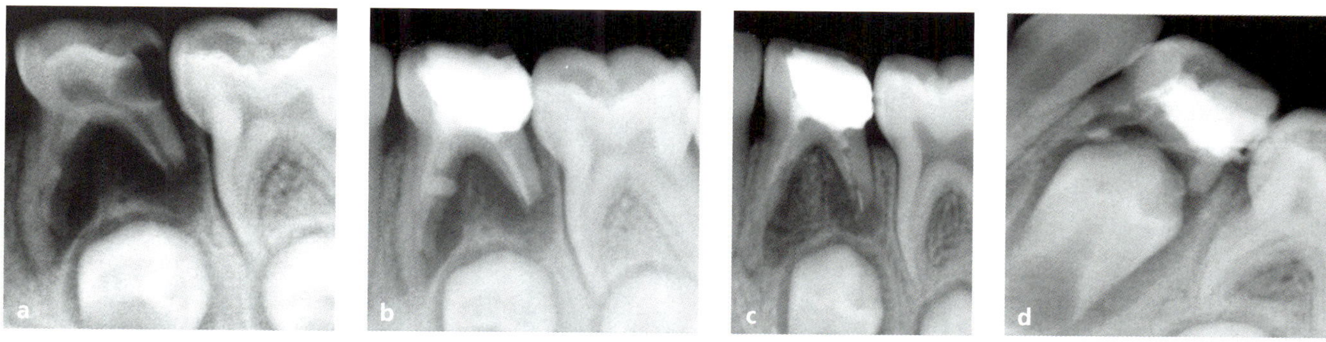

Figure 12.15 Pulpectomy with lesion. (**a**) Initial radiographic examination: it is possible to note a destroyed carious lesion at the level of the distal wall of 7.4. Furthermore, the image shows an area of radiolucency, which involves the root tips and furcation, whereas the bone cap is preserved. (**b**) The radiographic control after 30 days highlights the initial healing of the wound. (**c**) Control after 90 days from the previous control: it is possible to note further healing and reabsorption of the filling material. (**d**) With the subsequent control, it is possible to note the advanced resorption of the roots.

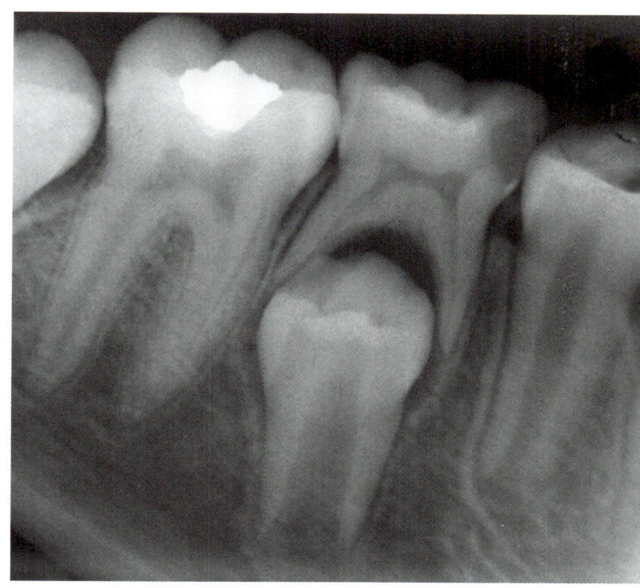

Figure 12.16 The intraoral radiograph highlights the carious lesion at the level of the mesial wall of 8.5, without preservation of the bone cap.

Pulpectomy involves several obligatory steps, which are necessary to obtain a positive treatment outcome. Before proceeding with the treatment, it is necessary to perform periapical intraoral radiography, which is necessary to assess the possible presence and extension of an apical lesion, the presence of a bony roof between the treated element and the corresponding permanent one (Fig. 12.16), and the degree of resorption. If even one of these variables is unfavorable, extraction must be performed.

After ensuring that the treatment is feasible, a locoregional anesthesia is performed, if necessary. The operative area must be isolated using a rubber dam. Then, the pulp chamber is opened, and the root canals are identified. Washing must be repeated with 5.25% sodium hypochlorite, with excess solution eliminated by suction.

The canals are initially probed with manual files 08, 10, and 15, which allow assessment of the working length using the apical detector, always taking into consideration the reference intraoral radiograph. This is followed by the shaping phase using Ni-Ti rotary instruments by adjusting the canal preparation length so that it moves a millimeter toward the coronal direction than the previously detected working lengths. The canals, duly shaped and cleansed, are dried with sterile paper cones and filled with filling material. If the treatment requires a dressing with calcium hydroxide, the material should have a solidity hard enough to be able to be placed inside the canal (Video 12.2, Video 12.3). In contrast, if definitive closure is indicated in one session, a canal filling with pure ZOE is performed, with a pasty texture, pushed up to the coronal third of the root. At the end of the endodontic treatment, filling with temporary materials is performed, and the patient is subsequently seen for clinical and radiographic follow-up. Only after healing is it possible to make the definitive reconstruction using composite materials or glass ionomer cement.

See clinical cases 1 and 3 shown in Figures 12.17 and 12.18.

Endodontic therapy of permanent teeth with immature apex

Unlike previous reports on deciduous dentition, one of the fundamental goals in endodontic treatment of permanent dentition is the degree of sealing achieved with the tridimensional filling of the canal system.
The methods used for canal filling require the compaction of the material inside the radicular system and therefore need an apical constriction. In dental elements with an immature apex, this characteristic is absent, and even the canal anatomy is different from that of dental elements with a mature apex, the course of a canal is wide, with parallel, or even divergent, thin radicular walls.
In such cases, the goal of endodontic treatment is twofold: on one hand, it is necessary to promote the thickening of endodontic canal walls; on the other hand, it is necessary to reconstruct or close the root apex to create the prerequisites for completing the treatment without risking excessive leakage of materials beyond the physiological limits of the radicular anatomy.
The treatment choices are especially indicated by the health status of the dental element being treated and, in particular, by the vitality or necrosis of this element. In young patients, the treatment of permanent teeth with immature apices affected by early and deep carious lesions or with pulp exposure caused by traumas requires a treatment intervention that maintains the vitality of the tooth concerned as much as possible to allow its complete morphological development.

The primary aim on the part of the clinician should be to avoid intervention with invasive techniques on the pulp by performing a direct capping. This involves decision-making regarding whether to initiate apexogenesis or apexification.

Clinical case 1

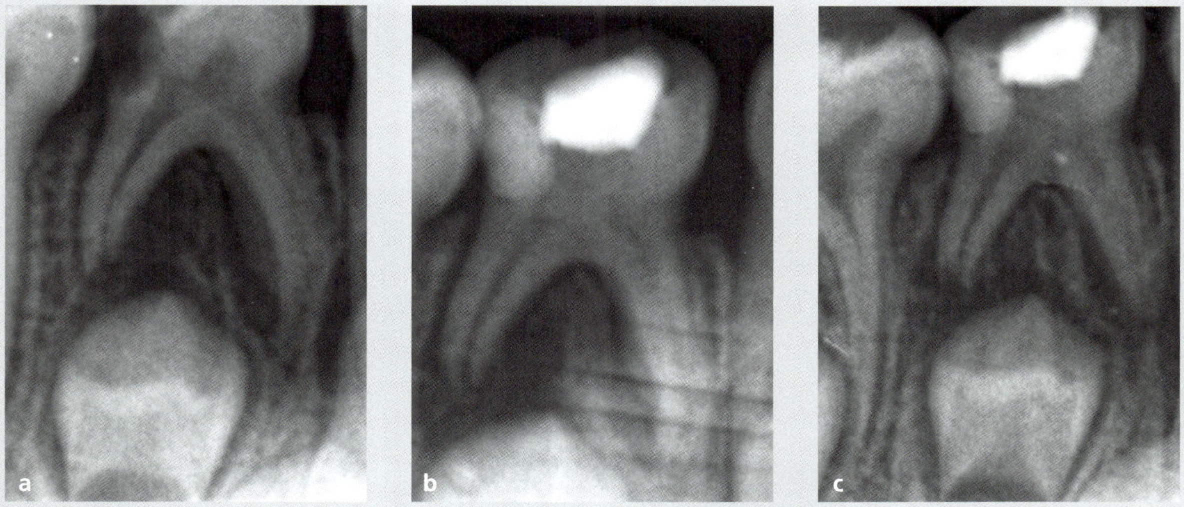

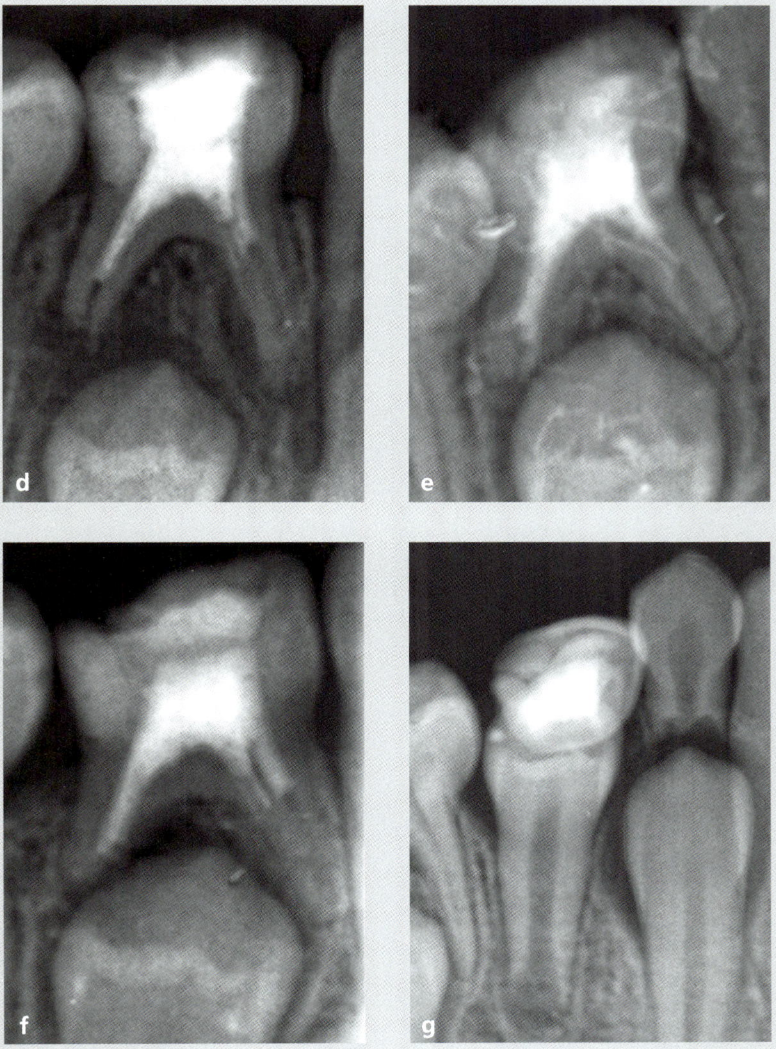

Figure 12.17 Pulpectomy of 8.4, which shows a fistulous lesion after clinical examination. (**a**) The preoperative radiograph shows a carious lesion that involves the pulp of a first deciduous molar and a wide periapical lesion. After performing preoperative reconstruction of the distal portion of the dental element and the intervention of pulpectomy with calcium hydroxide dressing (**b**), the radiographic examination in one mouth is performed (**c**). The radiographic examination shows the progressive healing of the periapical lesion; following clinical examination, it is possible to observe the disappearance of the previous fistulous path. After confirming the results, it is possible to proceed with the opening of the pulp chamber, removal of the intermediate dressing, adequate disinfection of the endodontic system, and creation of an adequate coronoradicular sealing with pure zinc oxide eugenol (**d**). After 1 week, the element is definitively reconstructed with a composite material. (**e**, **f**) The control radiographic examinations at 24 and 36 months show complete healing of the previous endodontic lesion and correct exfoliation of the treated deciduous element (**g**).

Clinical case 2

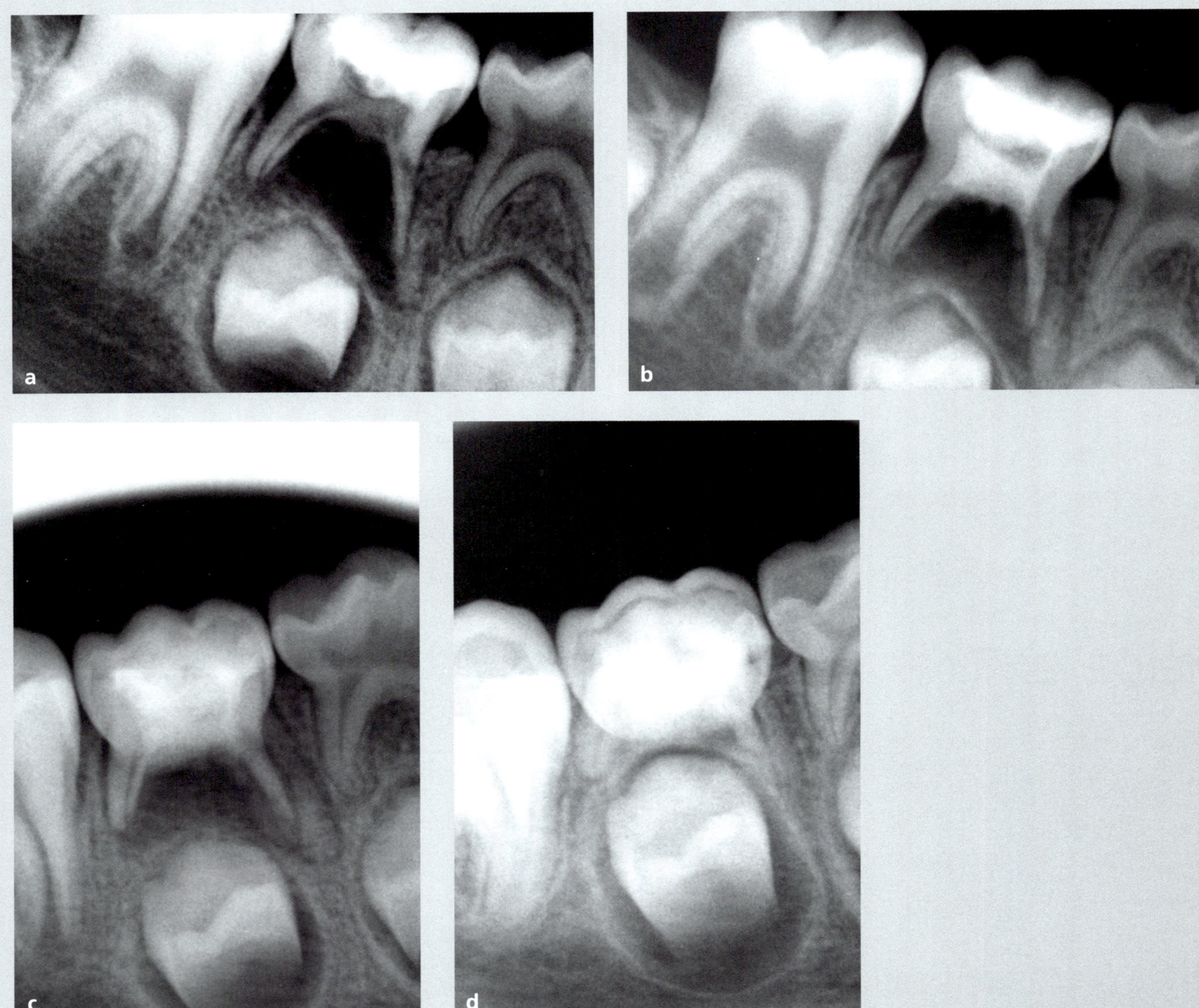

Figure 12.18 Pulpectomy with calcium hydroxide. (**a**) Preoperative radiograph showing a lesion at the level of the furcation of 8.5 caused by a floor perforation. (**b**) Radiograph after dressing with calcium hydroxide in root canals and reconstruction of perforation with MTA. (**c**) Control at 2 months, which shows partial improvement of the lesion. (**d**) Control at 6 months.

Apexogenesis

The preferred treatment for dental elements with open apices is apexogenesis, whose purpose is not just to guarantee the closure of the physiological apex, by preserving the tooth vitality, but also to improve the coronoradicular relationship, strengthening the radicular walls that otherwise would be extremely thin and fragile.
Dental elements that can undergo apexogenesis are those whose pulp exposure is iatrogenic or caused by accidental trauma, and thus, they show no irreversible pulp symptomatology.
To proceed with apexogenesis treatment, it is necessary to consider the age of the patient and the fact that complete radicular formation, as with the ensuing apex maturation, normally takes place 3–4 years after eruption.
The treatments, which are most indicated for young dental elements with compromised pulp, include direct pulp capping and partial or complete pulpotomy.

Direct pulp capping

Direct capping is indicated in cases of slight pulp exposure.
As previously described, direct capping of exposed pulp during the removal of carious processes is not recommended in deciduous dental elements but only in cases of small exposures in young permanent elements. Furthermore, the preoperative radiographic investigation must show no deep carious lesions that directly involve the pulp (Fig. 12.19a, b). Direct pulp capping is also indicated in cases of pulp exposure caused by traumatic events. The operative procedure requires local plexus and nerve block anesthesia, depending on the area concerned (Fig 12.19c). Furthermore, as it has been proved that the cause of pulp inflammation is invasion by bacterial contaminants, the operative area should be perfectly isolated by placing a rubber dam (Fig. 12.19d). The carious lesion must be eliminated, and the residual cavity and exposed pulp must be disinfected using appropriate substances such as chlorhexidine-based solutions (Fig. 12.19e, f). The most widely used materials in pediatric dentistry that are designed to stimulate reparation at the level of the dentin–pulp interconnection include calcium hydroxide and bioactive cements.
The most widely used material for permanent dentition is certainly calcium hydroxide as it is widely available and inexpensive. The alkaline pH induced by calcium hydroxide not only neutralizes the lactic acid of osteoclasts, thereby preventing the dissolution of the mineral component of dentin, but also activates alkaline phosphatase, which plays an important role in hard tissue formation. If clinicians consider the use of direct pulp capping with calcium hydroxide to be suitable, they will need to completely remove the enamel and dentin affected by the lesion by cleansing the surface and inspecting the bleeding with an imbued sterile cotton pellet. Subsequently, the clinician will need to place the material in contact with the area of pulp exposure (Fig 12.19g, h) and perform the temporary coronal restoration with glass ionomer cements or intermediate restorative materials, which can guarantee the per-

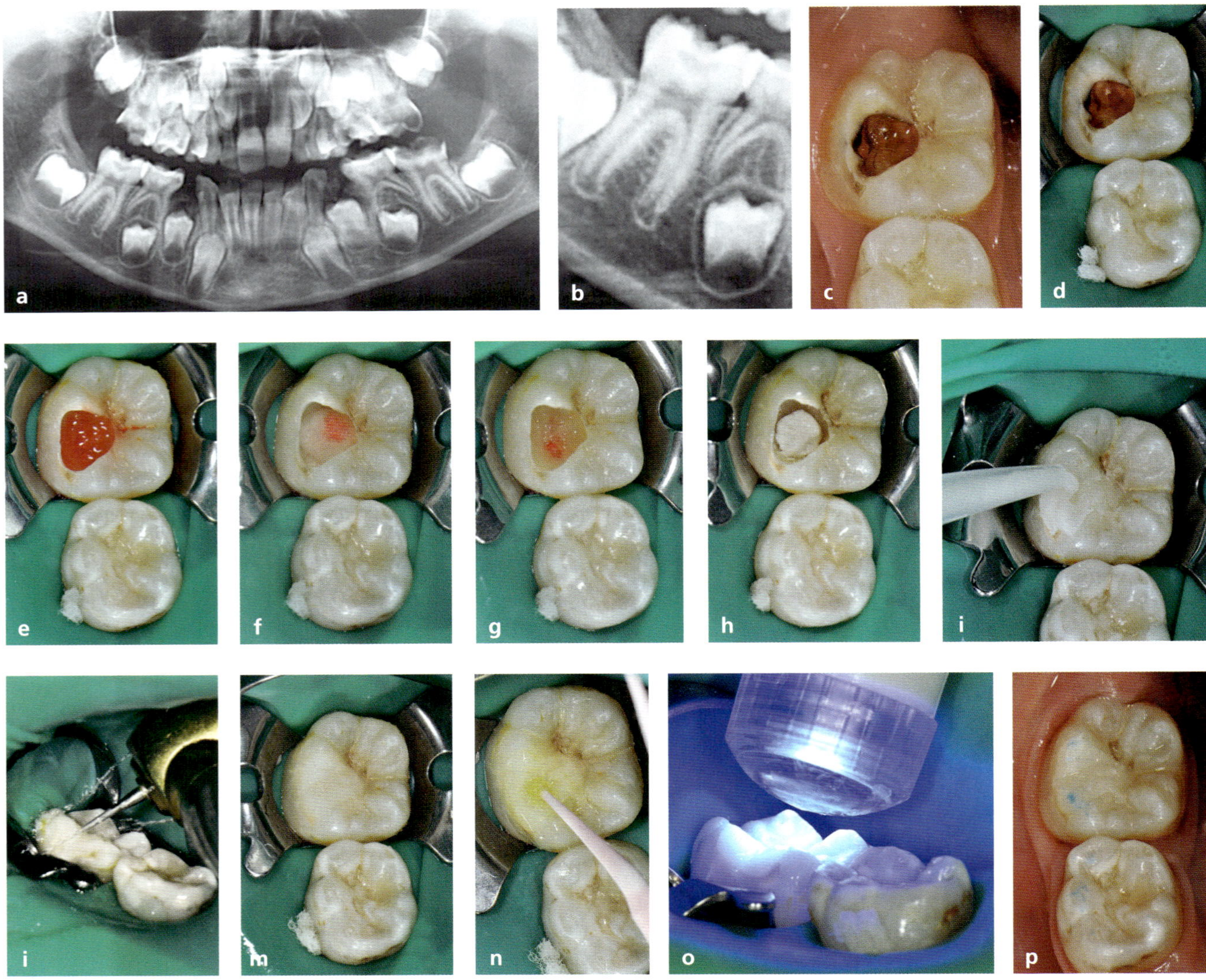

Figure 12.19 Direct capping of 4.6.

fect sealing of the dressing in relation to the external environment for the necessary time (Fig. 12.19i-p). It is essential to use vitality tests to assess pulp function and radiographic examinations to assess the absence of periapical lesions and therefore the progress of the physiological radicular formation. As soon as the formation of a dentin bridge is identified on radiographic examination, the definitive restoration is performed using composite resins after removing the previous restoration with calcium hydroxide.

The major limitations of this technique include the relatively long time required for formation of the dentin bridge and to perform the nondefinitive restoration.

A treatment solution that might allow the treated dental element to be reconstructed more quickly is direct capping using bioactive cements. The cavity preparation technique is as described above. After cleansing the exposed surfaces, the material is placed in such a way as to completely cover the exposed pulp. Coronal sealing is achieved via a definitive reconstruction using composite material, first in those cases where cements with short setting times are used and second with temporary filling using intermediate restorative materials and glass ionomer cements.

Pulpotomy

One apexogenesis procedure described in the literature is pulpotomy, which requires superficial or deep removal of the inflamed pulp tissue. Pulpotomy can be performed in clinical scenarios involving reversible pulpitis and in cases in which pulp exposure is large and/or in direct contact with a bacterial load for a sufficiently long time (trauma). The operative technique is as follows:

- locoregional anesthesia (plexus or nerve block)
- placement of a rubber dam
- cleansing of the cavity to avoid possible bacterial contamination of the pulp chamber
- opening of the access to the cavity under abundant irrigation
- removal of chamber pulp with a rotary instrument at high speed and under abundant irrigation
- control of hemostasis with imbued sterile cotton pellets for no more than 5 minutes
- application of the selected material (calcium hydroxide or MTA) in contact with the radicular pulp (2–4 mm thickness)
- filling with temporary reinforced ZOE cement, e.g., IRM
- definitive filling with composite resins at the coronal level
- radiographic follow-up after 3 months and subsequently every 12 months until apical maturation.

The newly formed dentin bridge is the product of the action of fibroblasts and those cells that have undergone differentiation into osteoblasts and odontoblasts. Immediately following apex closure, it is necessary to completely remove the pulp and perform a standard endodontic therapy after dentin bridge removal, as agreed in many studies in the literature.

In apexogenesis treatment procedures (Fig. 12.20 and 12.21), calcium hydroxide does not directly participate in dentin bridge formation but only exerts an alkalizing action that has antibacterial properties and is able to favor bone and dentin deposition.

As shown in the case indicated in Figure 12.20, if a trauma has caused a large pulp exposure in a young patient with immature apices and it is possible to perform immediate coronal restoration by attaching the concerned fragment, the authors suggest the use of MTA for the treatment of pulpotomy and the subsequent apexogenesis.

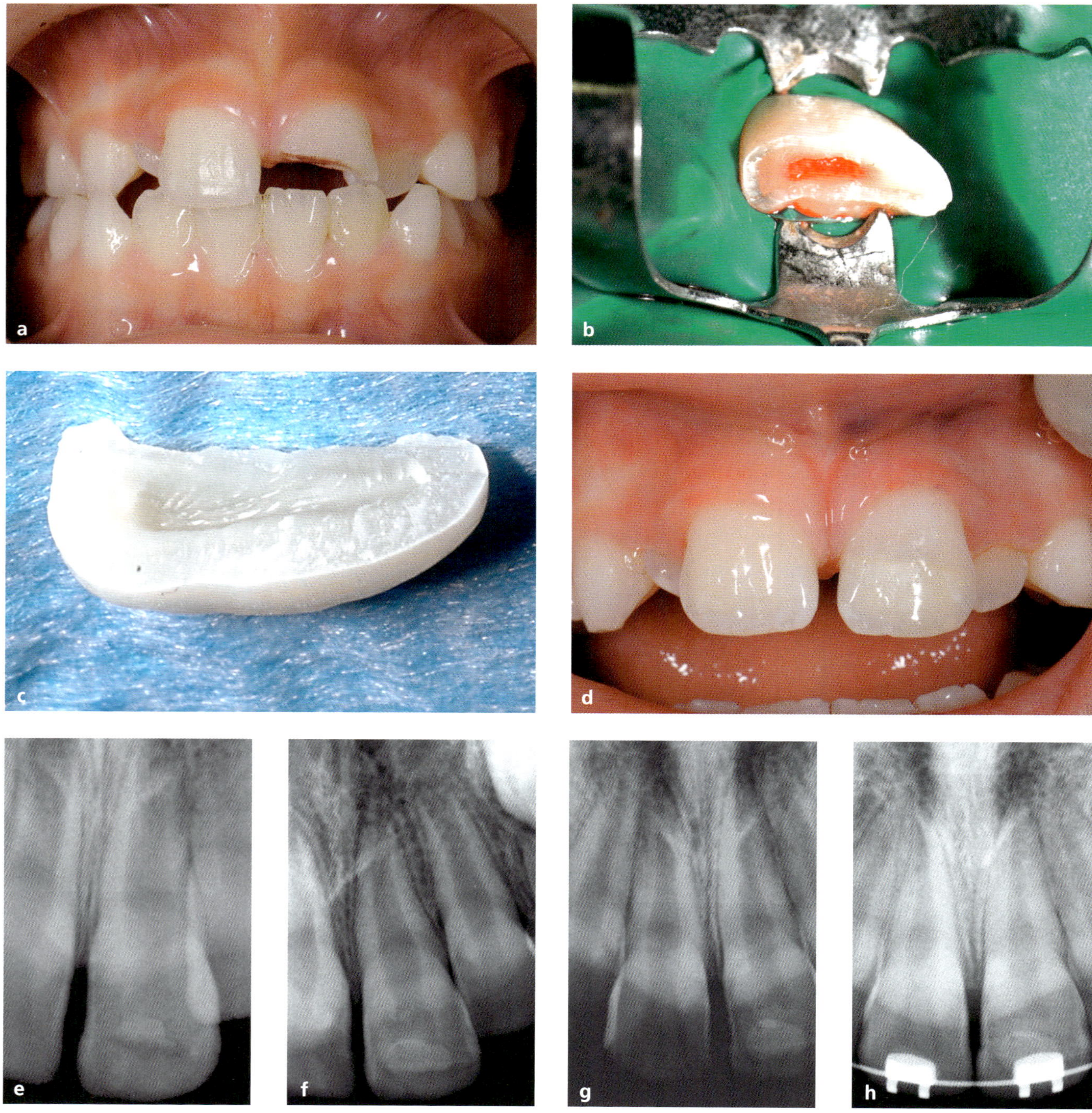

Figure 12.20 Apexogenesis with MTA and attachment of the fragment. (**a**) The patient was examined after a traumatic event that had occurred 48 hours earlier. Upon intraoral examination, it is possible to observe a coronal fracture complicated by a wide pulp exposure. (**b**) After performing adequate anesthesia for the affected dental element and isolating the area using a rubber dam, a partial pulpotomy is performed, and MTA is subsequently placed in contact with the pulp. (**c**, **d**) The immediate repositioning of the fragment allows creation of a good coronal sealing. (**e**) The radiographic examination shows the level of apical maturation and the correct positioning of the material. (**f**) After 10 months, it is possible to note how the dental element appears to be vital because of the physiological formation of the apical region. (**g**) The radiograph shows a complete radicular and apical arrangement with a good coronoradicular relationship. (**h**) A control performed 36 months after the start of the treatment confirms the positive prognosis and the stability over time of the treatment performed.

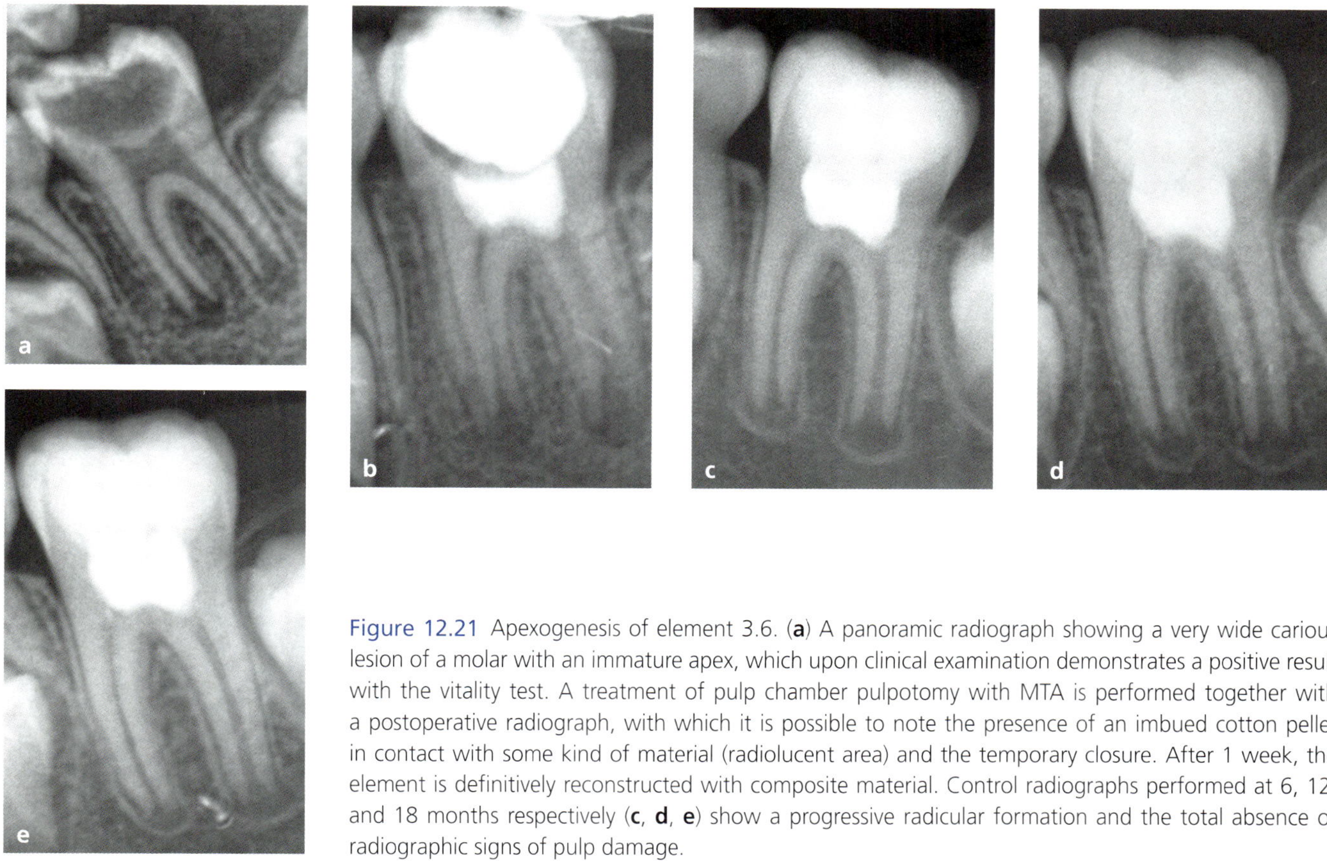

Figure 12.21 Apexogenesis of element 3.6. (**a**) A panoramic radiograph showing a very wide carious lesion of a molar with an immature apex, which upon clinical examination demonstrates a positive result with the vitality test. A treatment of pulp chamber pulpotomy with MTA is performed together with a postoperative radiograph, with which it is possible to note the presence of an imbued cotton pellet in contact with some kind of material (radiolucent area) and the temporary closure. After 1 week, the element is definitively reconstructed with composite material. Control radiographs performed at 6, 12, and 18 months respectively (**c**, **d**, **e**) show a progressive radicular formation and the total absence of radiographic signs of pulp damage.

Apexification

Apexification is performed when dental elements with immature apices have undergone pulp necrosis. In such cases, the goal of the treatment does not differ from that of apexogenesis, but as there is no vital pulp available, the results are not comparable. Good apexification cannot disregard the complete removal of the necrotic pulp and the establishment of an intracanal environment suitable for the formation of an apical stop.

The operative technique proceeds as follows:

- anesthesia, which is not indispensable but recommended for patient compliance: the less cooperative the patient is, the more they should not feel pain during treatment
- periapical intraoral radiography to assess maturation and detect working length
- monitoring of the rubber dam or isolation of the operative area using cotton rolls and surgical suction in the most extreme cases owing to noncooperation of the patient

- establishment of the access cavity
- abundant irrigation with 5.25% sodium hypochlorite
- equipment consisting of manual and rotary instruments up to 2 mm from the radiographically assessed working length to avoid further weakness for thin canal walls;
- drying of the canal and placement of calcium hydroxide within it
- placing of a sterile cotton pellet inside the pulp chamber
- closing of the access cavity to guarantee adequate sealing
- clinical and radiographic controls until the identification of apical barrier.

If the clinical and/or radiological control highlights pain or the absence of material inside the canals, and as calcium hydroxide can be absorbed by organic fluids, it is necessary to remove the residual part by washing and remove the dressing material, repeating all the steps previously described.
In the subsequent controls, it is necessary to radiographically check the formation of an apical barrier adequate enough to accommodate the endodontic filling materials (gutta-percha) and then to completely remove the dressing material and clinically check the formation of an apical stop. This procedure should be performed by using sterile paper cones inside the canal, gently resting them on the newly formed barrier, to probe for the presence of communication with the periapex.
The next step is the tridimensional filling of the canal system with thermoplasticized gutta-percha.

Clinical cases

The images provided illustrate some clinical cases treated by following the operative steps described above and show various types of apical closure, which differ among themselves by the presence or absence of the Hertwig sheath and the vital pulp tissue (odontoblasts).

Clinical case number 3 shows a Frank's Type I apical closure. Clinical case number 4 shows a Frank's Type II apical closure. Clinical case number 5 shows a Frank's Type III apical closure.

Considering the long time required for achieving the radicular apex formation and the definitive restoration of the tooth treated with calcium hydroxide, a treatment solution that uses MTA is proposed (Fig. 12.22). The first phases of the treatment procedure do not differ from those already described in the apexification technique (Fig. 12.22a, c), whereas the operative techniques differ in the phases of closure, during which it is necessary to perform the following steps:

- drying of the canal and placement of an MTA stop approximately 5 mm thick in the most apical position possible, with an imbued cotton pellet placed above to harden it (Fig. 12.22c)
- sealing of the access cavity with temporary cements, such as intermediate restorative materials and glass ionomer cements

- opening the access cavity after 4–5 days and using an MTA probe to ensure that hardening has been achieved
- filling of the canal with thermoplasticized gutta-percha (Fig. 12.22d)
- definitive restoration and radiographic follow-up.

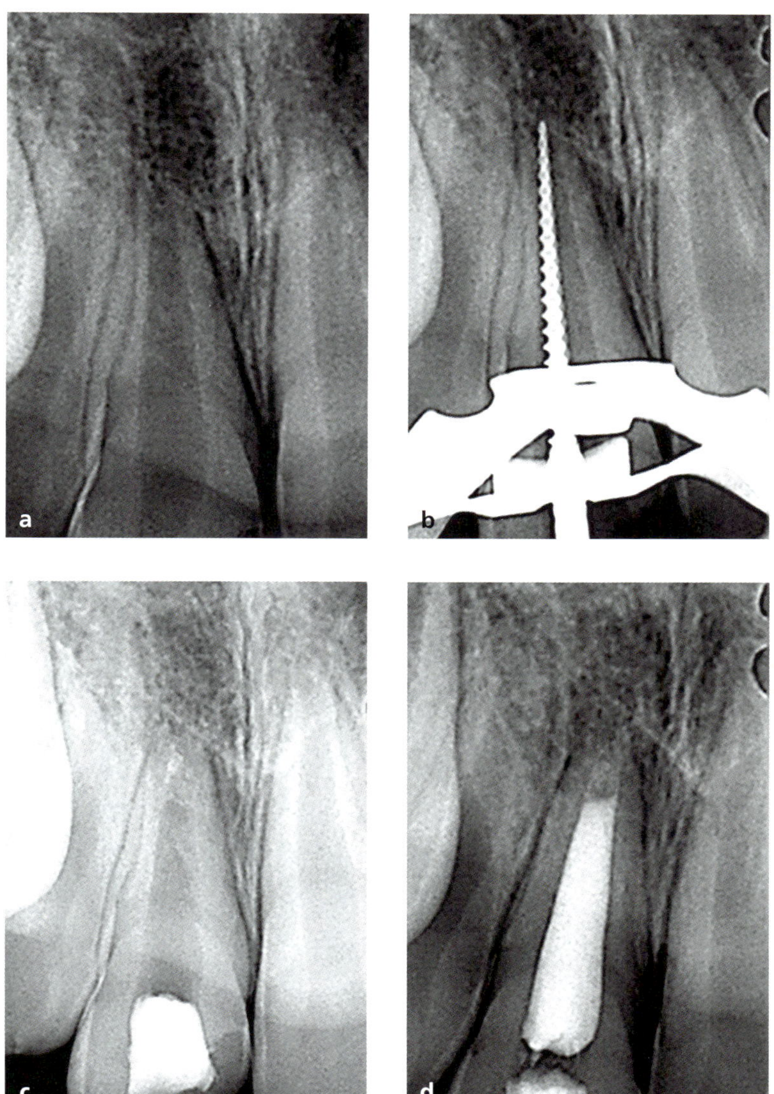

Figure 12.22 Apexification with MTA.

Clinical case 3

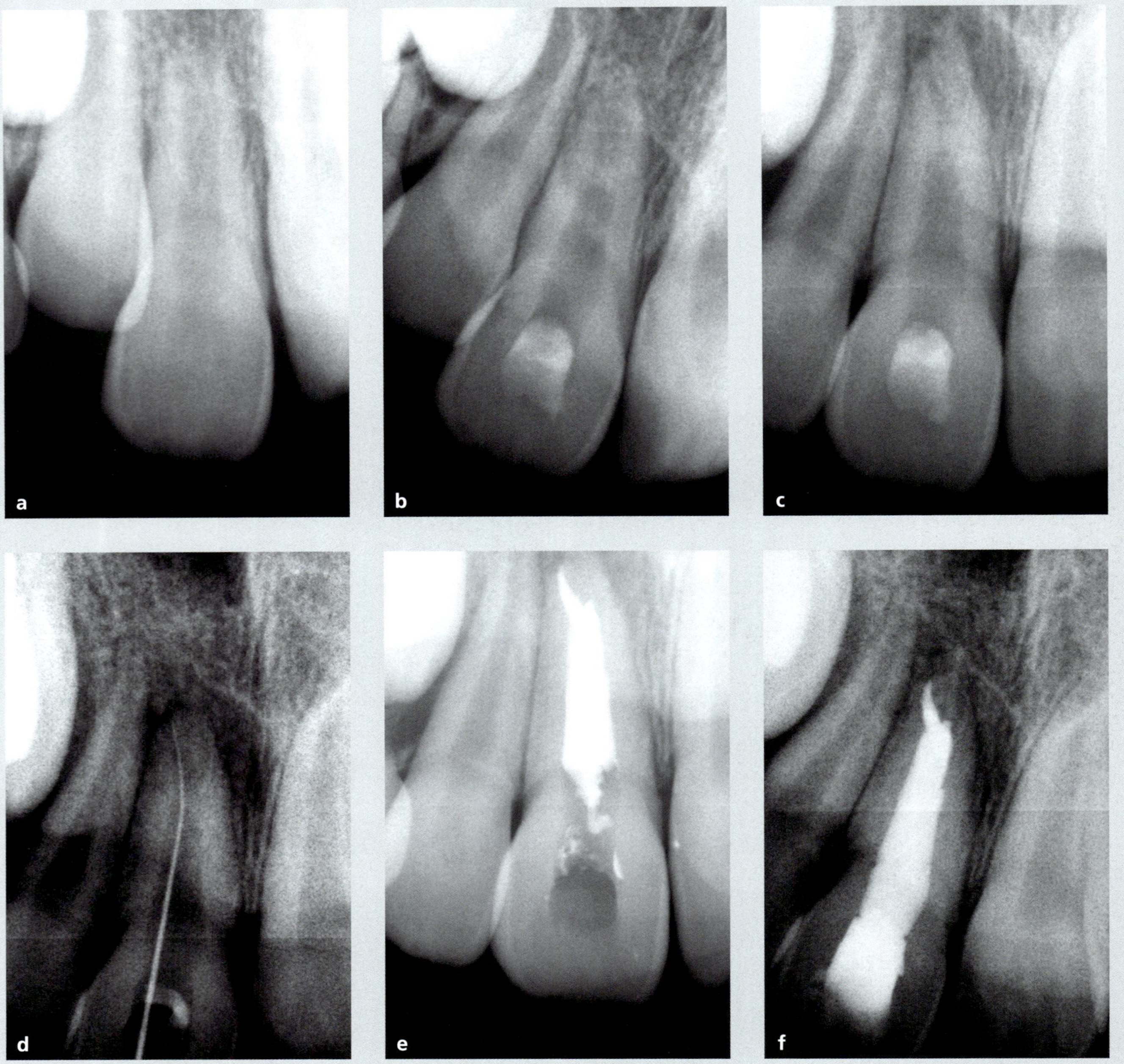

Figure 12.23 Following a trauma, the right upper central incisor was necrotic. (**a**) The radiographic image shows an immature apex with greater radicular diameters (trombone-shaped type). (**c**) Control radiograph 3 months after filling the canal with calcium hydroxide. (**b**) Control radiograph 9 months after filling the canal with calcium hydroxide. The apex shows a physiological closure derived from the presence of a Hertwig sheath and odontoblasts at the level of radicular flaring. The root is elongated, and it is possible to observe a narrowing of the canal in the apical third due to dentin application, which has caused wall thickening and formation of a radicular apex. (**d**) Assessment of working length. (**e**) Three-dimensional closure of the canal system with thermoplastic gutta-percha. (**f**) Control radiograph 12 months after the final closure of the radicular system.

Clinical case 4

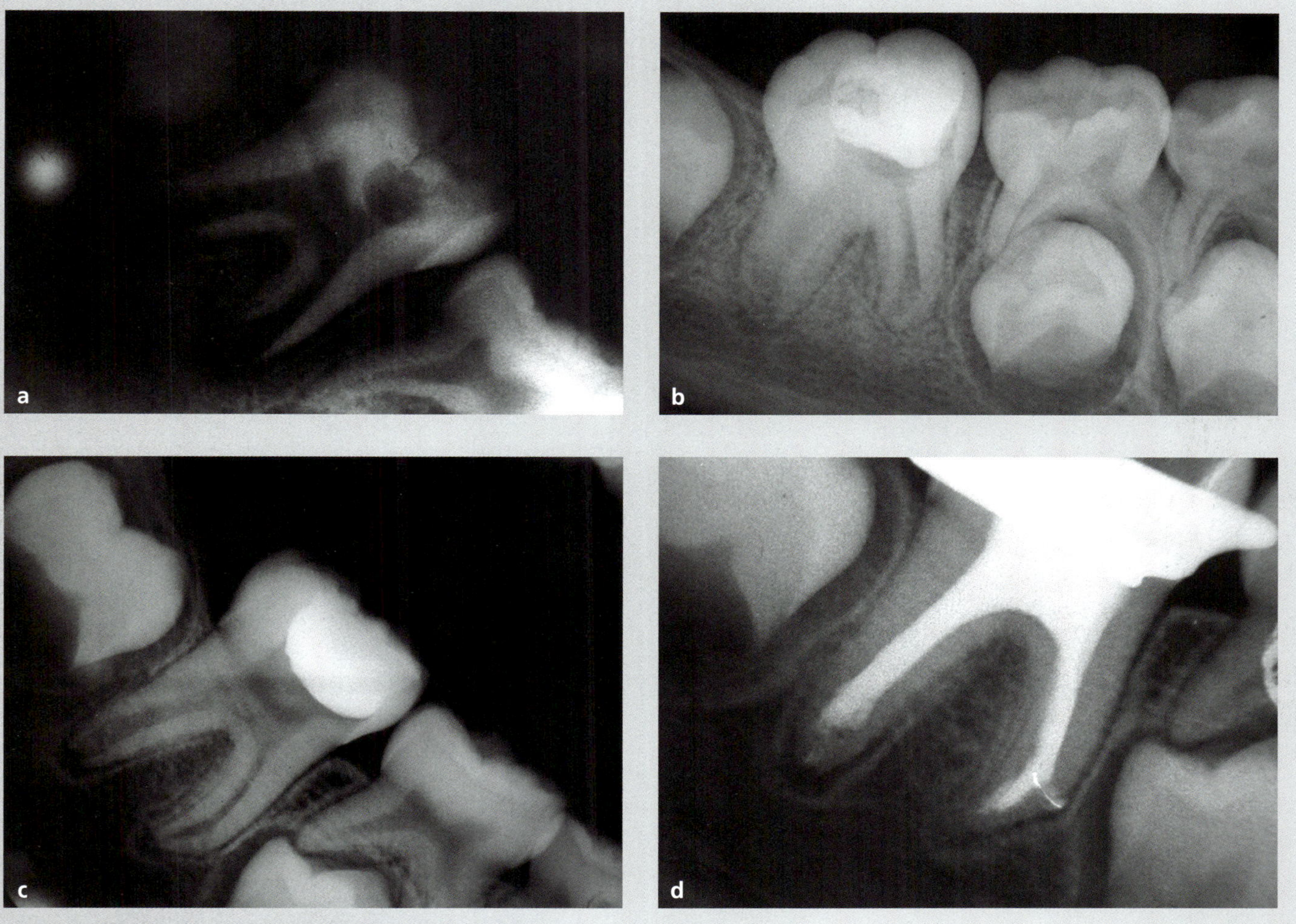

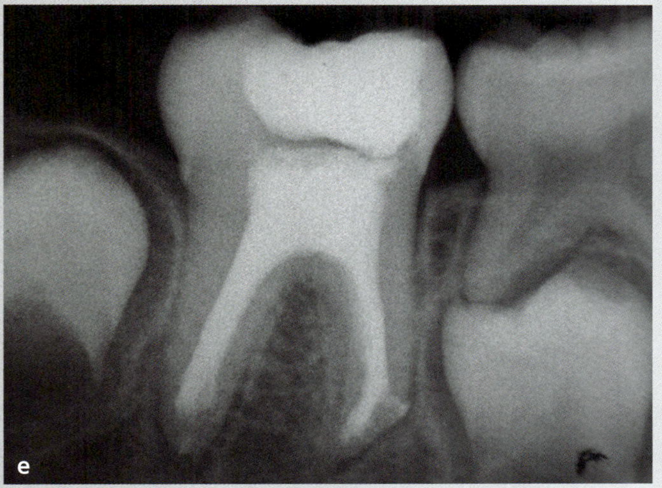

Figure 12.24 Apexification treatment of 4.6 (**a**) The preoperative radiographic shows a destroyed carious lesion of a necrotic molar with an open apex in a 6-year-old child. (**b**) Control radiograph 6 months before the dressing with calcium hydroxide. The root is elongated, but the apex is not closed. (**c**) After 18 months, it is possible to observe the formation of the radicular apex with an interruption of the radicular canal due to the absence of odontoblasts. (**d**) It is now possible to close the canal with filling material and perform a postoperative radiograph. (**e**) Control radiograph 1 month after closure of the canals.

Clinical case 5

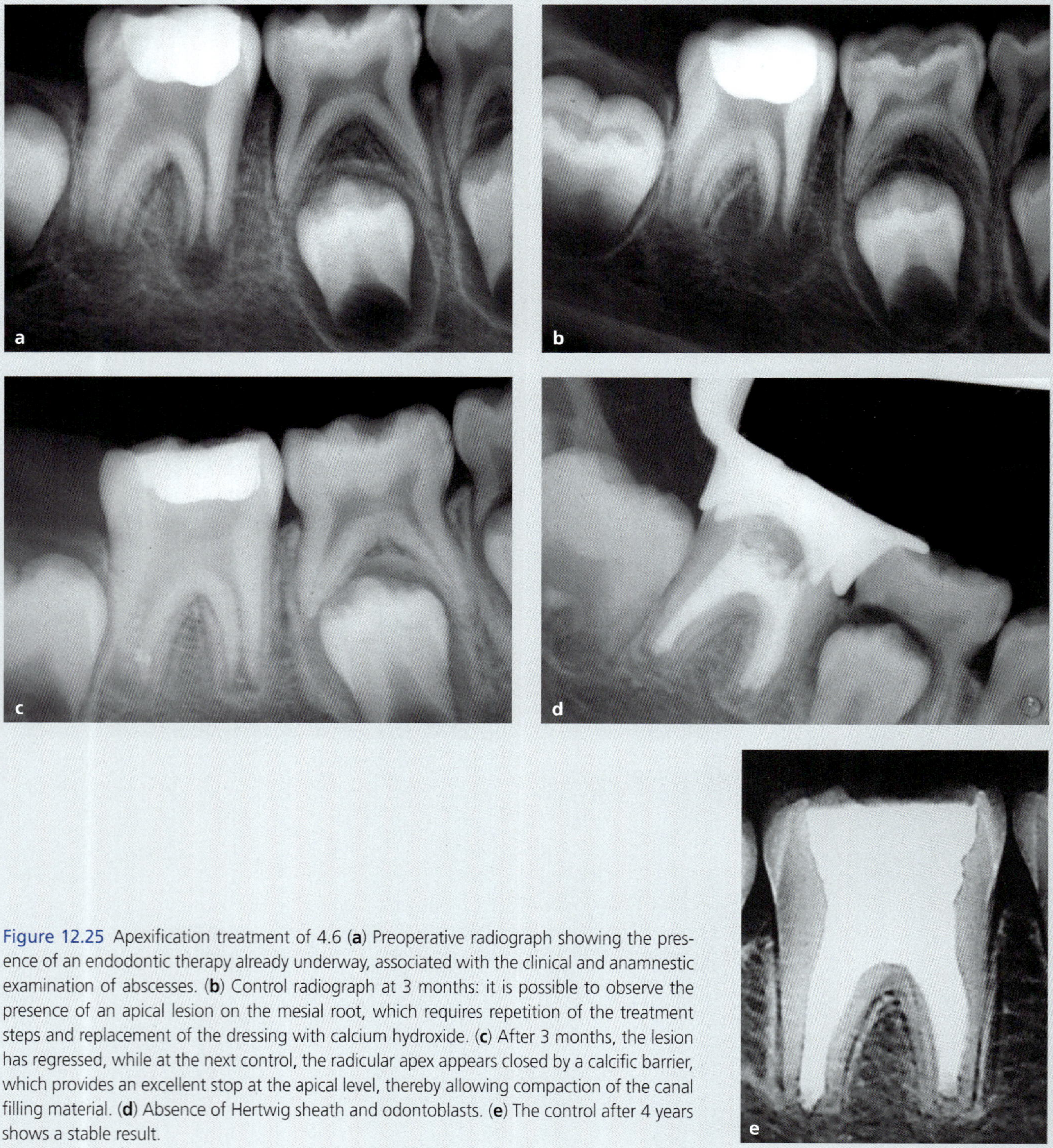

Figure 12.25 Apexification treatment of 4.6 (**a**) Preoperative radiograph showing the presence of an endodontic therapy already underway, associated with the clinical and anamnestic examination of abscesses. (**b**) Control radiograph at 3 months: it is possible to observe the presence of an apical lesion on the mesial root, which requires repetition of the treatment steps and replacement of the dressing with calcium hydroxide. (**c**) After 3 months, the lesion has regressed, while at the next control, the radicular apex appears closed by a calcific barrier, which provides an excellent stop at the apical level, thereby allowing compaction of the canal filling material. (**d**) Absence of Hertwig sheath and odontoblasts. (**e**) The control after 4 years shows a stable result.

References

Acs G, Lodolini G, Kaminsky S et al. Effect of nursing caries on body weight in a pediatric population. Pediatric Dent 1992;14:302-5.

Aeinehchi M, Eslami B, Ghanbariha M, Saffar AS. Mineral trioxide aggregate (MTA) and calcium hydroxide as pulp-capping agents in human teeth: a preliminary report. Int Endod J 2003;36:225-31.

Avram DC, Pulver F. Pulpotomy medicaments for vital primary teeth. Surveys to determine use and attitudes in pediatric dental practice and in dental schools throughout the world. J Dent Child 1989;56(6):426-34.

Block RM et al. Systemic distribution of ladeled paraformaldehyde incorporated within formocresol following pulpotomies in dogs. J Endodont 1983;9(5):176-89.

Carrotte P. Endodontic treatment for children. Br Dent J 2005;198(1):9-15.

Chacko V, Kukirose S. Human pulpal response to mineral trioxide aggregate (MTA): a histologic study. J Clin Pediatr Dent 2006;30:203-10.

Conti TR, Sakai VT, Camolese Fornetti AP et al. Pulpotomies with Portland cement in human primary molars. J Appl Oral Sci 2009; (17)1:66-9.

Di Nardo, Di Maio F, D'Arcangelo C, Varvara G. Canal filling in primary teeth. Description of two particular cases. Minerva Stomatol 2000;49(9):445-8.

Ford TR, Torabinejad M, Abedi HR et al. Using mineral trioxide aggregate as a pulp-capping material. JADA 1996;127:1491-4.

Fuks AB. Vital pulp therapy with new materials for primary teeth: new directions and treatment perspectives. JOE 2008;34(7s):18-24.

Fuks AB. Current concepts in vital primary pulp therapy. Eur J Paediatr Dent 2002;3(3):115-20.

Hommez GM, Coppens CR, De Moor RJ. Periapical health related to the quality of coronal restorations and root fillings. Int Endod J 2002;35(8):680-9.

Douglass JM, Douglass AB, Silk HJ. A practical guide to infant oral health. Am Fam Physicians 2004; 70(11).

Mani AS, Chawla SH, Tewari A, Goyal A. Evaluation of calcium hydroxide and zinc oxide eugenol as root canal filling materials in primary teeth. J Dent Child 2000;142-7.

Markovic D, Zivojinovic V, Vucetic M. Evaluation of three pulpotomy medicaments in primary teeth. Eur J Paediatr Dent 2005;3:133-8.

Mitchell PJ, Pitt Ford TR, Torabinejad M, McDonald F. Osteoblast biocompatibility of mineral trioxide aggregate. Biomaterials 1999;20(2):167-73.

Moretti ABS, Sakai VT, Oliveira TM et al. The effectiveness of mineral trioxide aggregate, calcium hydroxide and formocresol for pulpotomies in primary teeth. Int Endod J; 41(7):547-55.

Mortazavi M, Mesbahi M. Comparison of zinc oxide and eugenol, and Vitapex for root canal treatment of necrotic primary teeth. Int J Paediatric Dent 2004;14(6):417-24.

Nurko C, Garcia-Godoy F. Evaluation of a calcium hydroxide/iodoform paste (Vitapex) in root canal therapy for primary teeth. J Clin Pediatr Dent 1999;23(4):289-94.

Papagiannoulis L. Clinical studies on ferric sulphate as a pulpotomy medicament in primary teeth. Eur J Paediatr Dent 2002;3(3):126-32.

Polimeni A, Majorana A. Patologia cariosa e metodiche di prevenzione. Patologie parodontali e dei tessuti molli. Odontoiatria per il pediatra 2008.

Primosh RE, Glomb TA, Jerrell RG. Primary tooth pulp therapy as taught in predoctoral pediatric dental programs in the Unites States. Pediatr Dent 1997;19(2):118-22.

Ray HA, Trope M. Periapical status of endodontically treated teeth in relation to the technical quality of the root filling and the coronal restoration. Int Endod J 1995;28(1):12-8.

Tunç ES, Saroglu I, Sari S, Günhan O. The effect of sodium hypochlorite application on the success of calcium hydroxide pulpotomy in primary teeth. Oral Surg Oral Med Oral Pathol Oral Radiol Endodontol 2006;102e:22-6.

Ottolenghi L, Polimeni A, Bossù M, Salucci S. Uso di strumenti endodontici Ni-Ti nei decidui: studio in vitro. Dental Cadmos 2003; 4:105-112.

Taagger T et al. Pulpar reaction to glutaraldheyde dressing in monkey primary teeth. Endod Dent Traumat 1986;2:237-43.

Sadler TW. Embriologia medica di Langman. Milano: Masson; 1998.

Tronstad L, Andreasen JO, Hasselgren G et al. PH changes in dental tissues after root canal filling with calcium hydroxide. J Endod 1981;7:17-21.

Tronstad L, Asbjornsen K, Doving L et al. Influence of coronal restorations on the periapical health of endodontically treated teeth. Endod Dent Traumatol 2000;16(5):218-21.

Waterhouse PJ, Nunn JH, Withworth JM. An investigation of the relative efficacy of Buckley's Formocresol and calcium hydroxide in primary molar vital pulp therapy. Br Dent J 2000;188:32-6.

Chapter **13**

Oral surgery in pediatric dentistry

S. Annibali, GL. Sfasciotti

Dental extractions

Dental extraction involves the removal of teeth or their roots from the alveolar bone. It can be a simple or complex procedure. It is described as *complex* when the presence of certain local conditions or an accidental fracture of the crown or root make complete avulsion impossible, imposing a variation on the usual sequence of extraction steps. Extraction is described as "*surgical*" when it involves the creation of a mucoperiosteal access flap.

To accurately perform dental extractions, some indispensable conditions need to be met: precise medical history and clinical examination, radiographic assessment of the element to be extracted, visibility of and accessibility to the operating area, effective anesthesia, adequate equipment, and appropriate techniques.

In particular, the extraction maneuvers in pediatric patients must be performed with special attention, considering the high risk of uncontrolled movements in these patients; the narrowness of the surgical field; and, in case of a deciduous tooth extraction, the contiguity between the roots of the deciduous teeth and the buds of the permanent teeth, which might get damaged if maneuvering is not carefully performed.

Indications

The extraction must be performed only after excluding the possibility or suitability of standard treatments for the affected dental elements, even in case of the deciduous teeth, given their importance in the correct development of the stomatognathic system (Tab. 13.1 and 13.2).

Extraction equipment

The extraction equipment includes *forceps*, *levers*, and *syndesmotomes*.

The forceps used for the upper arch include the following (Fig. 13.1):

- straight type, with beak margins looking like convex circular segments, used for the incisors and canines

Table 13.1 Indications for the extraction of deciduous teeth

- Unrestorable caries in the presence of endodontic–periodontal lesions
- Radicular and periradicular lesions that are untreatable or that have not regressed even after appropriate treatment
- Untreatable periodontal lesions
- Endodontic or periodontal lesions that represent or may represent dental foci
- Untreatable corono-radicular traumatic lesions
- Unrestorable destructive caries
- Untreatable endodontic–periodontal lesions
- Lesions, including minor ones, in teeth that are close to transition or lesions in uncooperative patients that interfere with the functions of the stomatognathic system or with the development of dentition
- Persistence of a deciduous tooth beyond the physiological limits of tooth exchange in the presence of the homologous permanent tooth with at least two-thirds of the mineralized root
- Orthodontic reasons
- Prenatal or early teeth that adversely affect breast-feeding
- Persistence of a deciduous tooth beyond the physiological limits of exchange in the presence of the erupted or unerupted homologous permanent tooth if two-thirds of the root are already mineralized

Table 13.2 Absolute indications when extracting permanent teeth

- Destructive caries that do not allow conservative or prosthetic restoration of the dental element
- Endodontic and/or periapical lesions that are untreatable with root canal or surgical therapy
- Advanced periodontal lesions with significant loss of supporting tissue and impairment of masticatory function that causes discomfort to the patient
- Traumatic lesions with vertical or middle-third root fracture
- Supernumerary teeth that interfere with the correct development of dentition
- Orthodontic reasons
- Intratopic or ectopic teeth that are a result of functional changes or other conditions that cannot be recovered with orthodontic or surgical orthodontic treatment
- Lesions that require complex restoration treatments in uncooperative patients
- Roots that are not restorable with a prosthesis or residual roots
- Untreatable external or internal root resorption
- Teeth on the verge of bone fracture
- Teeth associated with bone or soft tissue lesions
- Teeth in the ectopic position or teeth that are so badly placed that they are not recoverable orthodontically

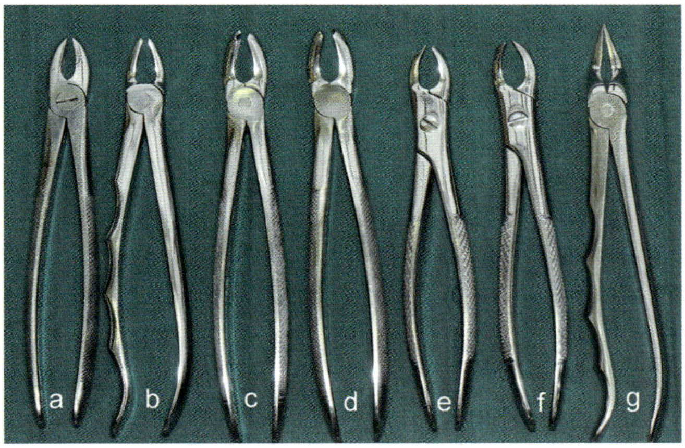

Figure 13.1 Forceps used for the upper arch: (**a**) for incisors and canines; (**b**) for premolars; (**c**) for right molars; (**d**) for left molars; (**e**) for right uncrowned molars; (**f**) for left uncrowned molars; and (**g**) for roots.

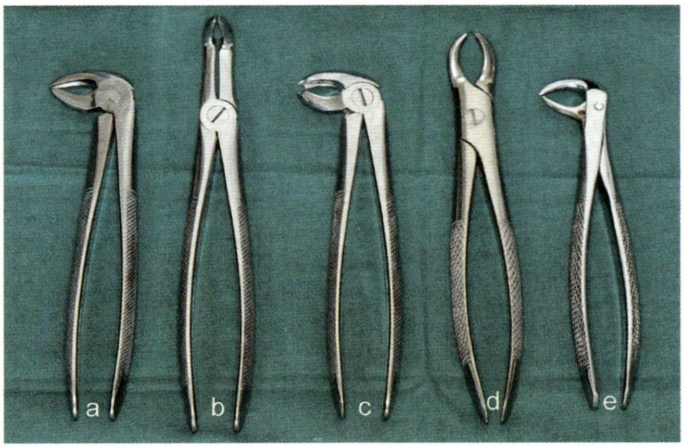

Figure 13.2 Forceps used for the lower arch: (**a**) for incisors, canines, and premolars; (**b**) for roots; (**c**) for molars; (**d**) cow horn type for uncrowned molars; and (**e**) parrot beak type for uncrowned molars.

- italic “S” type:
  - with beak margins looking like convex circular segments, used for the premolars
  - with the margin of the vestibular beak made of two semicircles joined at the center of a spur and the margin of the palatal beak looking like a convex semicircle, used for the first and second molars
  - with a conical and pointed vestibular beak and the margin of the palatal beak looking like a concave half-moon, used for the first and second uncrowned molars
- Bayonet-like type, with beak margins similar to convex circular segments, used for the roots in posterolateral areas.

The forceps used for the lower arch include the following (Fig. 13.2):
- those curved on the back, with beak margins looking like convex circular segments, used for the incisors, canines, premolars, and roots
- those curved on the back, with beak margins made of two semicircles joined at the center of a spur, used for the first and second molars
- those curved on the plate (cow horn type) or on the back (parrot beak type), with pointed cone-shaped beaks, used for uncrowned molars.

With respect to morphology, the forceps used for the deciduous teeth are identical to those used for the permanent teeth, although they are smaller to better accommodate the deciduous teeth and can be more easily hidden from the children’s view.
Straight levers are mainly used for the upper arch, whereas curved types are mainly used for the lower arch (Fig. 13.3).
Syndesmotomes are used to cut the dentoalveolar ligaments and are particularly indicated for the extraction of partially erupted, overlapped, or supernumerary teeth as they allow less traumatic avulsion, preserving alveolar bone and adjacent teeth (Fig. 13.4).

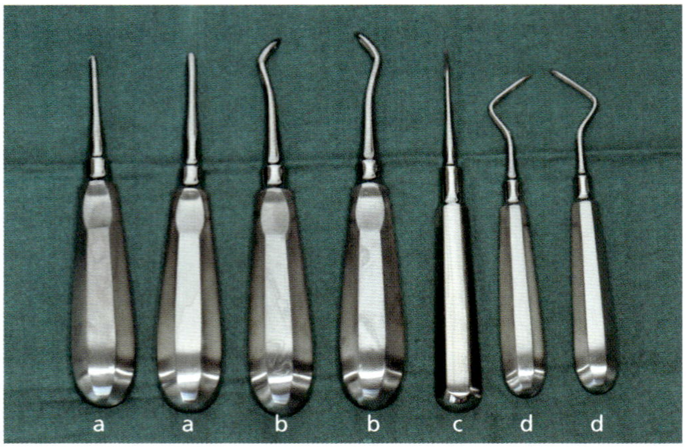

Figure 13.3 Levers: (**a**) straight, for the upper arch; (**b**) curved, for the lower arch; (**c**) apical straight lever; and (**d**) apical curved levers.

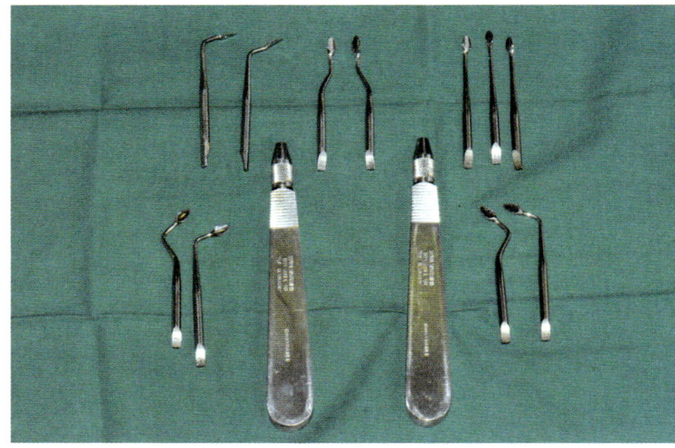

Figure 13.4 Syndesmotomes.

Surgical steps for simple extractions

The fundamental steps of extraction include the following:

- periotomy
- gripping with the forceps
- applying levers
- dislocation
- avulsion
- alveolus inspection
- suture
- hemostasis control.

Periotomy. It can be performed using syndesmotomes, levers, scalpels, periosteal elevators, or the beak margins of the extraction forceps; this procedure is used to detach the marginal gingiva from the tooth collar and cut the annular ligament of Koelliker, which constitutes the most coronal portion of the dentoalveolar ligament. This procedure allows inserting the beaks of the forceps deeply to improve the grip around the dental element, push the center of dislocation in a more apical position, and avoid crushing and lacerating the gingiva during avulsion maneuvers.

Gripping with the forceps. It requires positioning the beaks of the forceps parallel to the tooth axis as apically as possible so that beak margins, which are placed between the alveolar wall and the tooth, can perform a wedge action and expand the most coronal portion of the alveolar socket. To achieve an effective grip, which can uniformly transmit the force exerted on the handles to the tooth, the strongest contact between the dental crown and the beaks must be obtained during dislocation and avulsion steps.

A particular expedient of the related extraction technique must be adopted when dealing with deciduous molars with nonresorbed, thin, widely opened, and converging roots around the crown of the permanent tooth, and even more so if they are ankylosed. In such cases, to avoid damage to the permanent counterparts or to avoid their extraction, instead of using forceps, partial interradicular sectioning of the deciduous tooth should be performed using high-speed rotary tools so as to achieve radicular separation using a lever by breaking the thin layer of the residual dental tissue in a controlled manner. The removal of the single stumps thus obtained can safely be performed using forceps or levers, which should never be used at the furcation level to avoid any damage to the bud of the underlying permanent tooth (Fig. 13.5).
The presence of ankylosis can make this procedure more complex and may require the preparation of a mucoperiosteal flap as well as a cautious demolition of bone to avoid root fractures by helping overcome the tenacious resistance offered by the root cementum fused with the surrounding bone.

Applying levers. The lever tip must be placed between the alveolar wall and the dental root as parallel as possible to the tooth axis so that the tip can perform a wedge action.

Dislocation. This step can be performed using forceps or levers and can cause alveolar bone tissue expansion and periodontal ligament laceration, resulting in dentoalveolar space enlargement and subsequent mobilization of the dental element to be extracted.
The dislocation, achieved using forceps, must be performed in a vestibulo-oral direction and, in case of single-rooted teeth, can be completed by limited rotation around the dental element axis.
If levers are being used, the handle must be placed toward the dental crown so that the dislocation force is exerted on the crown itself and not on the margin of the alveolar process, which might otherwise break.

Avulsion. It implies the removal of the tooth from its alveolus and starts during the final step of dislocation; it is associated with the real traction movements in the direction of the least resistance offered by the tooth if the action is performed using forceps—in other words, the creation of a thrust in the coronal–apical direction if a lever is used.
The presence of a root apex fracture requires immediate surgical removal of the root using apical root elevators. The only exception is represented by the radicular residues of deciduous elements, whose removal can expose adjacent teeth or the permanent elements to the risk of damage. In such cases, it is better to leave them in situ because they mostly cause no complication, as they are often resorbed spontaneously or migrate toward the crest during permanent tooth eruption.

Alveolus inspection. This step involves clearing the residual cavity, i.e., the removal of pathological tissues or bone/dental fragments using spoon excavator or *curettes*, as well as digital compression of the alveolar wall, which favors hemostasis and healing.

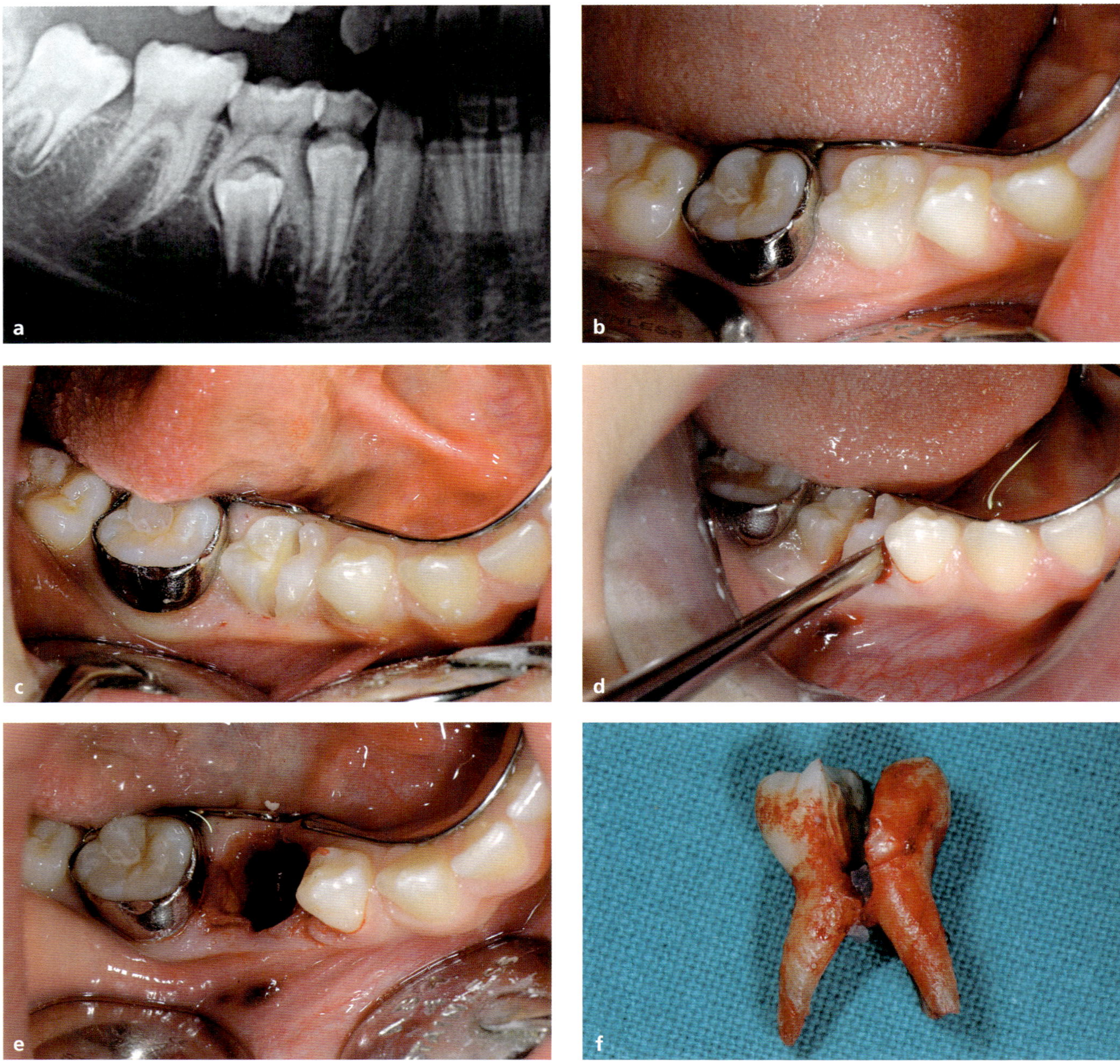

Figure 13.5 Extraction of a deciduous molar: (**a**) the details from the panoramic X-ray show the loss of resorption of 8.5, which prevented the eruption of the corresponding permanent tooth; (**b**) intraoral physical examination shows a slight infraocclusion of 8.5; (**c**) interradicular sectioning of the crown; (**d**) dislocation of the mesial portion; (**e**) postextraction alveolus; and (**f**) the extracted 8.5.

Suture. Suturing is performed to stabilize soft tissues and is necessary only if the marginal gingiva is mobile in relation to the underlying alveolar crest. In children, it can be performed using resorbable materials to avoid the removal of these materials that is eventually required.

Hemostasis control. It can be performed by pressing a gauze pad soaked in a physiological solution between the jaws in occlusion for around 10 minutes at the level of the alveolus in the posteruption phase.

Surgical steps for complex extractions

In complex extractions, the surgical steps can vary in terms of type and sequence depending on the features of the tooth or root to be extracted; the steps include the following:

- access flap
- ostectomy
- odontotomy
- dislocation
- avulsion
- bone margin adjustment
- suturing.

Access flap. Raising an access flap is aimed at accessing the underlying bone plane. The access flap is mucoperiosteal and intrasulcular in the presence of the dental element and may be envelope-, triangle-, or trapezoid-shaped depending on the complexity of the intervention. In certain situations, the detachment of the flap, with a more apical position for levers and forceps, is enough to complete avulsion.

Ostectomy or bone breach. It involves the removal of alveolar bone tissue, more frequently at the expense of the vestibular side, and is performed using bone milling cutters (a rosette or fissure cutter) mounted on a micromotor and with abundant irrigation.
In case of molar extractions, when interradicular odontotomy is required, it might be useful to extend ostectomy until the furcation opening is exposed, just as, in the presence of a particularly thick interdental septum, it might be useful to create a bone breach at the level of the root, to use the lever in the obtained groove, without involving the bone tissue of the adjacent teeth and the vestibular cortical bone.

Odontotomy. A single section or multiple sections may be defined on a dental element; it is possible to operate using high-speed rotary instruments and with abundant irrigation.
Odontotomy is indicated in single-rooted teeth in which there is marked radicular curvature because by allowing the elimination of the homolateral coronal portion of the radicular concavity, it eliminates the undercut that prevents the dislocation of the dental element.
In multirooted teeth with complex radicular morphology, because of the presence of divergent roots or apical hooks, interradicular sectioning is indicated as the division of the radicular trunks allows performing avulsion separately. In cases where the pulp chamber floor is affected by a destructive carious lesion, odontotomy can be performed using a lever at the furcation level.

Dislocation. It is basically performed using levers, which must be inserted between the alveolar wall and the root. In interradicular odontotomy, levers must be used in the created space and the procedure must start by dislocating the less curved, shortest or most movable root to ease the extraction of the less anatomically favorable root.

Avulsion. It can be performed using levers or root or hemostatic forceps.

Bone margin regulation. The trimming of sharp or irregular bone margins and the removal of fractured interradicular bone septum is performed using bone forceps, bone rasps, or rosette milling cutters mounted on low-speed rotary handpieces.

Suturing. Suturing is aimed at repositioning (in the initial position or in a new one) and stabilizing the detached soft tissue on the underlying bone plane to promote clot formation and healing.

Instructions for patients

The instructions to be followed during the postoperative period include several recommendations: not to chew at the extraction site for the first 6–8 hours, not to rinse and spit, consume a cold and liquid diet, and avoid oral hygiene procedures around the surgical wound. For the first 4–7 days, it is necessary to clean the wound using cotton pads or cotton swabs soaked in a 10-volume solution of hydrogen peroxide diluted by 50% with water and not to chew hard food on the affected side.

Odontomas and supernumerary teeth

Even though they are two different clinical entities, odontomas and supernumerary teeth show remarkable similarities such as follows: (1) they are frequently located in the anterior region of the upper jaw; (2) they exhibit a young age of onset; (3) the affected dental tissue is the same; and (4) they exhibit similar types of pathological manifestations. Particularly, the pathological manifestations include the following: (1) retention of deciduous or permanent teeth caused by the interposition of these entities along the physiological eruptive course; (2) eruption delay, ectopic eruption, or dental malposition (rotations or inclinations) caused by a lack of space due to the presence of these entities; and (3) possible dysplastic or inflammatory complications.
Supernumerary teeth and odontomas occur more frequently at the level of the premaxilla, where they hinder the eruption of the incisors, particularly that of the central incisor, with a higher incidence at this site than at other sites. Dental retention most frequently involves incisor-like and tuberculate supernumerary teeth due to their large size, as well as the composite variant of odontomas compared with the complex one because of the early onset and the more frequent occurrence of the former in the anterosuperior regions.

Diagnosis

For correct treatment planning, it is indispensable to perform the following: (1) panoramic X-ray, which allows the assessment of the morphological and spatial features of supernumerary teeth or odontomas, their relationships with the adjacent anatomical structures, and the presence of related pathological conditions; (2) intraoral periapical radiographs, which better define the mesiodistal and apico–coronal relations of the lesion with the adjacent teeth; and (3) intraoral occlusal radiographs, which clarify the oral and vestibular dimensions of the lesion.

Therapy

The therapeutic approach for supernumerary teeth and odontomas involves timely removal of these entities; identification of the onset of their pathological manifestations; and, if pathological manifestations are already present, preventing them from worsening.

Avulsion can be delayed only in the presence of deciduous or mixed dentition, when the supernumerary teeth or odontomas are not clearly identifiable, as they are still in an early phase of their formation, or when surgical trauma can interfere with the correct development of the involved dental elements. In such cases, periodic clinical and radiographic check-ups allow monitoring of the situation and help choose the best time for intervention.

The removal of erupted supernumerary teeth is not generally difficult, even though their eruption at an ectopic site or the presence of teeth crowding (which makes it more difficult to use forceps or levers), might make clinicians choose syndesmotomes.

Supernumerary teeth or odontomas in the bone structure of the jaws require surgical extraction, which involves the following: incision and detachment of mucoperiosteal flap; creation of a bone breach, followed by odontotomy; removal of the supernumerary element or odontomatous neoformation; inspection of residual cavity; and suturing (Fig. 13.6).

The incision direction, chosen in relation to the site and structure of the supernumerary teeth or odontomas, is intrasulcular and envelope-shaped at palatal and lingual sites and triangle- or trapezoid-shaped at vestibular sites.

Bone breach, created using rosette or fissure milling cutters mounted on a micromotor and with abundant irrigation, must be as small as possible to avoid any damage to the adjacent dental and anatomical structures and must simultaneously allow the identification and removal of new formations.

Odontotomy is indicated in the presence of supernumerary teeth with radicular anomalies, supplemental teeth, and complex variants of odontomas to fragment the mass of dental tissues they are made of that may prevent their enucleation. This procedure is usually not necessary for conoid supernumerary teeth due their reduced size, for tuberculate teeth without roots, and for composite odontomas comprising easily removable denticles.

Odontotomy is performed using rotary instruments mounted on high-speed handpieces and must be completed with the fracturing action of a lever to avoid damage to the underlying tissues.
Once the supernumerary tooth with its follicular sac or the odontoma is removed, the residual cavity is inspected, the surgical area is washed with a physiological solution, and sutures are placed.
If the presence of a supernumerary tooth or an odontoma has caused the retention of a dental element and this still shows *vis-a-tergo*, the incisal margin and at least a third of the crown should be exposed to favor spontaneous eruption, before suturing. On the contrary, if the tooth is far away from the alveolar crest or has an almost closed root tip (apex), an anchoring element should be applied to allow orthodontic traction.
At the end of the procedure aimed to remove an odontoma, it is necessary to perform a radiologic examination to ascertain complete enucleation.

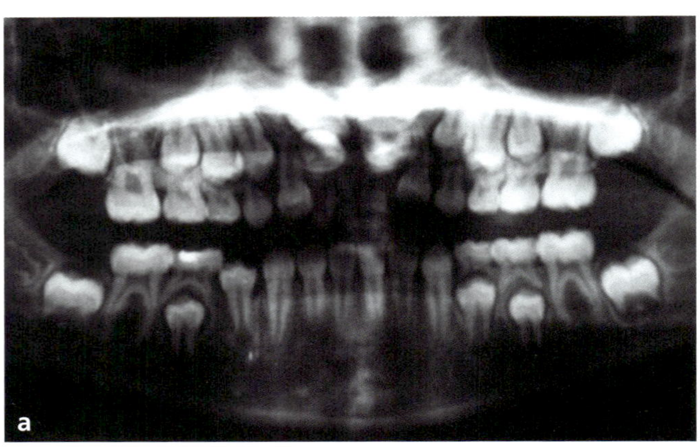

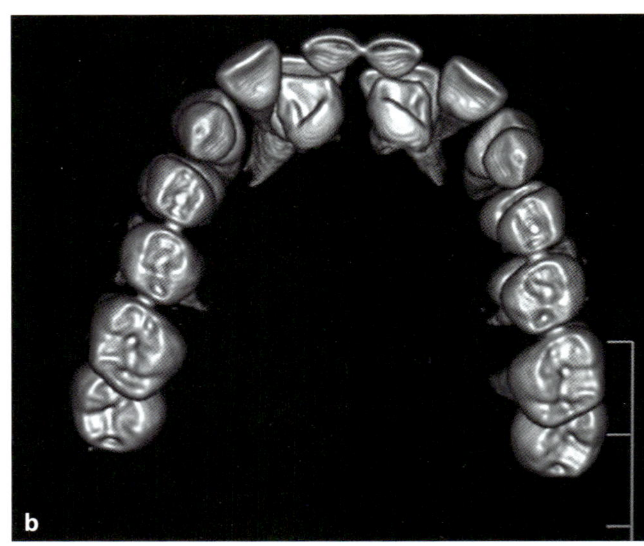

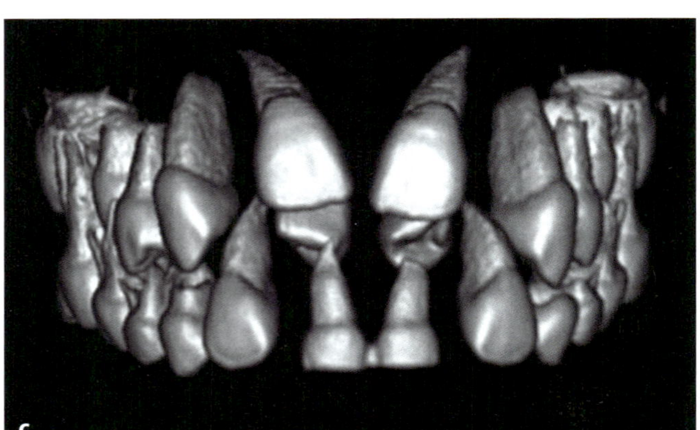

Figure 13.6 Removal of supernumerary teeth: (**a**) a panoramic X-ray of mixed dentition, in which it is possible to note the inclusion of central incisors, the persistence of the corresponding deciduous elements, and the presence of two impacted supernumerary teeth; (**b**) the 3D occlusal reconstruction by CT Dentascan shows a palatal protuberance of the supernumerary teeth; (**c**) the 3D frontal reconstruction by CT Dentascan shows vestibularly located impacted incisors (follows).

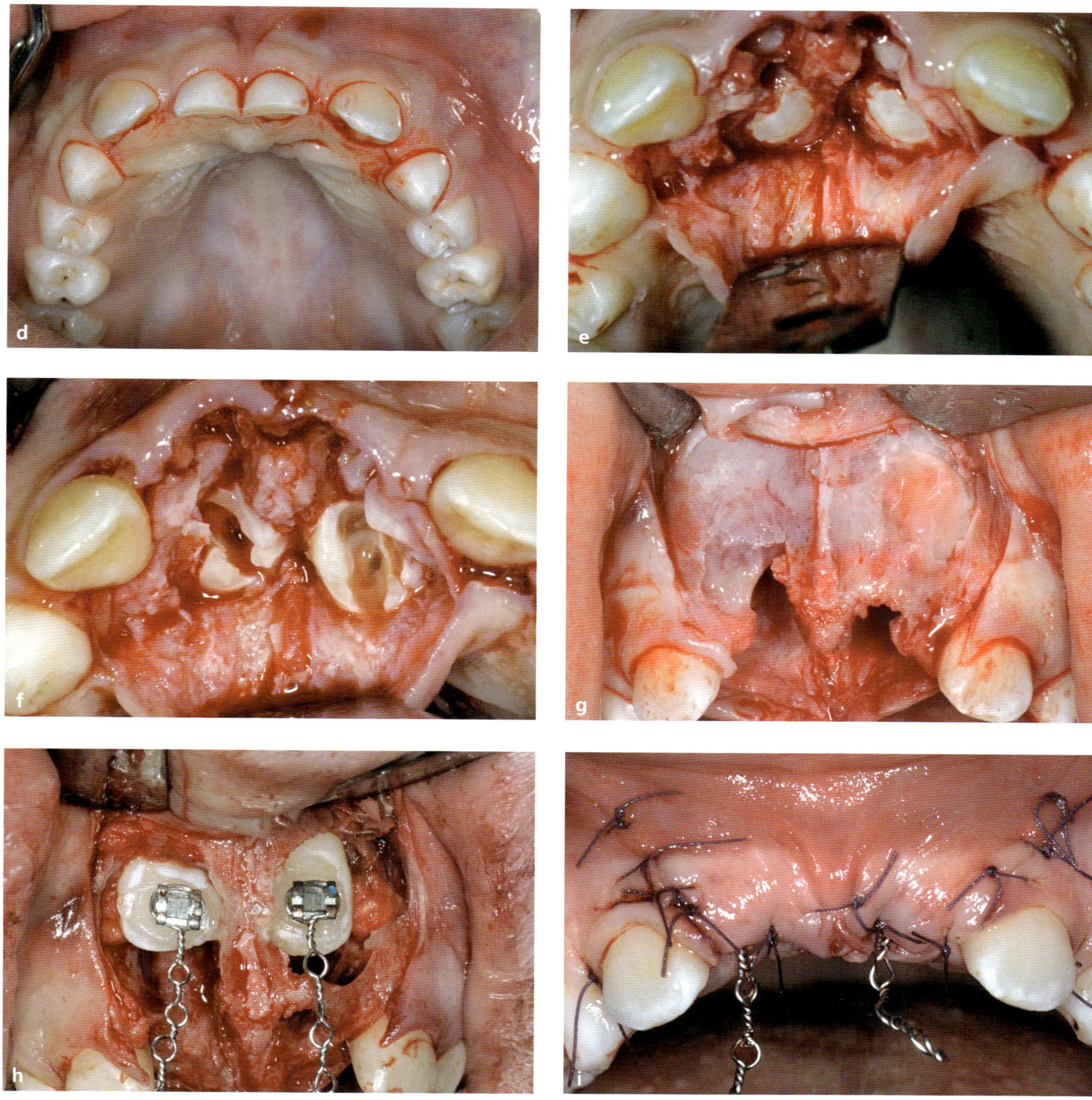

Figure 13.6 – Continued. (**d**) an intrasulcular linear incision on the palatal side extended to the medial side of the deciduous canines; (**e**) detachment of the palatal flap, performed before the extraction of the central deciduous teeth, and bone breach allow the exposure of supernumerary teeth; (**f**) odontotomy of supernumerary teeth, which facilitates their removal; (**g**) after the extraction of supernumerary teeth, it is possible to proceed with the incision and detachment of the vestibular trapezoidal flap; (**h**) exposure of the crown of the central incisors and application of orthodontic brackets; and (**i**) suture placement with detached stitches, with the traction thread coming out from the incision line.

Malformed teeth

Fusion and *gemination* are dental malformations classified among the developmental anomalies requiring surgical intervention, as they may lead to esthetic, periodontal, or orthodontic problems (such as lack of space, delayed eruption, or ectopic eruption).

Fusion. This is the consequence of the union of the enamel and/or the dental papillae of two (rarely more) dental buds that, after coming in contact at an early stage of their development, give rise to a single anomalous element that is characterized by the coalescence of the crowns, roots, or entire body of the teeth, as well as by different types of dental and pulpal connections. This malformation is more frequent in the deciduous dentition, particularly in the incisors, than in the permanent dentition and can involve two elements of the normal series (deciduous or permanent), one element of the normal series, and a supernumerary tooth or two supernumerary teeth.

Gemination. It occurs during the dental bud differentiation that, in response to local metabolic stimuli, undergoes partial or total *twinning*, giving rise to the formation of two dental elements that are partially or completely joined.

Therapy

The treatment of merged or geminated teeth is surgery and requires removal, odontotomy, or odontotectomy. The final choice is influenced by various factors, the most important being the type of dentition (primary or secondary).
In the deciduous dentition, the approach requires postponement of any type of intervention and implementation of periodic clinical and radiographic check-ups to monitor the regular resorption and exfoliation of the malformed tooth and eruption of the permanent tooth. Extraction is indicated only in the presence of anomalous radicular resorption of deciduous elements, which interfere with the eruption of the permanent ones, and should be performed when at least two-thirds of the mineralization process of the permanent root is complete.
In the presence of permanent teeth, the treatment should aim at the esthetic and functional recovery of the malformed tooth and is subject to a correct diagnostic approach, which together with the clinical and radiographic examination, should assess the level of union between the crowns and/or roots, their shape and orientation, and the configuration of endodontic space.
The choice of the surgical method is influenced by the following factors:

- the number of teeth within the arches, counting the anomalous tooth as two units, will be normal in the fusion between two permanent elements, whereas it will be increased by one unit in case of gemination or fusion with a supernumerary tooth

- the shape of the malformed tooth, whose corono-radicular section should allow separation, with the existence of endodontic spaces that do not communicate with each other or are not subject to root canal treatment.

Extraction. Regardless of the number of teeth within the arches, extraction is reserved for fused and geminated elements, with roots that cannot be surgically separated or that show a canal configuration that cannot be endodontically treated.

Odontotomy. Odontotomy requires splitting of the malformed tooth into two parts, which are both preserved. This procedure can be adopted in the presence of a normal dental series, when fusion has occurred between two permanent teeth that show separate roots or roots for which endodontic treatment can be performed.

Odontotectomy. It requires cutting of the anomalous element and avulsion of one of the parts thus obtained with the aim of restoring the normal morphovolumetric aspect. This procedure is indicated in case of fusion of a permanent tooth with a supernumerary one or in case of gemination, as the elimination of the excess part restores the normal dental shape. However, this method is subject to the possibility of recovering the residual part of the fused or geminated tooth, regardless of the necessity of endodontic treatment (Fig. 13.7).
To be successful, odontotomy and odontotectomy both require some technical expedients. Cutting of the malformed tooth should be performed under direct visual control, by exposing the root through an adequately sized bone breach and should be intraoperatively guided using intraoral periapical radiographs until it is finally completed. To avoid any damage to the part of the tooth that needs to be preserved, which might undergo resorption or ankylosis, cutting should be done at the expense of the dental region to be eliminated, which should be removed without using levers inside the created space.
The regular implementation of reparative processes at the level of the alveolar bone and periodontal ligament should be monitored through periodic clinical and radiographic check-ups until healing is completed. If there is no need for preoperative root canal treatment, it is important to check pulp vitality so as to establish an adequate therapy in the presence of pulp necrosis.
The therapeutic approach for fused and geminated teeth is multidisciplinary because, in addition to surgery, it might require orthodontic therapy, aimed at correctly aligning the recovered element within the arch, and a conservative or prosthetic treatment, aimed at restoring the normal coronal shape.

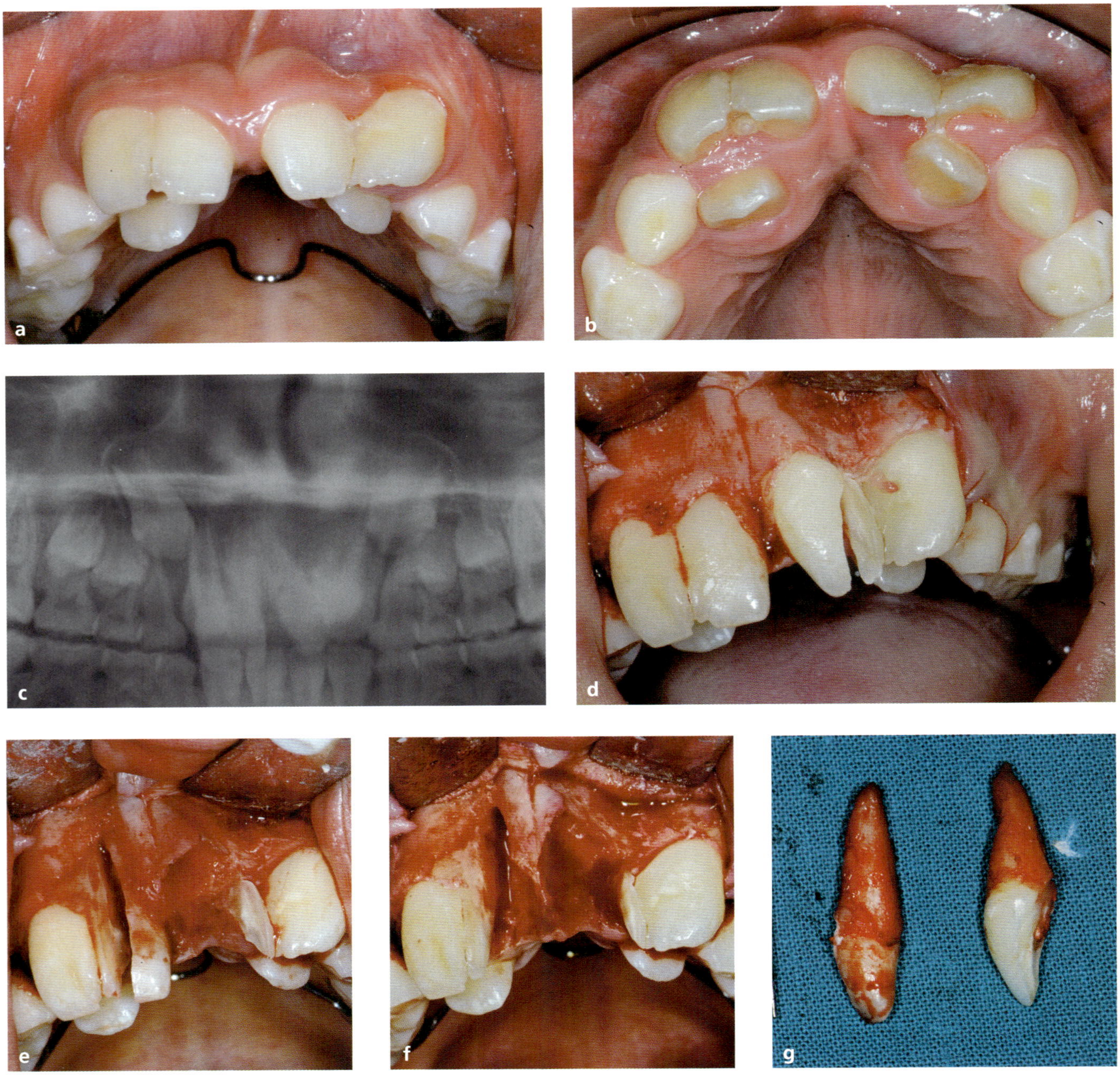

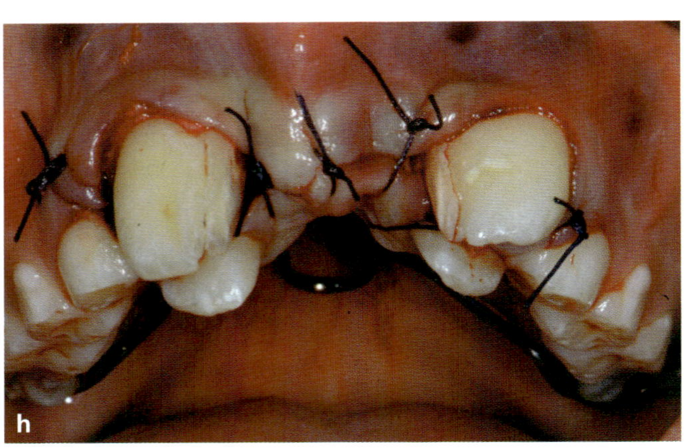

Figure 13.7 Odontotectomy of malformed upper central incisors: (**a**) after frontal intraoral physical examination, it was possible to note the fusion of 1.1 and 2.2 with the supernumerary teeth and the palatal eruption of 1.2 and 2.2; (**b**) physical examination of the occlusion confirmed the diagnosis; (**c**) detail from the panoramic X-ray that shows radicular morphology of the incisors, characterized by separated roots; (**d**) vertical odontotomy performed at the expense of the tooth portion to be eliminated; (**e**) after the avulsion of the mesial fragment of 2.1 corresponding to the supernumerary tooth, it was possible to perform the odontotomy of 1.1; (**f**) alveoli emptied after the avulsion of supernumerary teeth; (**g**) extracted fragments; and (**h**) suture placement.

Cystic lesions

A cyst is a newly formed cavity that is round or oval in shape; it may develop in the bone structure of the jaws. It has a lining that comprises fibrous connective tissue externally and a secreting epithelium internally, with fluid inside. Cystic lesions originate following a degenerative mechanism, from odontogenic or nonodontogenic epithelial residues (odontogenic and fissural cysts, respectively) inside the maxillary bones, and are recognized to have an inflammatory stimulus (inflammatory cysts) or an anomaly occurring during embryogenesis (developmental cysts) as a pathogenic moment.
The development of cysts can be subdivided into three main phases, depending on their slow and progressive growth at the expense of the surrounding bone tissue, as follows:

- **Latency**: the neoformation, when the cyst is still of modest size and gives rise to subjective or objective symptoms, unless it undergoes an inflammatory complication.
- **Deformation**: the progressive growth of the cyst causes the wear of the bone structure of the jaws, until the cortical bone becomes deformed, manifesting as a tumefaction frequently located in the vestibular area.
- **Fistulization**: overlapping of inflammatory processes can cause a sudden increase in the volume of the pre-existing tumefaction; edema and hyperemia of the overlying mucosa; pain with the involvement of local lymph nodes; and spontaneous opening of the cyst within the oral cavity, with leakage of seropurulent or purulent exudate.

Radiologically, the lesion appears as a radiotransparent, uniform, roundish, and usually unilocular image, with clear margins delimitated with a well-defined and thin border that is more intensely radiopaque than the surrounding tissue due to the bone reaction to the expansive process.
The currently accepted classification of cysts worldwide is the one formulated in 1992 by WHO on the basis of etiopathogenetic aspects (Tab. 13.3).
The most frequent odontogenic cysts in pediatric patients include the following:

- **Gingival cysts of newborns**: they affect newborns during the first 3 months of life and appear as nodules that are frequently multiple, located on the mucosa of the alveolar crest, white or yellow in color, and filled with keratin. They are asymptomatic and need no treatment, as they undergo spontaneous regression within 1–2 weeks.
- **Eruption cysts**: they appear as a bluish tumefaction at the expense of the soft tissues covering the crown of a dental element in eruption phase. This type of lesion heals spontaneously with the eruption of the tooth. However, healing may be favored by the removal of the operculum.
- **Follicular cysts**: they surround the crown of unerupted teeth, inserting themselves at the level of the collar, and are formed by the accumulation of fluids between the reduced epithelium of the enamel and crown or among the layers of the epithelium itself.
- **Radicular cysts of deciduous teeth**: they originate due to the proliferation of the epithelial cell rests of Malassez following an inflammatory stimulus induced by pulp necrosis.

Table 13.3 Classification of jaw cysts

Epithelial growth cysts	Inflammatory epithelial cysts
Odontogenic • Gingival cyst in children • Odontogenic keratocyst (primordial cyst) • Dentigerous cyst (follicular) • Eruption cyst • Lateral periodontal cyst • Adult gingival cyst • Glandular odontogenic cyst; odontogenic cyst **Nonodontogenic** • Cysts of the nasopalatine duct • Nasolabial cyst (nasoalveolar)	**Radicular cyst** • Apical and lateral cyst • Residual cyst **Periodontal cyst** • Inflammatory collateral cyst • Infected vestibular mandibular cyst

Source: Kramer IRH, 1992.

- **Infected mandibular buccal cysts**: they arise from the odontogenic epithelium as a consequence of an inflammatory stimulus starting from the superficial periodontium of a vital tooth under eruption and are frequently observed on the mandibular first molar in children aged between 6 and 8 years. These lesions, which are buccally located in relation to the molar roots, displace the roots lingually, resulting in the typical buccal inclination of the crown.

Therapy

The therapy for cystic lesions is surgery and comprises a conservative approach, called cystostomy or Partsch I method, and a radical approach, called cystectomy or Partsch II method.

Cystostomy, or marsupialization, is indicated in the deciduous or mixed dentition when a large cyst has involved permanent teeth in the phase of development. Indeed, the total enucleation of the cyst wall may both compromise the integrity or cause the avulsion of the affected dental elements and interfere with the eruption of dislocated buds due to the rapid bone healing process, which is its characteristic.

Therefore, in addition to minimizing the risk of damage to anatomical and dental structures, the conservative approach is particularly indicated in pediatric patients as it involves a minimally invasive intervention, which can easily performed even under local anesthesia. However, although it offers numerous undeniable advantages, this approach has several disadvantages: the relatively long healing time, need to wear resin obturator, need for frequent clinical and radiographic check-ups, and need for daily and accurate oral hygiene maintenance at home.

In all the other cases, the preferred intervention is cystectomy, which leads to the final removal of a cyst in a single surgical session and promotes rapid bone regeneration due to the formation of a clot that first tends to transform into connective tissue and then into bone tissue through metaplasia.

Cystostomy or marsupialization

It requires the opening of the cyst, drainage of its contents, and exposure of the epithelium to the oral cavity. This method eliminates the force within the cyst, which is responsible for bone resorption and promotes the activation of osteoblasts, favoring bone regeneration from the periphery to the center of the cystic cavity, which, in turn, undergoes a progressive decrease until its total disappearance. Furthermore, the slow and progressive ossification allows the teeth affected by the cystic lesion to reacquire their original position within the jaws and to spontaneously erupt.
The surgical technique involves the following steps (Fig. 13.8):

- incision of the mucosa over the cyst
- bone breach, in the presence of a preserved cortical bone
- removal of the most superficial portion of the cyst wall
- suturing of the cyst wall on the oral mucosa
- filling the cavity with gauze or other materials
- impression taking
- obturator placement.

Incision. Depending on the location of the lesion and the necessity of guaranteeing the obturator stability, the incision is performed on the vestibular side or on the peak and might not be necessary if the access is gained through the alveolus of extracted deciduous teeth. The incision is circular and simultaneously involves the alveolar mucosa and cyst wall in cases where the cortical bone is absent or very thin, and it is half-moon shaped with the concavity facing the fornix in cases where the cortical bone is intact to allow access to the underlying bone.

Bone breach. It can be performed using bone forceps or rosette milling cutters mounted on a micromotor.

Removal. The removal of the most superficial portion of the cyst wall, which should be sent to the pathologist for histological examination, allows access to the cyst cavity, which is emptied of its contents.

Suture. After trimming the bone margins and irrigating the area with a physiological solution, the residual cyst wall can be sutured to the oral mucosa, either immediately, in case of an operculum, or after removing the flap overlying the bone window. Suturing is not always necessary.
Filling the cavity with gauze or other materials. The goal of filling the cyst cavity with iodoform gauze is to maintain its patency and simultaneously prevent the penetration of food residue in the cavity. This situation may continue, with periodic replacement

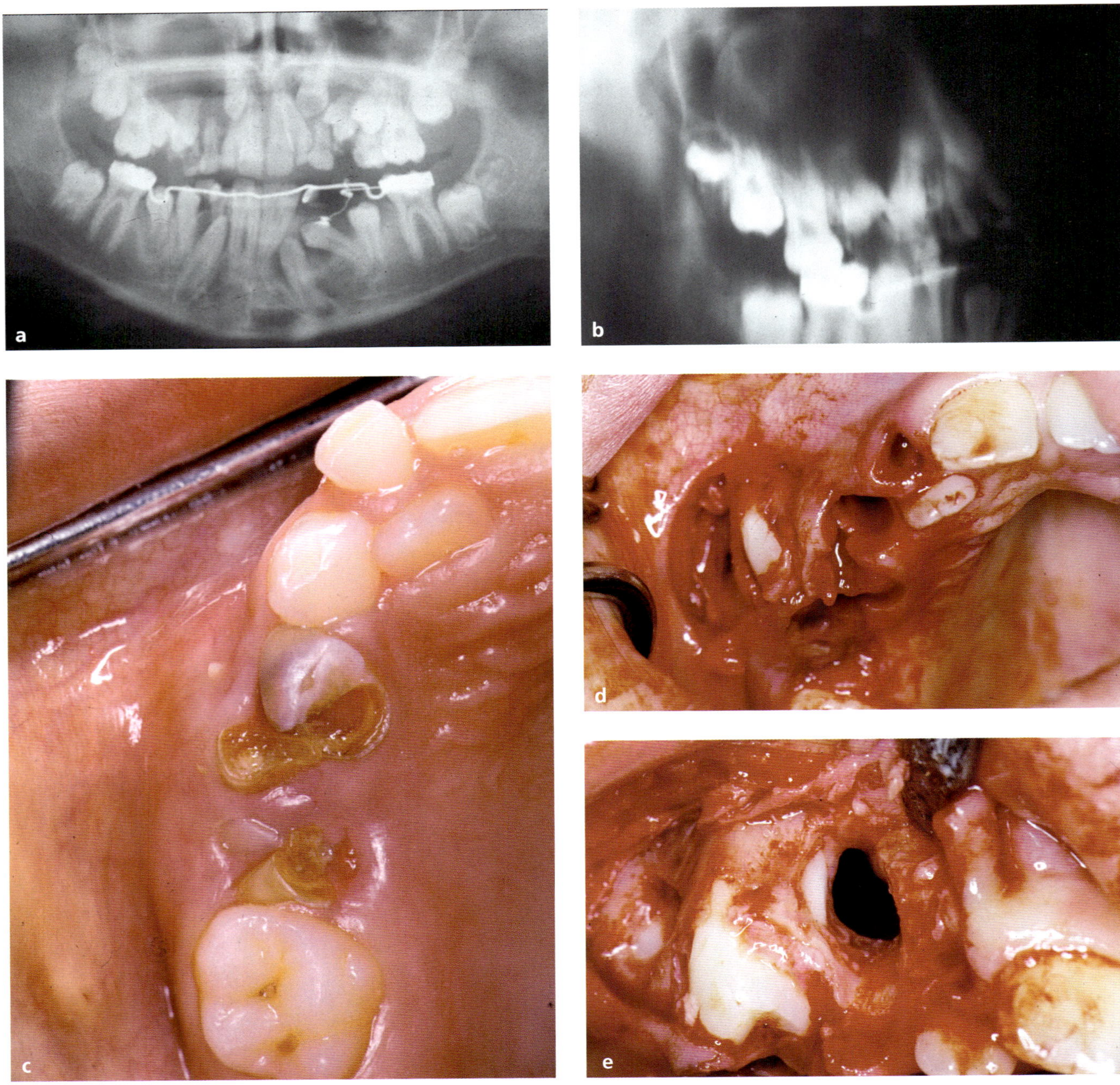

Figure 13.8 Marsupialization of a maxillary root cyst: (**a**) A panoramic X-ray shows a wide cystic radiolucency starting from the roots of the deciduous molars, which involves the entire right half of the jaw and the sinus space and which is responsible for the dislocation of the buds of the premolars and canine; (**b**) laterolateral stratigraphy confirms cyst expansion in the maxillary sinus up to the orbit floor; (**c**) after intraoral physical examination, it was possible to note a tumefaction of the vestibular fornix, the presence of 8.3, the radicular residues of 8.4 and 8.5, the persistence of 8.2, and the palatal eruption of 1.2; (**d**) after the extraction of 8.2, 8.3, and radicular residues, it was possible to proceed with the incision of a vestibular flap; (**e**) the detachment highlights the crown of 14 in vestibular position and allows to create a bone breach and a cyst opening; (**f**) a resin obturator fabricated to project inside the cavity; (**g**) the obturator placed in the oral cavity with the aim of maintaining the patency of the operculum and preventing the penetration of food residues; (**h**) intraoral physical examination after 12 months shows the obliteration of the cystic cavity and spontaneous eruption of the premolars. The goal of orthodontic treatment is to correct dental malpositions and recover the space for the eruption of the permanent canine; and (**i**) physical examination at the end of the treatment (*follows*).

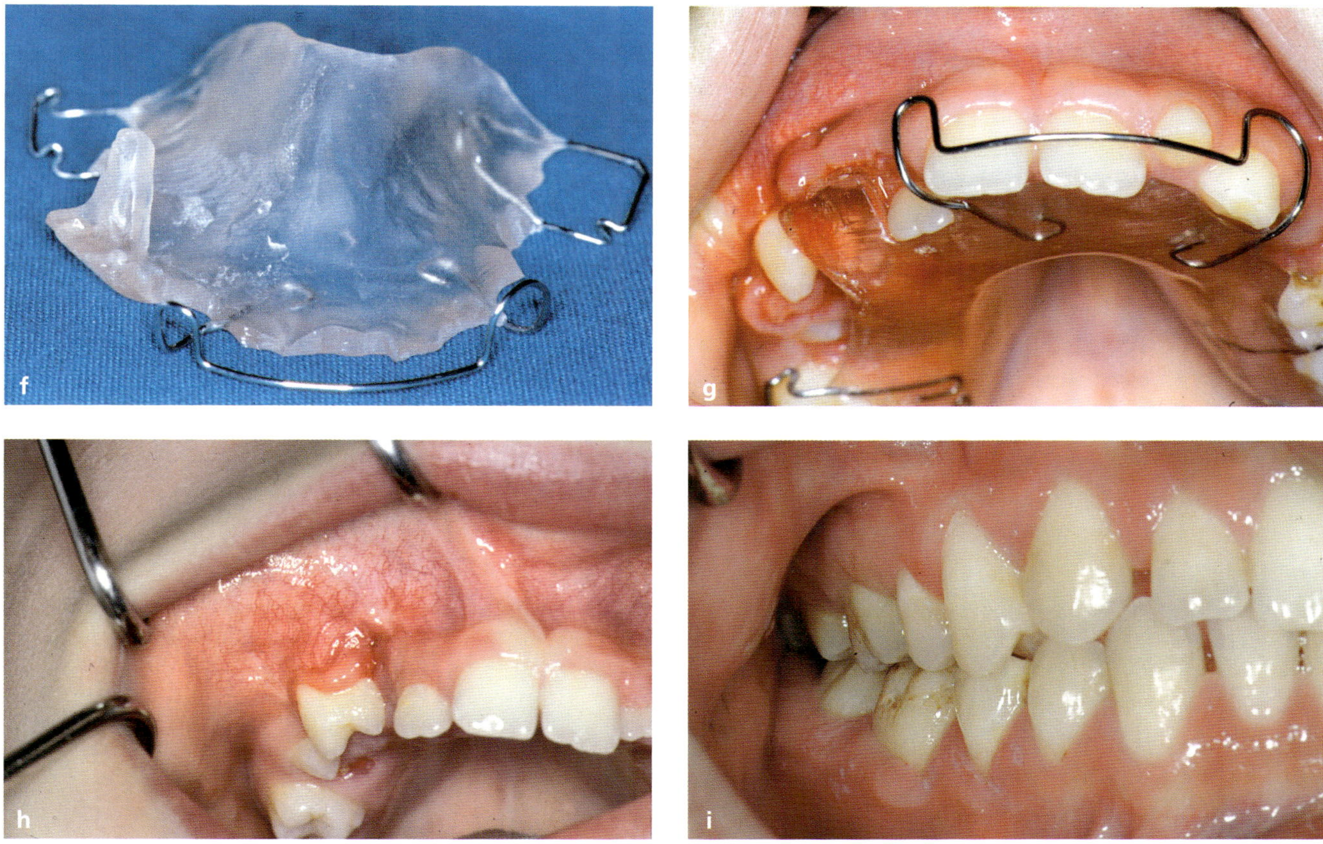

Figure 13.8 – Continued from previous page.

of gauze, for some weeks in case of small cysts or for a longer period by inserting an acrylic resin obturator, which should be worn for 24 hours and removed only after meals to perform oral hygiene procedures that include, in addition to teeth cleaning, irrigation of the cyst cavity with 3% hydrogen peroxide or 0.2% chlorhexidine solution.

Obturator fabrication. The obturator may be fabricated using the direct technique, which requires directly shaping the resin in the oral cavity, or the indirect one, which involves taking the impression of the dental arches using a silicon material and creating an opening to the cyst cavity. The second procedure is more desirable than the first one as it avoids the annoyance of the exothermic reaction of resin polymerization and the irritating action on the mucosa due to the spreading of the monomer. Another option is to fabricate an obturator based on the impression taken before the intervention, but in this case, it is necessary to proceed with relining to adjust the impression to the modified postoperative condition.

Cystostomy requires periodic clinical and radiographic check-ups to monitor the regular process of bone regeneration and to adapt the obturator size to the progressive narrowing of the cyst cavity so as to avoid interfering with healing and the eruption of the involved dental elements.

Cystectomy

Cystectomy involves enucleation of the cystic lesion and includes the following steps (Fig. 13.9):

- incision and flap detachment
- bone breach
- cyst wall removal
- checking residual cyst cavity
- flap repositioning and suturing.

Incision. It is a full-thickness incision and is determined by the shape of the cyst (linear, triangular, or trapezoidal), extension of the concerned area, and size of the lesion. The flap should (1) allow access to the operating area to avoid any traction and laceration of soft tissues, (2) not involve the surrounding anatomical structures, and (3) guarantee complete coverage of the operating area to obtain healing by primary intention. Finally, flap margins should be supported by intact bone to guarantee adequate support to the suture and to avoid dehiscence of the surgical wound.

Detachment. It should be performed with special care to avoid lacerations and perforations. It is relatively easy to perform in the presence of preserved cortical bone and becomes more complex if the cyst wall adheres to the overlying mucoperiosteal tissues, when it is possible to use scissors with blunt tips (Metzenbaum scissors).

Bone breach. Its size should be big enough to allow the removal of the entire cyst, and it should be performed in a way that helps preserve the integrity of the cyst wall as much as possible. In case of thin cortical bone, bone forceps can be used to delicately detach bone fragments; however, in case of thick cortical bone, it is necessary to use rosette milling cutters mounted on a low-speed handpiece, which should be used with a tangential sliding motion.

Removal. Cyst wall removal starts from the periphery of the bone breach and proceeds toward the cavity center. This step can be made easier via needle aspiration of the fluid inside, which requires the reduction of the pressure within the cyst and the placement of gauze soaked in a physiological solution between the level and bone plane. Once the most superficial part of the lesion has been removed, cleavage is facilitated by gentle traction exerted via hemostatic forceps on the mobilized portion of the cyst.

Checking the residual cyst cavity. It requires the removal of the cyst wall residues using *curettes* or spoon excavator, if the wall has not been completely removed; irrigation with a physiological solution; and trimming of the bone breach margins.

Repositioning and suturing. Repositioning the flap in its original position and suturing should guarantee an adequate level of hemostasis and healing by primary intention, before any postoperative complications.

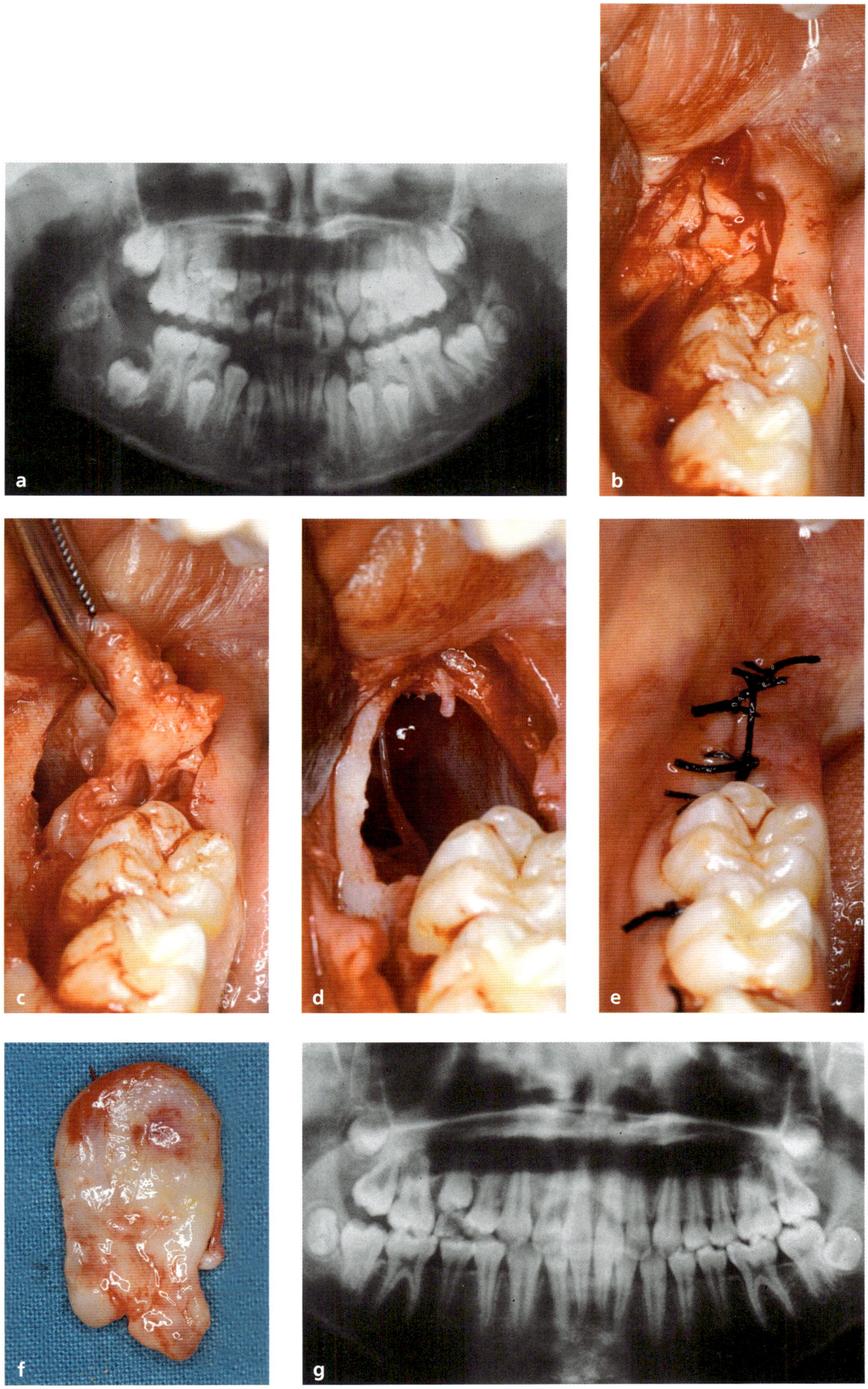

Figure 13.9 Cystectomy of a mandibular cyst: (**a**) On a panoramic X-ray, it is possible to notice a cystic area of radiolucency, spreading from the distal surface of the right first permanent molar to the mandibular ramus, that pushed the bud of the second molar downwards and that of the eighth molar distally; (**b**) the incision and lifting of an intrasulcular bag-like flap that highlights the upper cyst portion; (**c**) after detaching from the bone plane, the most superficial part of the cyst wall is removed by applying gentle traction using hemostatic forceps, and this contributes to move the deepest portion of the lesion; (**d**) the residual cavity after cyst enucleation; (**e**) silk suture placement with detached stitches; (**f**) surgical specimen; and (**g**) panoramic X-ray after healing.

Treatment of pathological frenula

Frenula are fibromucous folds of tissue that connect the lining mucosa of the alveolar processes to the submucosa of the lips (superior and inferior labial frenula) or cheeks (superior and inferior buccal frenula) and the ventral surface of the tongue to the oral floor (lingual frenulum).
Frenula are considered pathological when, due to anomalies in length, volume, texture, or insertion, they cause orthodontic; periodontal; prosthetic; esthetic; or functional problems, such as difficulties in breastfeeding, swallowing, or speech, as well as incorrect tongue postures.

The most frequently detected pathological frenula in pediatric patients include the following:

- Superior and inferior labial frenula that are hypertrophic or have an insertion in the adhering gingiva: these can create anomalous tractions on the free margin during the functional movements of the oral cavity (*pull syndrome*) and favor the onset of gingival retractions. The traction exerted by the frenulum is actually a contributing factor to the onset of this problem (which is favored by a thin periodontal biotype), scarce amount of residual adhering gum, and inadequate plaque control.
- Superior labial frenulum with an insertion on the vestibular side of the incisive papilla and on the transpapillary side (tectolabial): the deepest fibers pass through the intermaxillary suture and alter the physiological horizontal course of transseptal fibers interposed between the central incisors, which cause interincisive diastemas.
- Short lingual frenulum: it is responsible for ankyloglossia that, by forcing the tongue to rest more anteriorly, can exert an excessive pressure on the lower incisors, causing them to tilt. Furthermore, this anomalous thrust can cause anterior growth of the lower jaw and interfere with jaw development, leading to the appearance of an anterior open bite and lateroposterior crossbite.

Diagnosis

The goal of intraoral physical examination is to examine the clinical features of the frenulum; its insertion level, length, and texture (soft or fibrous); the type of insertion; and the amount of adhering gingiva. The distraction of the lip, which should be performed in the presence of labial frenula, induces tension in the frenulum and causes detachment and ischemia of the free gingival margin in medial or lateral pathological frenula and ischemia of the incisive papilla on the vestibular and/or palatal side in tectolabial frenula.
Ankyloglossia is diagnosed when the tongue is not able to touch the palatal vault due to a short lingual frenulum. Moreover, in the presence of an overly apical frenulum insertion, the tongue shows a bilobed appearance, which becomes more evident during protrusive movements.

In the tectolabial frenulum, the detection of a U- or V-shaped radiolucency at the level of the incisive bone septum in intraoral periapical or occlusal radiographs proves the existence of a parallel course of transseptal fibers within the median palatine suture.

Therapy

The approach is surgical and comprises frenulotomy or frenulectomy, which may be performed in association with other interventions such as circumferential supracrestal fiberotomy, sulcular gingivectomy, gingival graft placement, and vestibuloplasty. To treat the problems related to the superior labial frenulum, the most suitable age is between 9 and 22 years, after the eruption of the permanent incisors and canines, to avoid unnecessary interventions, such as spontaneous closure of an interincisive diastema, or too early interventions, which might result in relapses.
Regarding lingual frenulum, it is better to intervene as soon as possible if significant ankyloglossia is present.

Frenulotomy

It is indicated in the presence of short frenula and involves incision and disinsertion of their fibers with the purpose of eliminating tension. In labial frenula, the procedure includes the following steps: (1) making a half-thickness V-shaped or linear incision at the base of the frenulum at the level of the alveolar process; (2) disinsertion of the frenulum and muscle fibers starting from the periosteal plane from which they radiate; (3) suturing of the affected tissues on the labial side; and (4) application of a surgical wrap to protect and isolate the bleeding tissues, thus preventing relapse during healing (Fig. 13.10).
To avoid this problem and completely cover the surgical wound, a plastic surgery intervention with a Z-shaped incision has been suggested, which allows the transposition of the two triangular mucosal flaps and their suturing in an inverse position, with the modification of fiber orientation (from a vertical to a horizontal direction) (Fig. 13.11).
In the presence of short lingual frenula, frenulotomy can be performed: it involves performing a horizontal incision on the frenulum base, at the level of the ventral surface of the tongue, which, in turn, is blocked and duly held by grasping the tip with a gauze or via a suture passing at a distance of around 1 cm from the tip. If the margins of the diamond-shaped surgical wound are not sufficiently mobile to be handled and sutured with the detached points, it is possible to undermine them by inserting and opening the tips of surgical scissors between the mucosal plane and the underlying muscle plane so that movements can be facilitated.

Frenulectomy

It involves complete excision of the frenulum and its insertions and is indicated in the presence of tectolabial frenula, ankyloglossia, and gingival retractions. The removal of labial frenula can be performed using different techniques, the most commonly used of which include the V-shaped incision and parallel paramedian incision.

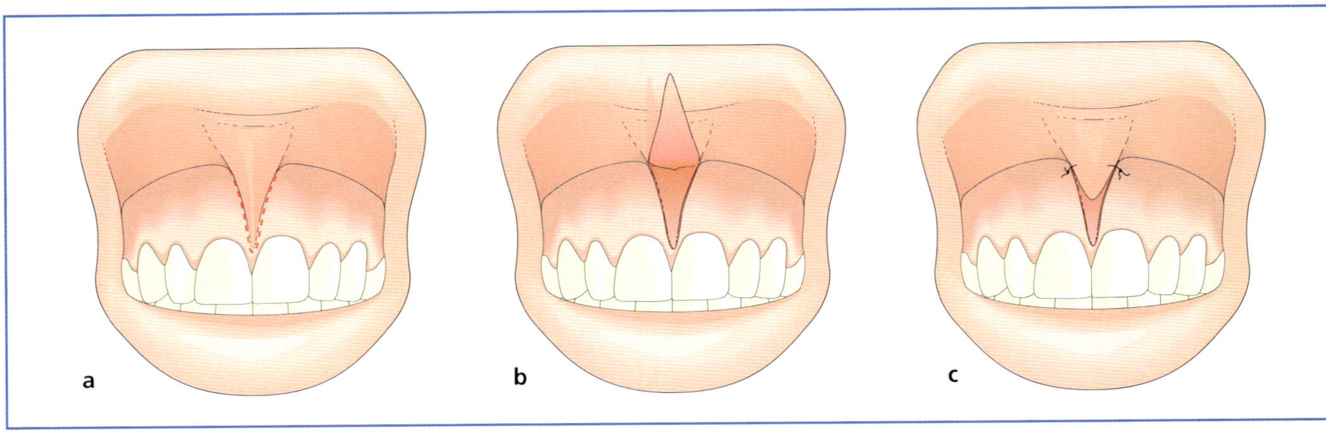

Figure 13.10 Frenulotomy: (**a**) the upper labial frenulum is inserted in the interincisive papilla; (**b**) a half-thickness incision, made at the base of the frenulum, that allows disinsertion from the periosteal plane of the frenulum and muscle fibers; and (**c**) suture placement with the detached tissues still on the labial side.

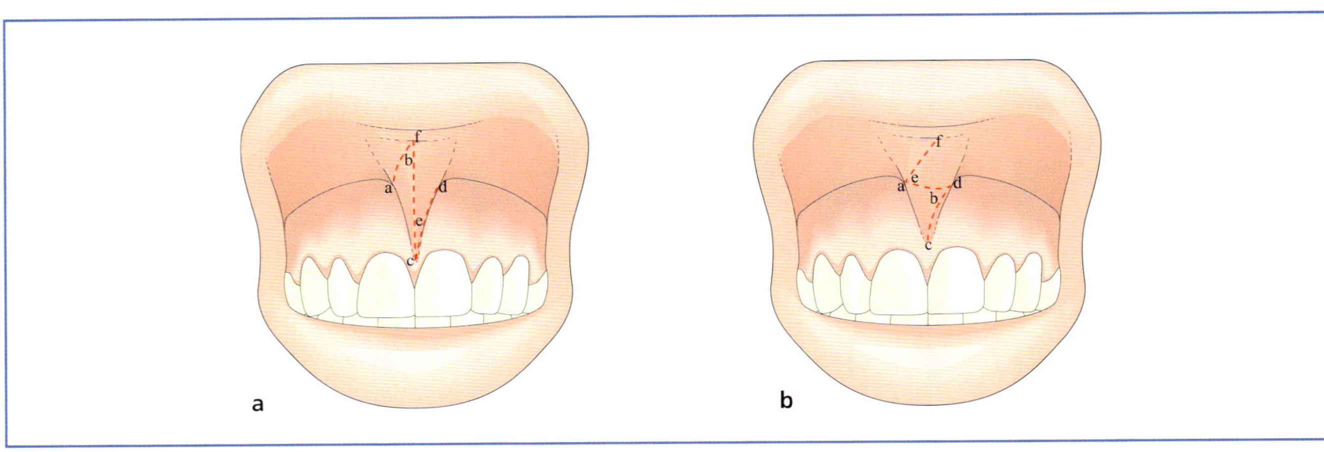

Figure 13.11 Plastic surgery using a Z-shaped incision: (**a**) from the end of the vertical incision, performed at the frenulum center, two secondary incisions depart, forming a 60° angle in a Z-shape structure; (**b**) the transposition of two mucosal triangular flaps and their suturing in a reverse position allow modification of the fiber orientation from a vertical to a horizontal one.

Using the V-shaped incision, frenulum removal is performed by sliding the scalpel over the surface of two hemostatic forceps, placed in a way so as to let the ends meet to form an inverted V, at the level of insertions on the inner surface of the lip and on the alveolar process. After removing the hemostatic forceps, a diamond-shaped wound remains, the margins of which must be undermined via blunt dissection using specifically dedicated scissors to create a tension-free suture and, consequently, facilitate healing by primary intention (Fig. 13.12).

Using parallel paramedian incisions, two vertical incisions are made on the sides of the frenulum and extended up to the retroincisive papilla, where they are joined by a short horizontal incision that allows separating the frenulum from the underlying periosteum, proceeding from the palate toward the fornix bottom. Sutures are placed by handling the incision margins along the midline without involving the adhering gingiva, which is protected with a surgical wrap and heals by secondary intention (Fig. 13.13).

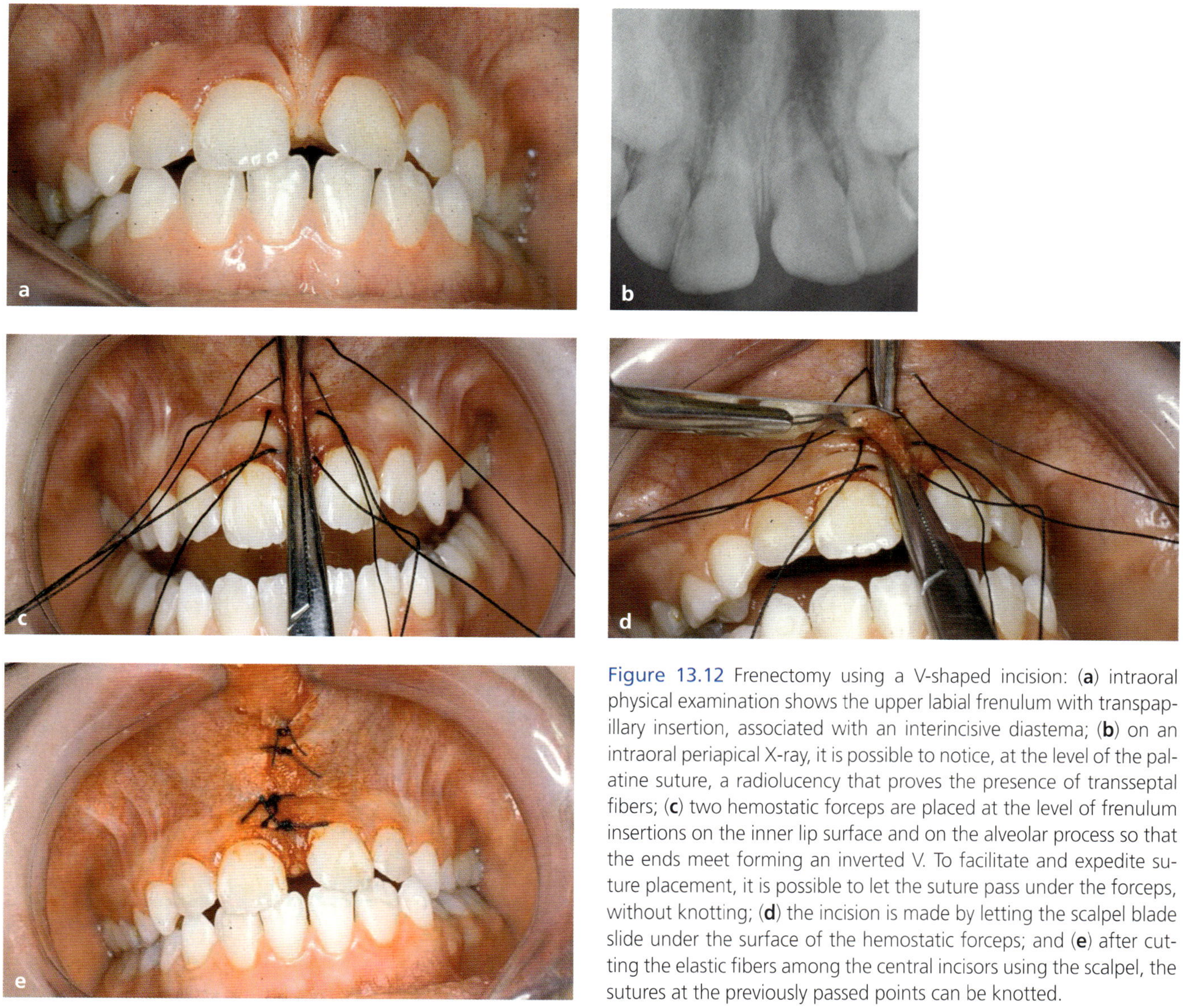

Figure 13.12 Frenectomy using a V-shaped incision: (**a**) intraoral physical examination shows the upper labial frenulum with transpapillary insertion, associated with an interincisive diastema; (**b**) on an intraoral periapical X-ray, it is possible to notice, at the level of the palatine suture, a radiolucency that proves the presence of transseptal fibers; (**c**) two hemostatic forceps are placed at the level of frenulum insertions on the inner lip surface and on the alveolar process so that the ends meet forming an inverted V. To facilitate and expedite suture placement, it is possible to let the suture pass under the forceps, without knotting; (**d**) the incision is made by letting the scalpel blade slide under the surface of the hemostatic forceps; and (**e**) after cutting the elastic fibers among the central incisors using the scalpel, the sutures at the previously passed points can be knotted.

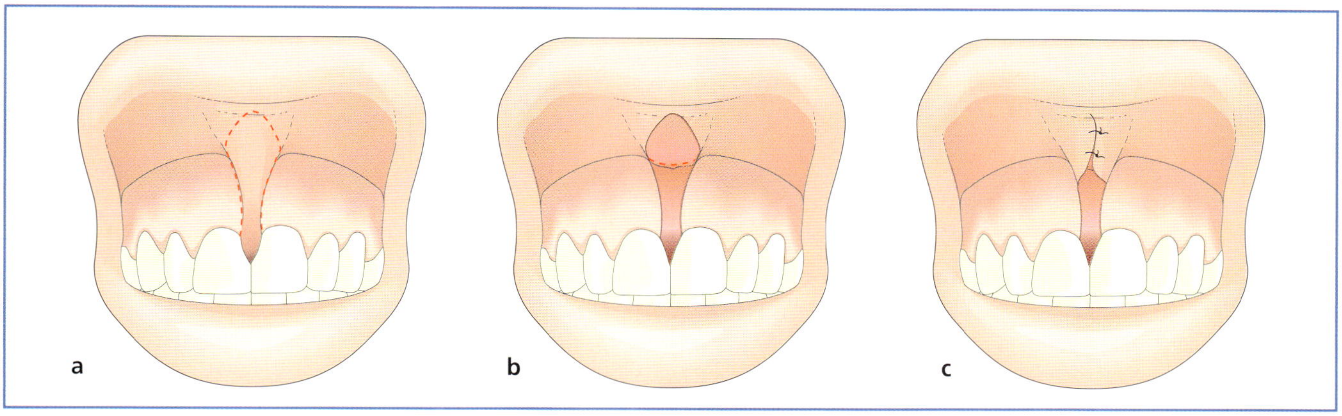

Figure 13.13 Frenulectomy with parallel paramedian incisions: (**a**) a transpapillary frenulum; (**b**) two vertical incisions made at the sides of the frenulum and extended up to the retroincisive papilla, where they are joined by a short horizontal incision, allowing the separation of the frenulum from the underlying periosteum; and (**c**) sutures are placed by handling the incision margins along the midline without involving the adhering gingiva, which, in turn, is protected by a surgical wrap and heals by secondary intention.

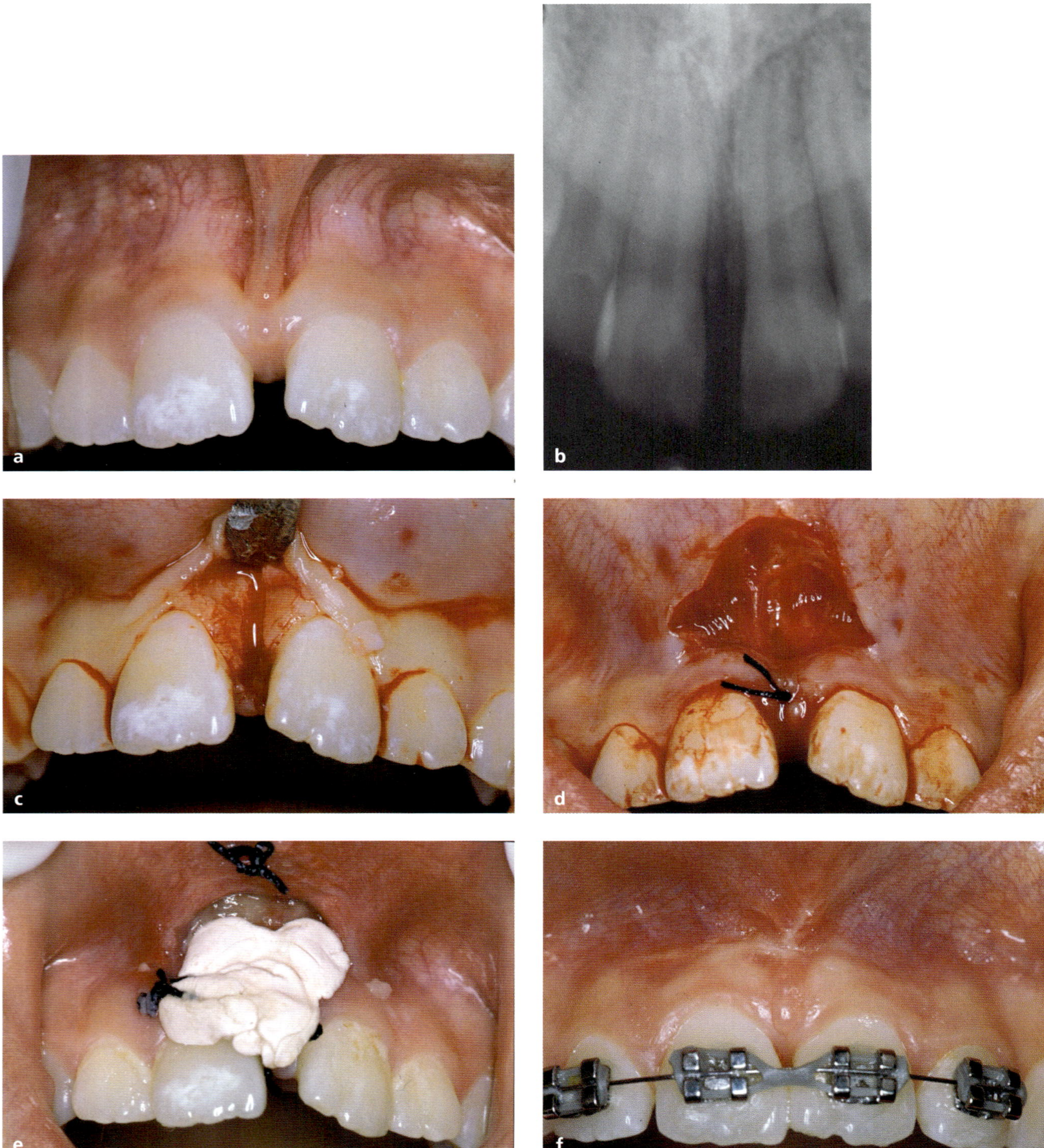

Figure 13.14 Frenulectomy in two operating phases: (**a**) on intraoral physical examination, it is possible to notice the transpapillary medial frenulum associated with the interincisive diastema; (**b**) intraoral periapical X-ray confirms the presence of transseptal fibers inside the palatine suture; (**c**) incision and detachment of an intrasulcular mucoperiosteal flap on the vestibular side of the central incisors that allow removal of transseptal fibers; (**d**) after positioning and stabilizing the flap with a suture over the intermaxillary bone wound, it is possible to cut the frenulum base; (**e**) suture placement in the upper part of the vestibular flap on the labial side, on which a periodontal wrap is positioned to protect the surgical wound, which, in turn, is left to heal by secondary intention; and (**f**) diastema closure is achieved with orthodontic therapy.

In cases of tectolabial frenulum, the excision of the frenulum is associated with the removal of transseptal fibers using a fissure bone milling cutter mounted on a low-speed handpiece or using a curette at the level of the median palatine suture.
All the methods described above lead to healing by secondary intention of the interincisive area, with long healing times and considerable discomfort among pediatric patients during the postoperative period.
To solve these problems, it is possible to adopt a surgical technique comprising two steps: the first step involves the removal of transseptal fibers, whereas the second step is a plastic surgery intervention on the fibromucous component of the frenulum (Fig. 13.14).
The first part requires the removal of transseptal fibers with a direct access to the median palatine suture, which is underlined through the incision and detachment of the mucoperiosteal flap with intrasulcular bags on the vestibular and palatal sides of the central incisors. The use of a full-thickness flap allows the repositioning of the flap and the placement of a suture over the intermaxillary bone wound, promoting healing by primary intention.
The second step comprises frenulectomy or frenulotomy performed following one of the previously described methods.
In cases of ankyloglossia, frenulectomy (Fig. 13.15) is preferably performed by making an incision over the hemostatic forceps, placed at the level of frenulum insertion on the tongue and oral floor, at a safe distance from the lingual caruncles and in a way so as to let the ends meet to form an inverted V. The margins of the diamond-shaped wound created after frenulum removal must be undermined by blunt dissection to allow the mucosal tissue to slide over the muscle plane and to place a tension-free suture, consequently allowing healing by primary intention. Furthermore, to obtain maximum tongue mobility, it is preferable not to proceed with the complete closure of soft tissues at the base of the tongue, at the level of the main transverse axis of the surgical wound, but to let them heal by secondary intention, interposing a roll of gauze fixed with a suture orientated in a laterolateral direction among the bleeding surfaces.
Regardless of the technique used, surgical treatment of frenula in children requires suturing to be performed using resorbable material because suture removal is frequently difficult and painful; furthermore, it is necessary to prescribe home exercises, focused on tongue mobility, in the postoperative period to improve functional recovery, especially for the lingual frenulum.
Circumferential supracrestal fiberotomy and **sulcular gingivectomy** are the procedures that, through the resection of transseptal fibers of the incisor group, can contribute to avoiding the risk of recurrence of midline diastema due to the elastic memory of the concerned fibers.
Free gingival grafts with samples taken from the palate or edentulous areas and laterally positioned pedicle grafts are indicated in the presence of periodontal lesions associated with the *pull syndrome* due to labial frenulum to increase the amount of adhering gingiva.
Vestibuloplasty allows to increase the width of the keratinized gingiva through the preparation of a periosteal surface that, with no muscle insertions under the frenulum, is left to heal by secondary intention.

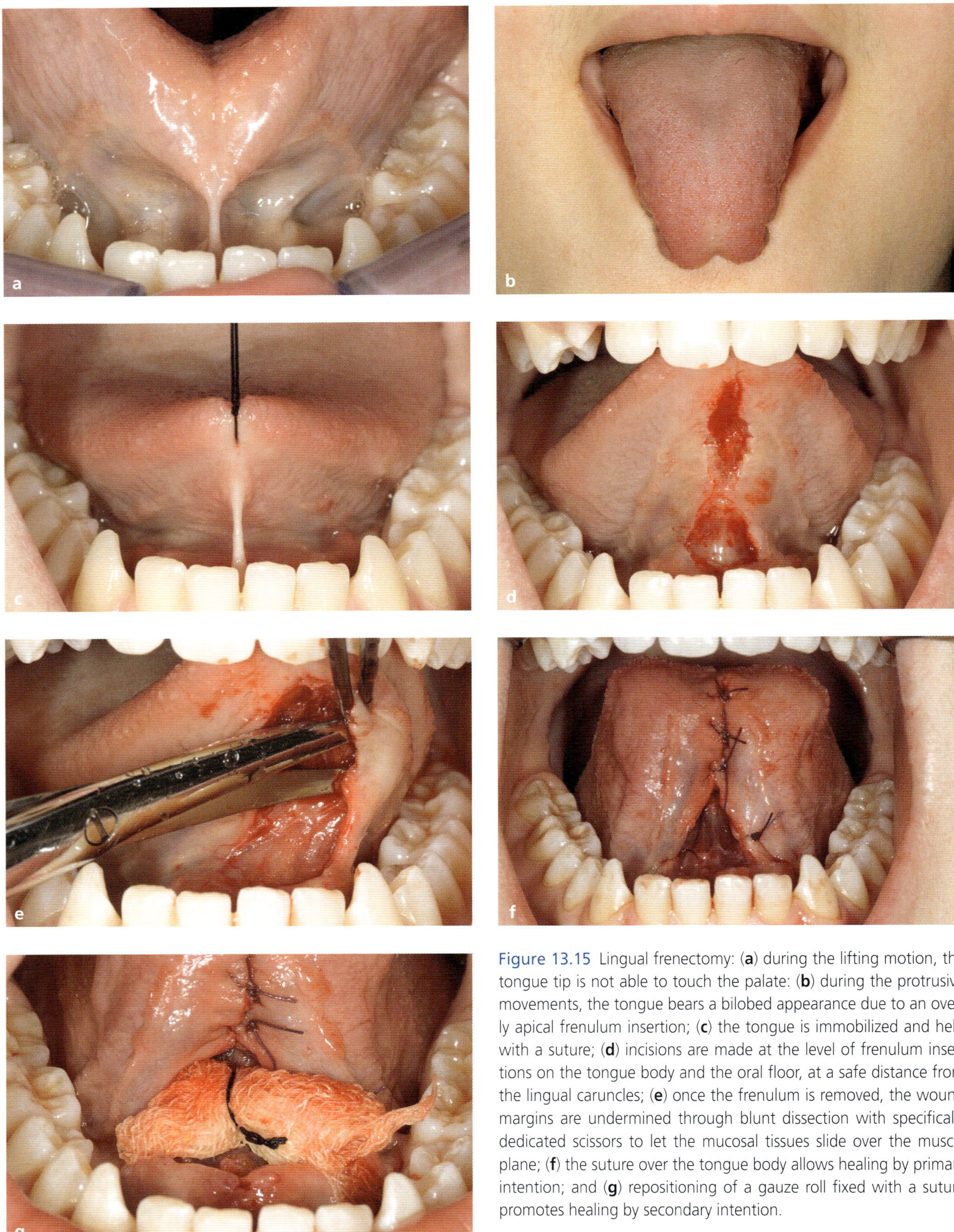

Figure 13.15 Lingual frenectomy: (**a**) during the lifting motion, the tongue tip is not able to touch the palate: (**b**) during the protrusive movements, the tongue bears a bilobed appearance due to an overly apical frenulum insertion; (**c**) the tongue is immobilized and held with a suture; (**d**) incisions are made at the level of frenulum insertions on the tongue body and the oral floor, at a safe distance from the lingual caruncles; (**e**) once the frenulum is removed, the wound margins are undermined through blunt dissection with specifically dedicated scissors to let the mucosal tissues slide over the muscle plane; (**f**) the suture over the tongue body allows healing by primary intention; and (**g**) repositioning of a gauze roll fixed with a suture promotes healing by secondary intention.

Cysts and pseudocysts of the minor salivary glands

Mucocele is a benign cystic neoformation characterized by a cavity filled with mucinous liquid that is secreted by minor salivary glands located in the lip submucosa, buccal mucosa, palate, and oral floor (ranula). There are two types of mucoceles: *extravasation* and *retention*. They are different in terms of etiopathogenesis and histological features but very similar in terms of clinical appearance and the treatment required.

Extravasation mucocele. It is the more frequently detected type and develops after a traumatic event that, after rupturing or sectioning a salivary gland duct, causes the extravasation of saliva into the submucosal connective tissue. It is a pseudocyst as the lesion has a fibrous connective tissue wall without epithelial lining.

Retention mucocele. It is a real cyst that develops due to the partial obstruction of a duct, which undergoes a progressive dilatation of its upstream portion, forming a cavity that is filled with secretions and is lined by epithelium.

Diagnosis

The diagnosis of mucocele is relatively easy and based on patient's medical history and clinical examination findings. The medical history is used to detect any history of trauma in the concerned area or bad habits such as lip or cheek biting; mode of onset (sudden); and clinical course, which alternates episodes of remission and relapse. The examination of the oral cavity highlights a tumefaction of round or oval shape, with size varying from a few millimeters to a few centimeters, whose color changes depending on the depth up to which the mucin is collected. The superficial lesions are bluish, smooth, and translucent, whereas the deeper ones are covered by mucosa with a normal appearance and color. The collections of mucus under the oral epithelium have a vesicle-like appearance instead. On palpation, the neoformation is painless, soft, floating, elastic, and mobile in the underlying planes.

Therapy

The therapy for mucocele is surgery and requires the excision of the mucoceles located on the lips, buccal mucosa, and palate, as well as marsupialization of ranula.
Removal (Fig. 13.16) can be performed by making an elliptical incision around the base of the neoformation, which is held using the Allis forceps and lifted from the underlying plane, or by incising the mucosa that covers the top of the mucocele without perforating it. Therefore, the lesion is isolated from the surrounding tissues through blunt dissection taking great care to avoid relapses due to operative trauma to the

neighboring salivary glands. Once the lesion is removed, the surgeon should remove all the salivary glands within the operating area to avoid relapses and to place a suture on the mucosal plane and on labial or buccal aspects. On the palate, the surgical wound is left to heal by secondary intention.

On the other hand, marsupialization is indicated for ranula because of its larger size in comparison to mucocele; the difficulties in identifying a cleavage plane; its association with the sublingual gland; and its contiguity with important anatomical structures such as the Wharton's duct, lingual nerve, sublingual vessels, and hypoglossal nerve branches.

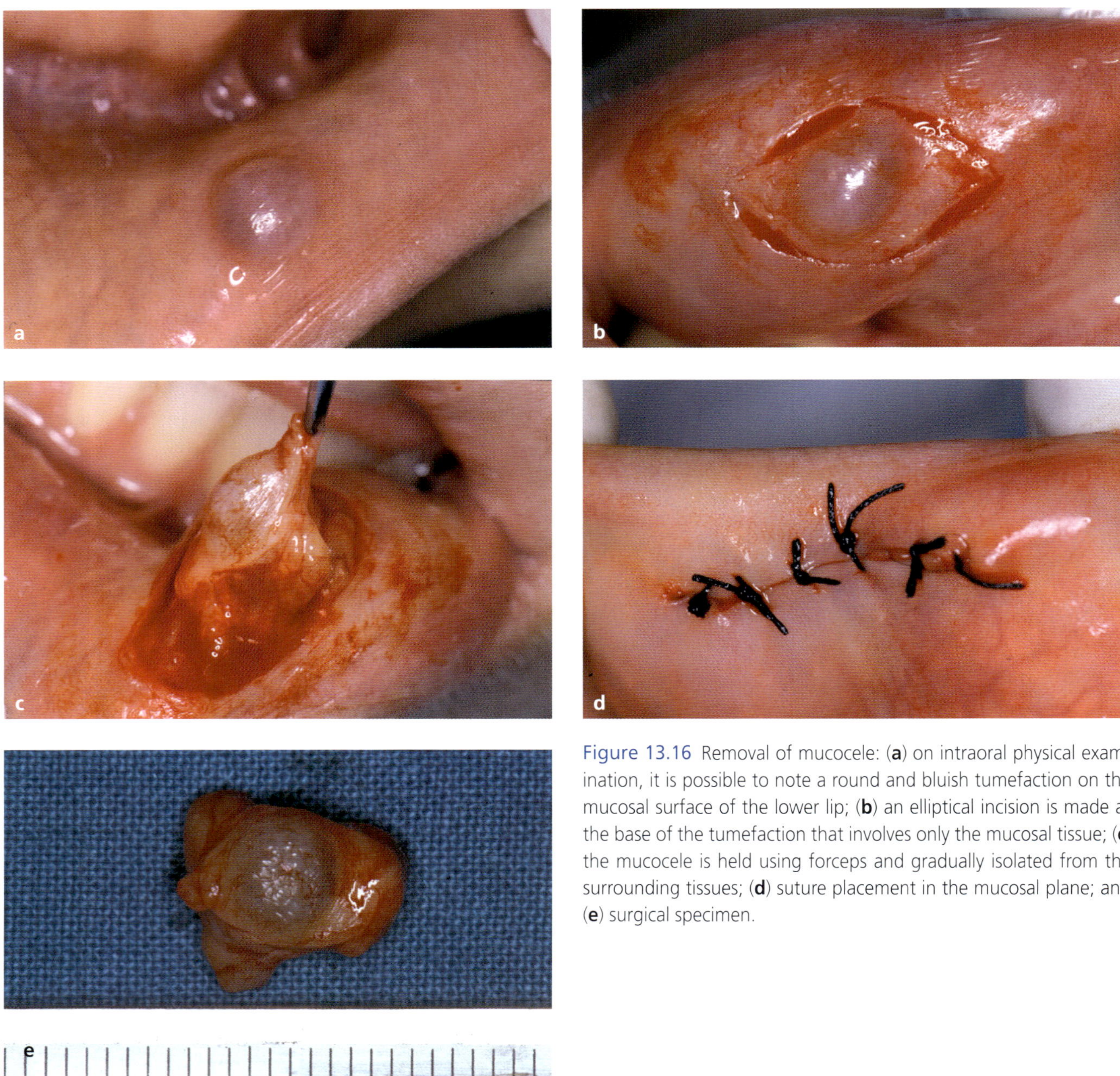

Figure 13.16 Removal of mucocele: (**a**) on intraoral physical examination, it is possible to note a round and bluish tumefaction on the mucosal surface of the lower lip; (**b**) an elliptical incision is made at the base of the tumefaction that involves only the mucosal tissue; (**c**) the mucocele is held using forceps and gradually isolated from the surrounding tissues; (**d**) suture placement in the mucosal plane; and (**e**) surgical specimen.

The technique requires simultaneous removal of the superficial portion of the neoformation and of the overlying mucosa after incising them on the periphery to remove a full-thickness, circular segment; the elimination of the mucous content; suturing the margins of the lower ranula wall to the surrounding oral mucosa using resorbable materials; and filling of the cavity with iodoform gauze, kept in place by sutures, which helps avoid the early opening of the surgical wound as well as the occurrence of relapses (Fig. 13.17).

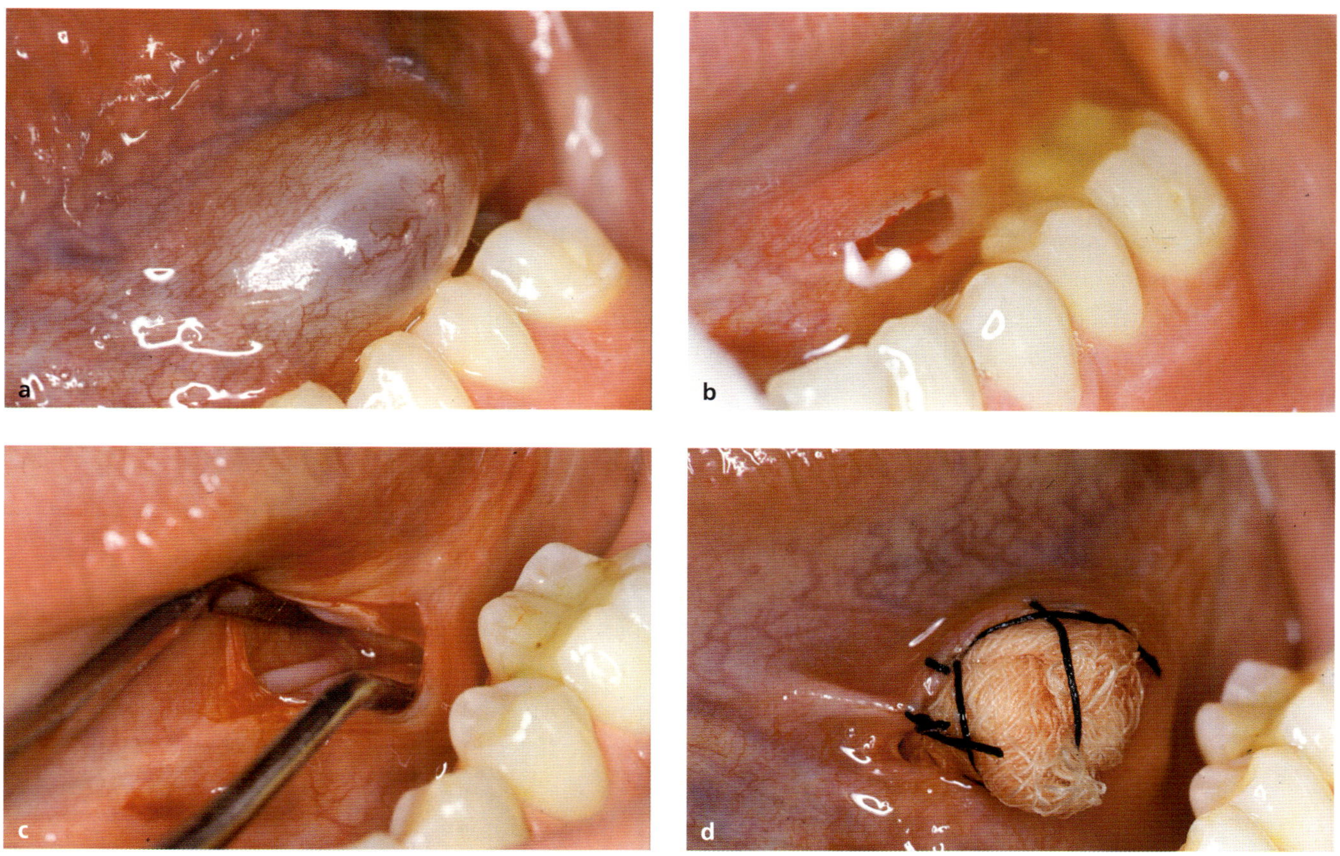

Figure 13.17 Marsupialization of ranula: (**a**) intraoral physical examination shows an oval tumefaction, covered by a mucosa of normal appearance and color, located on the oral floor on the left side; (**b**) making an incision on the ranula roof allows content leakage; (**c**) cavity opening; and (**d**) after suturing the margins of the lower ranula wall to the surrounding oral mucosa, a gauze pad is applied and kept in situ with sutures.

Odontogenic inflammations

Odontogenic inflammations are infectious processes of endodontic, periodontal, or pericoronal origin that might diffuse to the bone structure, soft tissues of the oral cavity, or skin of the face and neck. This term refers to the clinical pictures represented by periapical periodontitis, abscess, and phlegmon.
In pediatric patients, inflammation usually starts with the bacterial colonization of the periapical region after pulp necrosis caused by a carious lesion or trauma to the tooth. The subsequent developments depend on the virulence of the causative pathogenic microorganisms and the immune defenses of the host.
In the presence of a low and scarcely virulent bacterial load and inadequate immune defenses, the infection acquires a chronic course, with the appearance of apical granulomas, whose treatment requires endodontic therapy or the extraction of the concerned tooth. On the other hand, in the presence of a high and strongly virulent bacterial load associated with a poor host defense, inflammation turns into an abscess and a phlegmon. In an abscess, the purulent material is collected in a pathological cavity (bony, submucosal, or subcutaneous cavity) that is formed at the detriment of the adjacent destroyed or detached tissues and is delimited by a fibrous capsule; in a phlegmon, the collection of exudate is not delimited by reactive fibrous tissues, and therefore, it spreads in the superficial or deep connective tissues interposed among the teeth.

Diagnosis

Medical history has great importance in the diagnosis of odontogenic inflammations; in addition to identifying the patient's symptoms, as well as the time and modality of onset, it should help identify any previous use of antibiotics and the presence of systemic pathologies, which might influence the course of infection. Clinical examination has the purpose of highlighting a floating tumefaction with the presence of a liquefied abscess or a hard tumefaction in case of a phlegmon, as well as identifying the dental element responsible for the infective process.
For radiographic investigation, intraoral periapical radiography, panoramic X-ray, computed tomography, or magnetic resonance imaging can be used, depending on the inflammation extent, to confirm the diagnosis and origin of the infection.

Therapy

The therapeutic approach, which depends on the local and systemic clinical conditions, is divided into three phases:
- etiological phase
- surgical phase
- pharmacological phase.

Etiological phase. It is aimed at eliminating the cause of inflammation and requires extraction or endodontic treatment of the infected tooth.

Surgical therapy. It involves drainage of the exudate, which, in subperiosteal abscesses, occurs through the postextraction alveolus or the root canal; in submucosal or subcutaneous abscesses, it precedes the etiological phase and is performed by incising the covering of the purulent collection. Drainage might not be indicated for phlegmons, in which there is usually no delimited pus collection (Fig. 13.18).

The evacuation of an abscess requires administration of **anesthesia**, making an incision, deepening the abscess, and eventually drainage of the abscess. Regarding anesthesia, local approach at the level of the infected area is contraindicated; thus, surgeons prefer using truncal or refrigeration anesthesia, if possible, which turns out to be effective in the most superficial tissues, despite its short duration.

The **incision** is performed on the most declivous area, to promote exudate drainage, using a scalpel blade with a direct upward motion and without going too deep.

Deepening is performed through blunt dissection, inserting closed hemostatic forceps into the cavity, which subsequently is opened and pushed in all directions to facilitate the evacuation of the purulent material.

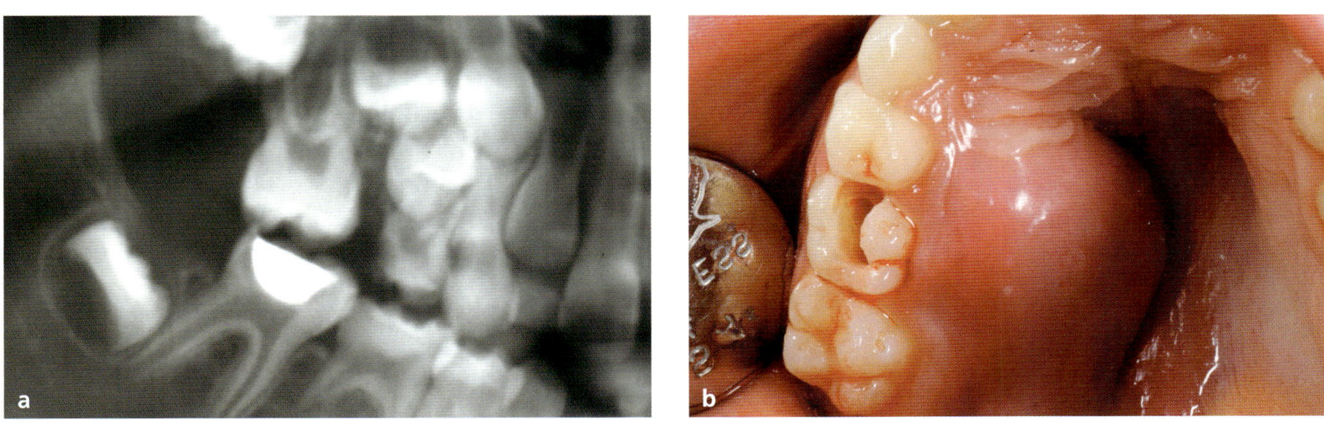

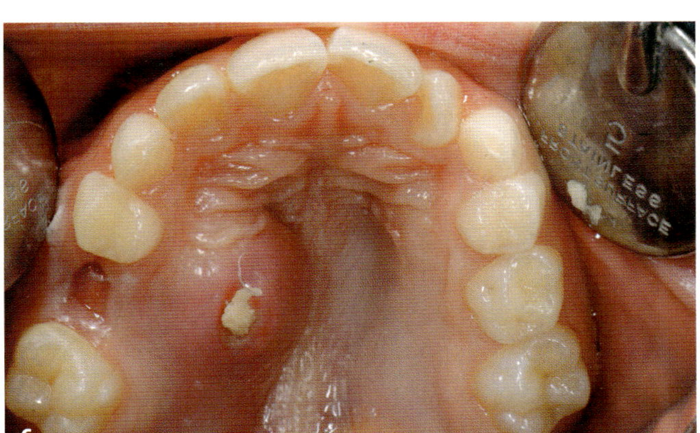

Figure 13.18 Drainage of a palatal abscess: (**a**) details of the panoramic X-ray show destructive caries in 8.5; (**b**) on intraoral physical examination, it is possible to note massive abscess collection on the right hemipalate due to the necrosis of 8.5, and the covering of the abscess has not allowed drainage through the root canal; and (**c**) after the incision of the abscess, drainage performed using iodoform gauze, followed by the extraction of 8.5, and it is now possible to note a progressive reduction in the healing tumefaction.

Drainage involves filling the cavity with iodoform gauze, which is replaced every other day, and serves to maintain the patency of the opening until acute inflammation is resolved.

Pharmacological therapy. It requires the following: (1) broad-spectrum antibiotics or, in the most severe cases, antibiotics selected on the basis of antibiograms; (2) nonsteroidal antiinflammatory drugs, such as antiedemics; (3) fibrinolytic drugs to speed up the healing process; and (4) muscle relaxants in case trismus is present.
In particular, antibiotic therapy is not indicated for all inflammations but indicated only in cases of a widespread and rapidly progressive infection, where it is not possible to perform surgical drainage or timely elimination of etiological factors, or simply in immunocompromised patients.

References

Annibali S, Pippi R. Semeiotica fisica odontostomatologica. Roma: Antonio Delfino Editore; 2002.

Annibali S, Pippi R, Sfasciotti GL. Chirurgia orale a scopo ortodontico. Milano: Elsevier Masson; 2007.

Chiapasco M et al. Manuale illustrato di chirurgia orale. 2a ed. Milano: Masson; 2006.

Covani U, Ferrini F. Chirurgia orale. Bologna: Martina; 2005.

Di Lauro F, Bucci E. Chirurgia odontostomatologica. Napoli: Florio edizioni scientifiche; 2000.

Kramer IRH, Pindborg JJ, Shear M. Histological typing of odontogenic tumours. 2a ed. Geneva: World Health Organization; 1992.

Santoro F, Maiorana C. Chirurgia speciale odontostomatologica. Milano: Masson; 1998.

Chapter 14

Orthodontic prevention

E. BARBATO, P. COZZA, C. CHIMENTI

The maxillary and mandibular bone bases, the dentoalveolar arches, the neuromuscular system, and the temporomandibular joints constitute the stomatognathic apparatus, a complex multifunctional system that plays a decisive role in functions such as swallowing, breathing, phonation, and chewing, which are essential for the life of an individual. In the presence of eugnathic skeletal growth, normal neuromuscular structure, and physiological development of dentition, the dental–maxillofacial relationship is harmoniously developed. Harmful factors can alter the normal evolutionary process of such a complex system with the establishment of malocclusions (Barbato and Leonardi, 2007).

Principles of prevention

Epidemiological studies have shown the role of genetic, environmental, and behavioral factors in the *etiopathogenesis* of malocclusions. The effects of various concurrent adverse factors on occlusion are greater than the sum of the effects of the individual factors, with implications on the severity and features of the malocclusion. However, in the absence of known factors, the occurrence of dysgnathia cannot be excluded.

To examine the various roles played by genetic and environmental factors, a distinction needs to be made between clinical conditions in which genetic influences play a predominant role and those in which environmental influences play a predominant role (Profitt and Fields, 2008). For malocclusions caused by genetic factors, preventive approaches are generally oriented toward early diagnosis and therapy, which, although not always decisive, can influence prognosis, for example, class III syndrome (Fig. 14.1). Environmental factors must be promptly eliminated to prevent their effects on occlusion in the absence of additional conditions that affect the normal growth process. Finger sucking, for example, can contribute as a hereditary component to a class II clinical condition, although it is difficult to assess the individual effects separately. The elimination of the bad habit does not always determine the resolution of dysgnathia, which is attributable to the hereditary component (Fig. 14.2) (Bishara, 2001; Profitt and Fields, 2008).

Considering occlusion as a dynamic process that continuously evolves, relapse might occur if the genetic or environmental factors responsible for dysgnathia continue to adversely affect the physiological development of the maxillary bases, even after an initial intervention.

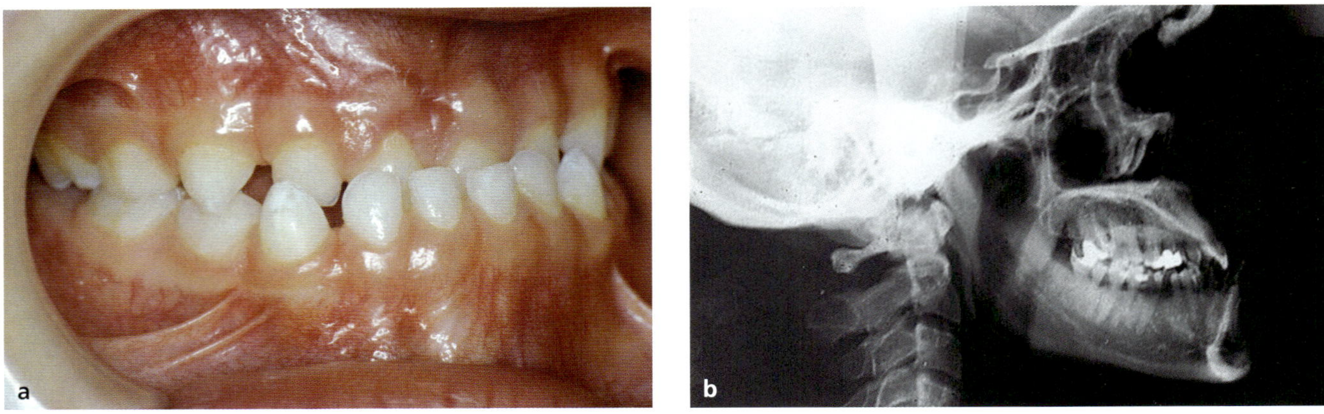

Figure 14.1 A.L., 5-year-old girl, deciduous dentition. Class III (**a**). Familiarity of this malocclusion confirmed on her father's dental x-ray of the skull in the lateral–lateral projection of the father (**b**). Early and timely intervention, although not always conclusive, can affect the prognosis, which remains guarded.

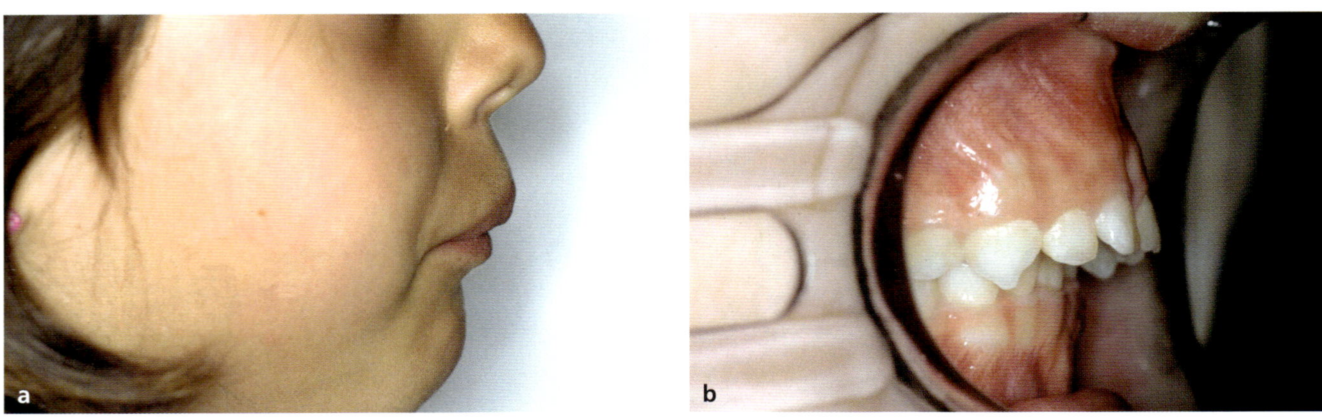

Figure 14.2 (**a**,**b**) L.D., 5-year-old girl, deciduous dentition. Class II malocclusion with maxillary protrusion aggravated by finger sucking. The elimination of the bad habit might not determine the resolution of the dysgnathia, which is attributable to the hereditary component.

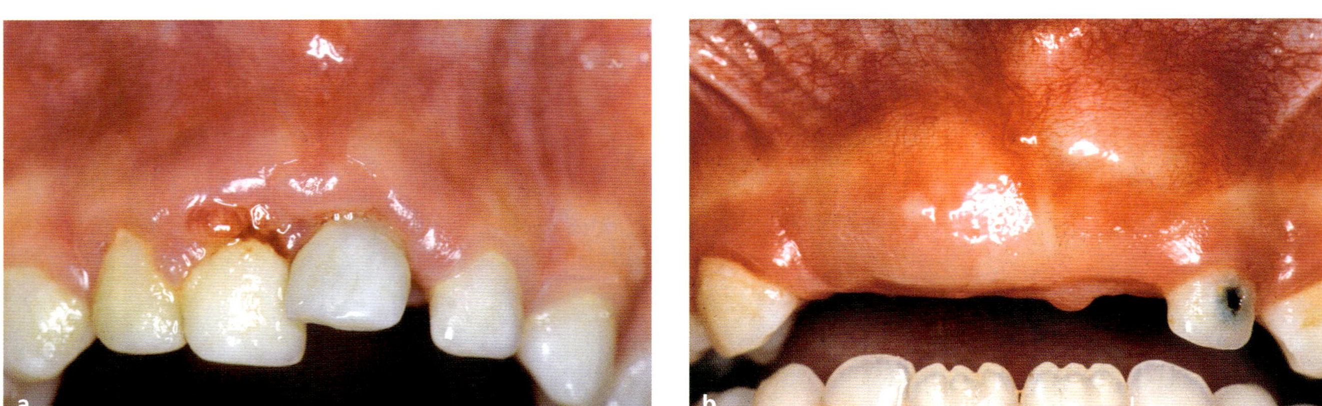

Figure 14.3 A traumatic event on the upper deciduous incisors may involve avulsion, dislocation, or possible inflammatory events (**a**,**b**). The permanent tooth bud may experience dislocation with subsequent retention and/or inclusion or ectopic eruption with orthodontic and mucogingival implications (**c–f**). A delay or failure to erupt can also result in implications in the lateral posterior regions with the mesialization of the entire homolateral hemiarch to the noneroded incisor, with the establishment of asymmetric occlusal relationships (**g**,**h**). Such a traumatic event may have mandibular implications, with repercussions for its physiological development and possible condylar fractures, which occasionally are not promptly diagnosed, and/or a potential risk of asymmetric growth (*continued*).

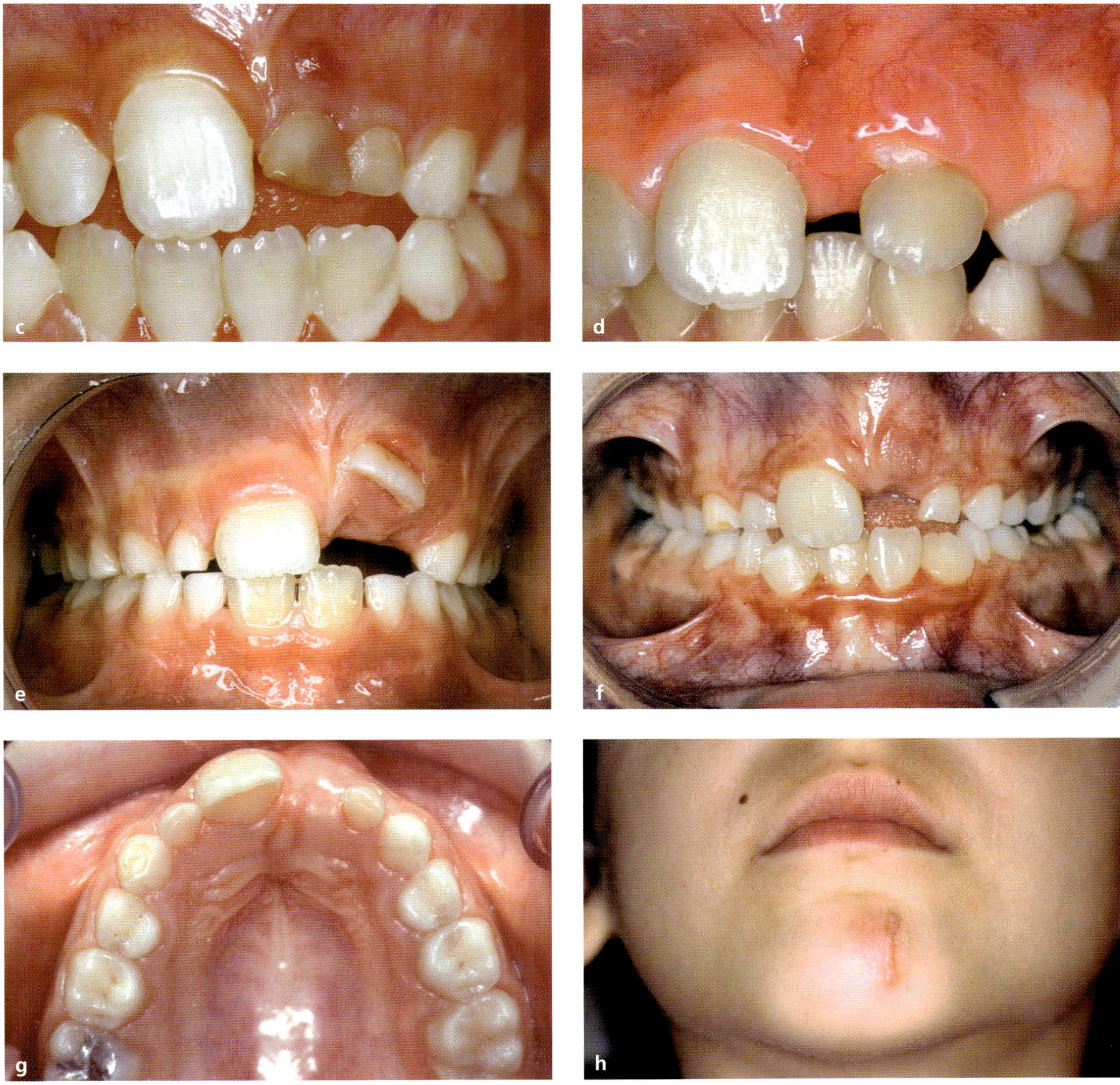

Figure 14.3 – Continued from previous page.

Primary prevention

Primary prevention is identified as the adoption of interventions aimed at avoiding the onset and development of malocclusions, avoiding risk factors, and promoting the physiological growth of the dental–maxillofacial complex (Fig. 14.3); in particular, the following interventions should be noted:

- early dental examinations aimed at preventing dental caries and monitoring oral hygiene and tooth and gum condition

- medical history (past pathological events, familiarity with orthodontic issues such as class III malocclusion, inclusions, and agenesis)
- periodic evaluation of the overall dental–maxillofacial structure, including monitoring of dentition change and growth
- control of dietary and behavioral habits and main functions of the stomatognathic apparatus, with the elimination of *bad habits*
- monitoring of auxological development
- prevention of traumatic events and monitoring of the possible consequences of traumatic events on the overall dental–maxillofacial structure.

Secondary prevention

Secondary prevention involves early detection of malocclusions, with the possibility of intervention, without, however, being able to avoid or reduce the occurrence but being able to avoid the progression of an initial abnormality to a more severe clinical condition. *Secondary prevention* is used in combination with interceptive therapy for the common purposes of "*identifying, evaluating, controlling, or neutralizing etiological or risk factors responsible for the initial malocclusion*." However, there is a thin line between primary and secondary prevention; *interceptive preventive orthodontics* consists of "*a set of preventive and corrective measures, procedures, and techniques designed to prevent a given causal event from causing a malocclusion or limit its effects on normal craniofacial growth*" (American Association of Orthodontists, 1971).

Evaluation of the occlusal disposition already present in the deciduous dentition allows identification of clinical conditions that could evolve into malocclusion of the teeth in the mixed and permanent dentition and requires targeted therapeutic strategies that, although not always decisive, can influence the growth process, thereby improving occlusal relationships and avoiding development into more serious forms. Additionally, clinical parameters such as diastemas and the absence of crowding in the deciduous dentition are not considered indicative of a physiological evolution of the arches in the mixed and/or permanent dentition; the absence of diastemas and the presence of crowding, on the other hand, are unfavorable prognostic indicators of a potential problem of crowding (Barbato and Leonardi, 2007).

An example of secondary prevention is panoramic x-ray, an investigative tool that is able to monitor the growth, development modalities, and development times of dentition and arches, as well as identify the actual or suspected predisposing conditions at an early stage, which particularly impose a risk to the development of normal occlusion (Fig. 14.4 and 14.5) (Barbato et al; 1999; King and Brudvik, 2010).

Tertiary prevention

Tertiary prevention involves the treatment of the outcomes and complications of malocclusion, of established and stable clinical conditions for which a corrective orthodontic

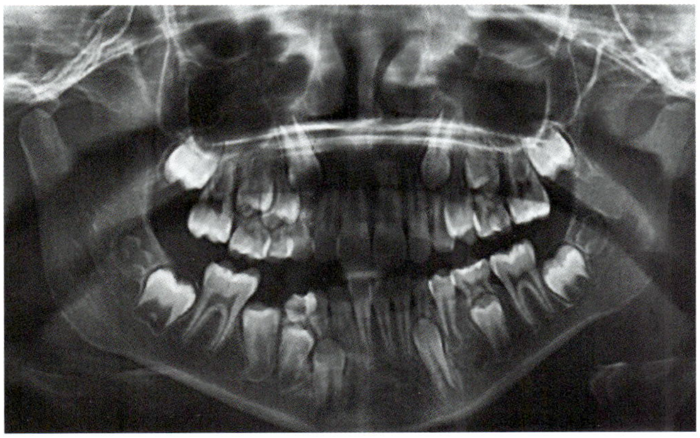

Figure 14.4 G.S., 7-year-old girl, panoramic x-ray, late mixed dentition. In addition to the absence of 8.5 because of early extraction due to for a carious lesion, it is possible to note a mandibular asymmetry with a separate development of the ascending branches.

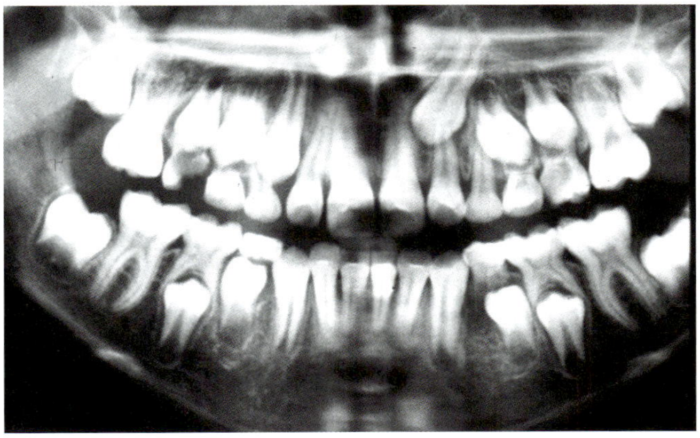

Figure 14.5 B.D., 9-year-old girl, panoramic x-ray, late mixed dentition. Altered position of 2.3 compared with those of 1.3 and 2.2; early sign of inclusion in a subject with positive familiarity to upper canine inclusion. Carious lesions noted in 5.5 and 6.5.

approach is required, or of cases in which the presence of maxillofacial discrepancies that are unresolved or unresolvable using common orthodontic–orthopedic procedures require a combined surgical–orthodontic approach as the only solution.

Functional issues

The dental arches develop within a *muscular corridor* comprising intra- and extra-oral muscles: a harmonious development of the arches is an expression of the balance between these components. The duration of the strength exerted by the muscles (*lips, cheeks, and tongue*) on the dental arches and on the maxillary bases is more relevant than its intensity in terms of the ensuing biological response (Engelke et al, 2011; Profitt and Fields, 2008).

Functional implications in malocclusions are primarily related to forces/pressures exerted during physiological activity. Variations of the occlusal balance are attributed neither to *masticatory forces* (which generate strong and intermittent pressures) nor to forces the exerted by the *lips*, *cheeks*, and tongue during *swallowing and phonation* (which exert slight and intermittent pressures) but to prolonged pressures over a period of time, such as the forces exerted by the resting *lips, cheeks, and tongue* and external forces due to *bad habits* or *orthodontic appliances*. Functional alterations, such as those caused by bad habits and breathing patterns, in modifying the balance between the intrinsic and extrinsic muscles can, therefore, determine and/or contribute to malocclusion. If a bad habit such as finger sucking causes prolonged pressure of more than a threshold value of 6 hours a day on the dental elements, it can have an effect at the dental level; however, it appears that forces of shorter durations do not produce any effect regardless of their intensity (Profitt and Fields, 2008).

Finger sucking

Finger sucking, considered a *transitional phenomenon*, is a primary habit acquired in the prenatal period. It is considered an expression of normal behavior up to 2 years of age (Bishara et al, 2006; Cozza, 2007).
The effects of finger sucking on the stomatognathic apparatus are related to various factors, including *duration, intensity, and frequency* (Gois et al, 2008; Montaldo et al, 2011). With the persistence of the sucking habit, the risk of malocclusion increases after 4 years of age; if it is prolonged up to 6 years of age, even though only occasionally, such a habit would not cause visible anomalies, which would resolve spontaneously. However, a duration exceeding the *threshold* would play a decisive role in the effects on arches. In terms of frequency, finger sucking can be intermittent or continuous; the presence of the finger in the oral cavity can be passive, without the participation of the perioral muscles, or active, when the contraction of the labial and buccinator muscles is detectable.

Diagnosis. The evaluation of medical history, intra- and extra-oral clinical features, and cephalometric parameters contribute to the diagnostic framework. Some clinical signs are pathognomonic of functional alteration (Fig. 14.6) (Cozza et al, 2005; Levrini et al, 1999; Melink et al, 2010; Montaldo et al, 2011; Warren and Bishara, 2002):

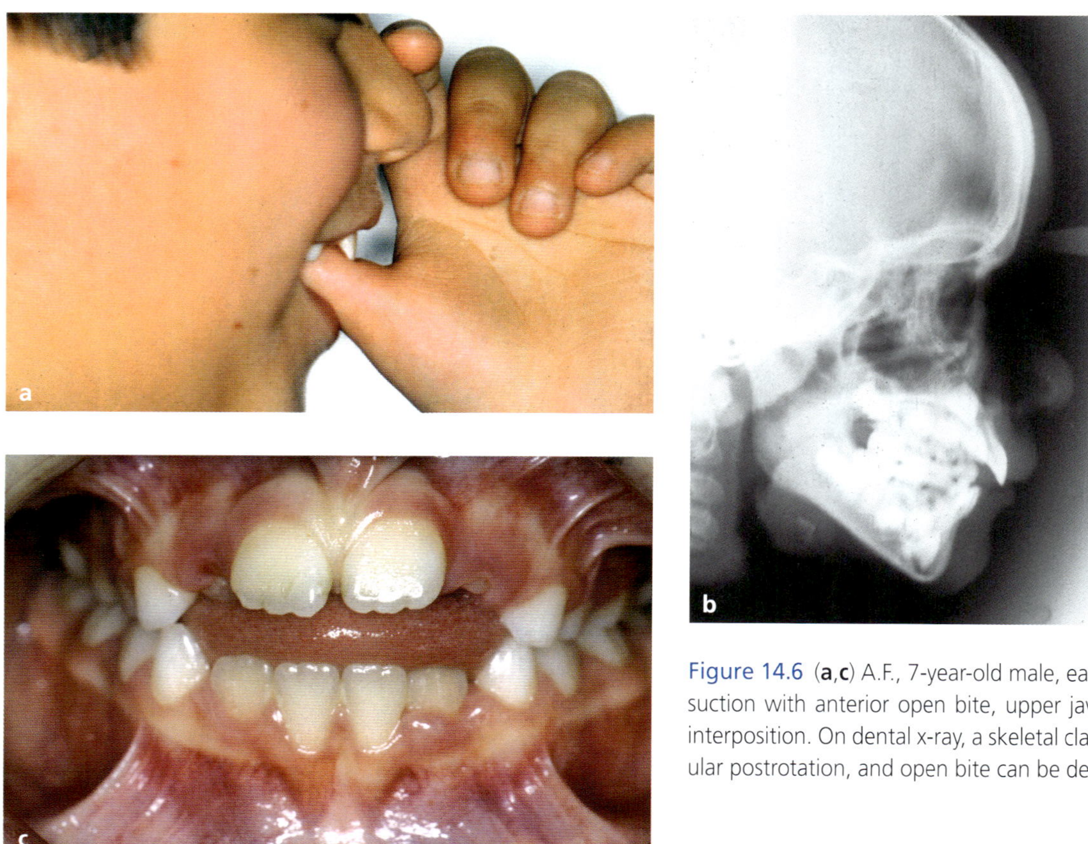

Figure 14.6 (**a**,**c**) A.F., 7-year-old male, early mixed dentition. Finger suction with anterior open bite, upper jaw contraction and lingual interposition. On dental x-ray, a skeletal class II malocclusion mandibular postrotation, and open bite can be detected.

- *open dentoalveolar bite* and expression of unfavorable factors: force exerted by the finger on the palate during sucking with the proclination and protrusion of the upper incisors and increase in overjet, reduced alveolar growth in the anterior region, and extrusion of the posterior teeth due to the absence of occlusal contact when the finger is inside the oral cavity
- *hypo-development*, *retrusion*, and mandibular *postrotation*
- *upper maxillary bone contraction* caused by the synergistic effect of the perioral muscles during finger sucking and, at the same time, the loss of the centrifugal growth function of the lingual muscles on the upper jaw because of the presence of the finger.

Keratin formation and morphological alterations of the finger involved in the sucking may occur.

Therapy. As a less harmful alternative to the finger, the use of a soother is sometimes recommended because it is used for less time and is not always available to the child. Interventions aimed at the removal of the bad habit, supported by positive behavioral and induced behavioral techniques, are also suggested to avoid side effects and additional habits resulting from deprivation, such as motivating and flattering the child when he/she does not suck the finger. Fixed and/or removable intraoral appliances equipped with structural elements that prevent finger sucking, e.g., grids, may occasionally be associated with additional orthodontic appliances to intercept the initial alterations induced by sucking and/or to control the effects of the application of these orthodontic appliances considering the overall dental–maxillofacial structure (Bishara, 2001; Levrini et al, 1999; Profitt and Fields, 2008).

Changes in respiratory function

Oral respiration is a pathophysiological condition characterized by the passage of the air mainly through the oropharyngeal channel rather than through the nasopharyngeal channel.

It is possible to distinguish *compulsory oral respiration* caused by the presence of an oral–rhino–pharyngeal obstruction that prevents or limits nasal respiration (e.g., adenoid or pharyngeal tonsil hypertrophy) from *usual oral respiration* (a bad habit) a real *habit* of oral respiration (in the absence of a mechanical impediment) owing to a previous respiratory pathology responsible for the acquired habit.

Diagnosis. Anamnestic, otorhinolaryngological, and orthodontic evaluations contribute to the overall diagnostic framework.

An early detection of respiratory complications with the possible aid of instrumental investigations and the identification of possible obstructive results in the establishment of the preliminary multidisciplinary diagnostic framework and in the restoration of proper respiratory function. Some intra- and extra-oral clinical features and cephalometric parameters are pathognomonic of the functional alteration (Fig. 14.7). The dolichofacial type is characteristic, with an increase in the length of the face, periocular venous stasis, labial incompetence, hypotonia of the upper lip, and *adenoid facies*. In addition, an altered cephalic posture can cause alterations in the craniofacial morphology and reduction in the nasopharyngeal space. Furthermore, it is possible to identify the tendency of anterior open bite due to a lack of contact between the dental arches with extrusion of the rear teeth; increase in the anterior facial height and post-

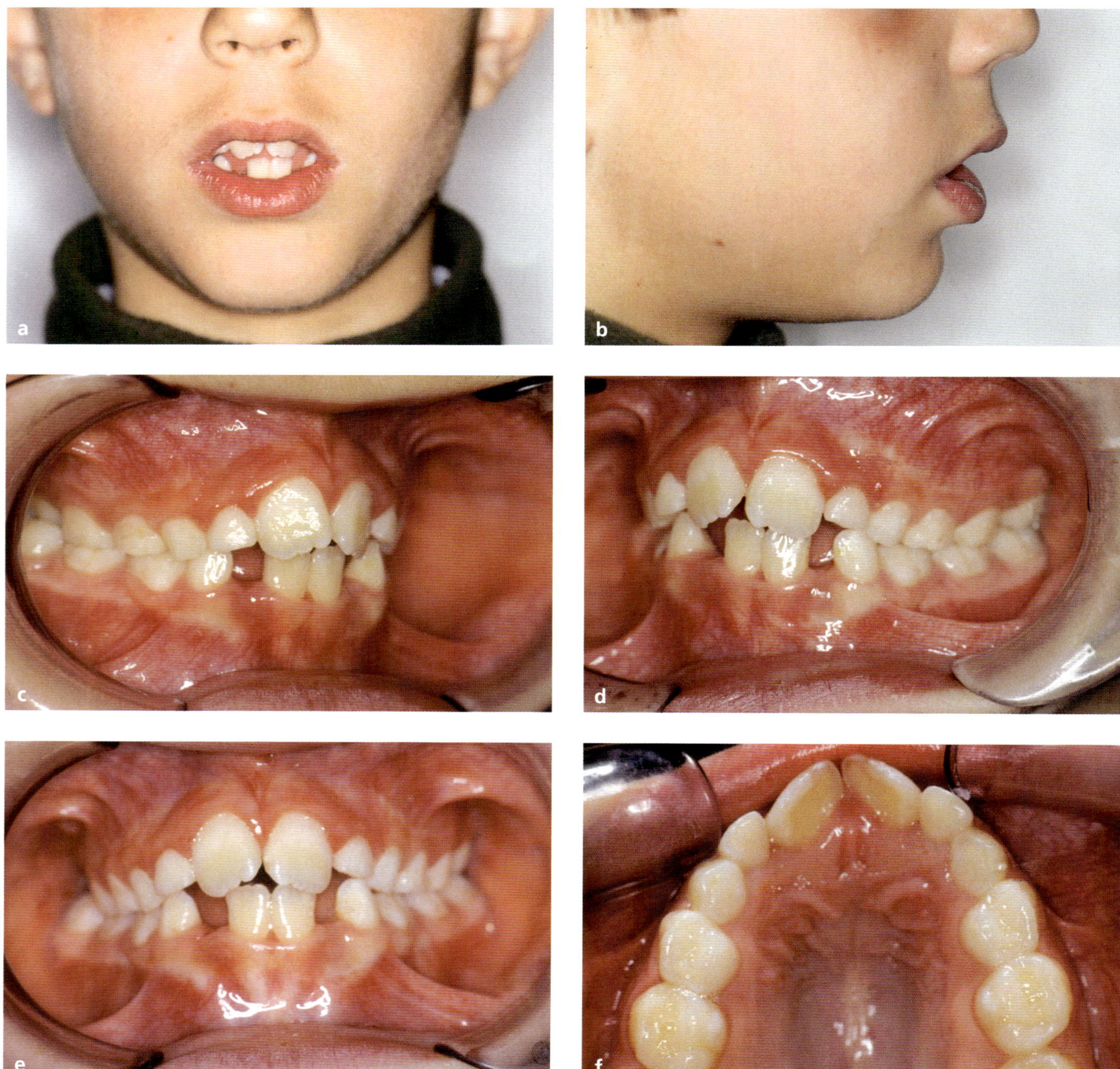

Figure 14.7 (**a**,**f**) A.P., 7-year-old boy, early mixed dentition. Oral breather, dolichofacial type, labial incompetence, convex profile. Class II molar, upper arch contracted, lower lingual posture.

mandibular rotation; *transverse hypoplasia of the maxillary arch with possible crossbite*, which is caused by alterations in the balance between intra- and extra-oral muscles; and stretching of the perioral musculature, which is a result of the various postures acquired to favor a respiratory space useful to guarantee a greater intake of air, with the loss of the incremental centrifugal *input* on the upper jaw due to the tongue placed in a lower position. In this context, a secondary atypical swallowing framework may be established.
Clinical examination may be supported by functional tests i.e., Rosenthal's, Gudin's, and Quinn's tests and Glatzel mirror test.

Therapy. The distinction between compulsory oral breathing and *usual oral breathing* is marked. Functional re-education can support the overall therapeutic approach, initially consciously, with breathing and swallowing exercises, and then transfer what is learned to the unconscious level. Orthodontic surgery involves the use of appliances to correct dental–maxillary–facial alterations after solving the functional problem to prevent possible relapses. The elective therapy is expansion, with appliances for slow or rapid expansion of the palate, to solve the transversal problem; the use of orthopedic appliances can be indicated to control the vertical component and intervene the sagittal implications.

Changes in swallowing function

The *swallowing* function changes in various stages of life (Cozza, 2007; Landouzy et al., 2009).
By the fourth month of intrauterine life, the tongue assumes a position similar to that of an infant during lactation, i.e., between the gum pads of the two arches. In infants, sucking milk requires the simultaneous involvement of the lingual and perioral muscular structures to promote the anterior seal; lifting the jaw supports the lingual action in promoting the sucking of milk that is directed posteriorly so as to be swallowed.
The transition to adult swallowing is gradual and is characterized by movements attributable to both infantile and adult patterns. This transitional evolutionary phase should coincide with the eruption of the deciduous incisors, which hinder the protrusion of the tongue between the arches; their eruption occurs at approximately 18–20 months, with the persistence of a swallowing pattern that is partially still infantile, which is considered physiological even in subsequent ages, up to 5–7 years. Weaning, dentition status, and neuromuscular maturation determine the transition from the infantile to the adult model, which is characterized by posterior lingual displacement, absence of anterior lingual thrust, presence of occlusal contact, and absence of participation of the perioral and genial muscles.
Swallowing is characterized by different phases (oral, pharyngeal, and esophageal) and is preceded by a phase of preparation for food intake, which can be swallowed if it has an adequate texture. The tip of the tongue comes into contact with the retro-incisive papilla and the lateral margins with the palatal surface of the teeth of the posterolateral

regions; the soft palate and the lingual posterior part ensure a rear seal that prevents food from proceeding into the pharynx ahead of time.
Regarding functional changes, *atypical swallowing* comprises the persistence of the infant swallowing pattern beyond the period considered physiological and is characterized by a *lingual thrust* in the anterior or posterior position, either monolaterally or bilaterally; the *perioral muscles*, particularly the lower and mental orbicular muscle, participate in the anterior seal, supporting the tongue in pushing the bolus toward the pharynx. Atypical swallowing can be distinguished as follows:

- primary atypical swallowing (actual atypical swallowing), which is caused by incoordination of muscle synergism or synaptic impulses or an immaturity of nerve centers
- secondary atypical swallowing (lingual interposition), which is subsequent to the presence of *hypertrophic tonsils* and *adenoids*, bad habits (for example, sucking of the finger or soother), and *local anatomical alterations* (macroglossia, short lingual frenulum, etc.); *hereditary factors*; and *protracted artificial lactation* (Cozza, 2007).

In *primary atypical swallowing*, the abnormal thrust of the tongue determines the occlusal morphological alteration; in *secondary atypical swallowing*, the function adapts to the pre-existing occlusal morphological anomaly.

Diagnosis. Clinical and functional evaluations, particularly of the participation of the perioral and masticatory muscle groups, are pivotal for the correct classification of the type of alteration (primary or secondary). There is an open anterior or posterior bite, of mono or bilateral type, depending on the lingual postural alteration, and a vestibular inclination of the dentition due to the predominance of the lingual musculature over the perioral musculature.

Therapy. The resolution of the dysfunction, with the restoration of an adequate lingual function, will support the preventive/interceptive orthodontic intervention to normalize the development and growth and restore the harmonious occlusal relationship.
Myofunctional therapy is the elective treatment aimed at eliminating atypical motor patterns and fixing new engrams, physiological neuromuscular patterns, which will then transform from acts of conscious and voluntary swallowing to habitual and unconscious ones. The most suitable age, also in terms of cooperation, is 7–10 years. The therapeutic cycle, which usually lasts a year, may include two phases of variable duration: *re-education* of the hypotonic muscle function until the restoration of the condition of muscle balance (usually 2–3 months with weekly sessions) and *maintenance* of the achieved results (in the following months, with monthly follow-ups).
Orthodontic surgery may involve the use of fixed and/or removable intraoral appliances equipped with structural elements, which prevent the interposition of the tongue between the arches (for example, grids), and occasionally involves additional orthodontic appliances in order to intercept initial alterations induced by sucking and/or to control the effects of the application of the same orthodontic appliances keeping in mind the overall dental–maxillary–facial structure (Fig. 14.8).

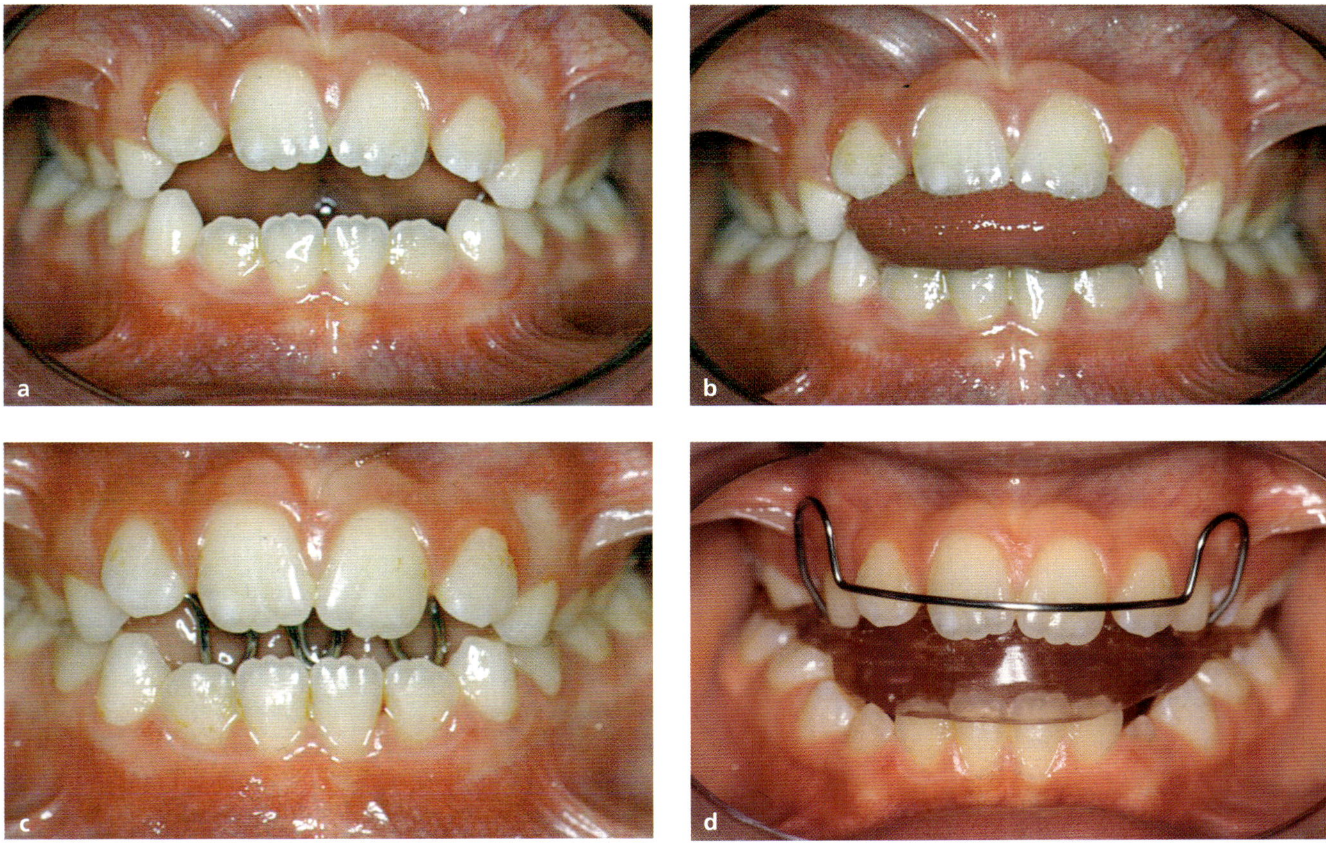

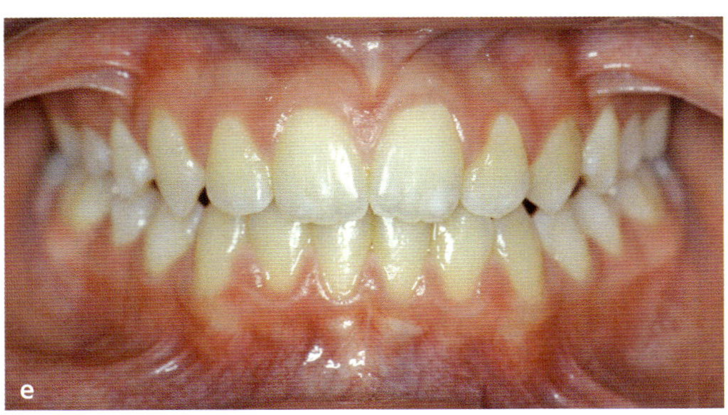

Figure 14.8 (**a**,**e**) F.B., 7-year-old girl. Anterior open bite caused by previous finger sucking and secondary lingual interposition. Functional alterations, language re-education, simultaneous application of a fixed palatal grid and subsequent functional appliance, and exchange monitoring were evaluated for the treatment of the clinical condition.

Interposition of the lower lip

The interposition of the lower lip is characterized by the absence of normal contact between lip fissures and can be classified as primary and secondary:

The primary form is caused by a structural and/or postural imbalance between oblique muscle belts (buccinator and orbicular muscle of the upper and lower lip). A hyperactive chin muscle can exert traction on the lower lip. Neuromuscular dyskinesia can affect skeletal and dental development that is associated with class II/I malocclusion (Frankel and Frankel, 1991).

In secondary interposition, the increased overjet, associated with a class II/I malocclusion, may favor the interposition of the lower lip in the absence of primary neuromuscular dyskinesia.

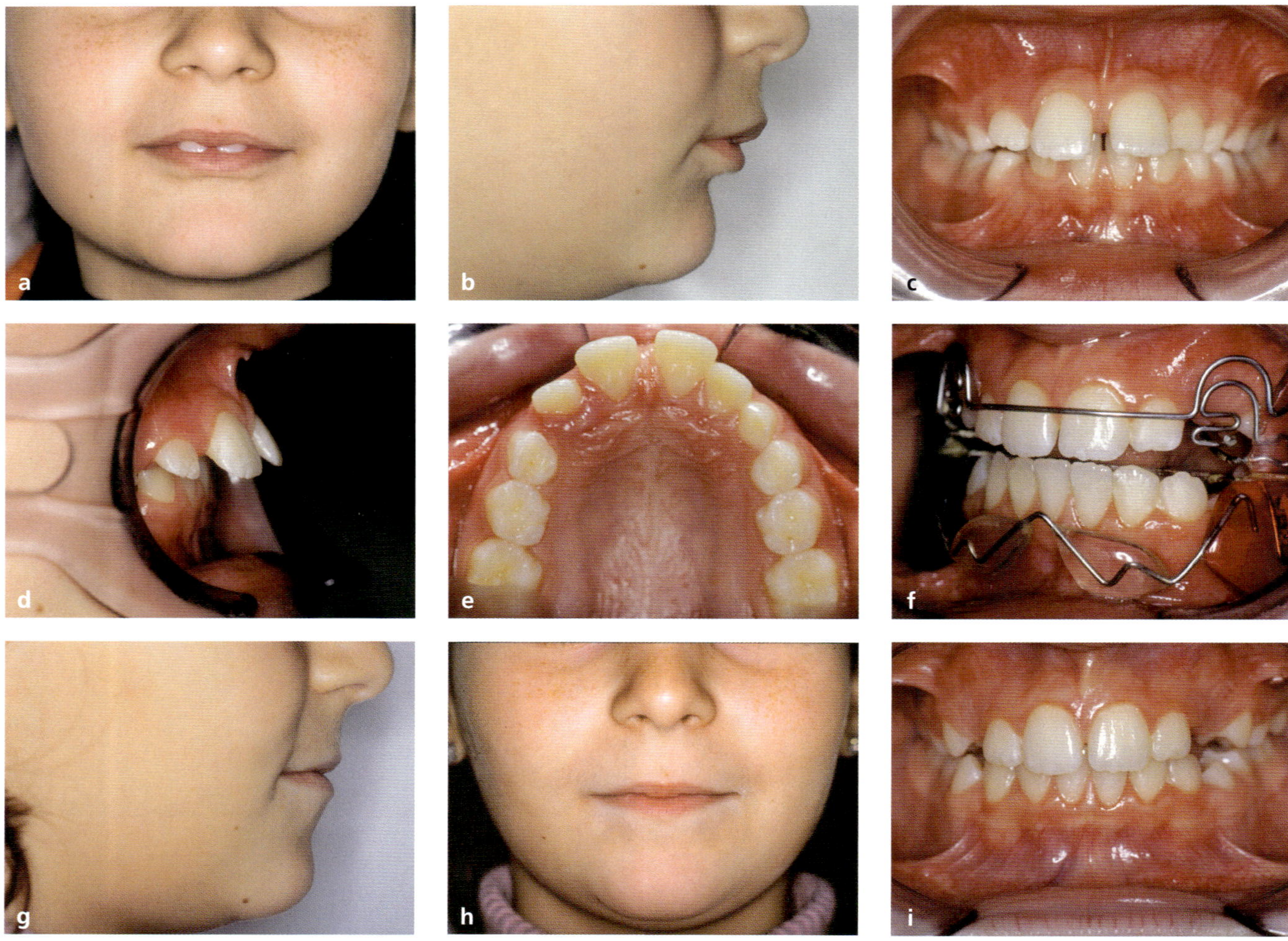

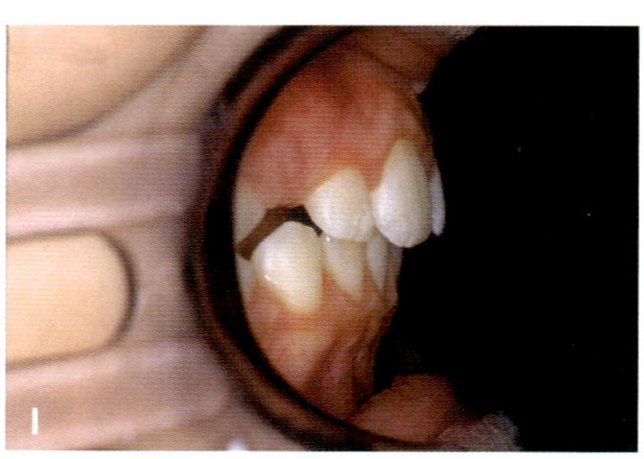

Figure 14.9 (**a**,**l**) S.F., 10-year-old girl, late mixed dentition. Brachyfacial typology, molar class II with mandibular retrusion, increased overjet with interposition of the lower lip; deep bite responsible for trauma of the palatal mucosa due to the incisors. The application of a function regulator (type 2) with a lip shield and a retro-incisive arch for correcting the malocclusion contributes to the resolution of the functional problem.

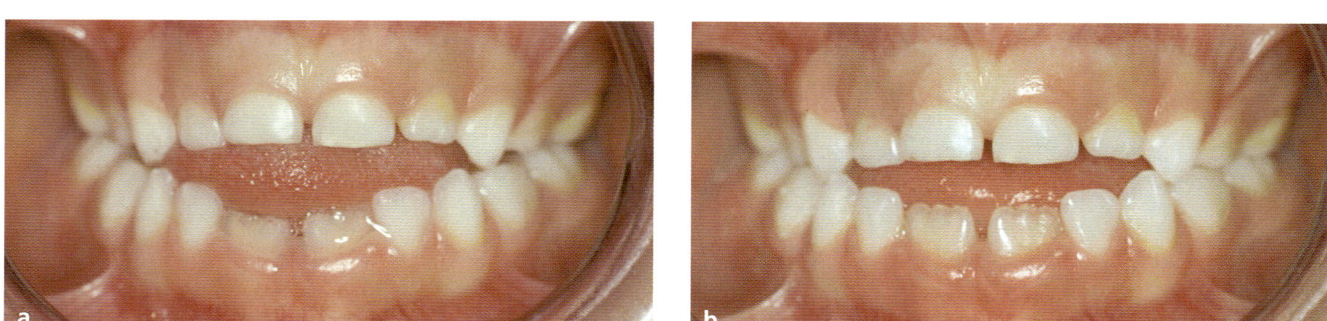

Figure 14.10 (**a**,**b**) V.G., 6-year-old girl, early mixed dentition. Anterior open bite with a class III growth pattern and low lingual posture. Anterior lingual interposition with phonetic implications.

Diagnosis. Functional, clinical, and if necessary, radiographic evaluations help identify the overall complication.

Therapy. Myotherapeutic exercises are indicated for the *primary forms*, with the use of lip buttons, to rebalance the neuromuscular function and establish an appropriate lip seal. For the *secondary forms*, the correction of the dysgnathia allows resolution of the structural cause responsible for the interposition of the lip (Fig. 14.9).

Language disorders

Knowledge of the physiological mechanisms that regulate the articulation of language and the pathological and physiological conditions that can impair or alter this function is decisive in determining the overall structure of the stomatognathic apparatus. Speech disorders can be classified as *phono-articular deficits* (dysarthria, dyslalia, and dysphonia) and *deficits of superior nervous functions* (aphasia, stuttering, and dyslexia). Peripheral phono-articular deficits due to organic causes (congenital or acquired morphological alterations of the structures involved in the oropharyngeal joint) or functional causes (altered coordination of the movements meant for the correct pronunciation of some phonemes) are related to the altered pronunciation of consonant phonemes. Articulation deficits of a greater orthognathodontic relevance include physiological or evolutionary dyslalia, transient phonation forms with altered pronunciation of consonants that occur during tooth development, and the organic or mechanical peripheral forms that occur as a result of anatomical or functional changes in the resonance cavities or speech organs (Barbato et al, 2000).
Based on the region where the altered articulation of the phoneme occurs, speech disorders are classified as *labial articulation deficits* (pronunciation of /p/, /b/, and /m/), which are rather rare and generally result from substance loss due to traumatic or surgical events, e.g., labial cleft and post-treatment scar tissues; *palatal articulation deficits* (decreased resonance of nasal phonemes /m/, /n/, and /gn/); and *dental–alveolar–maxillary articulation deficits*, which often occur due to malocclusion, e.g., open bite and diastemas: sigmatism (pronunciation of the consonant /s/s/) and zetacism (pronunciation of the consonant /z) are the most frequent deficits. *Lingual articulation deficits* are caused by alterations in the shape, volume, mobility, and posture of the tongue and involve modification of the functional patterns.

Diagnosis. Diagnosis is based on clinical and functional evaluation. The potential occlusal alterations are various, with implications in the various planes of the space (open bite, class II, class III, etc.), representing the cause, instead of the effect, of the functional problem (Fig. 14.10).

Therapy. Correction of structural dental and postural complications and functional re-education interventions contribute to the resolution of the phonetic deficit.

Dentition problems

Space management

Space management is a crucial problem in the orthodontic field, which assumes further importance in cases of early exfoliation of a deciduous element due to traumatic events, carious lesions, or crowding (Fig. 14.11). The early extraction of deciduous molars involves a mesial migration of the first permanent molar, with a decrease in the perimeter of the arch, difficult eruption of the permanent elements mesial to the first molar, and alteration of the occlusal relationships (Barbato and Leonardi, 2007; Bishara, 2001; Tunison et al, 2008).

Considering the absence of biological mechanisms intrinsic to the maxillary bases, the intervention must be timely, must be capable of increasing the length of the arch, and must consider the *radicular development of the permanent substitute*, the *distance between the permanent tooth and the alveolar crest*, and the *position of the contiguous teeth in the arch*. The assessment of *available space*, measured from the mesial surface of the first permanent molar on one side of the arch to the first permanent contralateral molar, is instrumental in assessing the possible positioning of all permanent teeth (Bishara, 2001).

In cases of *crowding* in the anterior region, it is important to identify the etiology.

Primary crowding is an expression of structural discrepancy between tooth size and available space; *secondary or symptomatic crowding* usually occurs due to environmental factors such as traumas, decay, avulsions, or early exfoliation; tertiary crowding occurs in the postadolescence period. Crowding can also be distinguished as follows:

- slight (2–3 mm): may undergo spontaneous correction for normal growth
- moderate or medium (4–6 mm): requires intervention aimed at preserving the length of the arch using fixed or mobile orthodontic appliances that are able to prevent the mesialization of the first permanent molars with the contextual possibility to use the *leeway space* until complete eruption of the permanent teeth mesial to the first molar (Fig. 14.12). Dentoalveolar expansion of the maxilla (using a *quad-helix*) can increase the width of the bone base and the perimeter of the arch, which is useful for the alignment of the permanent teeth in the upper arch (Barbato and Leonardi, 2007; Keski-Nisula et al, 2008)
- severe (7–10 mm): in early mixed dentition period, chronologically planned *elective extraction* protocols can be implemented for class I issues, with correct intermaxillary relationships and good neuromuscular balance (Bishara, 2001)
- extreme (>10 mm) (Profitt, 2008).

Some clinical conditions may simulate an excess of arch space due to the proclination and protusion of the incisors and the presence of a midline diastema.

The vestibular version of the incisal group, with the presence of diastemas, can be an expression of a physiological condition, such as "*ugly-duckling*" stage, or of more complex clinical conditions, such as class II/I malocclusion or anterior open bite due to functional alterations, and may be spontaneously resolved with the physiological development of the dental arches in the permanent dentition period or with the treatment of primary malocclusion. Similarly, an inter-incisor midline diastema can resolve physiologically once the canine change is completed in the absence of additional causes, such as the presence of supernumerary teeth (*mesiodens*), agenesis or altered morphology of the lateral incisors, oligodontia, dental–basal discrepancies, or abnormal insertion of the frenulum dentobasal (which requires frenulotomy/frenulectomy).

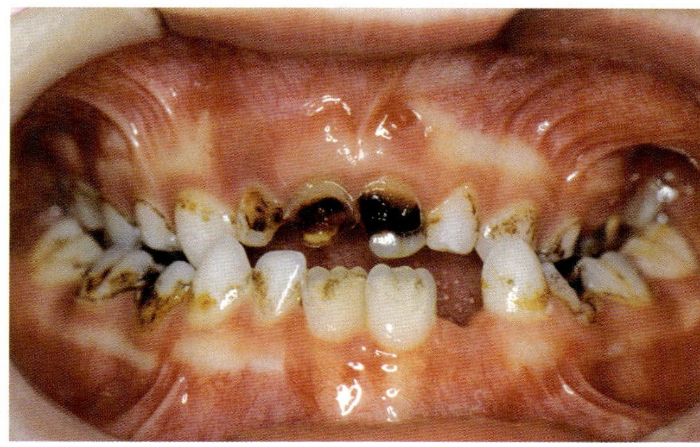

Figure 14.11 A.N., 6.5-year-old boy, early mixed dentition. Class III malocclusion; contraction of the upper sagittal and transverse maxilla. Presence of inflammatory events resulting from multiple carious lesions, which can exacerbate the overall dysgnathic condition, both at the dental (space loss) and skeletal (loss of incisal contacts, slipping, and lack of control of posture and/or mandibular growth levels).

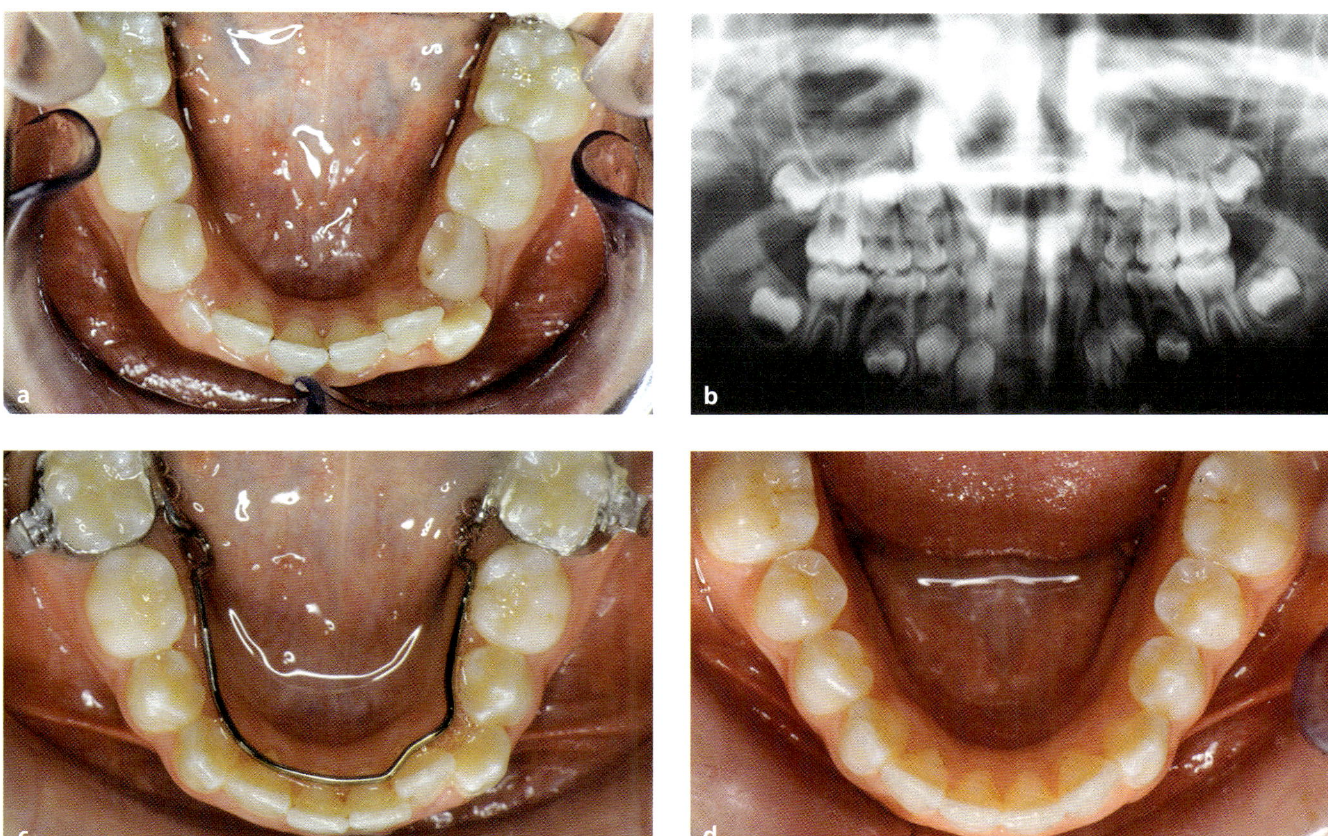

Figure 14.12 (**a–d**) C.A., 7.6-year-old girl. Dentobasal discrepancy previously detectable on panoramic x-ray and confirmed with the eruption of 3.3 in the arch. The application of a fixed space maintainer (lingual arch), exchange monitoring, and management or use of the *leeway space* enable the resolution of the clinical condition.

Infra-occluded or ankylosed teeth

Infra-occlusion usually affects the second deciduous molars, which are at a lower level compared with the occlusal plane and are often in continuity (*ankylosis*) with the surrounding bone. The consequent lack of exfoliation can involve complications related to the eruption of the corresponding permanent tooth, extrusion of the antagonist tooth, mesial inclination of the contiguous permanent molar, and reduction of the alveolar bone size (Fig. 14.13).

In the early mixed dentition period, the reconstruction of the clinical crown of an infra-occluded tooth guarantees a correct sagittal and vertical occlusal relationship. Extraction is indicated in the presence of coronal *tipping* of contiguous teeth and/or risk of dystopia or ectopic eruption of the corresponding permanent tooth. Radiographic monitoring allows determination of the most suitable time for the extraction of the infra-occluded tooth based on the position and radicular development stage of the corresponding permanent tooth.

Transposition of permanent teeth

This is a rare anomaly characterized by the inversion of the position of two contiguous teeth; it can be *complete* if it involves two elements *as a whole* (crown, root, or apex) or *incomplete if* the crowns are transposed but the apices are in their normal position. The most frequent form affects the maxillary canine and the first premolar, followed by the maxillary canine and lateral incisor. Early diagnosis is conclusive and requires targeted and timely clinical interceptive interventions in the mixed dentition period (Fig. 14.14) (Synodinos and Polyzois, 2011).

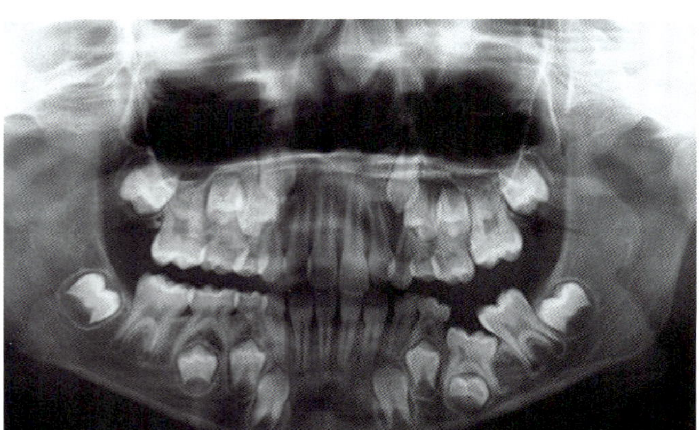

Figure 14.13 M.L., 7.5-year-old female, panoramic x-ray. Early mixed dentition, ankylosis of 7.5 with altered position of 3.5, mesial inclination of 36, distal inclination of 7.4, and extrusion of 6.5.

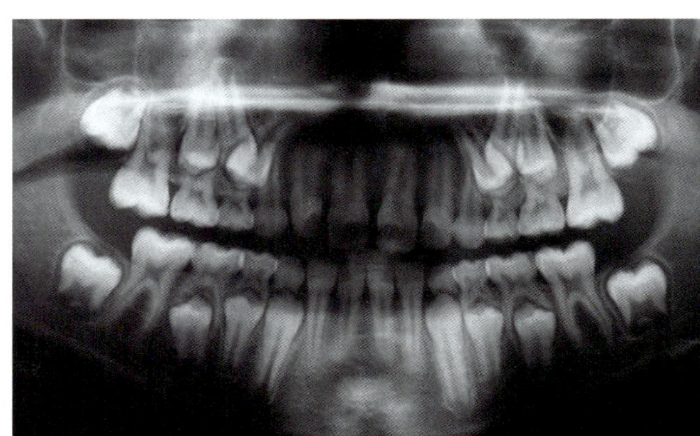

Figure 14.14 L.M., 8.6-year-old girl, panoramic x-ray. Inter-transitional phase of dentition. True full transposition of 1.3 and 1.4 with 2.3 and 2.4.

Dental agenesis

The absence of the buds of dental elements is related to genetic factors and is rarely found in the deciduous dentition; however, if present, agenesis of a deciduous tooth is usually associated with the agenesis of the corresponding permanent tooth. In the permanent dentition, agenesis primarily involves the third molars, maxillary and mandibular lateral incisors, and mandibular and maxillary second premolars. Early diagnosis requires an assessment of the overall dental–maxillofacial arrangement to determine whether to maintain the agenesis space or to proceed to its closure. The agenesis of the second premolar may be associated with the abnormal position of the contralateral tooth the eruptive pattern of which must be carefully monitored. The agenesis of the upper lateral incisor is frequently associated with the inclusion of the adjacent canine.

Supernumerary teeth

Deciduous teeth have a normal or conical shape (*eumorphic or additional*); permanent teeth may have a greater variety of shapes (dysmorphic, conical, etc.). The findings of a supernumerary dysmorphic conical *mesiodens*, usually among the upper central incisors, requires a prompt extraction intervention.

Persistence of deciduous teeth

Deciduous incisors. In case of abnormal eruption of a permanent tooth, usually in the lingual position, timely extraction of the corresponding deciduous tooth not that has yet exfoliated is indicated; the physiological action of the tongue contributes to the correct positioning of the permanent teeth during eruption in the arch. Occasionally, the persistence of the deciduous tooth can be associated with the presence of additional causal factors that hinder the physiological process of tooth exchange (Fig. 14.15).

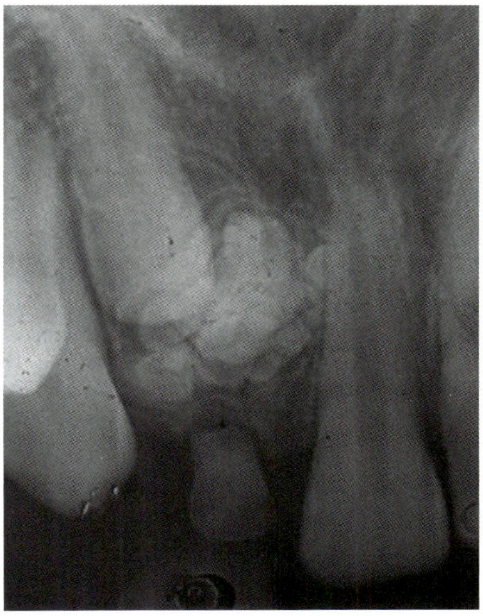

Figure 14.15 D.A., 12-year-old boy, intraoral x-ray. Inclusion of 12 due to the presence of multiple belatedly diagnosed odontomas.

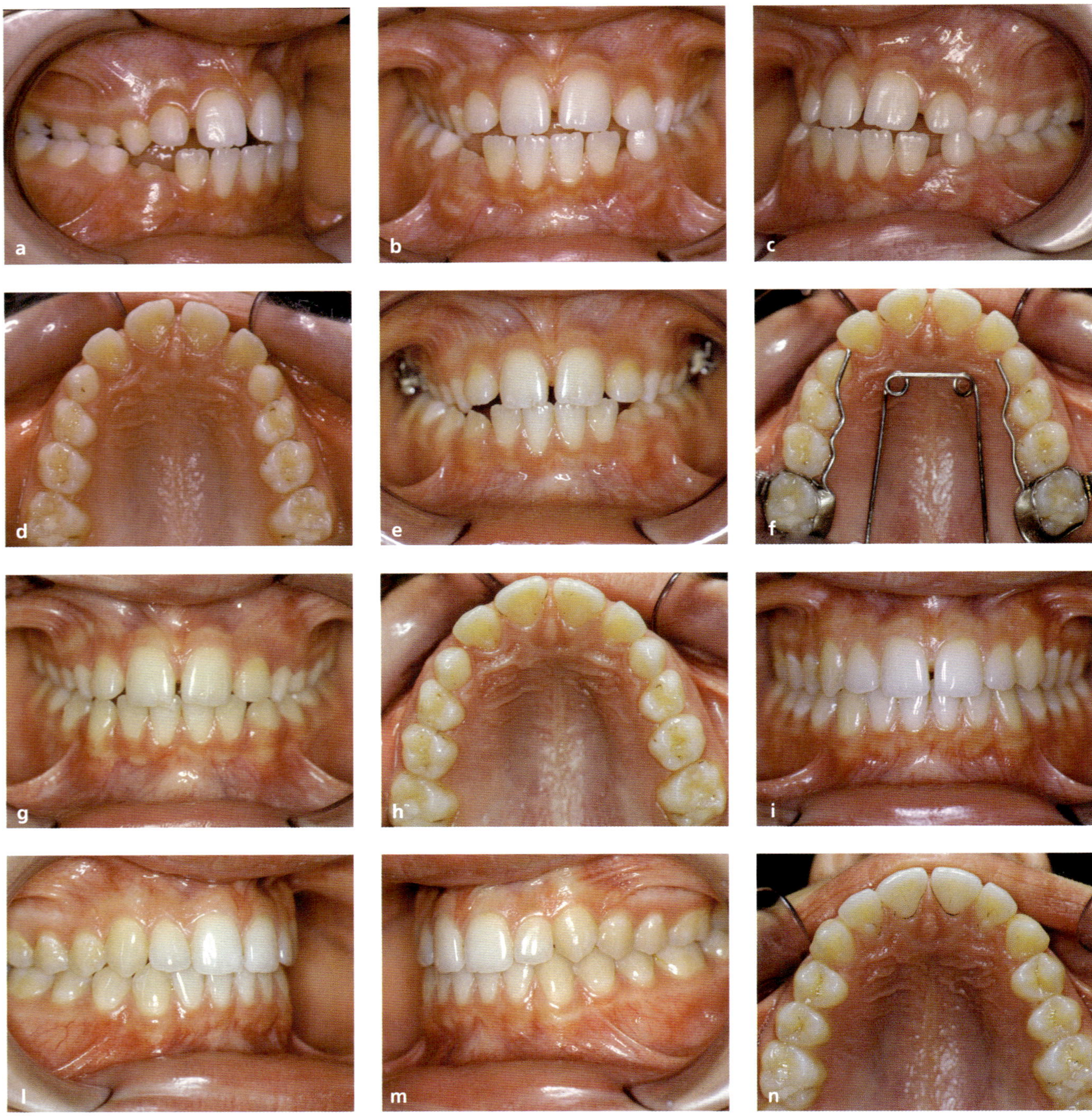

Figure 14.16 A.N., 10-year-old girl, late mixed dentition. Right molar class II, left molar class I. The midlines do not coincide, with the lower midline deviated to right due to mandibular lateral deviation, resulting in the contraction of the upper jaw (**a–d**). After the application of a slow expansion device in the upper jaw (*quad-helix*), correct transverse maxillary–mandibular and sagittal relationships are restored (**e–h**). Next, we proceed with the monitoring of tooth exchange until the completion of the physiological development of the dental arches. Timely interception of the mandibular lateral deviation also represented a preventive intervention of possible asymmetry (**i–n**).

Deciduous molars. Abnormal resorption of the roots of the deciduous molars can delay exfoliation, with possible altered position of the corresponding permanent teeth. Early diagnosis as well as clinical and radiographic monitoring of the development and position of the corresponding permanent tooth can suggest the most suitable time for the extraction of the deciduous tooth and any further preventive–interceptive interventions.

Deciduous canines. The extraction of the upper deciduous canine can at times represent an effective preventive measure for the inclusion for the permanent tooth with an abnormal eruptive path.

Transversal, sagittal, and vertical problems

Functional, genetic, and behavioral factors may be separately involved in determining structural alterations in the sagittal, transverse, and/or vertical plane. The solution of clinical conditions with implications in the different planes of space can, in turn, prevent more complex three-dimensional problems.

Alterations in the transverse plane

The correlation between the transverse dimension and the relation between the sagittal and vertical plane is a crucial aspect in orthodontics. The contraction of the upper jaw may be dentoalveolar, skeletal, or mixed. The maxillary transverse deficit is often associated with crossbite in the posterolateral, unilateral, or bilateral regions. The structural, dentoalveolar, or functional origin of the crossbite determines the therapeutic approach when it occurs due to a real intra-arch asymmetry, i.e., a bilateral maxillary contraction, in the presence or absence of lateral jaw deviation during closing; a recentering of the midlines at the maximum opening may confirm the suspicion of lateral–functional deviation. Thus, it is crucial to frame the maxillary–mandibular transverse relationship and identify the presence of possible laterally deviated previous contacts, usually referable to a single dental element in the deciduous dentition or a bilateral contraction of the jaw in the mixed dentition (Fig. 14.16).
Considering the low spontaneous correction rate of crossbite in the early deciduous and mixed dentition period following joint and neuromuscular adaptation caused by the acquired mandibular posture in lateral deviation, early treatment is indicated, with consequent alteration in maxillary–mandibular growth (Kecik et al, 2007; Kennedy and Osepchook, 2005; Silva Filho et al, 2000).
Selective grinding in the deciduous dentition allows the removal of occlusal interferences, leading to a resolution of the mandibular lateral deviation, with significant success (30%–50%), as a preventive/interceptive therapeutic intervention.

In unresolved cases, rapid or slow expansion may be used in the early mixed dentition period. In the presence of contextual mandibular retrusion, an early expansion measure can represent an endogenous functional therapy, which contributes to the normalization of maxillary–mandibular sagittal relationships (Baccetti, 2001; Guest et al, 2010; Harrison and Ashby, 2001).
Maxillary contraction can occur even in the absence of crossbite in the presence of dentoalveolar compensation of the transverse deficit. On the other hand, a unilateral crossbite can be detected in the presence of a normally developed maxilla due to an excessive transverse development of the jaw, resulting in relative insufficiency in the transverse diameter of the upper arch.
The analysis of potential discrepancies in condylar position between different occlusal relationships is a crucial component in the treatment of transverse complications.

Alterations in the sagittal plane

Alterations in the sagittal plane can be traced to *excessive maxillary development and/or mandibular deficit* (class II) or to *maxillary deficit and/or excessive mandibular development* (class III).
In *maxillary protrusion* forms (class II), the treatment is aimed at limiting maxillary growth using orthopedic appliances. If the protrusion is associated with a transverse discrepancy, it is advisable to proceed with maxillary expansion using targeted therapeutic appliances, with the possibility to also obtain sagittal improvements because of the expansion (endogenous functional therapy). Early treatment is decisive in the presence of increased overjet, such as trauma-prophylactic intervention (Barbato and Leonardi, 2007; Cozza et al, 2005).
In class II forms, because of *mandibular deficiency*, the elective treatment can be functional orthopedic treatment, with the use of appliances to stimulate mandibular growth and restore favorable environmental conditions. The peak of mandibular growth is the most indicated moment for the implementation of a functional therapy for class II conditions, which are identified via biological indicators of skeletal maturity (Fig. 14.17) (Guest et al, 2010; Martins et al, 2008; Profitt and Fields, 2008).
Class III clinical conditions are primarily attributable to maxillary deficiency associated with anterior crossbite. In general, this deficiency also affects the transverse plane; therefore, a preliminary expansion of the jaw using rapid-type appliances may be indicated to restore the correct transverse relationships and improve sagittal relationships, with the subsequent application of an inverse extraoral traction using functional appliances (Kilic et al, 2010). In any case, timely and early restoration of the correct maxillary–mandibular sagittal relationships is decisive, with the monitoring of the overall dental–maxillary–facial structure until the end of the growth.

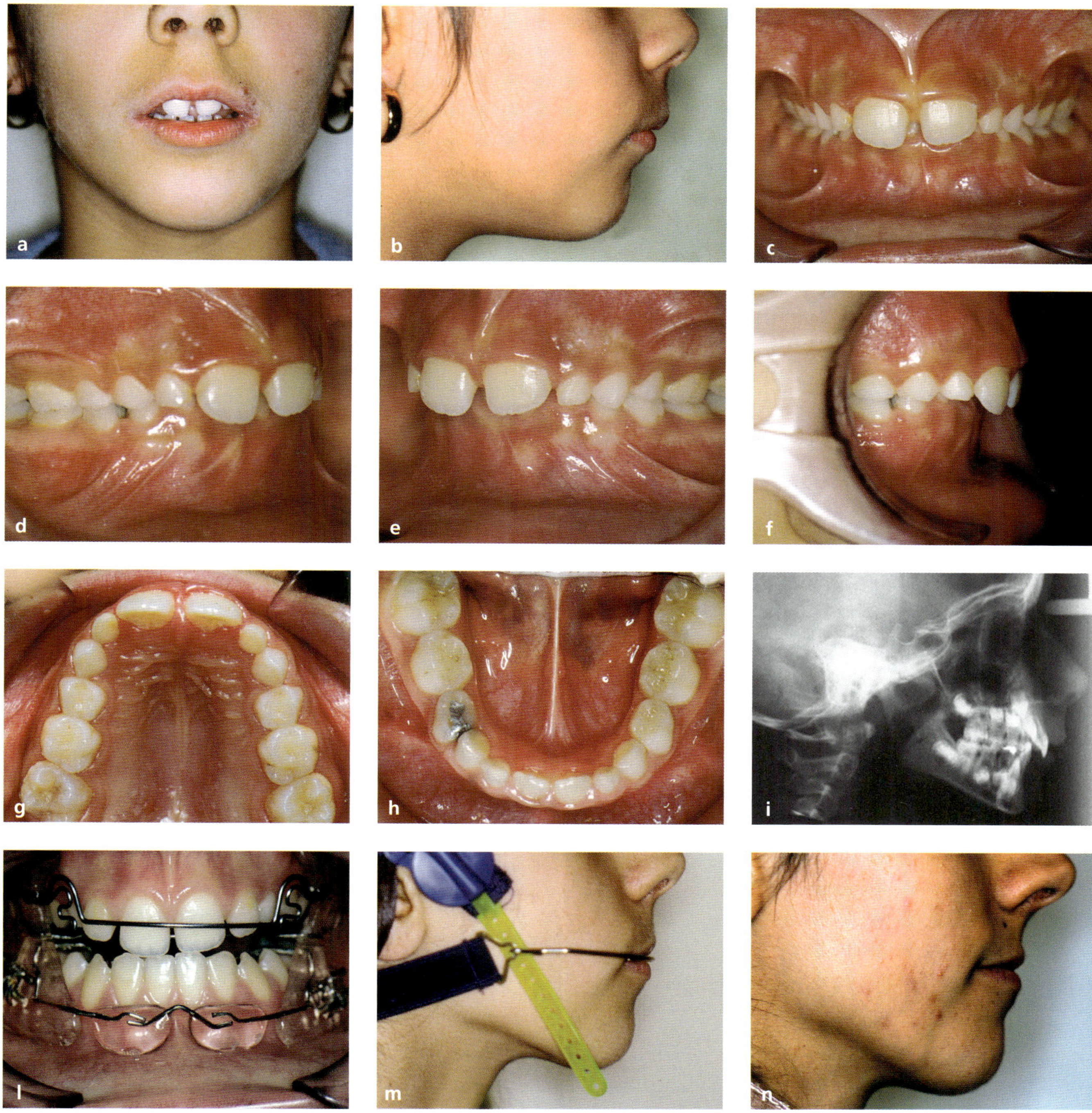

Figure 14.17 S.G., 8-year-old girl, early mixed dentition. Oral breather. Dolichofacial type, labial incompetence, convex profile. Bilateral molar and canine class II relationship and increased overjet and overbite (**a–h**). Maxillary protrusion associated with mandibular retrusion and postrotation (**i**). The therapeutic approach included application of a type II function regulator device that exerts effects in the three planes of the space and, later, a combined extraoral traction, which led to the resolution of the dysgnathic framework via exchange monitoring (**l–v**) (continued).

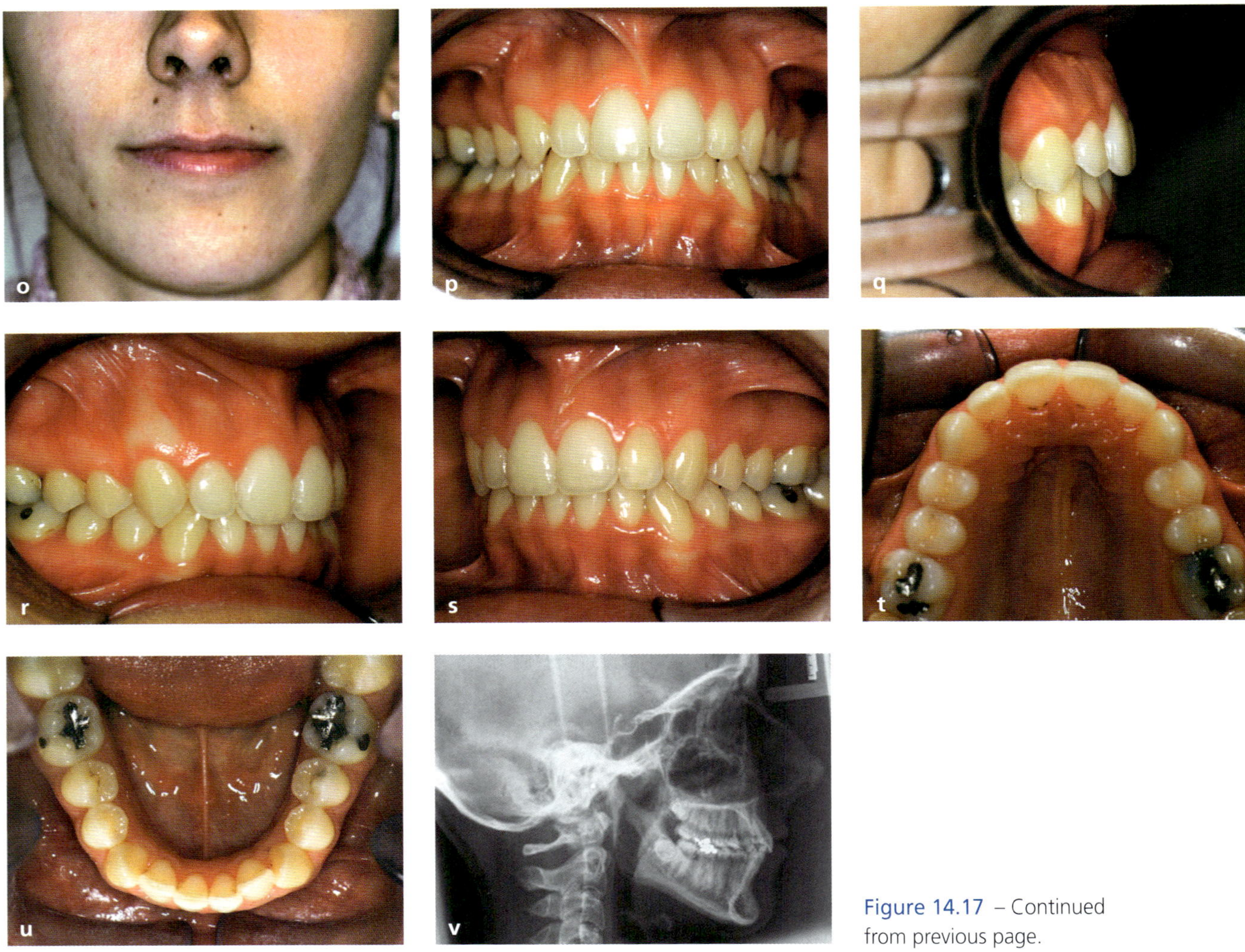

Figure 14.17 – Continued from previous page.

Alterations in the vertical plane

Open bite. This is a dental or dentoalveolar alteration that usually occurs due to functional alteration and tends to improve once the bad habit is eliminated. Clinical and x-ray examinations contribute to the diagnostic framework. If the open bite is associated with a *skeletal pattern*, in addition to eliminating the bad habit, it is necessary to intervene with an early and targeted orthopedic and/or functional therapy in the mixed dentition period (Cozza et al, 2005).

Deep bite. This is a dental, dentoalveolar, or skeletal alteration. Clinical and x-ray examinations contribute to the diagnostic framework. The upper incisors cover the vestibular surface of the lower incisors beyond 3 mm. The incisor margins occasionally leave an imprint on the palatal mucosa, with possible periodontal implications and the necessity for early treatment.

References

American Association of Orthodontists. Orthodontics: principles and polices, educational guidelines, organizational structures. St. Louisiana: American Association of Orthodontists, 1971.

Baccetti T, Franchi L, Cameron CG, McNamara JA Jr. Treatment timing for rapid maxillary expansion. Angle Orthod 2001;71:343-50.

Barbato E, Leonardi RM. Occlusione normale e patologica in dentizione decidua, mista e permanente. In: Sfondrini G, Giorgetti R. Odontoiatria per il pediatra. Pisa: Pacini; 2007. p. 39-48.

Barbato E, Proietti D, Conflitti B, Cannoni D. Ruolo diagnostico e prognostico dell'OPT nel soggetto in crescita. Dental Cadmos 1999;5:57-81.

Barbato E, Proietti D, Giancotti T. Disturbi del linguaggio nei quadri di malocclusione. Indagine preliminare. Dental Cadmos 2000;4:69-77.

Bishara SE, Warren JJ, Broffitt B et al. Changes in the prevalence of non-nutritive sucking patterns in the first 8 years of life. Am J Orthod Dentofacial Orthop 2006;130:31-6.

Bishara SE. Texbook of orthodontics. WB Saunders Company; Philadelphia 2001.

Cozza P, Baccetti T, Franchi L et al. Sucking habits and facial hyperdivergency as risk factors for anterior open bite in the mixed dentition. Am J Orthod Dentofacial Orthop 2005;128:517-9.

Cozza P, Mucedero M, Baccetti T et al. Early orthodontic treatment of skeletal open-bite malocclusion: a systematic review. Angle Orthod 2005;75:707-13.

Cozza P. Funzioni stomatognatiche principali: suzione, deglutizione, masticazione, fonesi, respirazione. In: Sfondrini G, Giorgetti R. Odontoiatria per il pediatra. Pisa: Pacini; 2007;56-76.

Engelke W, Jung K, Knosel M. Intra-oral compartment pressures: a bio- functional model and experimental measurements under different conditions of posture. Clin Oral Investig 2011;15(2):165-76.

Frankel R, Frankel C. Ortopedia orofacciale con il regolatore di funzione. Milano: Masson; 1991.

Gois EGO, Ribeiro Junior HC et al. Influence of non-nutritive sucking habits, breathing pattern and adenoid size on the development of malocclusion. Angle Orthod 2008;78:647-54.

Guest SS, McNamara JA Jr, Baccetti T et al. Improving class II malocclusion as a side-effect of rapid maxillary expansion: a prospective clinical study. Am J Orthod Dentofac Orthop 2010;138(5): 582-91.

Harrison JE, Ashby D. Orthodontic treatment for posterior crossbites. Cochrane Database Syst Rev 2001;2.

Kecik D, Kocadereli I, Saatci I. Evaluation of the treatment changes of functional posterior crossbite in the mixed dentition. Am J Orthod Dentofacial Orthop 2007;131:202-15.

Kennedy DB, Osepchook M. Unilateral posterior crossbite with mandibular shift: a review. J Can Dent Assoc 2005;71(8):569-73.

Keski-Nisula K, Hernesniemi R, Heiskanem M et al. Orthodontic intervention in the early mixed dentition: a prospective, controlled study on the effects of the eruption guidance appliance. Am J Orthod Dentofacial Orthop 2008;133(2):254-60.

Kilic N, Celikoglu M, Oktay H. Effects of the functional regulator III on profile changes in subjects with maxillary deficiency. Eur J Orthod 2010;32(6):729-34.

King GJ, Brudvik P. Effectiveness of interceptive orthodontic treatment in reducing malocclusions. Am J Orthod Dentofacial Orthop 2010;137(1):18-25.

Landouzy JM, Sergent Delattre A, Fenart R et al. The tongue: deglutition, orofacial functions and craniofacial growth. Int Orthod 20097(3);227-56.

Levrini L, Tagliabue A, Fabro S et al. Ideal treatment timing for thumb sucking. Italian Paediatr Dent 1999;2:31-4.

Martins RP, da Rosa Martins JC, Martins LP et al. Skeletal and dental components of Class II correction with the bionator and removable headgear splint appliances. Am J Orthod Dentofacial Ortop 2008;134(6):732-41.

Melink S, Vagner MV, Hocevar-Boltezar I et al. Posterior cross-bite in the deciduous dentition period, its relation with sucking habits, irregular oro-facial functions, and otolaryngological findings. Am J Orthod Dentofacial Orthop 2010;138:32-40.

Montaldo L, Montaldo P, Cuccaro P et al. Effects of feeding on non-nutritive sucking habits and implications on occlusion in mixed dentition. Int J Paediatr Dent 2011;21:68-73.

Profitt WR, Fields Jr. HW, Sarver DM. Ortodonzia moderrna. Milano: Masson; 2008.

Silva Filho OG, Ferrari Júnior FM, Aiello CA et al. Correction of posterior crossbite in the primary dentition. J Clin Pediatr Dent 2000;24:165-80.

Synodinos PN, Polyzois I. Maxillary canine-first premolar transposition in the permanent dentition: treatment considerations and a case report. J Ir Dent Assoc 2010 Dec-2011 Jan;56:264-7.

Tunison W, Flores-Mir C, El Badrawy H et al. Dental arch space changes following premature loss of primary first molars: a systematic review. Pediatr Dent 2008;30(4):297-302.

Warren JJ, Bishara SE. Duration of nutritive and non-nutritive sucking behaviors and their effects on the dental arches in the primary dentition. Am J Orthod Dentofac Orthop 2002;121: 347-56.

Chapter 15

Temporomandibular disorders in pediatric dentistry

C. Di Paolo, A. Michelotti, G. Galluccio

Temporomandibular disorders (TMDs) comprise a group of functional abnormalities, including pathologies of the temporomandibular joints (TMJs), masticatory muscles, and associated musculoskeletal structures of the head and neck that occur with a certain frequency during the pediatric age and adolescence.
Based on this classification and considering the strong implications between somatic and psychosocial factors underlying these disorders, Dworkin classified two conditions: (1) organic dysfunctions and pathologies (Axis I) and (2) psycho-compartmental pain implications (Axis II). Within Axis I, he distinguished three groups of disorders: (1) muscle, (2) joint, and (3) arthralgia, arthrosis, and arthritis. Dysfunctions have a significant negative impact on the quality of life of pediatric patients and are one of the primary causes of absence from school; 22% girls and 18% boys remain absent from school because of these dysfunctions. Studying these disorders in children is important to establish an early diagnosis for specific and timely treatments and prevent the possible development of craniofacial growth abnormalities and pain-related issues (headaches and cervicalgia) and/or more complex dysfunctions involving other components of the stomatognathic apparatus.

Epidemiological data

The literature provides extensive data on TMDs during pediatric age and adolescence and reports the onset of TMDs from the age of 4 years, followed by increasing onset between the ages of 6 and 12 years. In children aged less than 3 years, the symptoms are rare and it is very difficult to determine the level of risk. In the literature, cases of TMJ dysfunction caused by facial trauma, infection, or systemic disease have been reported. However, there is a case study of patients aged 3–6 years who developed dysfunctions caused by the onset of oral parafunctions, bad habits, or psychological stress.
Epidemiological data indicate that although the signs and symptoms of TMDs are more frequent during the second and third decades of life, they also start to occur, albeit less frequently, during early childhood; however, in this age group, early detection is difficult.
Niler reported clicking rates of 5% in children aged 3–5 years, 8%–13% in children aged 7 years, and 28% in children aged 10–13 years. A study by Egermark-Ericksson also found that among other clinical signs and symptoms, there was a considerable prevalence of joint sounds that increased with age.

The literature extensively focuses on children aged 6–15 years. Indeed, these children are mostly at risk because of the occurrence of predisposing factors that are primarily associated with tooth eruption and the manifestation of hereditary factors emerging therafter. The data show that the frequency of TMDs increases in the transitional phase from the deciduous to mixed dentition and, in adolescents, reaches a level similar to that in adults.

This was confirmed by an epidemiological study conducted in the south of Italy, in which approximately 27% of adolescents aged 12 years were found to require orthodontic treatment. Statistical data from an Argentine study showed that 78% of patients with oral parafunction present with signs and symptoms of TMDs at the age of 12 years. To confirm the global spread of TMDs, Luther, in an epidemiological analysis, reported that all the studies were in agreement that approximately 10% of the population aged more than 18 years experience pain and other dysfunctional symptoms that require therapeutic attention. Many develop predisposing factors during childhood. Another crucial point is the high number of comorbidities that these dysfunctional conditions have with other widespread pain phenomena such as headaches, cervical pain, and lumbar pain. The pathological course of these alterations, in particular headaches, also starts during the pediatric age.

From the analysis of epidemiological data, it is apparent that there is a need for in-depth evaluation of pediatric patients during diagnostics and screening, all signs and symptoms emerging from the TMJ and masticatory muscles, and the most frequent forms of comorbidities, such as headaches and cervicalgia, in order to establish adequate prevention systems. Indeed, these clinical manifestations not only affect millions of children but also large sections of the adult population worldwide, causing a significant increase in both social (absence from schools and workplaces) and economic costs (actual treatment costs in the United States are estimated at 4 billion dollars a year).

Etiopathogenesis

The etiology of TMDs is not completely clear at present. However, two schools of thought regarding the etiopathogenesis have developed over time, which in turn has generated two opposing theories: one refers to mechanical or structural causes of an occluso-articulatory nature and the other refers to neuromuscular causes. The integration of these two theories occurred in the late 1970s, leading to a multifactorial view of the etiology of TMDs. In 1977, De steno introduced a triad of factors potentially present in each individual: predisposition (occlusion and postural disorders), tissue alterations, and psychological dependence.

Currently, the most accredited etiological classification is the guidelines of the American Academy of Orofacial Pain (2008).

Predisposing, triggering, and perpetuating factors

The predisposing factors are represented by conditions that statistically increase the risk of disruptions in the balance of the stomatognathic apparatus and therefore, predispose to the pathology.

Dental malocclusion is undoubtedly among these conditions because it is a fundamental element that is required for appropriate harmony with the other structures of the system; occlusion is defined as a biomechanical-type morphological and functional relationship among all stomatognathic components. The major dental alterations that predispose children to TMD development are incorrect dental contacts, abnormalities in the anterior guides, class II, division II, increased overjet, compensated class III, and *crossbite*. Of these, crossbite seems to have a greater predisposition if present in the posterior unilateral form rather than in the anterior bilateral or anterior unilateral form, as found in a recent study (Tecco et al, 2010). In general, it is possible to affirm that occlusal anomalies that alter the mandible position in the distal and vertical directions lead to articular conditions favorable to the dislocation of the disc.

Parafunction or bad habits such as biting the lips, cheeks, or nails are among the most common factors in these patients; bruxism and tightening lead to dental wear, particularly of the front veneers, and muscular overload often favors the development of muscular tension, headaches, and migraines, occasionally of considerable intensity.

The behavioral, psychosocial, and emotional aspects of the individual must be considered because by altering the tolerance threshold, they also predispose the system to a loss of balance and functional harmony.

Other important factors include craniofacial dentoskeletal abnormalities and malformations that are congenital or sometimes following bone fractures, particularly of the mandibular condyle, which are not properly treated because they are not easily diagnosed in pediatric patients. In fact, these conditions can interfere with the correct course of craniofacial growth. Other factors to consider are postural issues that can contribute to a TMJ dysfunction or that can be caused by the latter. The assessment and treatment of such anomalies require an integrated specialist approach. Finally, predisposing factors include constitutional hereditary factors, such as the anatomy of the jaws, dental elements, joints, and ligaments with an increased number of elastic fibers (ligamentous laxity), as well as genetic and neuro-hormonal factors, which need further assessment.

Females have greater predisposition to the development of TMDs, with a ratio ranging from 3:1 to 9:1; moreover, caucasians seem to be the most affected by these diseases.

Triggering factors, on the other hand, are attributable to micro and macro traumas and/or occlusion overload, whereas perpetuating factors fall primarily within the domain of psycho-emotional features of the patient. However, a paradigmatic cause–effect view between certain factors and TMDs is not as appropriate because it depends on the subjective response.

The predisposing factors of TMDs are listed in Table 15.1.

Table 15.1 DTM predisposing factors

- Female gender
- Class II malocclusions, division 2
- Class III malocclusion, compensated
- Crossbite
- Increased overjet
- Clamping
- Systemic pathologies
- Bruxism
- Onychophagy
- Result of untreated condylar fractures
- Bad habits
- Contractions of dental arch
- Psycho-emotional conditions
- Structural alterations

Table 15.2 DTM symptoms

- Migraine
- Muscle-tension headache
- Neck pain
- Otalgia
- Dizziness
- Tinnitus
- Joint noises
- Periauricular pain
- Pain of chewing muscles
- Postural disorder
- Systemic pathologies
- Developmental alterations

Signs and symptoms

Among the signs and symptoms of the dysfunction, pain is the most frequently experienced; it can either be spontaneous or can occur during jaw movements. Other symptoms include headache or migraine and pain in the cervical region. Disorders involving the auditory system, such as tinnitus and vertigo, can also manifest. On the other hand, semiological analysis of the dysfunction includes mandibular movement anomalies that can be altered, limited, or asymmetric, such as the presence of joint noises, pain, and deficiency in functional movements of the stomatognathic apparatus, such as chewing, swallowing, and phonation. All occlusal factors described in the previous section may be visible. In some cases, the onset is acute with moderate symptoms that occasionally evolve positively in a spontaneous manner. In other cases, a condition develops; this condition manifests with more intense and persistent pain and physical, behavioral, psychological, and psychosocial symptoms similar to those of patients with chronic pain originating from other body regions. In all cases, medical history and accurate and appropriate examination according to current indications based on scientific evidence are essential for diagnosis.

The fundamental objective of the diagnosis is to exclude other diseases that cause orofacial pain or abnormalities in movement and oromandibular functions. Studies have shown that TMJ dysfunction may not manifest in children, whereas symptomatic cases may be confused with headache or otalgia by pediatricians and otolaryngologists. Therefore, with regard to the diagnosis of such conditions in children a formative dialog is essential between dentists and pediatricians who are the first to continuously monitor the health conditions of pediatric patients.

Therefore, the patient's medical history—besides being meticulous toward pain as a symptom and mandibular movements—must also take into account the psychological aspects and different tolerance levels in pediatric patients compared with adults.
The symptoms of TMDs are shown in Table 15.2.

Clinical examination of pediatric patients with temporomandibular dysfunction

Personal medical history

The young patient visits the clinic accompanied by one of the parents. The patient is asked about the nature of the problem, and the medical history is recorded, which includes the family, physiological, and past medical history, as well as history of the current illness.
It is important to investigate the presence of underlying diseases, such as systemic diseases, genetic syndromes, and malocclusions, as well as certain aspects of the child's life habits, such as trauma, sports, and exposure to cold, and the possible temporal link between particular events reported by the parent or the child and the occurrence of the disorder. The medical records may be collected via an interview or a questionnaire to record all relevant information for a complete medical history. In particular, medical history taking must be very accurate and systematic in the analysis of the symptoms reported by the young patient.
In case of pain, the child is asked to indicate the painful area and the intensity of discomfort using a visual analog scale (VAS) of 10 cm, in which the left extremity indicates no pain and the right extremity indicates the maximum pain imaginable.
If the child complains of pain in the TMJ and physical examination indicates a wide-opening mouth, the possibility of ligamentous laxity is assessed by asking the child to perform some directional movements for an initial assessment using the Beighton index.
Additionally, the parent should be asked whether any drugs have been administered and about the *course of pain over time*. To obtain information about the course of pain over time, the parent must fill in a daily report of the pain reported by the child with the indication of 10/10 intensity using the VAS. The evaluation of vegetative or reflex manifestations associated with the onset of seizures (nausea, vomiting, lacrimation, sweating, or others) is important in the differential diagnosis between pain resulting from oral pathologies and headaches. The pediatric patient's oral habits, both functional and parafunctional, should be investigated in the medical history.
Bruxism is a oral habit of great interest during the pediatric age; it initiates between 4 and 8 years of age with a maximum incidence between 10 and 14 years, and subsequently decreases. We distinguish between diurnal bruxism, considered by many as a voluntary parafunctional habit common during the phase of passage from decidu-

ous dentition to permanent dentition, and nocturnal bruxism, which is an involuntary parafunction of the masticatory system, also known as parasomnia in sleep medicine. Clinical diagnosis of bruxism includes evaluation of muscle signs (hypertrophy of masseters) and signs of dental wear.

The deciduous dentition undergoes a process of physiological wear during chewing with the cusps of canines and molar deciduous teeth. Natural tooth wear should be distinguished from signs of erosion, which are related to diet, i.e., the intake of acidic foods and drinks or gastric problems, such as gastroesophageal reflux, and from those of mechanical abrasion, which can be linked to improper brushing of teeth. The discriminatory element in diagnosis is related to the shape and location of the lesions (clear and matching surfaces in bruxism, cup lesions in brushing, and palatal wear of the incisors in reflux).

Clinical examination

General extraoral examination

The examination of the patient begins with careful observation of the face in frontal and lateral projection, paying attention to any facial abnormalities caused by swelling or asymmetry and evaluating the contour features (harmonic, convex, or concave), which indicate the presence of any alterations in the development of the bone bases; this should be followed by observation of the posture on the frontal and lateral side.

Intraoral examination

The intraoral examination begins with the assessment of the child's oral health status. At the dental level, in particular, we should examine the possible signs of erosion and wear interdental associations on the transverse (unilateral or bilateral *crossbite*), sagittal (molar and canine class and overjet), and vertical (open or covered bite) planes, connection of inter-incisive lines, and presence of dislocated precontacts.

Mandibular dynamics

Next, we should examine of the mandibular dynamics, instructing the child to make opening and closing movements of the mouth and sliding the jaw toward the right, left, and front, which, can be simulated by the clinician if necessary. While the child opens and closes the mouth, the trajectory of the movement is first recorded, observing whether it is straight (Fig. 15.1) throughout the movement, it has deviations during the movement, or the movement is on one side (deflection). Deviation refers to any variance from the median sagittal plane, which then disappears as the opening progresses (return to the median line). Deflection is indicated when there is a lateral displacement that increases with the opening and remains at the maximum opening, caused by the limitation of the movement of a joint.

The width of the opening is then assessed using a measuring instrument, such as a gage, millimeter ruler, and fingers of the hand.

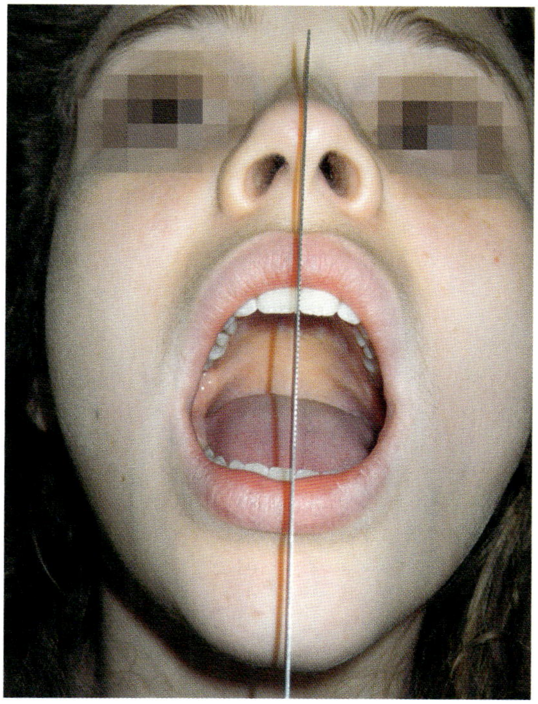

Figure 15.1 Straight opening.

Opening without pain. The patient is first asked to open the mouth as usual to a width so as to not feel any discomfort to evaluate the magnitude of normal opening. This is followed by the evaluation of the maximum excursion with and without effort.

Active opening. This is the measurement of the maximum opening of the mouth and is performed with a gauge or a millimeter ruler, referring to the margin of the upper incisors and the ideal line of the upper incisor overbite on the lower incisors. The normal value varies between 40 and 55 mm (Fig. 15.2).

Passive opening. After the child assumes the position of maximum active opening, the clinician places their thumb on the margin of the upper incisors and forefinger on the lower incisors and gently exerts pressure to increase the inter-incisive distance. The clinician then evaluates the objective sensation of elasticity or rigidity (*end-feel* and limit sensation) and the increment of the opening of the mouth, which is normally between 2 and 3 mm. Values greater than 2 mm with elastic *end-feel* lead to the suspicion of a muscular origin of the dysfunction. In contrast, if there is no increase in the opening and the *end-feel* is rigid, there is reason to suspect an intracapsular mechanical block (Fig. 15.3).

Laterotrusion. This is the measurement of the mandibular displacement during the movements of maximum right and left laterality. The amplitude of these movements is symmetrical and normally greater than 6 mm. A unilateral or bilateral limitation is an indication of joint or bilateral muscle contractures.

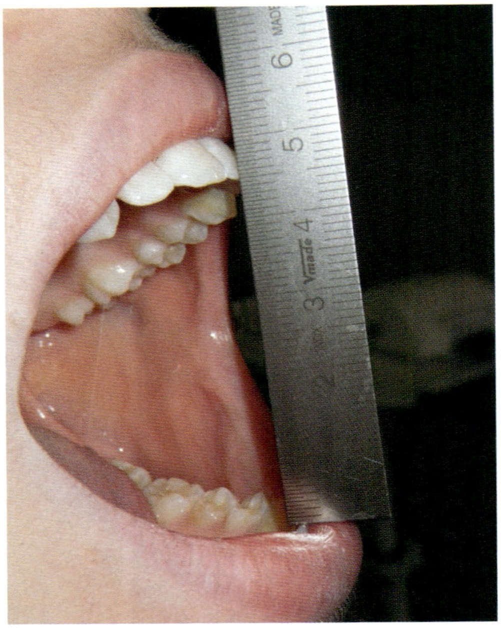

Figure 15.2 Active opening.

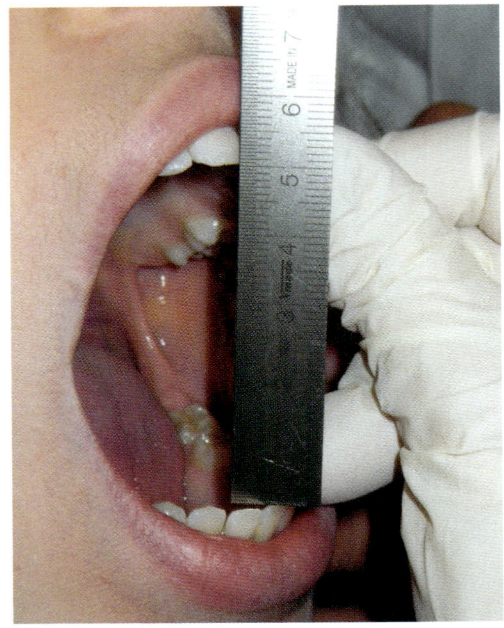

Figure 15.3 Passive opening.

Protrusion. The extent of the movement is obtained by adding the overjet value and the distance between vestibular surfaces of the upper incisors and incisal margin of the lower incisors after instructing the patient to perform the maximum level of protrusion. Under normal conditions, this value is greater than 6–7 mm, and the movement is straight.

Evaluation of temporomandibular joints

Palpation. Palpation is conducted simultaneously at level of the two joints and is performed laterally with the index finger placed on the preauricular area and then exerting a pressure in the anterior direction with the little finger in the external auditory meatus. This examination assesses the symmetry of the movements and the possible presence of pain.

Auscultation. Auscultation is performed at the same time as the palpation of the joint to detect any joint clicking or crackles. It is performed using the index or middle finger at the lateral pole of the condyle, instructing the patient to perform various movements of opening and closing, protrusion, and right and left laterality.
The anatomy of the jaw, which is a single bone in which the noise generated in one articulation can also spread to the other, must be considered to identify the side actually affected by the noise. A click is a clean and short noise that is detected during the opening and closing movement, indicating an alteration in the relationship between the condyle and joint disc. A crackle, on the other hand, resembles a gritty noise that accompanies the whole movement, indicating an alteration of the joint surfaces; in children, it may indicate rheumatoid arthritis. The presence of a single or reciprocal click noise or crackling orients the clinician in the diagnosis of TMDs of an articular nature.

Disc displacement with reduction

This is an alteration in the relationship between the condyle and disc, characterized by a click during opening as a clinical manifestation of the disc recapture by the condyle and a click, which is usually less evident, during the closing as a consequence of the anterior sliding of the disc (reciprocal clicking) (Fig. 15.4). The recapture of the disc (opening click) can be early, intermediate, or delayed; thus, the later the noises appear during the opening of the mouth, the more serious is the disc displacement. However, the closing click is generally much closer to the maximum intercuspation position. During opening, there is a mandibular deviation toward the joint affected by the pathological process, followed by a return to the medial line as the movement progresses. The opening speed modifies the position of the deviation appearance. Pain, when present, depends on the joint function.

Disc displacement without reduction

In the disc displacement without reduction, the normal condyle–disc relationship is lost during all mandibular movements (Fig. 15.5). The disc is not recaptured by the condyle but is forced forward by its progression. Pathology may be acute (acute *closed lock*) or chronic (chronic *closed lock*). In the case of acute joint lock, there is a limited opening capacity during the closing (20–30 mm) with a marked deviation toward the affected side, where pain intensifying with movement is reported. The laterotrusion toward the lateral side is limited and painful, while the protrusion is diverted toward the affected side. The opening cannot be passively increased by the clinician (rigid *end-feel*), and the patient also reports pain during bilateral manipulation of the jaw caused by the compression of the condyle on the retrodiscal tissues.

In the chronic joint lock, the pathological condition lasts for a long time; therefore, the pain is significantly reduced or even absent. The patient learns to perform mandibular movements that avoid forcing the condyles toward painful positions and, over time, a histological modification of the retrodiscal ligament may occur with a pseudo-disc formation that can functionally replace the dislocated disc. The opening of the mouth, counter-lateral movements, and protrusion are only slightly reduced. To accurately diagnose *chronic closed locks*, the patient's medical history should be referred. Typically, in the medical history, there is an initial phase with a click, followed by a second phase with a functional limitation without articular noise, and a third phase with normal opening without joint noise.

Subluxation

Subluxation is characterized by excessive opening of the mouth with a jaw snap at the end of the movement (Fig. 15.6). This click occurs in the terminal phase of opening and in the initial phase of closing at the same level. During the opening, there is a deviation and then a realignment from the median line of the mandibular route, which is much wider and occurs later than the deviation that occurs in case of disc displacement with reduction.

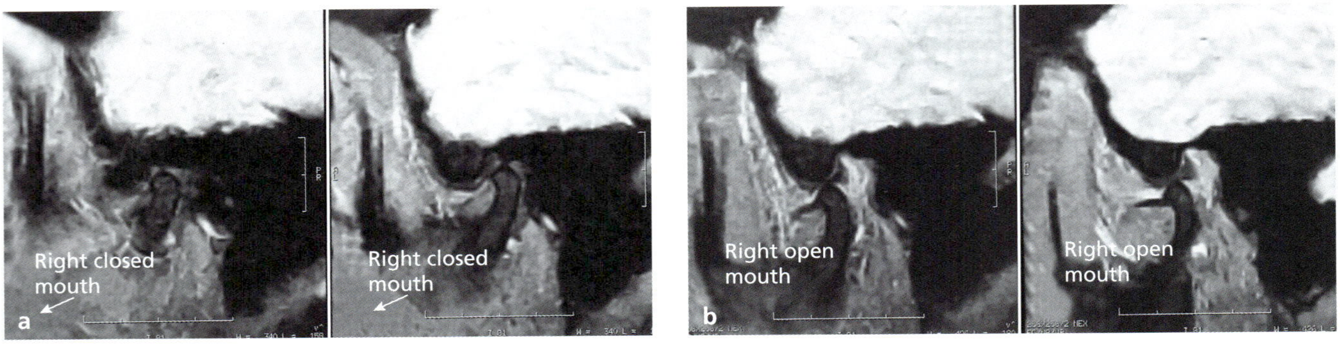

Figure 15.4 Nuclear magnetic resonance imaging showing disc displacement with closed (**a**) and open (**b**) mouth reduction.

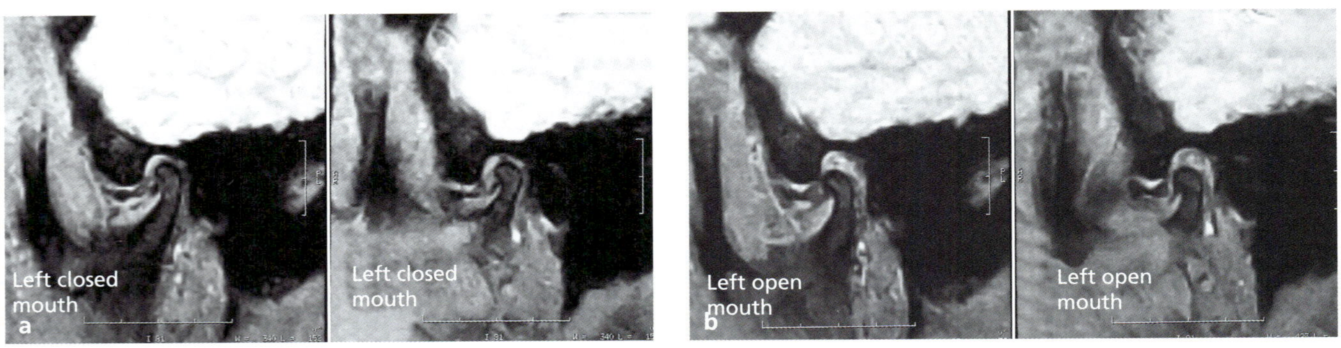

Figure 15.5 Nuclear magnetic resonance imaging showing disc displacement without reduction with closed (**a**) and open (**b**) mouth.

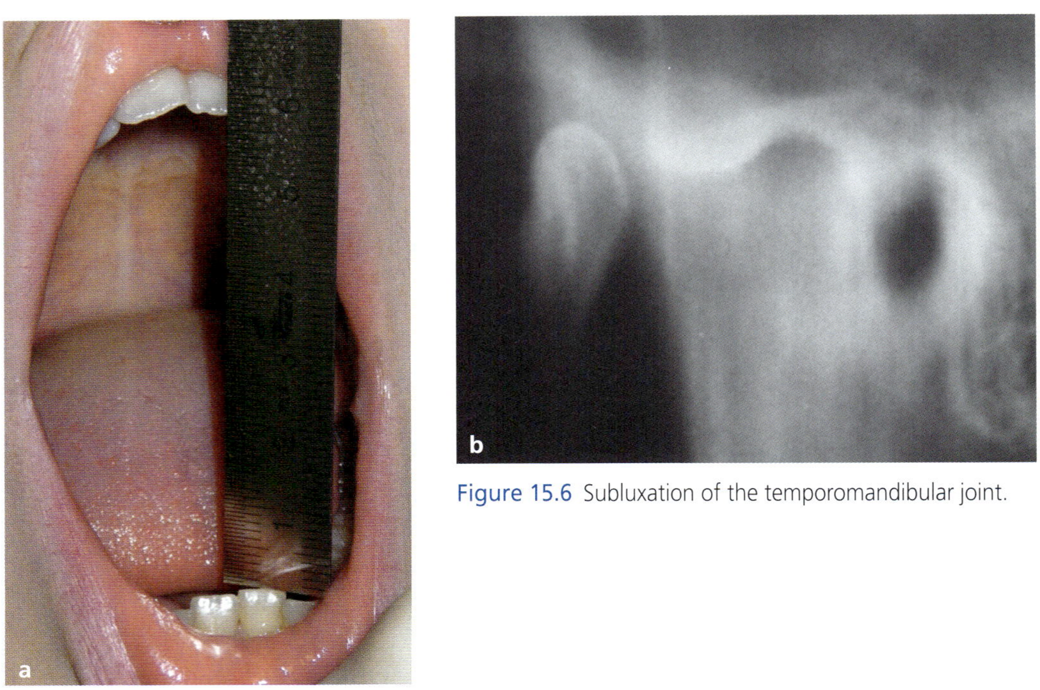

Figure 15.6 Subluxation of the temporomandibular joint.

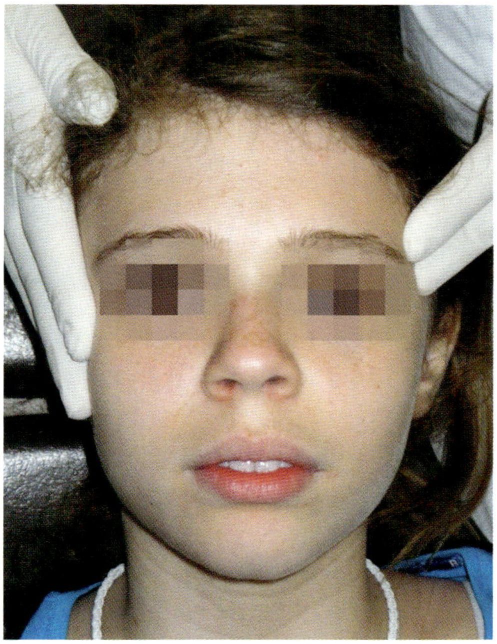

Figure 15.7 Palpation of the temporal muscle.

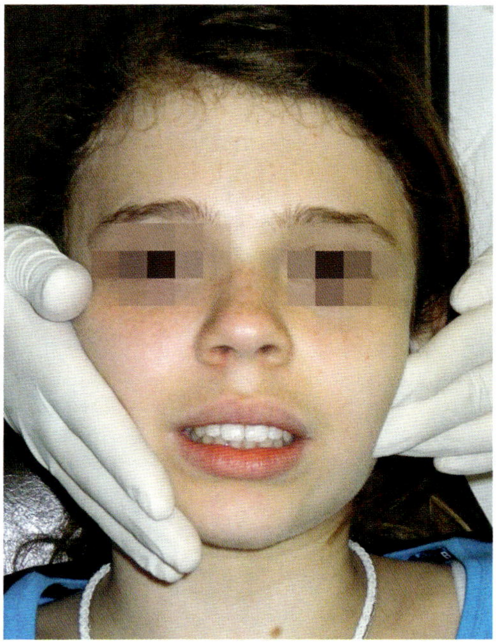

Figure 15.8 Palpation of the masseter muscle.

Palpation of the muscles

Under normal conditions, palpation of the masticatory muscles does not evoke pain. If this happens, it can be inferred that there is a tissue impairment caused by trauma or fatigue. During the examination, the pain intensity must be ascertained and recorded, instructing the child to report the extent of painful sensation on a scale (little, quite a lot, a lot). Any *trigger points* that constitute hypersensitive areas associated with remote-irradiated myofascial pain should be evaluated. The masticatory muscles (temporal, Fig. 15.7; masseter, Fig. 15.8), sternocleidomastoid, and trapezium are palpated; although these muscles do not directly intervene in mandibular movement, they are often considered as symptomatic in the presence of TMDs and the cause of headaches.

When the response is positive, the child is asked to quantify the degree of pain on a scale of 1-3 and to state whether the pain caused by palpation represents the pain he or she usually feels (familiar pain).

Treatment of patients with TMD: status of current knowledge

During the pediatric age, dysfunctional problems that may have a negative impact on the craniomandibular relationship, general posture of the individual, position of the teeth, and onset of pain, such as headache and cervicalgia, are common.

Treatment

The goals of TMD therapy in pediatric patients—not largely dissimilar to those in adult patients—should be both the recovery of joint function and correct occlusal conditions and appropriate neuromuscular rehabilitation because the resolution of painful and dysfunctional symptoms occurs with an adequate functional balance of stomatognathic components.

A characteristic feature of TMD treatment in children is also the timeliness of intervention; this is important to solve both objective and subjective symptoms and to prevent the eventual stabilization of such dysfunctional conditions resulting in anatomical damage.

As mentioned, tension, pain, and any functional limitations are often attributable to functional overload caused by altered occlusal conditions, parafunctions, bruxism, emotional tensions, or trauma; however, alterations in the osteoarticular relationship between the jaw and skull or between other craniocervical bone structures are possible. In the initial evaluation, however, the existence of other pathologies must not be excluded, e.g., inflammatory, autoimmune or infectious, and vascular or neurological pathologies and, although very rare, neoplastic pathologies.

Once these pathologies have been reasonably excluded, an appropriate treatment plan can be designed.

It is a good practice for the growing patient to opt for a treatment that is as conservative and noninvasive as possible, consistent with the present case, especially considering the dynamically changing structures.

The various treatment strategies should be evaluated after analyzing the main component(s) of the TMD, as well as the primary disorder reported by the young patient.

In the case of patients who are undergoing orthodontic treatment, the evaluation and treatment of the dysfunction, with the aim of recovering stable stomatognathic well-being, take priority over the occlusal recovery alone.

The various therapeutic approaches can be summarized as follows:

- functional therapies
- psychophysiological therapies
- occlusal therapies.

These therapies can be integrated with manual medicine treatments, such as the prescription of active exercises for neuromotor re-education or joint mobilizations, tailored according to the individual clinical case.

In some cases, drug therapy may be temporarily used, while surgical therapy may be administered only in rare cases, giving priority to less invasive forms, such as arthrocentesis of the TMJ.

Functional therapy

Pediatric functional therapy is based on the principle of redirecting growth via appropriate re-education of the functional activity of soft and neuromuscular tissues that constitute the "container" inside which the stomatognathic apparatus develops.

Because it is often possible to identify a functional problem (alteration of the physiological mechanism of swallowing, mouth breathing, lingual dyskinesia, and perioral tissues) in a growing patient, functional therapy appears to adequately correct the impaired functions with possible benefits for any pain. Indeed, according to the literature, it is more likely that dysfunctional aspects rather than specific relationships or conditions of malocclusion are predisposing to TMDs in the broad sense.

Functional pediatric therapy usually uses removable devices that require targeted exercises for muscular re-education. Removable devices also act on dysfunctional muscle structures.

The effectiveness of the functional equipment depends mainly on the cooperation offered by the patient both in terms of constant appliance use and in performance of the prescribed exercises, linked to the correct use of the devices, as well as connection to the biological potential of the patient and the initial severity of the problem.

Psychological–physiological treatments

Several authors have suggested a link between emotional factors, stress, and dysfunctional problems of the stomatognathic apparatus. Some studies have analyzed the relationship between psycho-emotional stress and parafunctions in the onset and persistence of TMDs; the classification of TMDs has been hypothesized in broader syndromes, such as *general adaptation syndrome* and *functional somatic syndrome*.

Recently, a predictive value has been attributed to psycho-emotional factors—which are part of the TMD genesis as perpetuating factors—in the onset of various dysfunctional syndromes, such as vertebral pain and TMDs.

From this perspective, the pediatric population is not immune to stress and emotional overload, which is involved in the onset of cephalic pathologies, parafunctions, and facial pain in patients with dysfunctions. Therefore, even if a strong correlation exists between bruxism and TMDs but not between TMDs and anxiety, the presence of depression or stress—in turn related to bruxism—in growing patients requires evaluation of these elements as well. However, the psycho-emotional factors in children appear to be in a positive relationship with the female sex and pain symptoms in the broad sense.

Moreover, from a therapeutic perspective, some treatment approaches associated with behavior and environmental reactions have demonstrated effectiveness in the treatment of pain originating from TMDs. In the literature, the effectiveness of pain-related psychological treatments for TMDs has been reported, including the combined treatments of electromyographic biofeedback and cognitive behavioral therapy. Therefore, any form of multidisciplinary management should always be considered.

Occlusal plates (bite plates)

In the pediatric population, the finding of TMDs in the RDC/TMD Axis I and in articular and muscular pathologies leads to the need to implement appropriate treatments after the previously indicated diagnostic pathway. Occlusal or *bite* plates are removable medical devices composed of customizable hard resin that are placed on a dental arch. They represent one of the most commonly used strategies in the initial approach to

patients with pain and functional limitations who present with an incorrect relationship between the joint heads. In the case of painful bruxism, especially during early childhood, preformed devices that play the same role of interposition between the arches and modification of occlusal relation can occasionally be used.
Occlusal plates can take various forms and may or may not cover the entire dental arch, offering support to the teeth of the other arch.
Occlusal plates are useful in the case of diagnostic uncertainties to confirm the diagnostic hypothesis.
As with adult patients, the types of devices vary according to the pathological condition. In extracapsular alterations of predominant muscular origin, the treatment aim should be deconditioning of the neuromuscular system. Therefore, occlusal covering equipment that can prevent any occlusal pathological contact that is able to determine a contracture muscle (release plates and neuromuscular plaques) should be indicated. In intracapsular alterations, on the other hand, the treatment aim should be a change in the ratio between joint heads. In this case, the therapeutic position is maintained by the presence of occlusal intercuspation on the device in the new position, which is often helped by a front ramp.
In case joint *lock* conditions have been diagnosed, the approach is oriented by the event duration, i.e., an acute *lock* characterized by a more evident symptomatology or a chronic *lock* in which the symptomatology tends to be less demanding for the patient; however, the risk that the pathology gives rise to more extensive damage because the joint surfaces are highly compromised.
While in the acute lock, it is possible to proceed to physiotherapy maneuvers of articular release with manipulation of the jaw. This approach has fewer possibilities of stable disc recapture than the chronic *lock*.
Alternatively, it is possible to use distracting plates or joint distractors, which allow the permanent recapture of the disc, decompression of the posterior bilaminar area, and a physiotherapeutic effect of stretching and decontraction of muscle fibers.
In addition to the primary therapies, it is possible to recognize some therapeutic "adjuvant" approaches to support the patient, which can be summarized as *pharmacological*, *physio-*, and *postural therapies*.

Pharmacological therapy. This therapy is proposed to act quickly and effectively in countering, as a first element, the painful symptomatology that characterizes TMDs of both joint and neuromuscular origin. The literature proposes the use of pharmacological combinations with anti-inflammatory and analgesic drugs combined with muscle relaxants with the dual purpose of interrupting the muscle contraction circuit that follows and causes the painful stimulus. However, it seems logical that in pediatric patients, prescription and administration of drugs should take place only to control acute pain and always with the utmost caution, avoiding anything that can extensively interfere with the balance of the organs of a growing individual.

Physiotherapeutic approach. This approach uses various methods that include manual therapy, in which the manual reoperation of the joint disc and muscular elongation

and decontraction are achieved, and postural therapy, which is effective through global muscle conditioning.
In addition to this approach, other adjuvant treatments to control pain, such as thermal therapy (thermotherapy or cryotherapy), ultrasound therapy, acupuncture, or transcutaneous electrical nerve stimulator, can be used.
If patients with TMJ dysfunctions exhibit concomitant and/or secondary changes in head and neck posture, physiotherapy treatment of *overall postural re-education* should be considered.
At the end of the treatment period, it is essential to conduct a new careful phase of diagnostic–therapeutic reassessment that ascertains the status of the dysfunction/pathology and simultaneously, the occlusal conditions of the subject, which, as mentioned, could be a condition of instability (dentition transition phase and pubertal peak of growth phase). If clinical well-being is achieved, it is necessary to evaluate the opportunity and modalities of possible finalization using primarily orthodontic therapies.

Malocclusion correction therapies in pediatric patients with a history of TMDs should be performed with careful attention to correcting occlusal conditions related to dysfunctions and should be prioritized over other treatment objectives.

Conclusions

TMDs primarily affect adults and females, most commonly those aged 25–45 years; they have a low prevalence in children aged 3–6 years, whereas in adolescents, they have the same frequency as that in adults with fewer differences between males and females and with the same prevalence of the muscle pain symptoms as joint disorders. Because of their cyclicity and duration, TMDs have a favorable prognosis.
Dentists play a key role in intercepting clinical cases of TMDs via accurate diagnosis, thereby preventing the occurrence of advanced dysfunctional or pathological conditions that would inevitably affect the growth of pediatric patients. These include the various occlusion anomalies, parafunctions, and bad habits. Moreover, it is recommended that patients with chronic pain, regardless of its origin, are treated in a multidisciplinary specialist setting. Thus, for the treatment of these patients, it is essential that gnathologists collaborate with other specialists who can provide treatment for all the side effects of TMDs, including physiotherapists, otorhinolaryngologists, neurologists, orthopedic specialists, speech therapists, physiologists, psychologists, and orthodontists.

References

AA VV. Treatment of temporomandibular disorders in children: summary statements and recommendations. American Academy of Pediatric Dentistry, University of Texas Health Science Center at San Antonio Dental School. J Am Dent Assoc 1990;120(3):265,267,269.

Aidar LA, Dominguez GC, Abrahão M et al. Effects of Herbst appliance treatment on temporomandibular joint disc position and morphology: a prospective magnetic resonance imaging study. Am J Orthod Dentofacial Orthop 2009;136(3):412-24.

Al-Ani Z, Gray RJ, Davies SJ et al. Stabilization splint therapy for the treatment of temporomandibular myofascial pain: a systematic review. J Dent Educ 2005;69(11):1242-50.

Auerbach SM, Laskin DM, Frantsve LM, Orr T. Depression, pain, exposure to stressful life events, and long-term outcomes in temporomandibular disorder patients. J Oral Maxillofac Surg 2001;59:628-33.

de Souza Barbosa T, Miyakoda LS, de Liz Pocztaruk R et al. Temporomandibular disorders and bruxism in childhood and adolescence: review of the literature. Int J Pediatr Otorhinolaryngol 2008;72(3):299-314. Epub 2008 Jan 3.

Bertolucci LE, Grey T. Clinical analysis of mid-laser versus placebo treatment of arthralgic TMJ degenerative joints. J Craniomand Pract 1995;13:26-9.

Bracco P, Deregibus A, Piscetta R, Ferrario G. Observations on the correlation between posture and jaw position: a pilot study. Cranio 1998;16(4):252-8.

Bracco P, Deregibus A, Piscetta R. Effects of different jaw relations on postural stability in human subjects. Neurosci Lett 2004;356(3):228-30.

Brage S, Sandanger I, Nygård JF. Emotional distress as a predictor for low back disability: a prospective 12-year population-based study. Spine 2007;32:269-74.

Brusati R. Trattato di tecnica chirurgica. Padova: Piccin; 1986. p. 245-51.

Clark GT, Seligman DA, Solberg WK, Pullinger AG. Guidelines for the treatment of temporomandibular disorders. J Craniomand Dis 1990;4:80-8.

Cortese SG, Biondi AM. Relationship between dysfunctions and parafunctional oral habits, and temporomandibular disorders in children and teenagers. Arch Argent Pediatr 2009;107(2):134-8.

Crider A, Glaros AG, Gevirtz RN. Efficacy of biofeedback-based treatments for temporomandibular disorders. Appl Psychophysiol Biofeedback 2005;30:333-45.

Cuccia AM, Caradonna C, Annunziata V, Caradonna D. Osteopathic manual therapy versus conventional conservative therapy in the treatment of temporomandibular disorders: a randomized controlled trial. J Bodyw Mov Ther 2010;14(2):179-84. Epub 2009 Sep.

Das UM, Keerthi R, Ashwin DP et al. Ankylosis of temporomandibular joint in children. J Indian Soc Pedod Prev Dent 2009;27(2):116-20.

Davis R, Brogden R. Pharmacotherapy. In: McNeill CH. Current controversies in TMD. Quintessence Publishing Co. Inc. 1991. p. 153-6.

de Andrade LH, Cavalcante MA, Raymundo R Jr, de Souza IP. Temporomandibular joint ankylosis in children. J Dent Child (Chic) 2009;76(1):41-5.

De Boever JA, Carlsson GE, Klineberg IJ. Need for occlusal therapy and prosthodontic treatment in the management of temporomandibular disorders. Part I. Occlusal interferences and occlusal adjustment. J Oral Rehabil 2000;27(5):367-79.

de Félicio CM, Freitas RL, Bataglion C. Effects of orofacial myofunctional therapy on temporomandibular disorders. Int J Orofac Myol 2007;33:21-9.

Deshayes MJ. Dentofacial orthopedics to treat facial asymmetries before six years of age. How to balance craniofacial growth and enhance temporomandibular function. Orthod Fr 2010;81(3):189-207. Epub 2010 Aug 17.

Dworkin SF. Perspective on the interaction of biological, psychological and social factors in TMD. J Am Dent Soc 1994;125:856-63.

Eberhard D, Bantleon HP, Steger W. The efficacy of anterior repositioning splint therapy studied by magnetic resonance imaging. Eur J Orthod 24:343-52.

Feine JS, Widmer CG, Lund JP. Physical therapy: a critique. Oral Surg Oral Med Oral Pathol Oral Radiol Endod 1997;83:123-7.

Ferrario V, Sforza C, Schmitz JH, Taroni A. Occlusion and center of foot pressure variation: is there a relationship? J Prosth Dent 1996; 76:302-8

Forssell H, Kalso E, Koskela P et al. Occlusal treatments in temporomandibular disorders: a qualitative systematic review of randomized controlled trials. Pain 83:549-560, 199.

Forssell H, Kalso E. Application of principles of evidence-based medicine to occlusal treatment for temporomandibular disorders: are there lessons to be learned? J Orofac Pain 2004;18:9-22. discussion 23-32.

Friedman MH, Weisberg J. Disturbi temporomandibolari. Diagnosi e trattamento. Quintessenza Book, Chicago, 1985.

Funt AL, Stack B, Gelb S et al. Terapia miofunzionale nel trattamento della sindrome craniomandibolare. In: Gelb H. Trattamento clinico del dolore e della disfunzione all'ATM, testa e collo. Roma: Marrapese Editore; 1999.

Gerber R. Okklusionslehre, okklusionsdiagnostik und im okklusionsbehandlung aspekte wandelunserer. Schweiz Mschr Zahnheilk 1970;80:447.

Glaros AG, Burton E. Parafunctional clenching, pain and effort in temporomandibular disorders. J Behav Med 2004;27:91-100.

Glaros AG, Glass EG, Hayden WJ. History of treatment received by patients with TMD: a preliminary investigation. J Orofac Pain 1995;9(2):147-51.

Glaros AG, Williams K, Lausten L. The role of parafunctions, emotions and stress in predicting facial pain. J Am Dent Assoc 2005; 136:451-8.

Gonçalves DA, Dal Fabbro AL, Campos JA et al. Symptoms of temporomandibular disorders in the population: an epidemiological study. J Orofac Pain 2010;24(3):270-8.

Gray RJ, Quayle AA, Hall CA, Schofield MA. Physiotherapy in the treatment of temporomandibular joint disorders: a comparative study of four treatment methods. Br Dent J 1994;176(7):257-61.

Gregg J, Rugh J. Pharmacological Therapy. In: Mohl et al (editor): a texbook of Occlusion. Quintessence Publishing Co. Inc. 1988. p. 351-356.

Henningsen P, Zipfel S, Herzog W. Management of functional somatic syndromes. Lancet 2007;369:946-55.

Henrikson T, Nilner M. Temporomandibular disorder and the need for stomatognathic treatment in orthodontically treated and untreated girls. Eur J Orthod 2000;22:283-92.

Hirsch C, John MT, Lautenschläger C, List T. Mandibular jaw movement capacity in 10-17-yr-old children and adolescents: normative values and the influence of gender, age, and temporomandibular disorders. Eur J Oral Sci 2006;114(6):465-70.

Intrieri RC, Jones GE et al. Masseter muscle hyperactivity and myofascial pain dysfunction syndrome: a relationship under stress. J Behav Med 1994;17:479-500.

Kato T, Thie NM, Huynh N et al. Topical review: sleep bruxism and the role of peripheral sensory influences. J Orofac Pain 2003;17:191-213.

Katsoulis J, Richter M. Efficacy of specific physiotherapy for temporomandibular joint dysfunction of muscular origin. Rev Stomatol Chir Maxillofac 2008;109(1):9-14. Epub 2007.

Klasser GD, Greene C. Oral appliances in the management of temporomandibular disorders. Oral Surg Oral Med Oral Pathol Oral Radiol Endod 2009;107:212-3.

Köhler AA, Helkimo AN, Magnusson T, Hugoson A. Prevalence of symptoms and signs indicative of temporomandibular disorders in children and adolescents. A cross-sectional epidemiological investigation covering two decades. Eur Arch Paediatr Dent 2009;10(Suppl 1):16-25.

Laskin DM. Etiology of the pain-dysfunction syndrome. J Am Dent Assoc 1969;79:147-53.

Leuin SC, Frydendall E, Gao D, Chan KH. Temporomandibular joint dysfunction after mandibular fracture in children: a 10-year review. Arch Otolaryngol Head Neck Surg 2011;137(1):10-4.

List T, Wahlund K, Wenneberg B, Dworkin SF. TMD in children and adolescents: Prevalence of pain, gender differences, and perceived treatment need. J Orofac Pain 1999;13(1):9-20.

Lobbezoo F, Soucy JP, Hartman NG et al. Effects of the D2 receptor agonist bromocriptine on sleep bruxism: report of two single-patient clinical trials. J Dent Res 1997;76:1610-4.

Lobbezoo F, Soucy JP, Montplaisir JY, Lavigne GJ. Striatal D2 receptor binding in sleep bruxism: a controlled study with iodine-123-iodobenzamide and single-photon-emission computed tomography. J Dent Res 1996;75:1804-10.

Luther F. TMD and occlusion part I. Damned if we do? Occlusion: the interface of dentistryand orthodontics. Br Dent J 2007;202:E2 (1-7).

Manfredini D, Lobbezoo F. Relationship between bruxism and temporomandibular disorders: a systematic review of literature from 1998 to 2008. Oral Surg Oral Med Oral Pathol Oral Radiol Endod 2010;109:26-50.

Manfredini D, Tognini F, Melchiorre D et al. Ultrasonography of the temporomandibular joint: Comparison of findings in patients with rheumatic diseases and temporomandibular disorders. A preliminary report. Oral Surg Oral Med Oral Pathol Oral Radiol Endod 2005;100(4):481-5.

McNeely ML, Armijo Olivo S, Magee DJ. A systematic review of the effectiveness of physical therapy interventions for temporomandibular disorders. Phys Ther 2006;86(5):710-25.

McNeill C. Management of temporomandibular disorders: Concepts and controversies. J Prosthet Dent 1997;77(5):510-22. Review.

Michelotti A, Iodice G. The role of orthodontics in temporomandibular disorders. J Oral Rehabil 2010;37(6):411-29. Epub 2010.

Mohlin BO, Derweduwen K, Pilley R et al. Malocclusion and temporomandibular disorder: a comparison of adolescents with moderate to severe dysfunction with those without signs and symptoms of temporomandibular disorder and their further development to 30 years of age. Angle Orthod 2004;74(3):319-27.

Motta LJ, Martins MD, Fernandes KP et al. Craniocervical posture and bruxism in children. Physiother Res Int 2011;16(1):57-61.

Nakagawa S, Sakabe J, Nakajima I, Akasaka M. Relationship between functional disc position and mandibular displacement in adolescent females: posteroanterior cephalograms and magnetic resonance imaging retrospective study. J Oral Rehabil 2002;29(5):417-22.

Nattero G. Mal di testa mestruale. I progressi della neurologia. 33:1982.

Negoro T, Briggs J, Plesh O et al. Bruxing patterns in children compared to intercuspal clenching and chewing as assessed with dental models, electromyography, and incisor jaw tracing: preliminary study. J Dent Child 1998;65:449-58.

Nidoli G, Torno M, Boriani R et al. Il significato della stabilometria nello studio dei cambiamenti indotti da quadri disfunzionali cranio-mandibolari. Ortognat It 1993;2(6):943-53.

Nilsson IM, List T, Drangsholt M. Prevalence of temporomandibular pain and subsequent dental treatment in Swedish adolescents. J Orofac Pain 2005;19(2):144-50.

Noimana M, Gartya A, Maimona Y et al. Acupuncture for treating temporomandibular disorder. Retrospective study on safety and efficacy. J Acupunct Meridian Stud 2010;3(4):260-6.

Palla S. Mioartropatie del sistema masticatorio e dolori oro facciali. Milano: RC libri; 2001.

Pedrotti L, Mora R, Bertani B et al. Association among postural and skull-cervico-mandibular disorders in childhood and adolescence. Analysis of 428 subjects. Pediatr Med Chir 2007;29(2):94-8.

Pereira LJ, Costa RC, França JP et al. Risk indicators for signs and symptoms of temporomandibular dysfunction in children. J Clin Pediatr Dent 2009;34(1):81-6.

Pereira LJ, Pereira-Cenci T, Del Bel Cury AA et al. Risk indicators of temporomandibular disorder incidences in early adolescence. Pediatr Dent 2010;32(4):324-8.

Pereira LJ, Pereira-Cenci T, Pereira SM et al. Psychological factors and the incidence of temporomandibular disorders in early adolescence. Braz Oral Res 2009;23(2):155-60.

Perillo L, Masucci C, Ferro F et al. Prevalence of orthodontic treatment need in southern Italian schoolchildren. Eur J Orthod 2010;32:49-53.

Peroz I, Hantel H. Stress, coping and craniomandibular disorders–a longitudinal study. Z Psychosom Med Psychother 2010;56:23-33.

Pessina E, Bosco M, Collesano V. Le placche occlusali nella terapia dei disordini cervico-cranio-mandibolari. Milano: Masson, 1998.

Pizolato RA, Silva De Freitas Fernandes F, Beatriz Duarte Gavião M. Deglutition and temporomandibular disorders in children. Minerva Stomatol 2009;58(11-12):567-76.

Ragonesi M. Conservative therapy for patients with temporomandibular disorders: preliminary results. D Cadmos 2011;2:6.

Ragonesi M. Le placche occlusali nei disordini temporomandibolari: analisi dei RCT. Dental Cadmos 2008;9:45-59.

Raymond Dionne A. Pharmacologic treatments for temporomandibular disorders. Oral Surg Oral Med Oral Pathol Oral Radiol Endod 1997;83:134-42.

Restrepo C, Gómez S, Manrique R. Treatment of bruxism in children: a systematic review. Quintessence Int. 2009;40:849-55.

Rodrigues-Garcia RC, Sakai S, Rugh JD et al. Effects of major Class II occlusal corrections on temporomandibular signs and symptoms. J Orofac Pain 1998;12(3):185-92.

Schiffman EL, Ohrbach R, Truelove EL et al. The research diagnostic criteria for temporomandibular disorders, V: Methods used to establish and validate revise axis I diagnostic algorithms. J Orofac Pain 2010;24:63-78.

Seyle H. Syndrome produced by diverse nocuous agents. Nature 1936;138:42.

Shirish I., Tarun G. Temporomandibular joint: Disorders, treatments, and biomechanics. Ann Biomed Eng 2009;(37)5:976-96.

Sonnesen L, Bakke M, Solow B. Temporomandibular disorders in relation to craniofacial dimensions, head posture and bite force in children selected for orthodontic treatment. Eur J Orthod 2001;23(2):179-92.

Stockstill JW, Bowley JF, Dunning D et al. Prevalence of temporomandibular disorders (TMD) in children based on physical signs. ASDC J Dent Child 1998;65(6):438, 459-67.

Suvinen TI, Reade PC, Kemppainen P et al. Review of aetiological concepts of temporomandibular pain disorders: towards a biopsychosocial model for integration of physical disorder factors with psychological and psychosocial illness impact factors. Eur J Pain 2005;9:613-33.

Syrop S. Pharmacologic therapy. In: Kaplan A, Assael L (editors). Temporomandibular disorders, diagnosis and treatment. WB Saunders Co.; 1991. p. 501-14.

Tecco S, Crincoli V, Di Bisceglie B et al. Signs and symptoms of temporomandibular joint disorders in Caucasian children and adolescents. Cranio 2011;29(1):71-9.

Tecco S, Festa F. Prevalence of signs and symptoms of temporomandibular disorders in children and adolescents with and without crossbites. World J Orthod 2010;11(1):37-42.

Torii KA, Chiwata IB. Occlusal adjustment using the bite plate-induced occlusal position as a reference position for temporomandibular disorders: a pilot study. Head Face Med. 2010;6(1):5.

Toscano P, Defabianis P. Clinical evaluation of temporomandibular disorders in children and adolescents: a review of the literature. Eur J Paediatr Dent 2009;10(4):188-92.

Tsukiyama Y, Baba K, Clark GT. An evidence-base assessment of occlusal adjustment as a treatment for temporomandibular disorders. J Prosthet Dent 2001;86(1):57-66.

Turk DC. Psychosocial and behavioural assessment of patients with temporomandibular disorders: diagnostic and treatment implications. Oral Surg Ora Med Oral Pathol Oral Radiol Endod 1997;83:65-71.

Tzaribachev N, Weber D, Horger M. Juvenile idiopathic arthritis: the silent killer of pediatric temporomandibular joints. Z Rheumatol 2010;69(2):124-9.

Vanderas AP. Relationship between craniomandibular dysfunction and oral parafunctions in Caucasian children with and without unpleasant life events. J Oral Rehabil 1995;22(4):289-94.

Vanderas AP. Synergistic effect of malocclusion and oral parafunctions on craniomandibular dysfunction in children with and without unpleasant life events. J Oral Rehabil 1996;23(1):61-5.

Viva E, Viva E. Postura e respirazione. Roma: Marrapese Editore; 2006.

Wahlund K, List T, Larsson B. Treatment of temporomandibular disorders among adolescents: a comparison between occlusal appliance, relaxation training and brief information. Acta Odontol Scand 2003;61(4):203-11.

Wahlund K. Temporomandibular disorders in adolescents. Epidemiological and methodological studies and a randomized controlled trial. Swed Dent J Suppl 2003;(164):inside front cover, 2-64. Review.

Weiler RM, Vitalle MS, Mori M et al. Prevalence of signs and symptoms of temporomandibular dysfunction in male adolescent athletes and non-athletes. Int J Pediatr Otorhinolaryngol 2010;74(8):896-900. Epub 2010 Jun 11.

Webography

http://blog.libero.it/craniofacciale/8999411.html

http://dspace.unict.it/jspui/handle/123456789/229-Tesi-Dottorato-G.Fichera

http://spazio.libero.it/craniofacciale/

Chapter 16

Mind mapping of myofunctional therapy during developmental ages

G. Laganà, S. Loberto, G. Migliardi, P. Cozza

Introduction

Myofunctional therapy is a re-educative method aimed at achieving a balance in the orofacial muscle tone and correcting the functions of stomatognathic relevance, such as swallowing, breathing, phonetic articulation, and chewing.
Its use in growing children in combination with traditional orthodontic therapy contributes significantly to the harmonious development of the jaws and maintenance of the obtained results.
It is currently recognized that most dentomaxillofacial dysmorphisms have a multifactorial etiology. Among the environmental causes, behavioral and structural abnormalities of the orofacial muscles are the most frequent their elimination plays a decisive role in the resolution of malocclusions.
Myofunctional therapy acts on muscle function, a key element in determining the jaw growth pattern. Form and function are closely interrelated and mutually conditioned; correct function results in the harmonious development of the shape of the jaws, whereas abnormal function can negatively affect the shape of the jaws and dental arches.
Similar to functional orthodontic therapy, myofunctional therapy can be defined as physiotherapy of the orofacial muscles; it is based on the principle of neuromuscular re-education and muscular gymnastics using natural biological forces.
Speech therapists are usually the professionals who deal with the muscular and functional rehabilitation of the oromaxillofacial region; they are also responsible for the assessment of the following:

- various phases of swallowing, from the evolutionary to the involutionary
- upper airways as a region of respiratory flow management, voice resonance, and phoneme articulation
- orality as a privileged area of knowledge, relationships, communication, and evolution
- education, retraining, and learning.

Speech therapists should not only provide exercises and request repetitive practice of the exercises but also offer a personalized approach to care and treatment. Apart from understanding the origins of the problem, they support learning by selecting the most appropriate activity and the way to approach it, considering the variables that the treatment presents, such as the patient's motivation, attention span, and cooperation from family members.

A close cooperation between speech therapists and orthodontists is fundamentally important to work synergistically to achieve a common goal. Depending on the pathology to be treated, cooperation with other professionals, such as pediatricians, otorhinolaryngologists, neuropsychiatrists, and physiologists should not be overlooked.

Historical background

The development of myofunctional therapy has received significant contributions from various branches of medicine, such as from medical gymnastics to orthopedics and from orthopedic-functional therapy to physiokinesitherapy.

In fact, myofunctional therapy has no specific origin. The evolutionary stages of orthodontics are combined with the basic concepts of myofunctional therapy, together following a path of development, leading to clearly distinguished roles and competences of both disciplines.

In 1839, P.J. Le Foulon affirmed that "neither the palatine vault nor the dental arches are unchangeable in their dimensions as has been believed for a long time". Therefore, in subsequent studies, an increasing effort was made to evaluate the relationships between the "functions" that occur within the dentomaxillary complex and its "development."

During their experiments around 1893, W. Roux and J. Wolff noticed that especially during the early years of life, the growth of the jaws is closely linked to the various functions that occur within it, such as chewing, phonation, swallowing, and breathing; therefore, they developed one of the fundamental theoretical principles of functional therapy: "the function models the bone and directs its growth and also guides the direction of the bone trabeculae."

The new function model may refer to different components of the orofacial system, including the tongue, lips, muscles, ligaments, and periosteum. These structures participate in the development of a eugnathic morphological model that includes not only an improvement in occlusion and an adequate relationship between the jaws but also changes in their direction and growth so as to determine alterations in size and facial proportions.

Functional appliances appeared in orthodontic settings between the late 19th and early 20th centuries. American dentist N.W. Kingsley introduced a device called the "bite-jumping appliance," which allowed the sagittal relationships between the arches to be modified by moving the jaw and keeping it in the correct position.

French dentist P. Robin, in an article published in 1902, described the use of "monobloc" to treat the syndrome named after him, which is characterized by microgenia of the jaw, glossoptosis, and respiratory failure due to airway obstruction. According to Robin "...the base of the tongue, which falls back and downwards in front of the spine, hinders the airflow from the nose to the lungs and laterally compresses the neurovascular bundles of the neck..." The main objective was to improve the patient's breathing function. In fact, the appliance produced bimaxillary expansion and mandibular and lingual protrusion with consequent widening of the esophageal and tracheal ducts. According to Robin, respiratory gymnastics was an integral part of the treatment of glossoptosis syndrome.

Danish dentist V. Andresen adopted P. Robin's concepts in 1908 and designed a device very similar to the monobloc, which he initially called *retention activator* and he experimented with it for the first time on his daughter. The device was a bimaxillary system composed of vulcanite that was administered as a retainer to pediatric patients after a fixed treatment. During the application period, Andresen had the opportunity to observe unexpected improvements in occlusion and favorable dental movements probably caused by the activation of the masticatory system muscles. He then decided to modify Kingsley's device to one that stimulated jaw development in young orthodontic patients.

In 1934, German dentist K. Haupl used Andresen's device, which he called "activator," to obtain, according to Roux's hypothesis of functional adaptation, a clinical confirmation of functional philosophy.

From the collaboration between Andresen and Haupl in 1936, the theories of modern functional therapy were consolidated and confirmed in the book *Functional Jaw Orthopaedics*. The objective was to move the jaw forward to cause certain bone and cartilage remodeling and to modify not only the position but also the structure.

Andresen and Haupl replaced the common devices that used mechanical forces to induce the displacement of teeth with a new type of equipment with inclined planes that used functional stimuli from muscle activity. The activator, consisting of a vulcanite palatine plate with front and side inclined planes, caused contraction of the masticatory muscles, forcing the patient to close the mouth and bring the arches into contact, thereby forcing the teeth to slide and attain the appropriate position. Subsequently, the underlying bone structures were modeled according to the shape of the equipment.

After moving to Oslo, Andresen had the opportunity to develop and spread his thoughts about the therapeutic applications offered by the activator through the "Norwegian system."

The devices used in this system are activators of the muscles and blood circulation; the exploited forces result from alterations in the muscle tone and are transmitted to the teeth and jaws by inducing structural changes in the latter. Unlike that with fixed devices, functional therapy influences function and growth more than dental elements, which are considered as simple mediators between the bone and device.

In Europe, it was considered certain that the removal of obstacles would allow unrestricted growth and that the growth direction and response of the bone tissue could be affected this response could also occur in areas far from those adjacent to the teeth.

In the United States, however, there was no belief in the possibility of stimulating growth: the equipment used was exclusively mechanical and the teeth were primarily worked upon, while the neuromuscular function remained unchanged.

When it had already been spreading across Europe for several decades, functional therapy had just begun to arouse interest in America; in particular, the works of A.P. Rogers, a student of Angle's, published for the first time in 1918, which is considered the official year for the birth of myofunctional therapy.

His work focused on determining the role of neuromuscular behavior in dentoskeletal development and orthodontic therapy. His theories, which later spread across Europe, were based on the belief that orofacial muscle stimulation could partially or completely correct certain dental dysmorphisms; he stated that "...muscles are living orthodontic devices..." and should therefore be re-educated to stabilize and improve results that can be achieved by initial orthodontic treatment to create the necessary conditions for normal jaw growth. Rogers presented myofunctional therapy as an indispensable accessory and, in particular, proposed the treatment of muscle imbalances via repetitive exercises aimed at improving muscle tone.

According to these principles, F. Watry (1933) used the bimaxillary monobloc along with exercises for functional re-education of the orofacial muscles to correct the anomalies and stabilize the obtained results.

H.P. Bimler was the first to modify the classic activator by designing an elastic device called the "functional elastic modeler" in 1949. Its remarkable elasticity was meant to transfer muscular activity, particularly that of the internal pterygoid muscles, to the stomatognathic apparatus more effectively. From the results, he understood that it was possible to expand the jaws by transferring the muscular forces in a cross-sectional manner.

In Great Britain, in the 1940s, R.E. Rix, C.F. Ballard, W.J. Tulley, and E. Gwynne-Evans studied swallowing from the etiopathogenic and therapeutic perspectives.

In the 1950s, Germany was a protagonist in the development of a series of functional orthodontic theories: W. Balters and R. Fränkel designed their functional devices during this time, recommending muscle exercises as an integral part of the therapy.

In particular, Balters focused on the etiology of malocclusions considered as components of a general pathological situation. Using a new device known as "Bionator," he proposed to restore the crucial functional balance between the muscles of the tongue and the perioral muscles of the lips and cheeks. The Bionator was created following a careful study on the *dynamic space*, which is defined as the empty space inside the mouth anatomically surrounded by the lips and cheeks but functionally represented by what fills it: the tongue and the oral muscles, which are capable of producing a defined force of filling. The Bionator was constructed only after an accurate patient diagnosis using plaster models to study the occlusal relationships and analyzing the muscle function of the tongue.

According to Fränkel, some functional muscle processes are genetically determined at birth, and abnormal situations that interfere with normal function and consequent development can occur only during growth.

Referring to Roux's theory of "functional adaptation," he turned his attention primarily to the elimination of any functional or mechanical anomaly and particularly to the analysis of disorders related to lip seal, chewing, swallowing, and breathing.

Fränkel established the principle that a large proportion of dentoskeletal dysfunction on the sagittal level are derived from the functional imbalance of the "perioral muscular slings" composed of the orbicular lip and buccinator muscle fibers. Based on these concepts, he devised an apparatus known as "Function regulator."

In 1951, H. Stockfisch modified Bimler's functional elastic modeler by creating a biodynamic device called a "Kinetor," consisting of a double plate with buccinator loops, which was capable of receiving muscle impulses in the sagittal, vertical, and transverse directions.

Myofunctional therapy has also been enriched by corrective gymnastics, physiotherapy, and kinesiotherapy, which have contributed enormously to the development of methods for the rehabilitation of orofacial muscles. In particular, the "neuromuscular proprioceptive facilitation technique" was introduced and disseminated in the 1950s by M.S. Rood.

In the 1950s and 1960s, M.L. Moss and his wife L. Salentijn conducted important experiments on craniofacial growth that formed the basis of the "functional matrix theory" (1962), which remains to be one of the fundamental principles of functional orthopedic therapy of the jaws.

According to this theory, each cranial component comprises a skeletal unit and functional matrix. The functional matrix is represented by the cavities and soft tissues, which are necessary for specific functions, while the skeletal unit, represented by bones, cartilage, and tendons, serves to protect and support the functional matrix. It is evident how the functional matrix guides the development of the skeletal unit, which is, therefore, susceptible to adaptation.

On the basis of this concept, it is also clear how myofunctional therapy—a treatment aimed at rebalancing the muscular tone and re-educating the functions—must accompany orthodontic treatment. In contrast, it is also true that to re-educate a function, it is often necessary to restore the correct form; thus, orthodontic therapy may be useful in combination with myofunctional therapy.

In the 1960s and 1970s, various methods of orofacial myofunctional therapy were proposed. In the early 1960s, research on atypical swallowing by W.J. Straub received considerable attention. Straub proposed the first method of myofunctional therapy based on performing many exercises that were later used by other authors, in particular those that involve the use of elastic bands to re-educate the position of the tongue during swallowing.

In the United States, R.H. Barret and M.L. Hanson, two specialists in language pathology, were actively involved in research; they were convinced of the need for re-education of all orofacial muscles and not only of the swallowing muscles.

A.D. Garliner proposed an easy and practical method from the clinical perspective and shared his own experience in an enthusiastic and lively manner, demonstrating the effectiveness of this type of therapy; in addition, the foundation of the first institute of myofunctional therapy conducting therapeutic and research activities can be attributed to this researcher. The large number of publications, courses, and conferences has established this method as the best known in the world.

In the mid-1970s, M. Fournier's method, which is still potent today in support of the need for the re-education of orofacial functions, began to spread in France.

His method was devised on the basis of Professor M. Bouvet's previous experiences; he was a kinesiotherapist who already practiced this re-education in 1967. Fournier's re-education program was inspired by a professional collaboration with J. Delaire.

Myofunctional therapy in Europe is also based on Barret-Hanson's experiences, especially with regard to N. Maurin's French speech therapy school.
At the same time, interest in functional and myofunctional therapy spread throughout the rest of Europe.
In Italy, several schools have followed and explored this discipline: the School of Bologna with G. Maj and E. Muzj, the School of Turin with A. Hertel, and the School of Milan with O. Hoffer and E. Giannì.
Garliner himself facilitated this interest by conducting courses in Italy; he was welcomed by the most famous Italian functionalists, among these was A. Levrini, one of the first supporters of myofunctional therapy in Italy.
Important contributions of the Italian school were published by Cozza P et al. in 2002 in a text that clearly highlights the indications and benefits of the myofunctional therapy in the present day.

Presentation of the method

The aim of myofunctional therapy, as already illustrated, is to achieve proper orofacial muscle function and swallowing, breathing, chewing, and phonetic patterns. Several factors contribute to dysfunction in one of these patterns and may be related either to malocclusion or to "emotional stress," which affects the muscles. Therefore, the importance of an accurate differential diagnosis permitting establishment of a targeted, effective, and, above all, lasting rehabilitation treatment is evident.

There are essentially two myofunctional therapeutic models used worldwide:

- the American method, which belongs to D. Garliner's school, in which the main focus is on re-education of swallowing and rehabilitation of the muscles involved. It is based on the use of auxiliary devices, elastic bands placed on the tip of the tongue and held by it to make contact with the retro-incisive papilla, to help the patient better understand the correct position
- the European method, which belongs to M. Fournier's French school, in which the use of elastic bands is not recommended because they would prevent the correct proprioception of the palate by the tongue and, vice versa, the proprioception of the tongue by the palate mucosa. Re-education of breathing is critical in Fournier's method, which Garliner did not analyze.

Both these methods have proven to be extremely effective and have produced excellent results till date.
The method we present summarizes the features of both methods, focusing on the concept of proprioception, an essential element in the learning of the correct neuromotor patterns at conscious and unconscious levels.
The therapeutic cycle comprises a series of sessions conducted by the clinician and routine daily exercises by the patient.

Exercises should be performed for a minimum of 10 minutes and a maximum of 30 minutes without tiring the patient. The progressive increase in time and effort in performing therapeutic practices is essential.
Therapeutic sessions should have a maximum duration of 20–30 minutes. Approximately 10 sessions are recommended for 5–6 months with regular follow-ups throughout the following year (treatment may differ considerably from case to case).
The therapeutic cycle consists of a 3–6-month active re-education phase, followed by a maintenance phase of the same duration; in total, the myofunctional re-education program occurs over approximately 1 year.
In the active phase of therapy, we usually start by assigning proprioception and muscle strengthening exercises for the orbicular, buccinator, and masticatory muscles. Simultaneously, we initiate proprioception and mobilization exercises for the tongue, continuing progressively with specific exercises for all the oral functions, beginning with the nasal respiratory re-education.
It is good to assign only three or four exercises at a time, providing the patient with worksheets (for example, for lingual posture training and swallowing) and reminders.
During the maintenance phase, in which the sessions are conducted less frequently, the state of automation of the neuromuscular corrections is evaluated.
The timing of the intervention, whether before, during, or after orthodontic therapy, depends greatly on the type of treatment planned.
Indeed, it is necessary to restore anatomical normality, where this is severely altered by malocclusion, until it is not possible to provide sufficient detection points or a front seal to establish a proper swallowing pattern.
Examples include severe skeletal problems, inadequate upper jaws, and uni- and bilateral crossbite, in which intercuspation does not allow proper masseter activity.

Aims of myofunctional therapy

Myofunctional rehabilitation is a treatment aimed at rebalancing the tone of the orofacial muscles and re-educating the postures of stomatognathic interest to achieve appropriate recovery of the functions (Fig. 16.1).
The aim of this therapy is the re-education of the functions of swallowing, articulating, chewing, and breathing via the elimination of bad habits and detection of dysfunctions that need correction.
The speech therapist first evaluates, and using observation and testing, collects detailed information that helps the imbalance and muscles involved in the incorrect execution of a certain function.
The first step, therefore, is identification of the dyskinetic and deficient muscles.
Dyskinetic muscles do not have suitable mobility and/or control over their kinetics; the restoration of their function is achieved using a proper learning pathway. This type of anomaly primarily affects the functions of the tongue. In the most serious cases

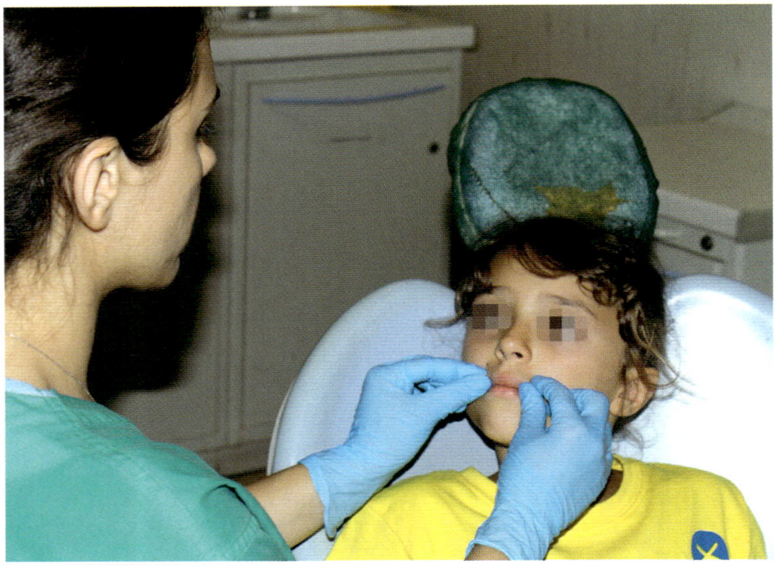

Figure 16.1 Examination. Clinical examination includes evaluation of the tone of each region and analysis of the functions of the stomatognathic apparatus.

of motor immaturity—for example, when the patient is instructed to slide the tip of the tongue on the surface of the palate—having no points of reference, the tongue is thrusted out of the mouth or moved from cheek to cheek.

Deficient muscles are those that do not have an adequate tone, and their restoration is achieved by muscle strengthening via specific exercises. This type of abnormality is often found in the orbicular muscle of the lips, which is frequently hypotonic on preliminary examination, both in oral breather patients and in patients with atypical swallowing. When the patient is asked to maintain a lip seal, the muscles contract to keep the lips in contact.

Some muscle components in the orofacial complex work in synergy or antagonism with other muscular structures to perform a movement or function. For these movements or functions to be executed properly, the strength developed by these muscles must be equivalent. Therefore, when this does not occur, the synergy of movement should be achieved. This type of problem often occurs in mouth-breathing patients in whom the upper lip is usually hypotonic and clinically short while the lower lip is hypertonic. Therefore, the recovery of correct postures is the final stage of therapy, in which balance and automation of functions replace previous habits.

Learning pathway

Myofunctional therapy is fundamentally based on two essential concepts that are closely interdependent: proprioception with the acquisition of a correct oral motor pattern and muscle re-education.
Proprioception is the means by which it is possible to replace poor postural and functional neuromuscular patterns with correct patterns by acquiring awareness of the dysfunction.
This type of sensitivity provides information about the position of the body or its parts in relation to the external environment and the position of one part of the body in relation to the others; it also allows the adjustment of body posture or parts.
The information is collected by specific receptors called proprioceptors that are located in the muscles, tendons, and joints.
The proprioceptors are mechanical receptors, i.e., receptors that are stimulated by the stretching of the structures in which they are located.

The proprioceptors are as follows:

- neuromuscular fuses, mainly distributed in the small muscles (responsible for the finest movements), which indicate the current length and any variation in the length of the muscle fibers
- *Golgi's tendon organs*, mainly in the periarticular ligaments, which signal the tension to which the tendons are subjected during muscular contraction.

The spatial position of the jaw, for example, is regulated by these specific receptors that are present in the masticatory muscles themselves and in the periarticular ligaments, which communicate the state of tension of muscles and tendons to the central nervous system, allowing a continuous adjustment of the tone of gravitation and anti-gravitation muscles.
Proprioceptive sensitivity is essential for the re-education of functions and a correct oral motor scheme because it represents the instrument that allows replacement of both static and dynamic incorrect neuromuscular patterns with correct movements.
In addition to the stimulation of the reflected arches, the stimulation of the proprioceptive pathways, both conscious and unconscious, allows the achievement of posture and praxis automation.
The reacquisition of *conscious proprioceptive sensitivity* allows the patient to be aware of the posture he is adopting.
The development of *unconscious proprioceptive sensitivity* is even more important because it stimulates the pathway of cerebellar reflex to respond to a given impulse following a correct neuromuscular pattern.
Furthermore, the improvement of the epicritical sensory capacity of the oral mucosa, particularly at the labial, lingual, and palatal levels, leads to greater control of the lingual posture according to the hypotheses outlined previously.

The exercises that are assigned retrace the movements that comprise a function or determine a posture. In the beginning, they will be performed voluntarily; thereafter, they will become progressively automatic and then reflexes.
For instance, this applies to the re-education of atypical swallowing: the first step is to determine the area where the tip of the tongue rests on the palate, at rest, during swallowing, or at the level of the retro-incisive papilla. The contact with the tip of the tongue at this level generates proprioceptive impulses to the central nervous system, which are necessary to establish the new neuromuscular pattern related to its position.

Muscle re-education is aimed at achieving the correct muscular tone of the orofacial region via strengthening exercises and muscle relaxation techniques and aims to optimize the strength, size, and tone of the muscles. To some extent, it can be considered a means by which a function or postural attitude can be modified.

The re-education of functions and rehabilitation of orofacial muscle tone can be performed in two ways: classical and reflex re-education.

- Classical, voluntary, or cortical re-education is based on the conscious learning of function and correct postures through the repeated execution of exercises that slowly and progressively conditions the subcortical regions, thereby allowing the automation of the correct praxis and postures. D. Garliner and M. Fournier proposed a functional re-education based on the continuous and ongoing repetition of specific exercises aimed at progressive conditioning of the incorrect neuromuscular pattern, both consciously and unconsciously. The exercises assigned repeat partially or completely the movement of a certain muscle in the execution of a praxis: for example, the raising of the tongue toward the hard palate to "imitate" the second phase of swallowing.
  This method obviously requires a great deal of cooperation on behalf of the patient, who often does not understand the usefulness of the assigned task.
- Reflex re-education uses various sensitive stimuli, which allow the development of a particular sensitivity related to the control of the lingual muscles.

Reflex re-education was developed from the "proprioceptive neuromuscular facilitations technique," conceived by M.S. Rood for the orofacial rehabilitation of patients with hypotonic or spastic muscles.
Proprioceptive neuromuscular facilitation has been defined by M.S. Rood as "the activation, facilitation, and inhibition of muscular activity, voluntary and otherwise, through the reflex arc." The means used in this method stimulate the sensitive receptors to obtain a motor response through the reflex arc. Thus, results can be achieved without the need for voluntary cortical control by the patient. For example, the application of a thermal-type sensitive stimulus at the level of the retro-incisive papilla draws the tip of the tongue into the same position without active patient participation.

The proprioceptive impulses induced by counter-resistance exercises and stretching facilitate the muscular response, in addition to the exteroceptive receptor stimuli, following cortical stimulation.

Currently, the technique of proprioceptive neuromuscular facilitation is employed not only for the correction of imbalances in the orofacial muscles and re-education of swallowing but also for the treatment of algo-dysfunctional craniocervicomandibular syndromes. The most important advantage of this type of rehabilitation is that active patient cooperation is not required. Moreover, teaching a new type of swallowing at a subcortical involuntary level seems more reasonable because the swallowing function is a subcortical function. Conversely, the patient gaining awareness regarding the correct postures and praxis is an important step and undoubtedly means that re-education that is exclusively unconscious is clearly more elaborate.

The combination of the two methods in myofunctional therapy is probably the best solution and ensures the best results for automation of the new neuromuscular patterns (Fig. 16.2).

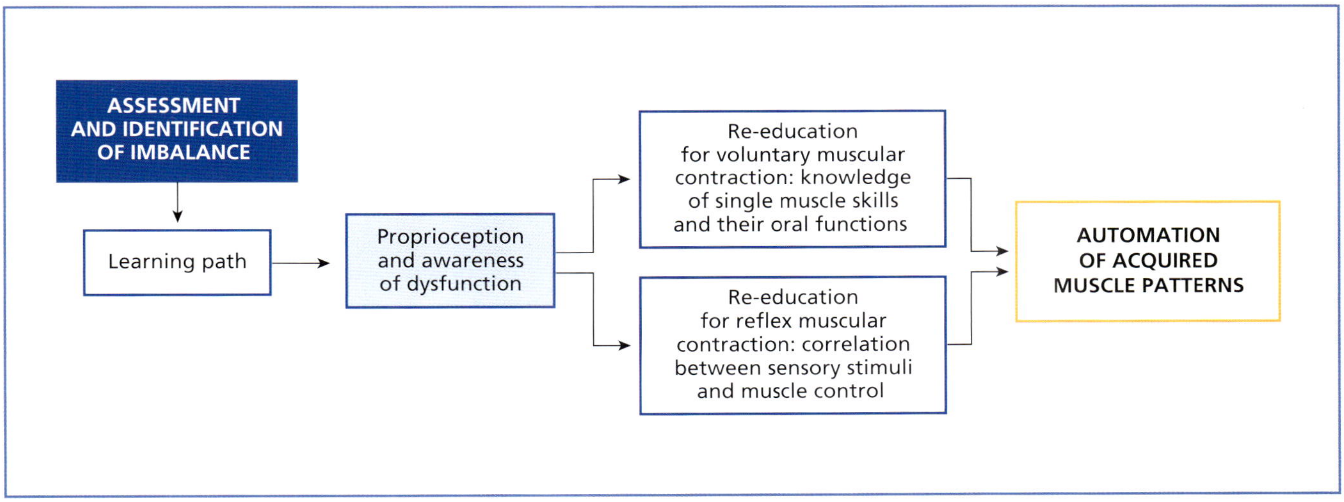

Figure 16.2 Mind mapping of myofunctional therapy.

Breathing

There are three muscular regions involved in respiratory function: nasal muscles, diaphragm, and peridiaphragm muscles. Their correct function is essential to purify, heat, filter, and humidify the air that will then be ready to reach the lungs.

Imbalance assessment and identification

The examination of the patient in relation to the type of breathing is performed in three stages: preliminary interview, clinical observation at rest, and functional examination.
The *preliminary interview* with the parents aims to gain information on the patient's breathing habits: to understand if he/she frequently adopts an open-mouthed position, snores, wets the pillow at night, complains of dryness of the oropharyngeal mucosa, has obstructive diseases of the upper respiratory tract, or has previously visited an otorhinolaryngologist or an allergist.
Clinical observation at rest is used to assess the type of upper airway breathing by simply observing the patient during the preliminary interview with the parents and examining his/her habitual attitude while listening and looking around.

It is important to note, however, that having an open-mouthed postural behavior does not mean experiencing mouth breathing. Therefore, the tests described below are necessary to confirm or invalidate the preliminary assessments. Clinical observation at rest is supplemented by an assessment of the presence or absence of the following features in a mouth breather:

- an increase in the face length, especially at the middle and lower third
- the appearance of the lips, which are incompetent and often characterized by dryness of the semi-mucosa covering them
- the closed-mouth posture, which appears evidently forced and accompanied by a contraction of the perioral and mental muscles
- the nasal morphological structure with small and visibly hypofunctional or obstructed nostrils or even a deviated nasal septum
- a malocclusion that is frequently characterized by a transversal contraction of the upper jaw with a broad or regular mandibular arch
- continuous atypical swallowing
- the typical presence of the *facies* of the mouth breather with dark circles, labial incompetence, and narrow nostrils.

Respiratory capacity is then examined via a *functional examination* that is carried out using various tests, which may distinguish between dysfunctional and structural mouth breathers:

- *Gudin's nostril reflex*: the examiner instructs the patient to close the mouth, and with the thumb and forefinger of the hand, occludes both nostrils for a few sec-

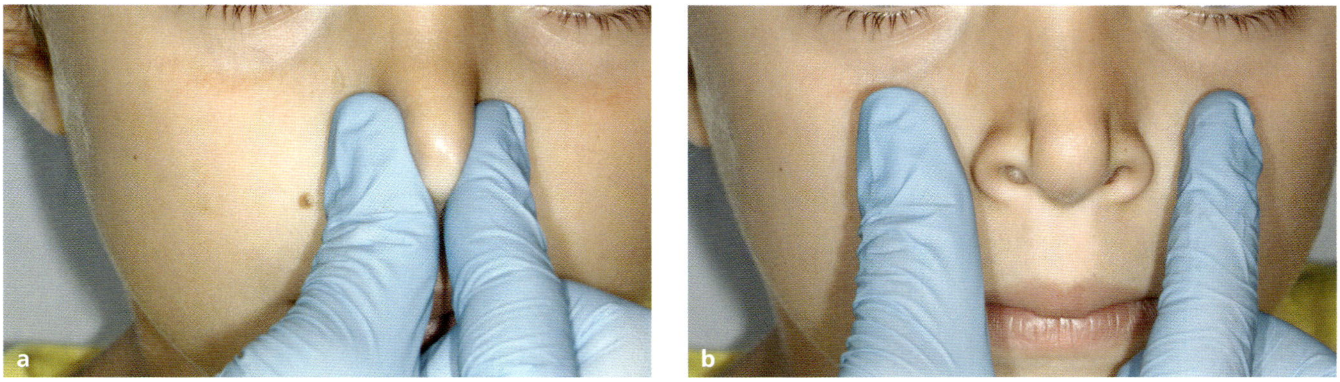

Figure 16.3 Gudin's nostril reflex: the reflex response consists of an immediate dilation of the wings of the nose.

onds, subsequently releasing the fingers. The reflected response is an immediate dilation of the wings of the nose, leading to the collection of air. In mouth-breathing patients, there is either no movement at the nostril level or this movement occurs very subtly, accompanied by the opening of the mouth, which has the equivalent purpose of inhaling air (Fig. 16.3)

- *Rosenthal test*: the patient is instructed to take approximately 15 slow and deep breaths, inhaling and exhaling with the mouth closed. The examiner monitors the heart rate and the patient's pulse and invites them to stop in case of dizziness, a sign of an initial state of alkalosis. The test is negative in the absence of respiratory fatigue, mouth opening, or increased heartbeat. The test is positive when the patient makes an evident effort during the test, opens the mouth before the end of the test, or experiences an increase in heartbeat
- *mirror test*: the patient is instructed to breathe with the mouth closed, placing a small mirror under his nostrils. Thus, we can evaluate the extent of opacification of the mirror at the passage of the exhaled air and whether this is symmetrical between the two nostrils. For this purpose, it is practical to use the *Glatzel* mirror, on which concentric circles are drawn to evaluate the quantity of exhaled air from the two nostrils and, therefore, the expiratory capacity.

For diaphragmatic activity, the type of prevalent respiration is assessed, referring to the lower tract of the airways.
The respiratory mode at the level of the lower airways should be observed simply by moving the hand on the thoracic–abdominal region while the patient is instructed to inhale and exhale normally. Possible findings are as follows:

- apical respiration
- costodiaphragmatic respiration
- abdominal respiration.

The nose and its functions

Learning pathway

Proprioception and dysfunction awareness

The following series of exercises aims at achieving the physiological competence of the nasal respiratory function.

Nose blowing. Many mouth breathers have no perception of their nose, unable to even blow it, thereby preventing the passage of normal airflow at this level. To start breathing re-education, it is essential that the nose is pervious. Therefore, they must learn to blow one nostril at a time and then both at the same time. It is important to explain to them that blowing the nose with the tip of the tongue in contact with the palatine papilla is much more effective.
After achieving patency of the nostrils, some exercises aimed at emptying the retro-pharynx and the paranasal sinuses of mucus, which can be easily eliminated through swallowing, are indicated.

The candle. This consists of expirations through the nose in front of the flame of a burning candle. The patient is able to appreciate the movement of the flame, which can be visually associated with the escape of air from the nose.

The mirror. A mirror is placed below the nostrils of the patient, who is encouraged to exhale through the nose. With the use of the mirror, the patient is able to appreciate the airflow, which can be seen on the fogged-up glass (Fig. 16.4).

The tissue paper. A small sheet of tissue paper rests on the nostrils. The patient is invited to inhale deeply in order to hold the paper in this position.

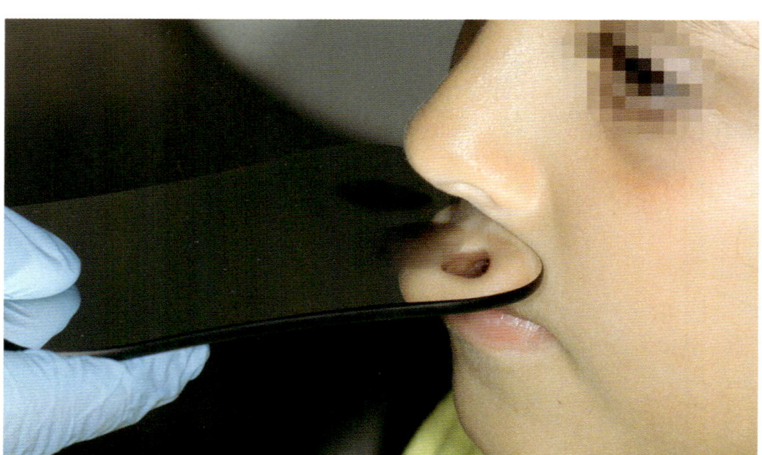

Figure 16.4 The mirror: the patient can notice the airflow, which can be visualized due to the fog on the mirror.

The dragon. A thin straw is gently inserted into one nostril, with the other end immersed in a container of water. The patient is instructed "boil" the water.
In this phase, it is very useful to perform nasal washes in the morning, evening, and before the exercises using commercially available devices.

Voluntary muscle re-education

The dilating muscles of the nostrils, which are responsible for opening the nostrils during inhalation, are often hypotonic; for this reason, muscle toning is indicated.
Binary gymnastics consists of inhaling and exhaling acts that are performed alternately by the right and left nostrils. In particular, the thumb of the right hand is placed on the right nostril to stop the airflow, and then the patient is instructed to exhale and inhale through the left nostril. The same steps are performed with the left nostril (Fig. 16.5).

Reflex muscle re-education

The objective of this rehabilitation process is to achieve normal nasonasal respiration at rest during the day and night as well as during physical exertion. During the act of inhalation, the nostrils dilate and the wings of the nose open. To stimulate this opening, M. Fournier suggests the following methods of facilitation:

- correct posture of the tongue on the palate, which can sometimes cause opening of the nose wings, so that re-education of swallowing may be sufficient to rehabilitate the patient to a nasal respiration, particularly when the Rosenthal test is negative in the preliminary analysis
- the *smile exercise*, which favors the opening of the wings of the nose by stretching the labial commissures and upper lip (Fig. 16.6)
- exercises for the *toning of the upper lip and lower lips*; the stretching of the upper lip causes opening of the wings of the nose.

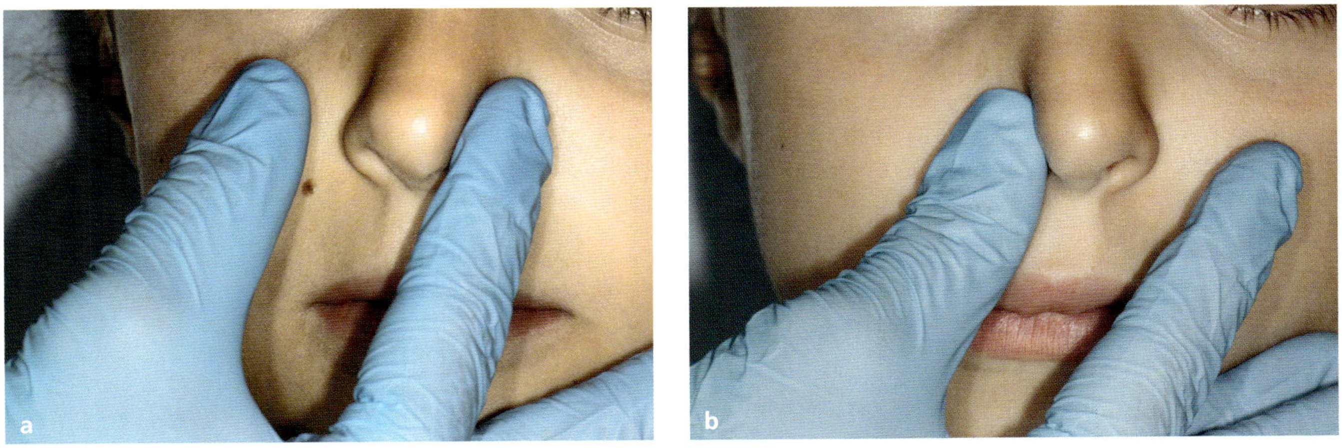

Figure 16.5 Nostril gymnastics: development of nasal respiratory function and respiratory proprioception.

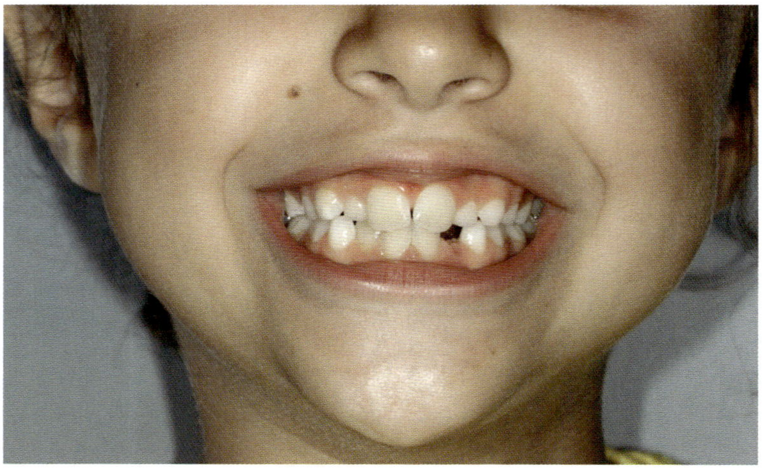

Figure 16.6 Smile exercise: toning the buccinator muscle and opening the wings of the nose.

The diaphragm and its functions

Learning pathway

Proprioception and dysfunction awareness

These exercises are prescribed to help the patient establish a better awareness of breathing and refine the perception of the sensations during breathing. A patient exhibiting apical respiration must gain familiarity with costodiaphragmatic respiration to achieve adequate re-education. For this purpose, the re-educator proposes himself as a model so that the patient learns to imitate the correct execution of the following breathing movements.

Vital respiration. Performing nasal inhalation, followed by a "sound" exhalation through the oral cavity (sc…sc…sc).

The "sniff test". The patient is asked to perform three small consecutive nasal inhalations; this causes the movement of the diaphragm.

The balloons. The patient is asked to inflate a balloon, and placing an already inflated one on the abdomen, to concentrate on the movement of the diaphragm during inhalation and exhalation. This exercise improves proprioception at the diaphragmatic level and tones the buccinator muscle by training nasal inhalation.

Automation of acquired neuromuscular patterns

The automation phase of the newly learned mechanism involves a correct function at rest and during normal daily activities.
The pattern is programmed with frequent sessions initially to allow the patient to become familiar with the newly acquired skills and then have less frequent sessions during the maintenance phase, which is aimed to automate the mechanism, bringing it to the subconscious level.

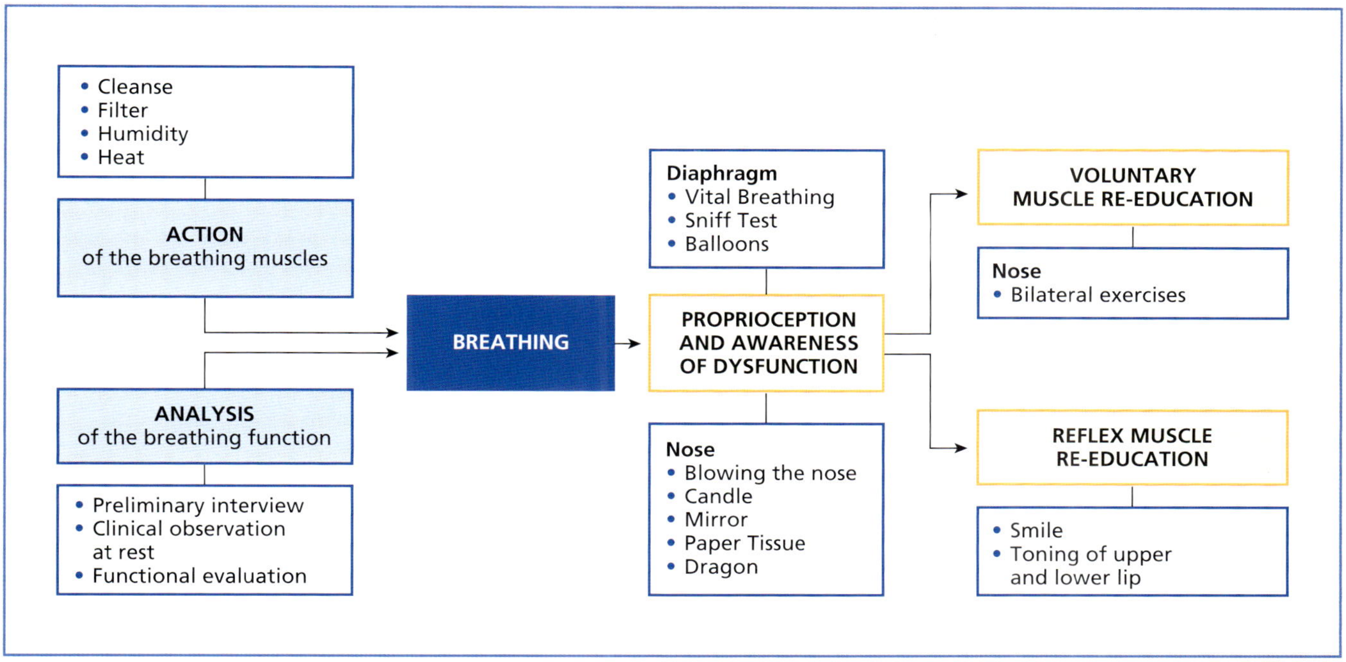

Figure 16.7 Mind mapping of the respiratory function.

The maintenance phase is considered complete when the patient, after acquiring good voluntary control of the learned patterns, is able to perform the respiratory function correctly and spontaneously. This will occur if the function is re-educated in association with other oral functions: the orofacial region must be considered *as a whole*, and each function acts as a catalyst for the automation of the other (Fig. 16.7).

Chewing

The masticatory muscles are responsible for mandibular movements and therefore, play an important role during masticatory function:

- the masseter, temporal, and internal pterygoid muscles determine the elevation of the jaw, thereby achieving occlusal contact
- posterior bundles of the temporal muscle produce retraction of the jaw
- external pterygoid muscles determine protrusion of the jaw
- external pterygoid muscle of the balancing side and internal pterygoid muscle of the working side are responsible for the lateral movement of the jaw.

The contraction and tone of the masticatory muscles also play a determining role on the various modes of growth of the facial bones.
Variation in the tone of some muscle groups can, therefore, allow regulation of bone growth, converting potentially pathological conditions into harmonious facial development patterns.

Imbalance assessment and identification

Many patients, particularly young patients, are unable to easily perform mandibular movements.
The tests should be conducted by performing the simplest movements.

- *Opening and closing*. The maximal mandibular excursion must be of approximately three fingers, and such movements must be performed without lateral deviations or circular jaw movements. Abnormal mandibular movements occur more often during this exercise. The closure should be as linear as possible
- *Left and right laterality*. The patient is instructed to move the chin alternately to the right and left. The lateral excursion of the jaw is usually asymmetrical, but the differences between the two sides should be slight
- Protrusion. The patient should carry the chin forward; in this movement, deviations in laterality should not be observed.

In the evaluation of these movements, a resistance can be applied to the mandibular displacement; for instance, it is possible to place a closed fist and exercise a force in a direction opposite to that exercised by the patient while moving the jaw. Thus, the strength produced by the masticatory muscles can also be verified.
For each movement, the following considerations are needed:

- the path followed by the jaw: whether it is straight or abnormal or if it has lateral or curved deviations
- motor maturity: the movement may be normal, rigid, or difficult to perform (although in younger patients, it is likely that immediate nonperformance of the required movement is because of a lack of comprehension)
- possible evocation of pain
- presence of joint sounds.

These two incidences can be identified in very small children, even if the feedback in adult patients is more common.

Learning pathway

Proprioception and dysfunction awareness

Given the frequent difficulty in understanding the exercises, particularly among children, the re-educator must propose himself as a model to imitate and explain the exercises to be performed as appropriate for the patient's age. The exercises for proprioception of the masticatory muscles are aimed at the automation and awareness of the correct position of mandibular resting.
These exercises coincide with those for toning of the masticatory muscles performed according to the principle of counter-resistance: the proprioceptive impulses induced by this type of work facilitate the muscle response as a result of cortical stimulation.

Voluntary muscle re-education

Muscle gymnastic exercises should be assigned on the basis of the preliminary analysis of the masticatory muscle region. The following two types can be distinguished:

1. *muscle toning exercises*
2. *muscle relaxation exercises.*

1. *Muscle toning exercises*

Protrusion. The patient is instructed to push the jaw forward, encouraging him to observe the movement in front of a mirror, so that any errors can be corrected. Generally, it is difficult for the patient alone to notice possible lateral deviations in the movement of mandibular protrusion, but he can be aided by the re-educator who, by correcting the patient, accustoms him to perform the movement properly.
At this point, isometric contraction is performed, i.e., a static counter-resistance with the purpose of "releasing" muscle tensions and toning the protrusion muscles specifically (particularly the external pterygoid muscle). The patient is instructed to push the jaw symmetrically and exercise resistance to this movement, opposing his fist at the chin level for a duration of 5 seconds. The development of two equal but opposite forces results in a static situation in which the jaw is immobile. A complete relaxation is performed immediately after, and the patient then repeats the exercise. If pain is experienced during this movement, the breadth of the mandibular progression should be limited, and the duration of the isometric contraction should be reduced to 1 second. According to M. Fournier, "a free jaw must be obtained in 15 days" (Fig. 16.8).

Retrusion. Still with an isometric working mode, the patient is instructed to move the jaw back and to oppose resistance to this movement, exerting a traction in the posterior–anterior direction, which is achieved by placing an index finger as a hook inside the lower arch. The contraction should be continued for 3–5 seconds, after which the muscles are released.

Retrusion part 2. Starting with the occlusion arches, the patient is instructed to withdraw the jaw, sliding the teeth of the lower arch on those of the upper arch. By positioning the fingers in association with the condyles, it is possible to sense their displacement in the posterior direction. The exercise must be repeated 10 times.

Laterality. During these movements, there is a difficulty in understanding for the patient, who is often able to move the jaw only on one side, continuing to move it from the same side even when the opposite movement is required. Therefore, using a mirror, the patient should visually monitor the exercise. Occasionally, the amplitude between the right and left side excursion can be asymmetrical; in such cases, recourse is made to muscle work in counter-resistance, in which the patient perform insufficient lateral movement and is instructed to place his hand at the level of the body of the jaw, thereby exerting a force that is opposite to the mandibular movement for 5 seconds; the combination of the two forces must determine a situation of static jaw.
Care should be taken to not conduct asymmetric muscle work for an extended period of time to avoid a condition of rigidity of the counter-lateral side. In general, a period

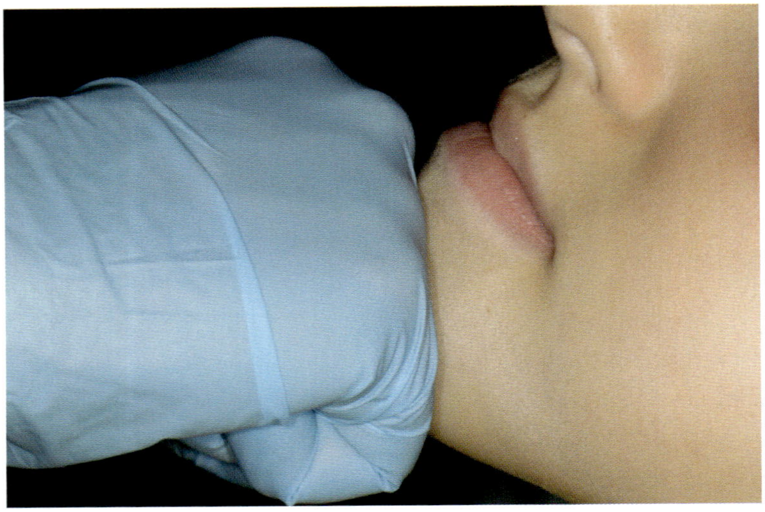

Figure 16.8 Protrusion: toning the masticatory muscles.

of 2 weeks is sufficient to attain balance, following which the patient should continue practicing on both sides.

Opening. In this type of mandibular movement, it is possible to identify deviations in the lateral direction, of which the patient must become aware. The exercise involves the application of the counter-resistance principle, realized through of lowering of the jaw, to which a force exercised by the fist of the patient himself is exerted in the opposite direction below the chin, which instead pushes up in an attempt to close the mouth. The isometric contraction is maintained for 5 seconds before moving to a state of muscle relaxation, followed by a new contraction.

Closure. The patient is instructed to close his mouth and oppose this movement by leaning his fingers on the lower incisors, thereby facilitating counter-resistance work. The contraction should be maintained for approximately 5 seconds.

Closure part 2. The jaw-lifting muscles can be stimulated by simply closing the patient's mouth until tooth contact is achieved, which must be maintained for 10 seconds while strongly clenching the teeth. The contraction of the masseters must be felt by the patient by positioning the fingertips at their level.

Chewing. This consists of chewing each bite of food (preferably of hard consistency) for 10 seconds before swallowing. Chewing must take place on one side, alternating sides each time. It is essential to create competence and strength of the posterior seal (masseter) to abandon the atypical dysfunction (lips or tongue).
This is one of the first exercises in the rehabilitation pathway of oral functions.

Masseter exercise. With open lips, comfortable and firm, the patient is instructed to tighten and relax the masseters while performing nasal respiration.

2. *Muscle relaxation exercises*

Passive exercises. These are performed by the re-educator and consist of massages and mobilizations.
During passive massages, the patient is placed in a dorsal decubitus position while lying on a bed, and the re-educator massages the masseters and temporal, pterygoid, and digastric muscles of the periarticular region and scalp to achieve complete relaxation of these regions.
Conversely, passive mobilization of the jaw consists of reproduction of all mandibular movements, this time guided by the re-educator, which is provided to achieve a sufficient state of muscle distension.
Food with a hard consistency should be introduced gradually because the use of solid food (hard, dry, and fibrous) is a stimulus for the mastication reflex that helps develop and coordinate all masticatory muscle chains.
The chewing function should be alternated involving premolar and molar teeth, and should be carried out with continent and inactive closed lips along with the possibility of comfortable nasal respiration.
The continued use of feeding bottles, which is often linked to a wider picture of relational educational disorder, can hinder the child's food emancipation; without training of the masticatory muscles, the child will continue to prefer soft foods.
Moreover, some references of "occlusal stability" should not be overlooked; this itself is the starting point of the correct speech therapy approach in order to help the child evolve toward adult oral functions. From a chronological point of view, the passage from an infant swallowing to the physiological one begins to be observed with the exchange of the first dental elements (Fig. 16.9).

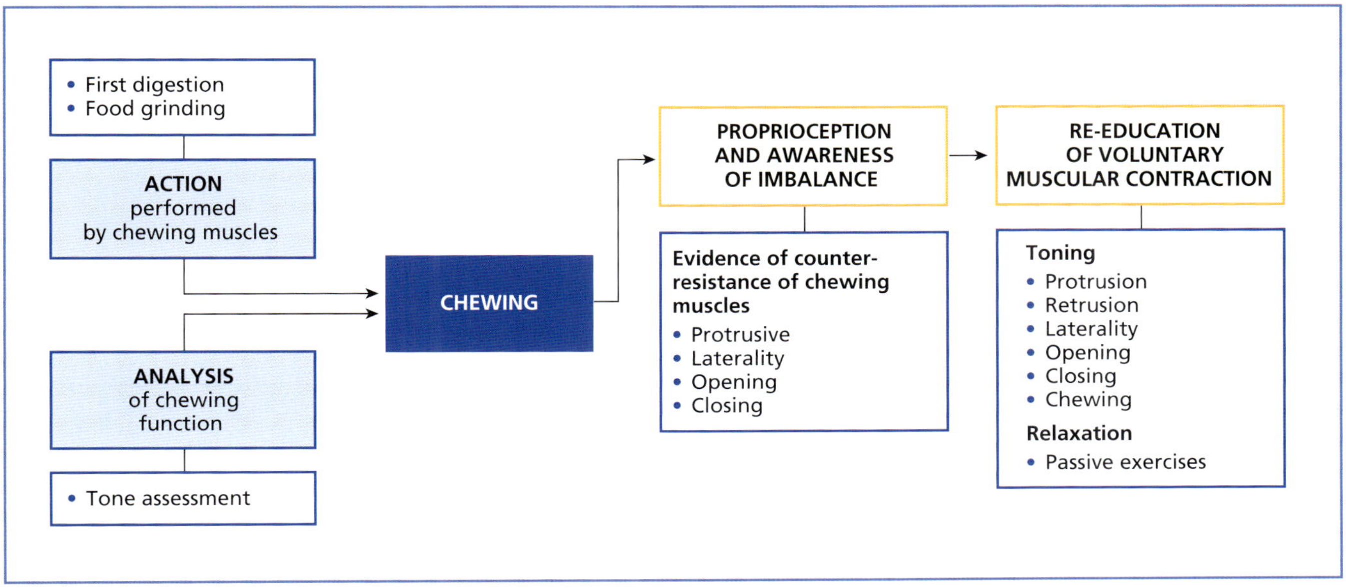

Figure 16.9 Mind mapping of the masticatory function.

Swallowing

Swallowing is a very complex act, both voluntary and involuntary, that is performed thousands of times a day; when it is properly carried out, it performs the function of transporting food and saliva from the mouth to the esophagus, eliminating nasal secretions, cleansing the auditory tubes, and transporting waste substances from the esophagus and oropharynx with a protective mechanism.

Imbalance assessment and identification

To evaluate the act of swallowing, the examiner, lowering the lower lip of the patient during inspection, instructs him/her to swallow trying to slightly open the lips. It is desirable to wait for the patient to do so spontaneously, avoiding conditioning him/her during the test, especially in the case of children.
In addition to experience, the most important parameters in the evaluation of swallowing and orofacial muscular imbalance are observation of perioral muscles, verification of the type of laryngeal elevation, verification of mylohyoid activity, and verification of masseter and temporal contraction.
Instrumental methods may be used to manifest swallowing activity, especially when there are no spaces between the arches or because the hyperactivity of the perioral muscles prevents the person from opening their lips.
The Payne technique allows greater precision in detecting the position of the tongue at rest and during the act of swallowing or phonation. This technique involves positioning of a fluorescent substance on the tip of the tongue (and subsequently on other tongue regions), which marks the areas of the oral cavity with which it comes into contact. By illuminating the oral cavity with an ultraviolet lamp, the marked areas are revealed, thereby highlighting the position taken by the tongue during swallowing. The following positions are possible:

- contact with the retro-incisive papilla
- contact with the palatal surface of the upper incisors
- contact with the lingual face of the lower incisors
- anteriorly, laterally, or posteriorly inserted between the arches.

However, the position of the tongue during swallowing often coincides with the position usually attained at rest.
To evaluate the status of the lip muscles, the examiner relies on observation. The examiner may also attempt to part the lips with the thumb and forefinger, considering the degree of resistance offered by these muscles, but a secondary contraction reflex may still be present.
Note that during swallowing, the lips should be slightly in contact, without any muscle contraction.
The following cases may occur:

- normal lip tone

- clenching/hyperactivity of the lips during swallowing, which occurs following the need to create an anterior seal, typical of a swallowing dysfunction
- closure of the lips with contraction of the mental muscle, which occurs when the lips alone are unable to create such a seal.

The lips and their functions

Learning pathway

Proprioception and dysfunction awareness

In some patients, abnormalities in lip posture can be observed; these abnormalities can be corrected by proprioceptive training combined with exercises to strengthen the labial muscle.

In opening. The patient is instructed to smile with the teeth clenched, with a symmetrical opening of the lips to their maximum extension, without any protrusion of the chin. The position should be maintained for 5 seconds.

In closing. The patient is asked to keep the lips closed in the normal position and correct any faults observed with the help of a mirror. The corrected position should be maintained for 5 seconds.

Voluntary muscle re-education

The purpose of exercising the muscles around the lips is to obtain good lip closure without visible contraction. The following exercises can be performed:

1. *muscle toning exercises*
2. *muscle relaxation exercises*.

1. *Muscle toning exercises*

This series of exercises is indicated if partial or complete hypotonia of the lips has been observed during clinical examination. To perform such exercises, it is advisable to use an *oral screen*, which is a removable elastic device that consists of a vestibular intraoral screen and an external hook.

Traction on the ring. The patient must hold the oral screen to the lips while exerting a traction on the ring with sufficient intensity to extract the device with a "popping" sound. This exercise strengthens all the facial muscles, in particular the labial muscles, and must be repeated as many times as possible.

Practice in front of a mirror. Positioned in front of a mirror, the patient must try to swallow with the oral screen in the mouth with the lips contracted and the tip of the tongue positioned on the palate. This exercise should be repeated several times a day at every instance of swallowing, even while digesting meals and drinks.

Retention exercise. This exercise is particularly indicated in cases of weak lip muscles. The patient must hold the oral screen actively using the lips, as if giving a kiss. Remodeling of the arches will be achieved owing to the pressure exerted on the teeth by the device, as well as retrusion of the frontal group.

Sucking the oral screen. This exercise generates a depression in the oral cavity, and the contraction of the cheek muscles adapts the screen to the dental arches and gums, favoring their remodeling into the ideal form. If the patient fails to create the right depression in the mouth, the labial and cheek muscles will stay away from the jaws. The exercise consists of an active phase, during which depression and muscle activity cause the arches to adopt an ideal shape, and a passive phase, which allows the tongue to adopt the correct position by favoring the remodeling of the arches.

Licorice exercise. A licorice wheel is attached at the end of a 30-cm-long string. The patient is instructed to stand with the torso bent at 90° to the legs and to hold the other end of the string only with the lips and pull it toward the mouth in order to approach the licorice. By increasing the weight to be lifted, the patient will have to progressively increase the amount of muscle exercise. A licorice wheel will then be added every 3 days.

Grimace exercise. This exercise aims to tone the inner part of the orbicularis muscle, thereby developing forces with a predominantly horizontal direction. The patient inserts two fingers into the corners of the mouth and is instructed to exert traction toward the outside; this force must be opposed by contracting the inner part of the orbicularis. The traction is maintained until muscle fatigue or pain is experienced or for a maximum of 15 seconds.

The labials. This exercise is indicated in cases in which the patient can barely attain a good degree of lip closure while pronouncing labial phonemes. He/she will have to repeat the syllables MA, BA, and PA in front of the mirror several times in succession and with force, paying particular attention to the reciprocal movement of the lips approaching each other. This exercise can also be useful in cases where only one lip moves during pronunciation; the patient is asked to pronounce such phonemes, striving to use only the hypotonic or less mobile lip.

Kiss/smile exercise. The patient is instructed to alternate the forward contraction of the lips (kiss position) with the retraction of the lips by stretching them over the dental arches and thrusting them toward the inside of the mouth (smile position) (Fig. 16.10).

Right/left exercise. The patient should push the corner of the mouth forward as much as possible to the left and then to the right.

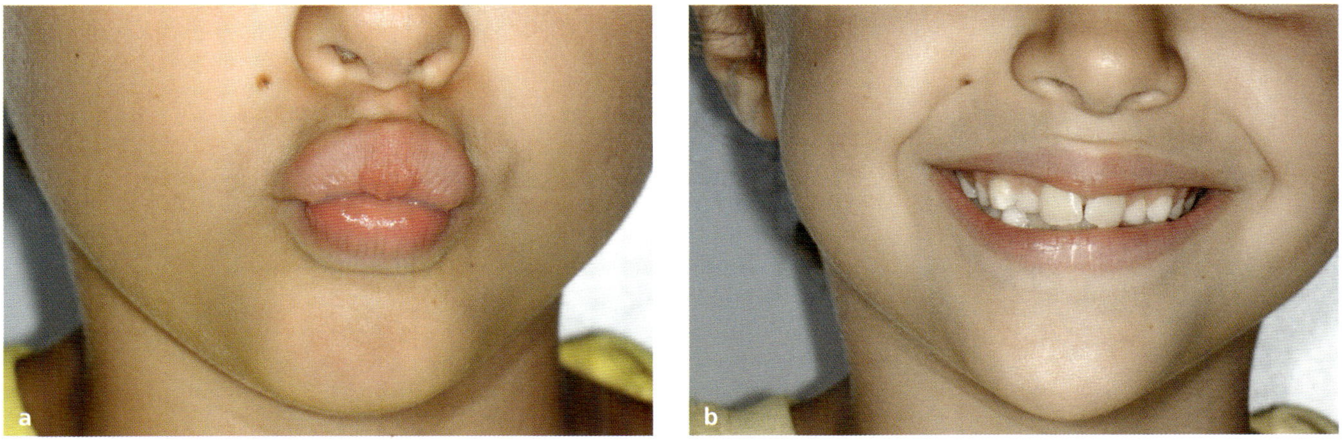

Figure 16.10 Kiss/smile exercise: toning the orbicularis oris muscle.

Muscle relaxation exercises

These exercises are indicated if there is a partial or complete state of hypertonia of the lips.

The guard dog. The patient is asked to raise the upper lip, displaying the gums and thus imitating a growling dog. This exercise should be performed with occluded arches.

Lipstick exercise. The lower lip should be positioned as high as possible on the upper lip and slowly return to its resting position, pressing the upper lip. The patient must make the movement in occlusion (Fig. 16.11).

Reflexive muscle re-education

Active massage. With the index finger resting transversely just below the base of the nose, the patient massages the upper lip downwards, rotating the finger until it reaches the upper margin. The mouth is semi-opened, and all muscles must remain relaxed (Fig. 16.12).

Passive massage. This exercise is performed by the clinician or by a second person who stands behind the patient, places the tips of his/her thumbs on the lips and makes circular movements, associated with a slight compression directed toward the center, down, and front.
In association with this, the clinician—still positioned behind the patient—holds the upper lip with the thumbs and forefingers of both hands at one corner of the mouth. The clinician then stretches this from top to bottom, alternating the right and left hand and moving the fingers gradually toward the opposite side. However, dysfunctions in contraction of the lips cannot be resolved with any specific exercise if the tongue does not manage to swallow autonomously without the "help" of the lips (Fig. 16.13).

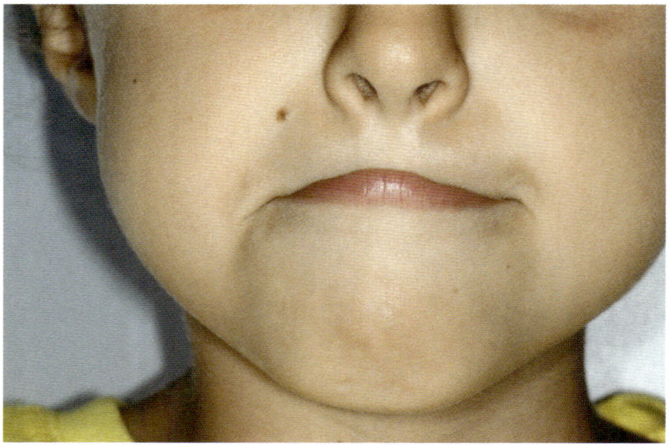

Figure 16.11 Lipstick exercise: muscle distension, recovery of the proprioception of the mandibular protrusion, and extension of the upper lip.

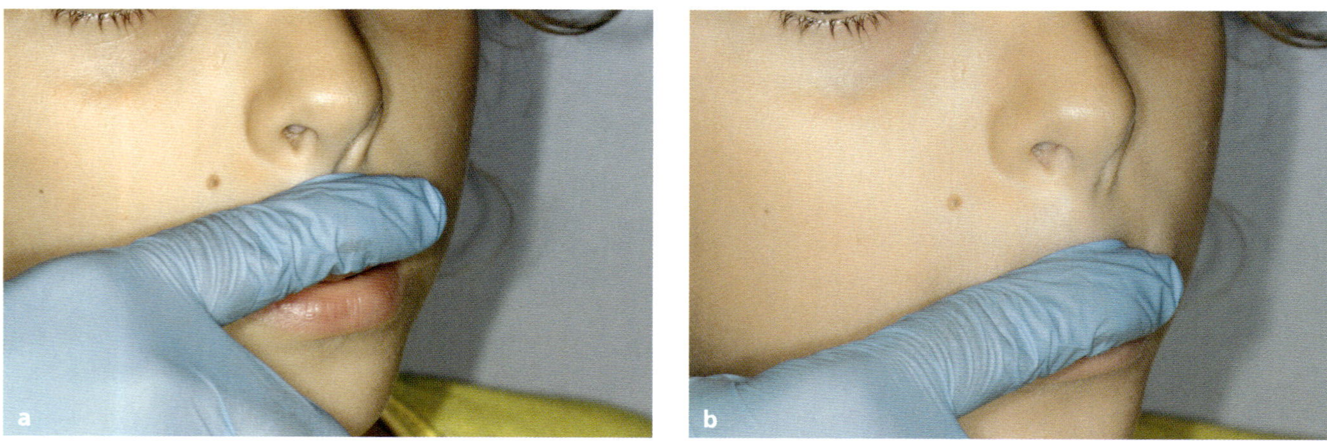

Figure 16.12 Active massage: muscle relaxation for upper lip hypertonia.

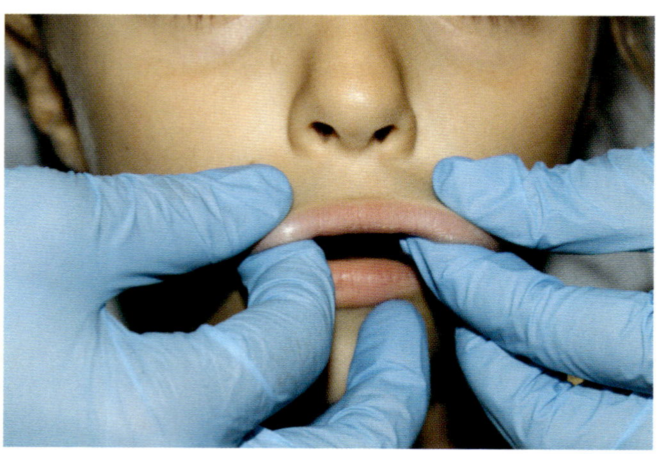

Figure 16.13 Passive massage: muscle relaxation for hypertonia of the orbicularis oris muscles.

The tongue and its functions

Learning pathway

Proprioception and dysfunction awareness

Proprioceptive work is fundamental as it allows the patient to become aware of the morphology of the oral cavity, particularly the palate. The sensations from the receptors of the palatine mucosa and that of the anterior two-thirds of the tongue reach the central nervous system, thereby modifying the lingual posture and the initial position for swallowing.
It is important that the change in the swallowing mode is based initially on the conscious and voluntary learning of the learned principles, and then gradually becomes reflexive.

The tip of the tongue. The patient is encouraged to slide the tip of the tongue across the palate, from right to left and from back to front and vice versa. He/she is also asked to distinguish between smooth and ridged areas of the palate; the latter is recognizable with the use of a mirror.
In *proprioceptive neuromuscular facilitation*, the motor response evoked by various types of stimulations is independent of conscious learning. The neuromuscular response is achieved through the stimulation of proprioceptors as well as of the free nerve endings and receptors that regulate the tactile and thermal sensitivity of the tongue. The method developed by M. Rood was later modified by M. Falk and M. Wells and comprises the following exercises.

Cooling. The exercise consists of the application of a thermal stimulus (the extremity of a small ice cylinder). The muscular response evoked consists of the reflexive elevation of the tongue toward the stimulated zone. This exercise also aims to improve the sensitivity of the mucosa, muscle tone, and lingual posture (Fig. 16.14).

Brushing. A superficial stimulus acting on the free nerve endings is used to assess the tactile sensitivity of the tongue. The lateral edges of the tongue protruding outside the oral cavity are brushed using a thin brush for approximately 10 minutes. The result is evident after a short time and consists of an increase in the muscle tone of the tongue and a simultaneous reduction in its volume.

Voluntary muscle re-education

The myofunctional re-education of the tongue can be achieved with the following exercises:

1. *muscle gymnastics*
2. *functional recovery*.

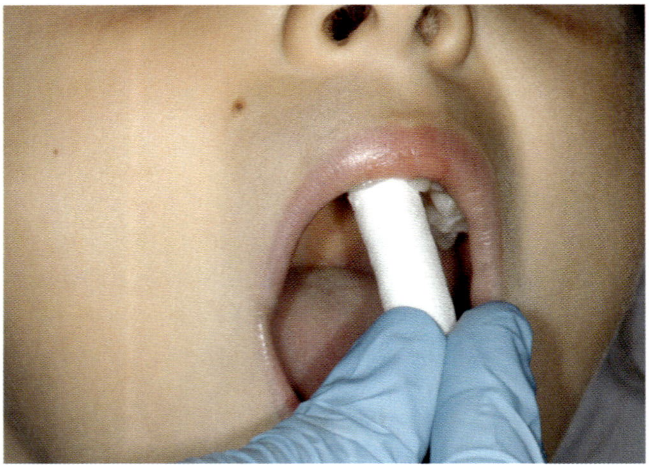

Figure 16.14 Cooling: proprioception of the retro-incisive papilla.

1. *Muscle gymnastics exercises*

The re-education to correct swallowing should be accompanied by the simultaneous restoration of the balance between various muscles of the tongue. The strength developed by the protrusive muscles of the tongue must be equal to that developed by muscles responsible for the opposite movement as the strength of the muscles that contract the tongue transversely must be equal to that exerted by the muscles that lengthen it. In fact, lingual posture is greatly influenced by muscular tone because swallowing and pronunciation of certain phonemes cannot occur without adequate lingual muscle tone.
Therefore, the aims of rehabilitation of lingual muscles are the toning and strengthening of the tongue.

Toning of the tip of the tongue

Tongue depressor. The patient is instructed to push the tip of the tongue against a wooden tongue depressor placed in front of the mouth and to oppose the push by applying a counter force to the depressor, thereby exerting counter-resistance. The tongue must be positioned horizontally to the tongue depressor so that the tip performs the work and not the body or the posterior portion of the tongue (Fig. 16.15).

"R". This exercise involves pronouncing the letter "R" for as long as possible, making the tip of the tongue vibrate against the anterior portion of the palate.

Toning the body of the tongue

The gallop. This exercise involves imitating the noise produced by a horse galloping. The tongue, initially positioned with the tip in contact with the palate, is then moved away, performing a large movement toward the oral floor.
If the tongue is not well toned, the snap is weak; sometimes the performance of this exercise is tiring for the patient; in such cases, it is necessary to reduce the amount of muscular work.

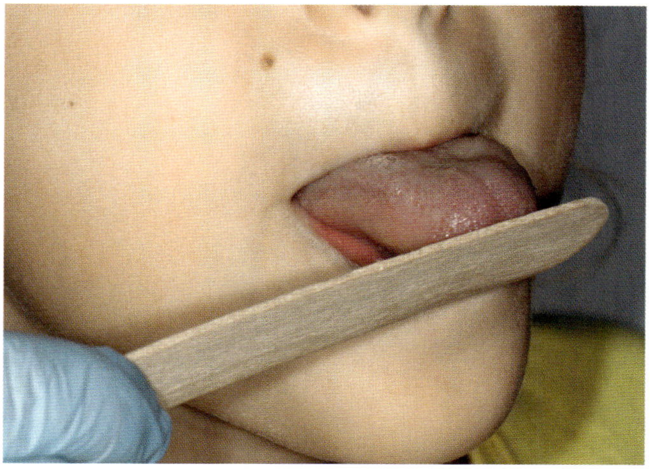

Figure 16.15 Tongue depressor: toning of the tip of the tongue and contraction of the external pterygoid muscles.

Improving the ability to transversally restrict the tongue

Some patients place the tongue so wide transversally that it remains imprinted with the indentation of the teeth at the edge. In these individuals, the presence of open lateral and posterior bite is often observed.

The tip. The patient is instructed to poke the tongue outside the oral cavity, make it pointed, and contract it along the whole of its length.

2. *Functional recovery exercises*

These exercises are performed for posture, elevation, tongue mobilization, and re-education of swallowing and phonation.

Exercises for lingual elevation

"Behind the teeth" (or "the papilla" or "L") exercise. The patient is encouraged to rest the tip of the tongue in contact with the retro-incisive papilla and to open the mouth without changing the position of the tongue. It is important that the patient does not feel pain in the oral floor and slightly limits the opening of the mouth. The mouth must remain open for approximately 3 seconds, and the patient should breathe through the nose (Fig. 16.16).

Exercises for mobilization of the tongue

In the preliminary analysis, a difficulty in moving the tongue and controlling the movements—which may seem imprecise, not fluid and slow—can be observed.

Chocolate. Chocolate is placed on the patient's lips and he/she is asked to lick it by moving their tongue along the lip surface. The exercise should be repeated by performing the movement slowly.

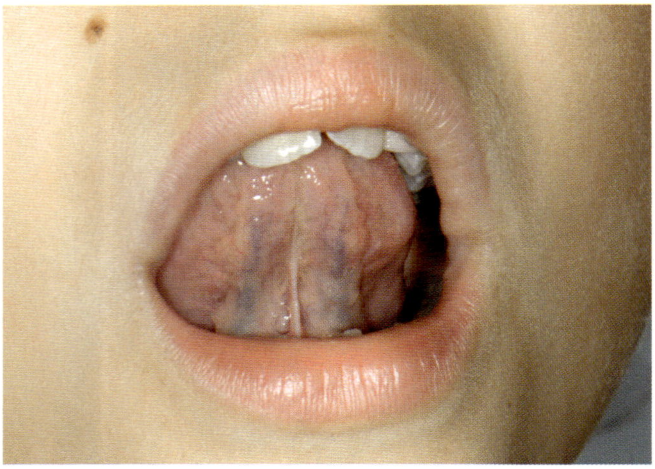

Figure 16.16 "Behind the teeth" exercise: elevation of the tongue and improvement of the proprioception of tongue and palate.

The movements. The patient is asked to move the tongue toward the tip of the nose and toward the chin, move it laterally toward the right and left cheek, slide it inside the fornices and on the inner surface of the cheeks, touch the oral floor with the tip of the tongue, and slide it along the surface of the palate, first making contact with the lingual surfaces of the teeth and then along the palatine suture from front to back.

Exercises to improve discriminatory tactile sensitivity of the tongue and palate

Because the tactile sensitivity of the tongue and palatal mucosa is important in controlling the lingual posture, these exercises are indicated if abnormalities are observed in the tongue's position at rest and during swallowing.
They coincide with the exercises of "*cooling*," "*brushing*," and "*pressure*" of proprioceptive neuromuscular facilitation.

Lingual posture re-education exercises

After working on proprioception and indicating the correct position of the tongue, with the tip resting on the "ridged part" of the palate, the patient is instructed to take this position; minor corrections are usually necessary, and it is useful if the patient becomes visually aware of this position with the help of a mirror.
The following two exercises belong to Garliner's method and involve extensive use of elastic bands (orthodontic elastic bands for intermaxillary traction) for the rehabilitation of posture and swallowing. According to some authors, however, the interpositioning of a foreign body between the tongue and palate hinders or prevents proprioception at a conscious and unconscious level.

One elastic band. An elastic band is placed on the tip of the tongue, which is brought into contact with the palatine ridges. The patient is instructed to move the arches into occlusion, keeping the elastic band in position (Fig. 16.17).
The exercise should be performed first with open lips and then with closed lips.

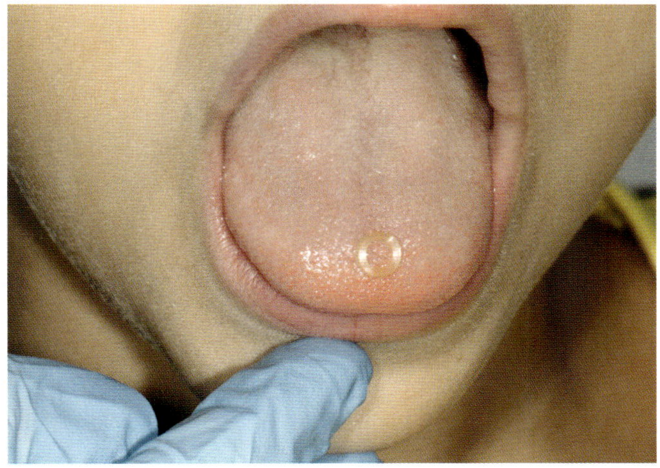

Figure 16.17 Elastic band: re-education of the posture of the tongue and contraction of the masticatory muscles.

Two elastic bands. Using two elastic bands, after a few days of exercising with one elastic band and when the tongue is freed from the lips to swallow, one band is placed between the lips and the other on the tip of the tongue. The patient is instructed to close the lips without any visible effort and bring the tongue into contact with the retro-incisive papilla; the arches are in slight occlusal contact. This position should be initially maintained for 5 minutes; the time should be gradually increased to 60 minutes until, within 2–3 months, the resting position is automatically assumed.
This is usually achieved in 5–6 months.

Exercises for swallowing re-education

It is essential that the patient is aware of the differences between his/her swallowing pattern and the physiological swallowing pattern.

The following three points should are important for proper swallowing:

- support of the tip of the tongue on the retro-incisive papilla: after performing proprioception exercises, this rule is usually easily understood
- arches in slight occlusal contact
- no contraction of lips, cheeks, and chin.

A mirror can be used to clearly indicate errors during the patient's usual swallowing. Once the initial position of swallowing is understood through proprioception and lingual posture re-education exercises, the subsequent movements of the tongue during swallowing should be explained to the patient.

"Tongue on the palate" exercise. After achieving a good performance in all previous exercises, the motor sequence is completed by encouraging the patient to bring the dental arches into contact and swallow saliva, keeping the position unchanged; this increases patient awareness of the pressure exerted by the back of the tongue on the back of the palate. The clinician should check that there is no contraction of the buccal and mental muscles; moreover, closing of the lips must not be accompanied by hy-

percontraction of the lips so that the clinician can open them without effort to check that the position of the tongue is maintained and there is no tongue interposition in any space between the arches.
The following exercises belong to Garliner's method; similar to the previous ones, they involve the use of elastic bands that must be placed on the lingual apex and brought into contact with the palate, resulting in the complete act of swallowing, after which the clinician must check the position of the elastic bands. If the positions are different from the initial one, it means that the patient has not maintained the correct position but has moved more or less markedly depending on the distance of the elastic bands from the previous position.

Reflex muscle re-education

The aim of this re-education is to combine the correct pattern with the swallowing of liquids and solid food.

The sips. This exercise involves the swallowing of liquids that pose more difficulty in execution than that of saliva owing to the amount of material present in the oral cavity. The patient starts by introducing only small amounts of water into the oral cavity. If the patient is unable to place his tongue against the palate, the water tends to come out of the mouth. Therefore, he/she will be forced to contract the orbicularis oris strongly and suck the liquid. This exercise should be performed initially at lunch and dinner for 5 consecutive times; gradually, the patient should be able to increase the amount of water introduced into the mouth and swallowed, and perform this exercise even outside of mealtimes. Finally, solid food should also be properly swallowed, combining bilateral alternating of chewing and proper swallowing.

Automation of acquired neuromuscular patterns

Automatic swallowing consists of achieving correct function at the conscious level, at rest, and during food intake.
Myofunctional treatment during mixed dentition allows good functioning of the oral system to be achieved while waiting for the completion of teeth growth and development. This is accomplished with a favorable orientation of growth and because of the decisive cooperation of the patient. It also offers opportunities for establishing a harmonious relationship between the various facial components with the definite objective that growth can proceed in a coordinated manner (Fig. 16.18).

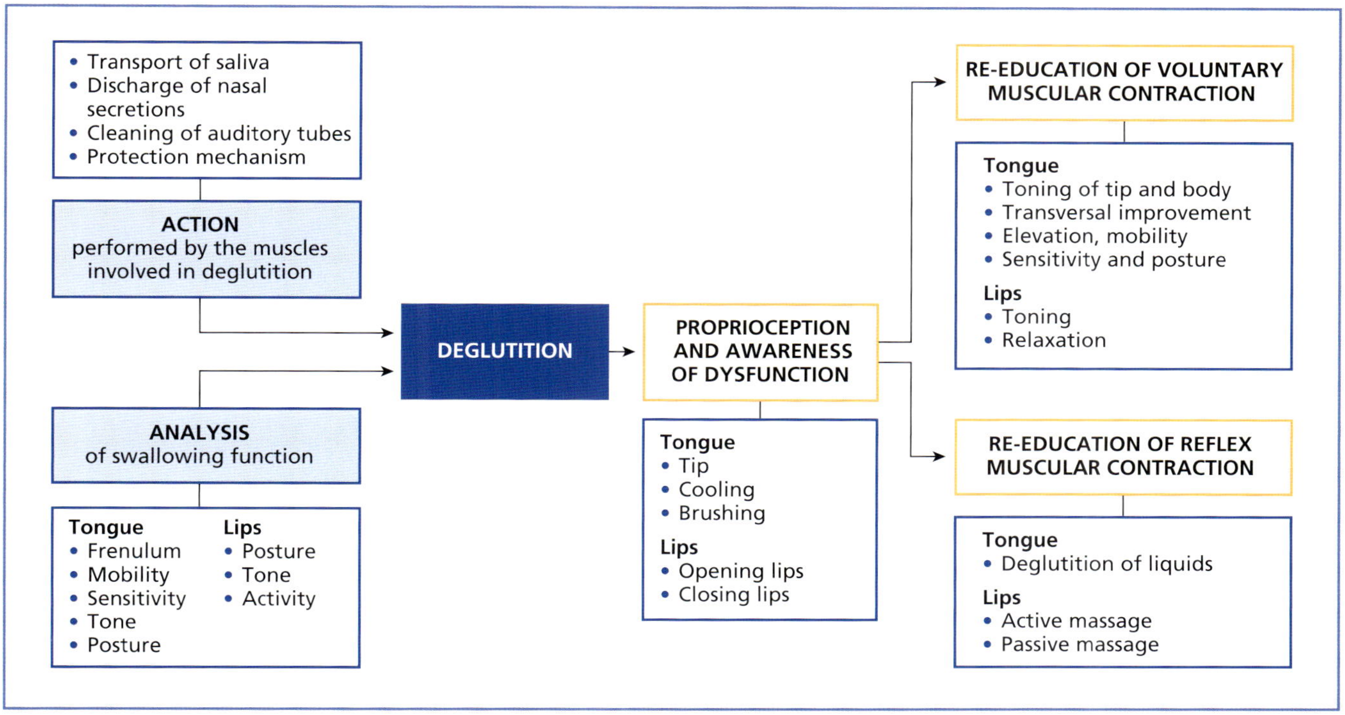

Figure 16.18 Mind mapping of the swallowing function.

Phonation

The phonatory function is responsible for the production of sounds and articulation of words and phonemes and is the fundamental basis for communication.

Correct function is achieved with the anatomical–functional integrity of the organs involved, such as the tongue, palate, soft palate, lips, jaw, and occlusion. In particular, physiological functioning of the following muscle regions is necessary to properly perform phonatory activity:

- orbicularis oris muscle (intrinsic and extrinsic bundles)
- intrinsic (longitudinal lower, longitudinal upper, and vertical) and extrinsic (genioglossus, hyoglossus, palatoglossus and styloglossus) lingual muscles.

Changes in the phonetic articulation give rise to *dyslalia*, which may be the direct consequence of an orofacial muscular imbalance, therefore, requiring a broader diagnostic framework.

When *orofacial muscular imbalance* occurs, the "destructive dysfunctional force" is usually low.

Conversely, if the "dyslalic weight" is greater, a more suitable rehabilitation course should be used.

Imbalance assessment and identification

The logopedic evaluation of phonetic articulation is conducted through observation during spontaneous speech, reading, and repetition. It involves administering specific tests that analyze the production of individual sounds.
Analysis of the *distinguishing features* allows further data to be obtained on the state and functionality of the muscle regions that require treatment.

Particular attention should be paid to the following:

- interdentality (i.e., the tongue is interposed between the upper and lower incisors)
- laterality
- lingual elevation during the alveolar and palatal phonemes /gl, /ci, and /gi/
- lingual regression during the velar phonemes /k/ and g/
- harmonization of lip, lingual, and mandibular movements.

In the case of the evaluation of dyslalia as a symptom of orofacial muscular imbalance in relation to dental malocclusion, phoneme production is not considered as much as the *articulatory pattern* that can be dysfunctional for the orofacial balance, although unperceived at the auditory level.
On the other hand, some dyslalias (similar to some sigmatisms), although audibly detectable, have no harmful effects on the dental shape.
Therefore, it is necessary to evaluate the functionality of orofacial muscles to verify the presence of a deviated oral pattern in relation to other functions, such as resting position, swallowing, breathing, and the parafunctions.

Learning pathway

Proprioception and awareness of dysfunction

During the pronunciation of some phonemes, the tongue is placed precisely at the level of the palate in the same position as that adopted at rest. If this does not happen, the articulation of some phonemes, and in particular of the palatal and sibilant sounds, is somewhat altered.
For the correct articulation of palatals (L, N, D, T, and R), the tip of the tongue must rest on the palatine ridges. The point of support is minimal for the pronunciation of L and progressively wider for N, D, and T, for which the contact between the tip of the tongue and palate is achieved at the level of the palatal mucosa, from canine to canine.
R is defined as multi-vibrating, and for its correct pronunciation, the tip of the tongue must produce repeated vibrations coming into contact with the alveolar region, however, avoiding contact with the dental elements.
In general, S and Z are considered to be correctly articulated when the lateral edges of the tongue are in contact with the molars, the back is flattened, and the tip remains free and not in contact with the lingual surface of the dental elements of the anterior group, thereby allowing the exit of air.

The pronunciation of the "SC" sound involves the same type of lingual support, the only difference being that a groove is formed on the back of the tongue in the anterior–posterior direction. An important distinction also concerns the position of the lips: during the pronunciation of sibilants, the labial commissures are slightly stretched; however, during the pronunciation of the "SC" sound, the lips are not distended but rounded.

Voluntary muscle re-education

Considered as an oral function, phonetic articulation is closely associated with swallowing because, in rehabilitation, these functions often have associated abnormalities in a *cause–effect* relationship.
Therefore, muscle gymnastic exercises related to the lingual re-education for phonatory activity are similar to those already described for swallowing.

Muscle reflex re-education

In proprioceptive neuromuscular facilitation, the motor response evoked by various types of stimulations is independent of conscious learning of postures and praxis. The neuromuscular response is achieved through the stimulation of proprioceptors as well as of the free nerve endings and receptors that regulate the tactile and thermal sensitivity of the tongue.
The pressure applied to the back of the tongue during the "*pressure*" exercise results in the movement of the tongue in a posterior direction; this movement reflects the pressure exerted by the tongue during the pronunciation of the "S" sound.
The pressure applied on the margins of the tongue increases muscle tone, accompanied by a decrease in tongue volume. This exercise is particularly useful in cases of hypotonia and hyposensitivity of the tongue.
The pressure exerted by a finger at the level of the oral floor, at the insertion of the geniohyoid muscle, before the patient swallows, induces the tip of the tongue to position itself against the palate after the removal of the stimulus.

Automation of acquired neuromuscular patterns

The re-education of dyslalia in the presence of an orofacial muscular imbalance requires a proprioceptive approach and myofunctional therapy aimed at recovering the competence of the musculature involved in the deviated motor pattern.
In pediatric age, work on the articulation of phonemes is motivating for the patient and improves the level of patient cooperation, as the child has a better understanding of the need for good phonetic skills rather than correction of posture and swallowing (Fig. 16.19).

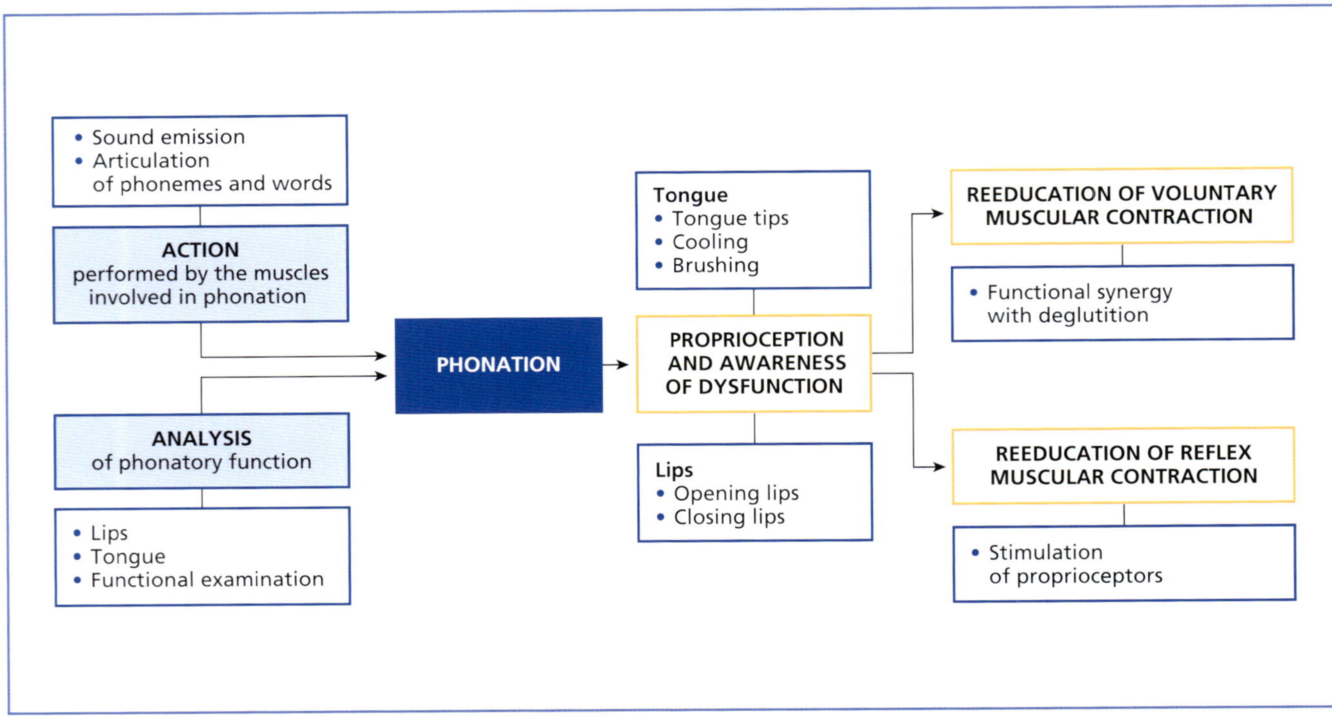

Figure 16.19 Mind mapping of the phonatory function.

References

Andresen V, Haupl K, Petrik L. Funktionskieferorthopaedie. Muenchen: Barth; 1957.

Asbell MB. A brief history of orthodontics. Am J. Orthod Dentofacial Orthop 1990;98:206-13.

Ballard CF. Some observation on variations of tongue posture as seen in lateral skulls radiographs and their significance. Tr Europ Orthod Soc 1955;31:155-58.

Balters W. Il Bionator e i suoi limiti. Milano: Ed. Pro Stomatologia; 1967.

Barret RH, Hanson ML. Oral Myofunctional disorders. St. Louis: C.V. Mosby; 1974.

Bimler H. Die elastischen Gebissformer. Zahnaerztl Welt. 1949;4:499-503.

Bondevik O. Viggo Andresen: a pioneer in orofacial orthopedics. J Orofacial Orthop 1997;58:181-89.

Carels C, Van der Linden FPGM. Concepts on functional appliances' mode of action.

Am. J. Orthod Dentofacial Orthop 1987;92:162-8.

Chauvois A, Fournier M, Girardin F. Rieducazione delle funzioni nel trattamento ortodontico. Verona: Ed. C.I.S.C.O; 1994.

Cozza P, Fidato R, Germani C, Santoro G, Siciliani G. La deglutizione atipica. Mondo Ortodontico 1992;17:141-59.

Cozza P, Polimeni A, De Toffol L. Manuale di terapia miofunzionale. Roma: Elsevier; 2002.

Falk M, Wells M. Treatment of deviant swallow patterns with Neuromuscular Facilitation. Int J Oral Myo 1977;1:27-9.

Fraenkel R, Fraenkel C. Orofacial Orthopedics with the Function Regulator. Basel: Karger; 1989.

Garliner D. Myofunctional Therapy. Philadelphia: W.B. Saunders; 1976.

Gwynne-Evans E. The orofacial muscles: their function and behaviour in relation to the teeth. Eur Orthod Soc Trans. 1947.

Hoffer O. La terapia gnatortopedica con apparecchiature rimovibili. Minerva Stomat 1959;6:375.

Hotz R. Application and appliance manipulation of functional forces. Am. J. Orthod Dentofacial Orthop 1970;58:459-78.

Kingsley N.W., A treatise on Oral Deformity with Appropriate Preventive and Remedial Treatment. New York, Appleton & Co, 1880.

Le Foulon PJ. Orthopedic denture. Gaz. Hop. 1839.

Leighton BC, Howard RD. Orthodontics – the last hundred years. Br. Dent. J. 1981;151:14-19.

Levrini A. La terapia miofunzionale. Milano: Ed. Masson; 1997.

Moss ML, Salentijn L. The primary role of functional matrices in facial growth. Am J Orthod Dentofacial Orthop 1969;55:566-77.

Moyers RE. Manuale di Ortodonzia. Scienza e tecnica dentistica. Milano: Ed. Internazionali; 1991.

Muzj E. Terapia ortopedica funzionale della faccia. Bologna: Ed. Cappelli; 1950.

Rix RE. Deglutition and Teeth. Dent Record 1946;66.

Robin P. La glossoptose. Paris: G. Doin Ed.; 1928.

Rogers AP. Muscle training and its relation to the orthodontia. Int J Orthod 1918;4:555-77.

Rood MS. Neurophysiological mechanisms utilize in the treatment of neuromuscular dysfunction. Am J Occup Ther 1956;10:220-4.

Rosenthal G. Manuel des exercices respiratoires. Rapporteur Congres de Liège. 1904-1930: Ed. Alcan.

Roux W. Beitrage zur morphologie der functionellen ampassung. Arch Pathol Anat 1870;9:120-58.

Schindler O. Manuale operativo di fisiopatologia della deglutizione. Torino: Ed. Omega; 1990.

Stockfisch H. Der Kinetor in der Kieferorthopaedie. Die Praxie des polyvalenten bimaxillaeren Apparates und seine rationelle Technik mit Plastik-Fertigteilen. Heidelberg: A. Huethig; 1966.

Straub WJ. Malfunction of the tongue. Part III. The abnormal swallowing habit: its cause, effects, and the results in relation to orthodontic treatment and speech therapy. Am J Orthod Dentofacial Orthop 1962;48.

Subtelny JD. Malocclusion, orthodontic corrections and orofacial muscle adaption. Angle Orthod. 1970;40:170-201.

Tulley WJ. Adverse muscle forces – Their diagnostic significance. Am J Orthod Dentofacial Orthop 1956;42:801-14.

Watry F. Die physiotherapeutische Behandlung der Kieferdeformitaten. Fortschr Orthod 1933.

Wolff J. Uber die innere architecturen der knochens. Virchows Arch Anat 1870;50:389-453.

Chapter 17

Obstructive sleep apnea in pediatric patients

E. Cretella Lombardo, G. Laganà, P. Cozza, A. Polimeni

Definition

The term sleep-disordered breathing (SDB) refers to breathing difficulties that occur during sleep. SDB is a breathing disorder characterized by partial or complete obstruction of the upper airways, which interrupts pulmonary ventilation and oxygenation, thereby worsening sleep quality.

There is a considerable variability in the symptoms of patients affected by SDB, which is directly proportional to the resistance that the upper airways offer to air passage when they are obstructed.

SDB represents a continuum of respiratory disorders; in other words, SDB comprises several complications ranging from primary snoring to obstructive sleep apnea (OSA) (Fig. 17.1).

Primary snoring occurs when normal breathing is replaced by a ventilatory pattern in which the nasal component is integrated by oral respiration. All children aged approximately 3 years tend to snore during the deepest stage of sleep; this behavior can be considered "physiological" at this age.

Upper airway resistance syndrome (UARS) is an intermediate condition that includes daytime symptoms caused by breathing disorders without apnea or hypopnea. UARS is caused by a reduction in the passage of air, which forces the chest muscles and diaphragm to make an intense effort to collect air and push it into the lungs.

Obstructive hypoventilation or *obstructive hypopnea* involves airflow reduction of at least 30% and can manifest with or without waking and/or a 3%–4% oxygen desaturation.

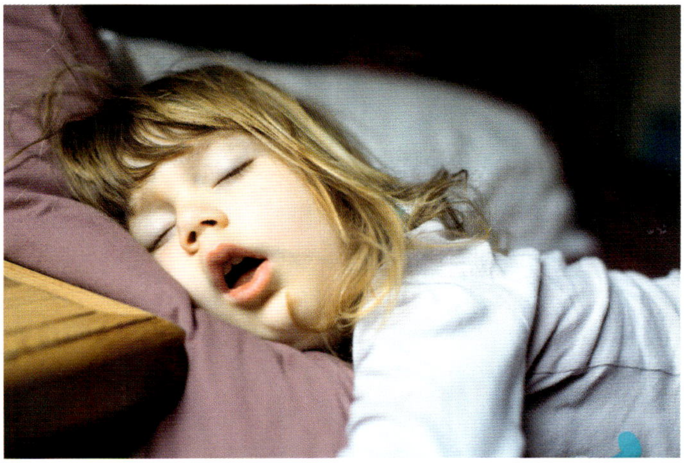

Figure 17.1 Obstructive sleep apnea.

The last stage of SDB is OSA. This involves narrowing of the upper airways caused by local and systemic factors, which occurs during sleep and partially or completely blocks air passage. This can cause a respiratory block lasting 10–20 seconds or more and can occur several times during the night. Symptoms of OSA include heavy snoring, suffocation, or panting during sleep, nighttime hyperactivity, and daytime sleepiness.

Epidemiology and etiopathogenesis

The prevalence of sleep disorders in children of school-going age is highly variable:

- The percentage of children that snore during school-going age is 3.2%–27%.
- The percentage of children affected by OSA during school-going age is 1.2%–5.7%.

In terms of ethnicity, it is interesting to note that African American children show a higher frequency of SDB than Caucasian children. According to a study by Ong in 1998 in the United States, Asians are statistically more likely to have OSA than Caucasians. In adolescents, it is possible to note differences in terms of gender, with a higher incidence in males than in females.

Breathing disorders during sleep can occur at any age, but they seem to occur more commonly in children aged 2–6 years because of hypertrophy of the lymphatic tissue, which is typical of this age group; from 6 years of age, the lymphatic tissue undergoes regression, which in turn reduces the resistance to airflow resistance to airflow, leading to leading to the appearance of respiratory symptoms.

The etiology of OSA in pediatric patients is multifactorial and can be classified on the basis of three main causes for the sake of simplicity: *anatomical-structural, functional, and concomitant factors* (Fig. 17.2).

Anatomical and structural factors

Anatomical and structural anomalies reduce the patency of airways caused by anatomical changes and, therefore, are also present when patients are awake. However, they become obstructive during sleep because of muscle hypotonia, which physiologically occurs during this phase.

Craniofacial anomalies

The presence of craniofacial abnormalities is an important risk factor for the development of respiratory disorders. In fact, craniofacial structures represent a scaffold that protects the upper airways. The presence of anomalies such as mandibular retropositioning, micrognathia, and hypoplasia of the upper jaw can predispose a person to an obstructive clinical condition. Micrognathia occurs in at least 60 genetic syndromes, such as Pierre Robin, Treacher Collins, and Goldenhar, in which other malformations, such as macroglossia, volumetric reduction of the oropharynx, and dorsal displacement of the tongue, frequently coexist.

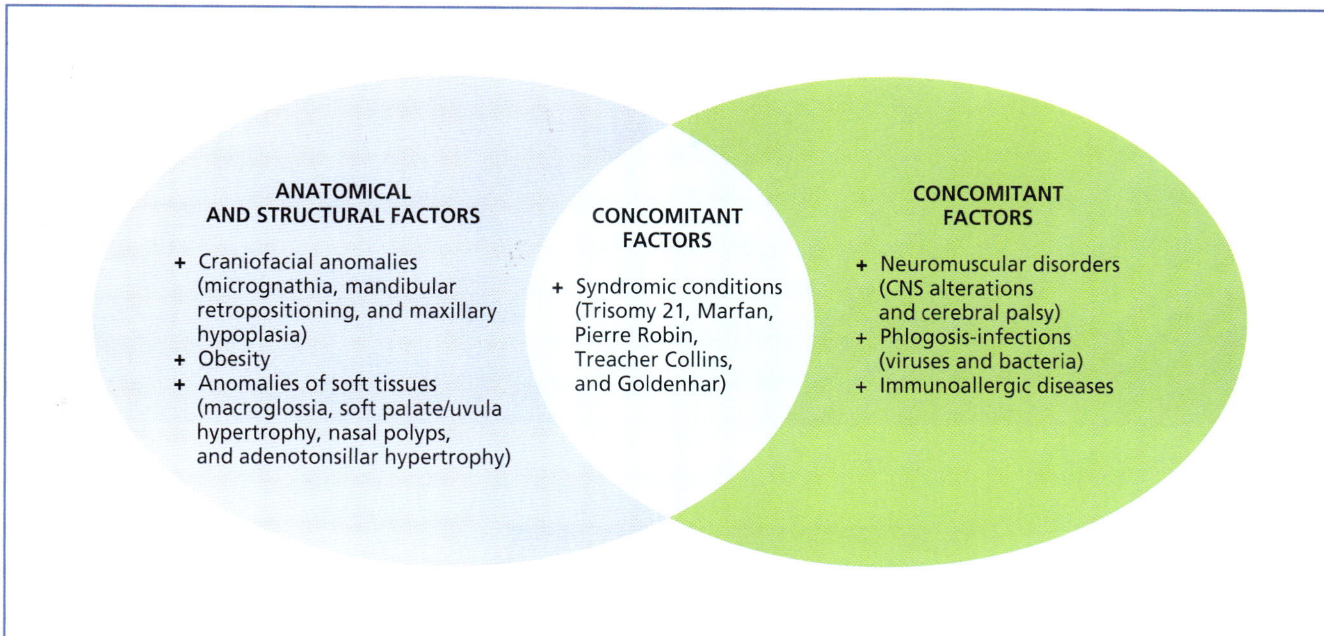

Figure 17.2 Etiological factors of obstructive sleep apnea.

Soft tissue anomalies

Conditions such as macroglossia, hypertrophy of the soft palate and uvula, nasal polyposis, and tumors lead to obstruction of the air passage, ultimately resulting in respiratory complications. In particular, adenotonsillar hypertrophy (Fig. 17.3 and 17.4) constitutes the physiological condition that most frequently underlies OSA in pediatric patients. As mentioned, an increase in the incidence of nighttime obstructive apneas can be observed in children aged 2–6 years; in fact, in this age group, the upper airways are small in terms of volume and cross-section, and the ratio between the volume of the airways and that of the adenotonsillar tissue favors the latter. Subsequently, after the age of 6 years, this ratio reverses and the volume/cross-section of airways increases without general association with the increase of adenoid and/or tonsillar volumes (adenotonsillar volume frequently tends to reduce until normalization). Excessive obstruction of choanal spaces by adenoids and excessive obstruction of the hypopharynx by tonsils are important obstructive components affecting the upper respiratory tract. However, not all children affected by adenotonsillar hypertrophy suffer from breathing disorders during sleep, and it is commonly believed that there is no close correlation between the degree of hypertrophy in lymphatic structures and the severity of obstructive clinical condition due to the role played by other factors. Therefore, it is easy to understand the importance given to a correct surgical indication and the knowledge of anatomical and functional factors, from which it is possible to predict a partial resolution in the postsurgical phase with the use of complementary treatment.

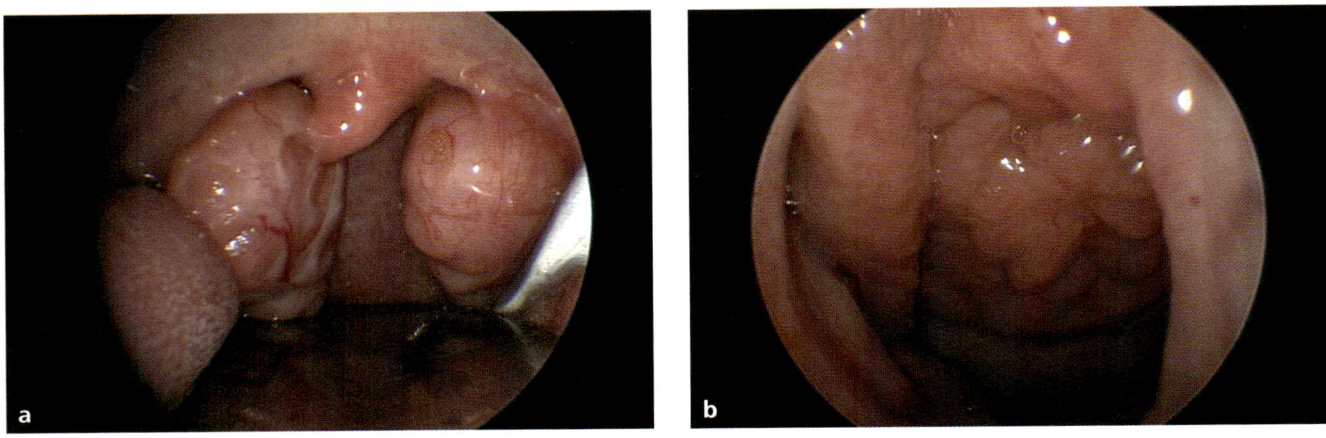

Figure 17.3 Endoscopic section of tonsils (**a**) and hypertrophic adenoids (**b**).

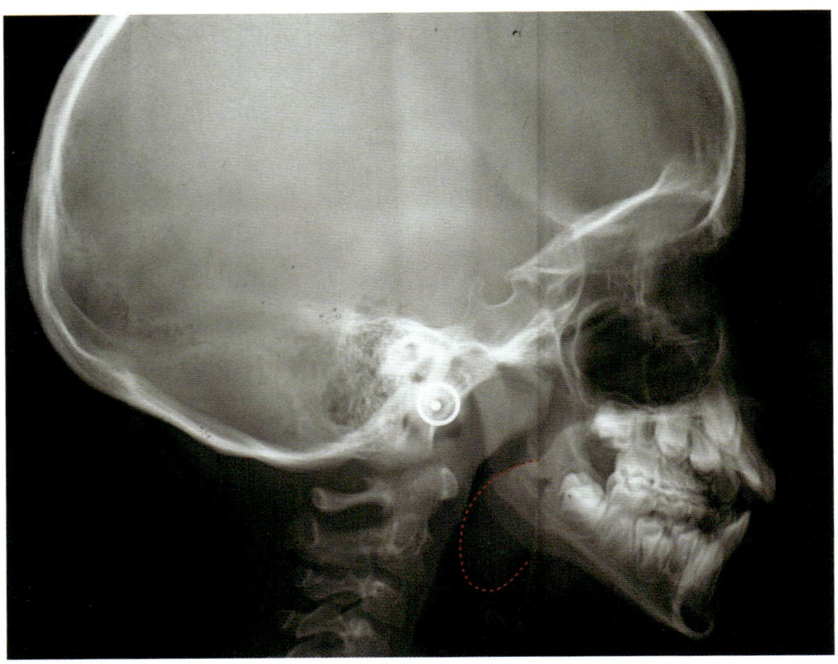

Figure 17.4 Tonsillar hypertrophy observed through teleradiography of the skull performed in laterolateral projection.

Obesity

An additional risk factor observed in growing patients with respiratory disorders is obesity (Fig. 17.5). The prevalence of obesity at an early age is a constantly increasing phenomenon. In children with obesity, the risk of developing OSA can vary from 30% to 60%.

The buildup of adipose tissue can favor the development of apnea through several mechanisms: this condition favors anatomical narrowing at the pharyngeal level, and therefore, the onset of an apneic event. In patients with severe obesity, it is possible to observe an upward thrust of the diaphragm, with the subsequent reduction of contraction capacity and consequent reduction of lung volumes. Furthermore, visceral fat increases the activity of respiratory muscles, leading to the production of a negative progression with the final collapse of the upper airways during inhalation.

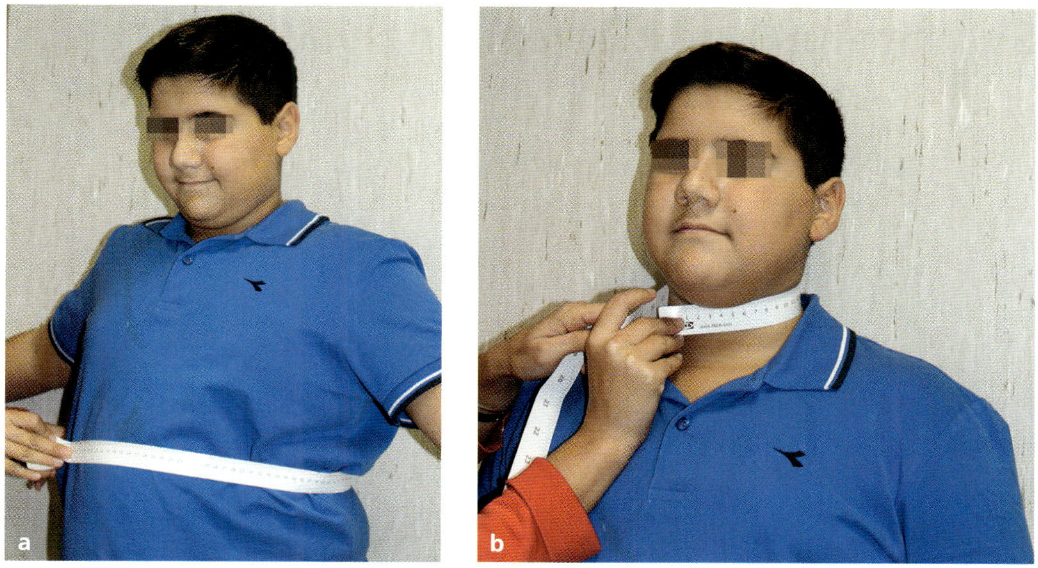

Figure 17.5 Pediatric patient with obesity and OSA of mild severity (AHI = 6.2); measurement of neck (**a**) and waist (**b**) circumferences.

Functional factors

In addition to anatomical factors, functional factors increase airway collapsibility. Functional anomalies, as opposed to structural anomalies, only occur during sleep. These conditions include reduced muscle tone of the airways, neuromuscular disorders, and inflammatory conditions affecting the respiratory tract, such as allergic rhinitis and asthma. Furthermore, children with neuromuscular disorders caused by generalized hypotonia (muscular dystrophy) or incoordination (cerebral palsy) are at a greater risk of developing severe apnea.

Concomitant factors

In some syndromic conditions, the anatomic and functional factors can coexist. In addition to the aforementioned Pierre Robin, Treacher Collins, and Goldenhar syndromes, other syndromes are associated with OSA owing to the combination of these factors. The syndromes most frequently associated with obstructive events include trisomy 21, in which there is a marked muscle hypotonia associated with macroglossia; achondroplasia, characterized by muscle hypotonia, maxillary hypoplasia, and nerve compression of respiratory muscles; and Marfan syndrome, in which the characteristic craniofacial alterations are associated with an increased collapsibility of the upper airways.

Therefore, OSA pathophysiology appears to be the result of a complex interaction among anatomical structures, neuromuscular tones, and other factors, such as inflammatory events, which can contribute to the onset of respiratory pathology.

Symptoms and clinical analysis

SDB in children shows variable symptoms that are frequently difficult to diagnose.
Only 7% of children affected by SBD suffer from daytime sleepiness. In adults, this symptom is very common; in comparison, children tend to be hyperactive. Furthermore, some symptoms can continue for many years, such as snoring and nighttime waking, while others are observed only in certain age groups.
The obstruction of the respiratory tract can manifest not only because of anatomical factors such as enlarged tonsils but also because of anatomical changes in the airways itself caused by the increased respiratory effort associated with repeated snoring every night for years. These anatomical changes can include mandibular morphological alterations, hypertrophy of the tongue, and descent of the hyoid bone because of the negative pressure that tends to push the laryngobronchial tree downward.
Furthermore, children with mouth breathing can also develop language disorders, craniofacial alterations, and postural anomalies.
Many authors have described the alterations of the growth pattern and craniofacial system in children with respiratory complications.
In fact, mouth breathing modifies the growth pattern of the face and causes various morphological and functional alterations in the patient. The main alterations caused by SDB affect the upper jaw, face, muscle tone, and mandibular position.
Children with respiratory complications tend to compensate for the obstruction by adopting specific postures during sleep, e.g., cervical hypertension or the so-called "*knee-to-chest*" position to guarantee airway patency and raise the hyoid level.

The tendency to adopt abnormal sleeping positions during the growing phase results in the alteration of occlusal development and modification of growth patterns.

During mouth breathing, the tongue cannot shape the palate, and this results in a constricted and deep palatal vault and poor jaw growth, which in turn can cause further reduction in air passage through the nasal cavities, constriction of the arches, and anterior crossbite.
The tongue can play an important role in the development of the jaws.
A more anterior tongue position can lead to mandibular prognathism, whereas a more posterior position can lead to mandibular underdevelopment.
In patients with respiratory disorders, it is possible to observe an increased gonial angle because of the hourly rotation of the mandibular plane in relation to the skull base. This leads to increased lower anterior facial height and total anterior facial height.
Many studies have used the cephalometric approach to analyze the anatomical characteristics of patients with respiratory complications.
There are limited data available regarding the craniofacial morphology and oropharyngeal dimensions in children with SDB. A study by Cozza et al. in 2004 assessed the differences in craniofacial morphology between children with OSA and a healthy control group. The children with OSA showed a class II skeletal pattern with reduced

mandibular length and increased overbite. The analysis performed using plaster models showed greater maxillary and mandibular constriction than the control group. The intermaxillary space, in which the tongue is naturally accommodated, appeared diminished. Based on these findings, it is reasonable to believe that the tongue can compensate for the reduced inter-arch size by assuming a more posterior and superior position, which would justify the implementation of treatment based on mandibular advancement.

Patients with respiratory complications keep their mouth constantly open; this makes the correct development of perioral muscles difficult. The alteration of the muscle tone occurs with the following events: interpositioning of the tongue during phonation and swallowing, orbicular tension, short upper lip, hyperactivity of the lower lip, and lack of labial seal.

Furthermore, significant differences have been found in craniofacial characteristics between patients with adenoid hypertrophy and those with tonsillar hypertrophy.

Hypertrophic adenoids lead to a reduced branch length, more vertical growth direction, reduced mandibular body length, an increased retrognathic mandible, and a marked discrepancy between the upper and lower jaw on the sagittal plane.

Hypertrophic tonsils lead to an increased branch length, more horizontal growth direction, increased mandibular body length, more anterior position of the mandible, and a reduced discrepancy between the upper and lower jaw on the sagittal plane.

Diagnosis

Respiratory sleep disorders in children have recently gained more attention because of a series of implications caused by the lack of early diagnosis and interceptive therapy. Polysomnography (PSG) is considered the gold standard for accurate SDB diagnosis.

During PSG, skin detectors are used to detect several parameters: brain activity, eye movement, muscle tone, oronasal flow, respiratory efforts, and oxygen saturation. An electroencephalogram records brain activity and allows the detection of sleep stages, distinguishes between sleep and wake states, and identifies anomalous brain activities such as seizures. Electrooculogram and electromyogram enable the identification of the rapid eye movement phase because during this phase it is possible to distinguish characteristic eye movements and loss of muscle tone.

Furthermore, thoracoabdominal movements, body position, and snoring are also monitored. Due to the quantitative parameters provided by PSG, it is possible to define the apnea–hypopnea index (AHI), the most commonly used and well-known parameter, on the basis of which the level of OSA severity has been established.

AHI is classified as follows in children:

- mild: 1–5 AHI
- moderate: 5–10 AHI
- severe: +10 AHI

AHI is defined as the sum of apneas and hypopneas for each hour of sleep considered in the examination and is assessed upon the diagnosis of OSA in a child, even in the presence of a single apneic event per hour of sleep.
Polysomnographic recording usually lasts for approximately 6–7 hours and requires hospitalization for at least one night.
Currently, there are different types of small-sized devices to perform PSG, even at home. However, because of the high costs, the complexity of implementation (both for children and their parents) and the difficulty of early identification of people at risk, several authors have attempted using alternative diagnostic methods: medical history associated with physical examination, audio recordings, video recordings, pulse oximetry, and validated diagnostic questionnaires.
Among these methods, the questionnaires and overnight oximetry are assumed to possess a very high diagnostic value.
A meta-analysis conducted in 2004 by De Luca Canto et al. assessed the diagnostic value of the questionnaires and clinical examinations used by the authors for diagnosis of SDB.
This study showed that among the questionnaires published in the literature, the Pediatric Sleep Questionnaire (PSQ) in its reduced form of 22 items (PSQ-SRBD Scale) has the best diagnostic accuracy with a sensitivity of 0.81% and a specificity of 0.83%.
This questionnaire can be easily answered by the parents of subjects between 2 and 18 years of age, exclusively using the following simple answers: "Yes," "No," and "I do not know." It is divided into 10 sections and accounts for the different aspects of sleep quality, from snoring to daytime and nighttime behavioral habits.
On the contrary, overnight pulse oximetry was the first screening test that allowed the detection of sleep-related diseases. Pulse oximetry measures the quality of oxygen (O_2) present in the arterial blood (hemoglobin saturation – Sat. % Hb) using an electronic device called oximeter. This device is connected to a finger with a clamp (digital probe) and detects the cardiac frequency and oxygen saturation level of hemoglobin using a noninvasive, painless method.

Consequences

OSAs are associated with substantial morbidity; decreased neurocognitive development, poor school performance, and behavioral anomalies are the most commonly reported consequences in pediatric patients with OSA, but the complications related to the presence of this disorder can be detrimental to several systems. Therefore, the health of these patients is compromised at several levels.

Intermittent hypoxemia and sleep fragmentation caused by SDB can, in fact, underlie inflammatory responses, and increased levels of these responses can lead to cardiovascular, cognitive, and behavioral pathologies.

At the *cardiovascular* level, the worst OSA sequela is pulmonary hypertension; however, this pathology is not commonly observed in children, who tend to develop less severe cardiovascular dysfunctions such as blood pressure abnormalities, cardiac remodeling, and endothelial dysfunction.

As mentioned OSAs and snoring in pediatric patients have been associated with *behavioral and neurocognitive changes*. Children with OSAs frequently exhibit marked hyperactivity, concentration difficulties, attention problems, and impulsivity, all signs attributable to clinical pictures of attention-deficit hyperactivity disorder.

Such children are irritable and exhibit depressed mood and little interest in daily activities.

Nocturnal enuresis is another condition frequently detected in these patients, probably because of an inhibitory effect of this pathology on the body's responses to changes in bladder pressure.

Furthermore, associations between OSA and *metabolic syndrome* in postpubertal adolescents have also been detected, whereas among the pediatric population, the presence of OSAs has shown a significant correlation with reduced insulin sensitivity in obese children.

Lastly, OSAs are associated with *growth delay*, which also compromises physical development; the increase in respiratory effort and the load supported by the heart because of the obstruction result in a greater demand for energy. Therefore, the body uses more energy to sustain the cardiovascular system, thus decreasing the amount of available energy for physiological growth. Many of these children secrete lower levels of growth hormones, are underweight, and show a less than normal height compared with their peers.

However, it has been observed that this growth deficit normalizes after adenotonsillectomy.

Arterial hypertension and cardiovascular abnormalities have also shown improvement or complete regression after adequate treatment.

If OSAs in preschool-age children are not adequately treated, they can induce irreversible learning disabilities.

Treatment

Surgical therapy

In 1986, a study was conducted by Linder-Aronson et al. on patients with adenoid hypertrophy by analyzing cephalometric values before and after adenoidectomy. After comparing these subjects to a control group, they reported an increased lower anterior facial height, increased inclination of the mandibular plane, and more retrognathic mandible. A significant improvement was observed in the angular values assessed 5 years after adenoidectomy.
A subsequent study conducted in 1991 by Hultcrantz et al. assessed the facial growth and arch shape in children undergoing tonsillectomy; the assessments were made before and after surgery by analyzing plaster models and teleradiography of the skull with laterolateral projection.
Two years after surgical intervention, it was possible to observe 77% resolution of the open bite and 50%–65% resolution of the crossbite with better outcomes in children who had undergone surgery before 6 years of age.
Therefore, there is an improvement in growth direction and occlusal alterations after surgery; this seems because of the normalization of the ventilatory pattern, as well as oral and nasal respiration.
Furthermore, studies have shown that occlusal and craniofacial alterations tend to improve after the correction of airway obstruction, especially in preschool-age children.
Therefore, adenotonsillectomy is the most frequently performed surgical intervention in children, and its main goal is to re-establish nasal respiration, thus improving lives and strengthening the myofunctional facial state after surgery.
Surgery was shown to be effective in reducing symptoms and determining favorable changes in the behavioral profile and polysomnographic findings.
However, full recovery was not observed in any of these studies.

Mechanical ventilation treatment (continuous positive airway pressure)

Mechanical ventilation is a palliative treatment aimed at improving symptoms but not eliminating their underlying cause. It involves the use of a continuous positive airway pressure device that supports mechanical ventilation at a continuous positive pressure. This is a ventilation therapy that creates a continuous air insufflation through the nasal pathway at a positive pressure and during the night, using a specially designed mask. The pressure is generated by a minicompressor, which acts as a pneumatic dilator for the upper airways, avoiding pharynx obstruction and canceling the event that generates apnea. In any case, not all patients manage to continue this treatment due to the discomfort involved; in fact, several side effects may appear, such as nasal congestion, claustrophobia, and skin abrasions on the face.

Orthodontic treatment

For some time now, the scientific community has been highlighting the central role played by dentistry not only in detecting obstructive pathology but also, especially, treating mild-to-moderate forms. In this context, it is necessary to collaborate with a sleep center, which involves specialists of what is now called sleep medicine. The first to introduce this issue in dentistry was Pierre Robin (1867–1950) in the last century, who first used the monobloc for mandibular advancement and soft tissue conditioning.
On March 15, 2016, the Italian Ministry of Health published *national guidelines for the prevention and treatment of snoring and OSAs in children*, which include *evidence-based* recommendations and indications for the management of snoring and OSA syndrome. These *guidelines* read that "dentistry, through regular checks, can identify snoring and OSAs and can provide timely intervention with the application of related oral devices. During clinical examination, dentists should pay attention to craniofacial features related to mouth breathing, elongated faces, small and retruded chin, dental crowding, and high and narrow palate, and while collecting data regarding the patient's medical history, they should also collect information related to school performance, concentration capacity, possible presence of nocturnal enuresis, poor appetite, obesity, and recurrent airway infections" (Haviv et al, 2014).
As specifically designed oral appliances are used in orthodontic treatment, they can be considered an important support for improving respiratory problems in pediatric patients.
Oral appliances can improve the patency of the upper airway during sleep by widening them and/or decreasing their collapsibility.
After confirming the presence of snoring or apnea in a pediatric patient along with a related craniofacial morphology, orthodontists can intervene using specifically designed orthodontic appliances, especially if the otorhinolaryngological component is not considered predominant in the etiopathogenesis of snoring or obstructive syndrome.

Orthodontists can eliminate some craniofacial features that represent a risk factor for the development of respiratory issues.
Several orthodontic therapies have been proposed for reducing respiratory symptoms.

Upper jaw expansion

Expansion has proved to be highly effective in increasing the transverse size of the upper jaw from the skeletal and dental point of view. Rapid maxillary expander (RME) is a device largely used in patients with respiratory problems and jaw constriction (Fig. 17.6 and 17.7). This device acts at the level of the median palatine suture, inducing its opening and determining the correction of the transverse deficit.
The enlargement of the nasal cavities, obtained after the opening of the median palatine suture, has proved to be able to reduce the resistance of the nasal airways and improve the respiratory pattern in pediatric patients (Fig. 17.8).

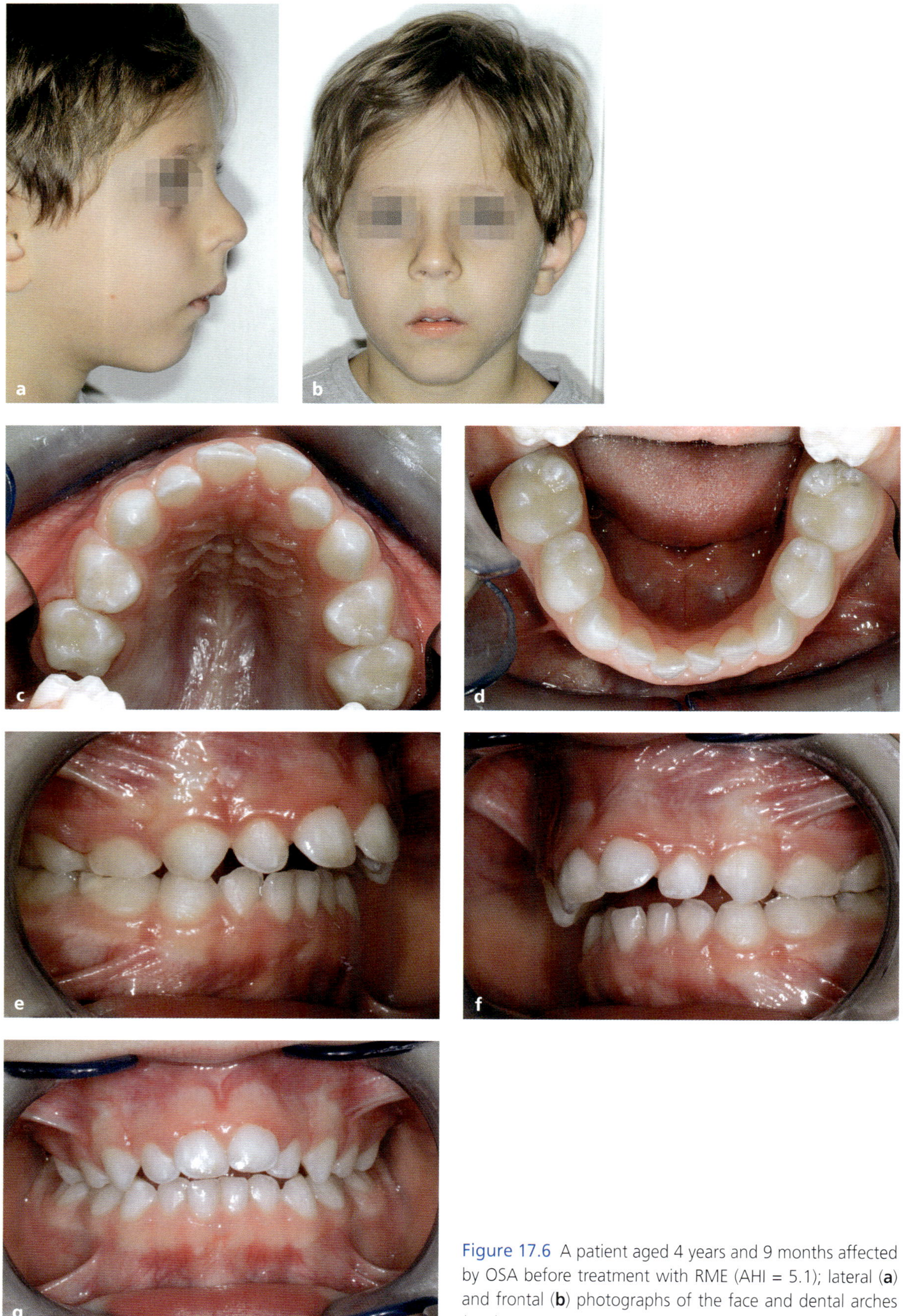

Figure 17.6 A patient aged 4 years and 9 months affected by OSA before treatment with RME (AHI = 5.1); lateral (**a**) and frontal (**b**) photographs of the face and dental arches (**c–g**).

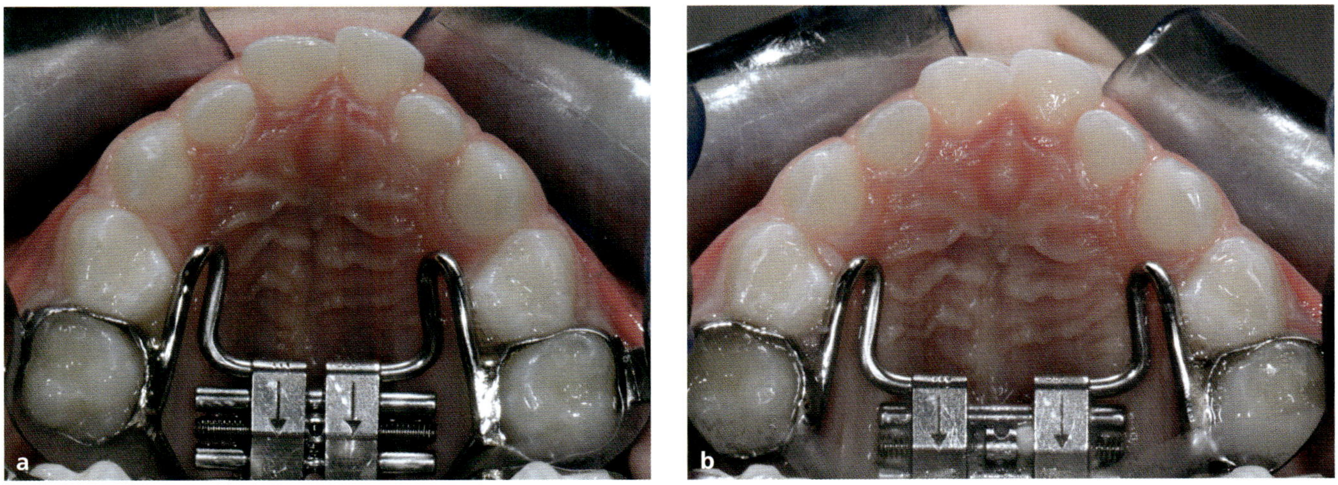

Figure 17.7 Clinical application and intraoral view of the rapid maxillary expander; photographs of the upper arch before (**a**) and after (**b**) expansion.

In fact, it is well known that the lateral displacement of the nasal cavities is associated with enlargement of the upper airways.
The positive effect of this orthopedic–orthodontic maneuver on the symptoms reported by children with OSA was proved a long time ago using both respiratory function tests and polysomnographic recordings.

Furthermore, many studies have shown that early interventions using this device reduce tonsillar hypertrophy. This effect is due to both the enlargement of the pharyngeal lumen, in which the tonsils appear smaller, and to the improvement of nasal respiration, which reduces the incidence of diseases affecting the respiratory tract.

The results obtained with palatal expansion are manifold: increased diameter of the upper pharyngeal airways, reduced nasal resistance, increased nasal volume, positive effects on maxillary system growth, improved lingual posture, and improved middle ear functionality.
Therefore, it is clear that early intervention in the developmental age is important to reduce the risks associated with obstructive events, obtain an improved effect on the nasal cavities, and promote a harmonious craniofacial growth.

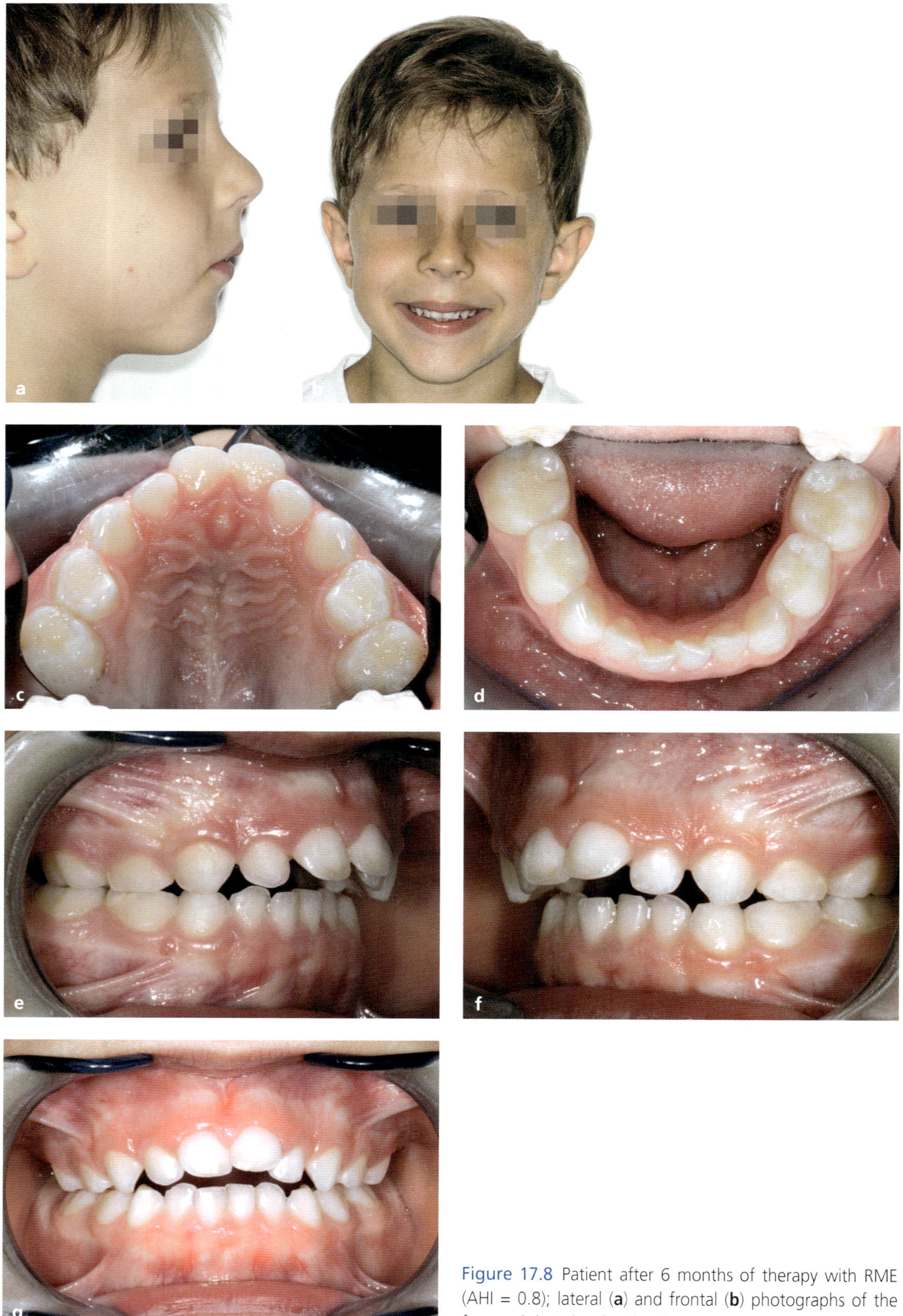

Figure 17.8 Patient after 6 months of therapy with RME (AHI = 0.8); lateral (**a**) and frontal (**b**) photographs of the face and dental arches (**c–g**).

Mandibular advancement

Oral and functional orthopedic appliances have been used in children to move the mandible forward, enlarge the upper airways, and improve respiratory function in patients with OSA and craniofacial abnormalities (Fig. 17.9 and 17.10).
This approach can permanently modify nasal respiration in children, lowering the risk of OSA onset in pediatric age.

Orthopedic–orthodontic treatment using functional appliances is a further valid therapeutic approach for respiratory problems in pediatric patients. Functional therapy for mandibular advancement not only improves the skeletal base relationship but also reduces the risk of collapse in the upper airways (Fig. 17.11). The therapeutic approach is based on the concept that all orthodontic abnormalities related to mandibular retropositioning benefit from a functional advancement therapy that can expand the space posteriorly to the tongue, simultaneously promoting mandibular advancement. The anterior mandibular displacement obtained using functional devices influences the position of the hyoid bone and, consequently, the position of the tongue, increasing the intermaxillary space in which the tongue itself is accommodated, and improves the shape of the upper airways. With mandibular advancement, it is possible to obtain both the resolution of class II skeletal malocclusions and the improvement of retropharyngeal relationships.

In any case, the choice of appliance is directly dependent on the clinical picture. Therefore, it is possible to perform only the expansion of the upper jaw in patients with respiratory disorders not associated with mandibular retropositioning; on the contrary, in the presence of a class II malocclusion and correct transverse diameter, the treatment of choice is functional therapy. In certain more complex cases, it is also possible to perform a combined treatment comprising expansion and advancement. Therefore, two approaches can be identified, both of which are valid for the treatment of respiratory disorders in pediatric patients. These therapeutic indications can be used in combination to perform a complete therapy aimed at eliminating all craniofacial abnormalities that are predisposing factors for the development of respiratory problems.

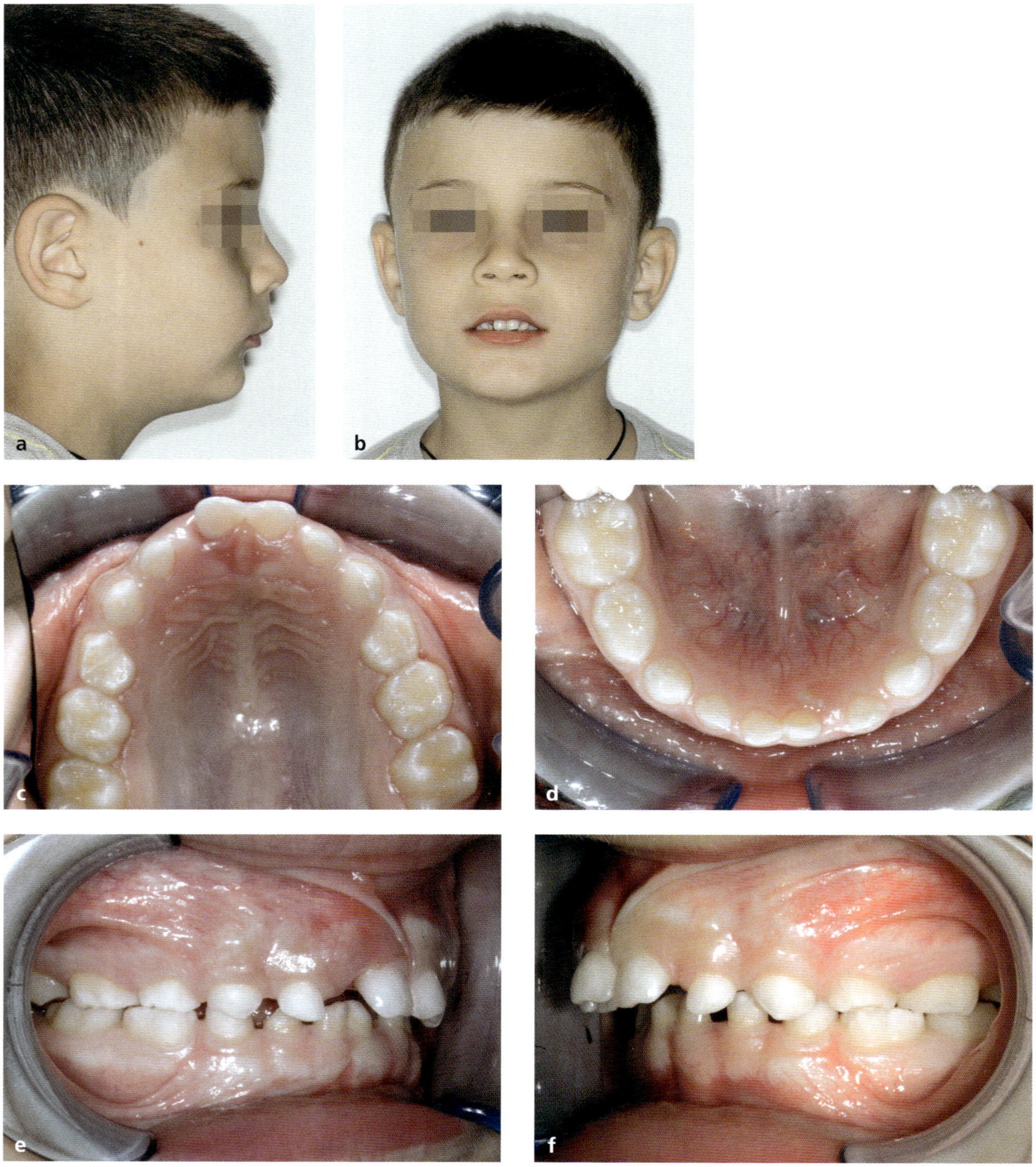

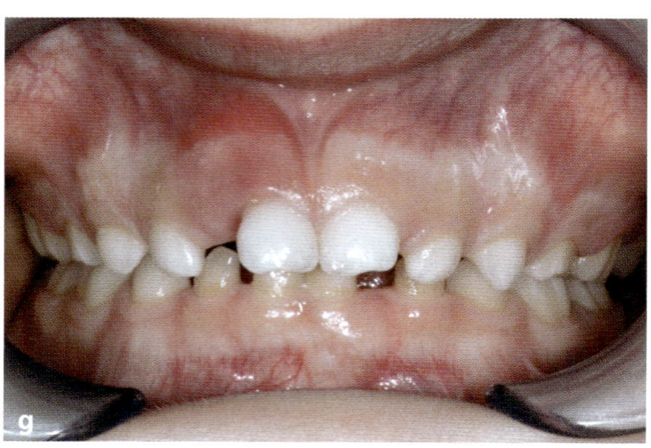

Figure 17.9 A patient aged 5 years and 4 months affected by OSA before the treatment of mandibular advancement (AHI = 3.2); lateral (**a**) and frontal (**b**) photographs of the face and dental arches (**c–g**).

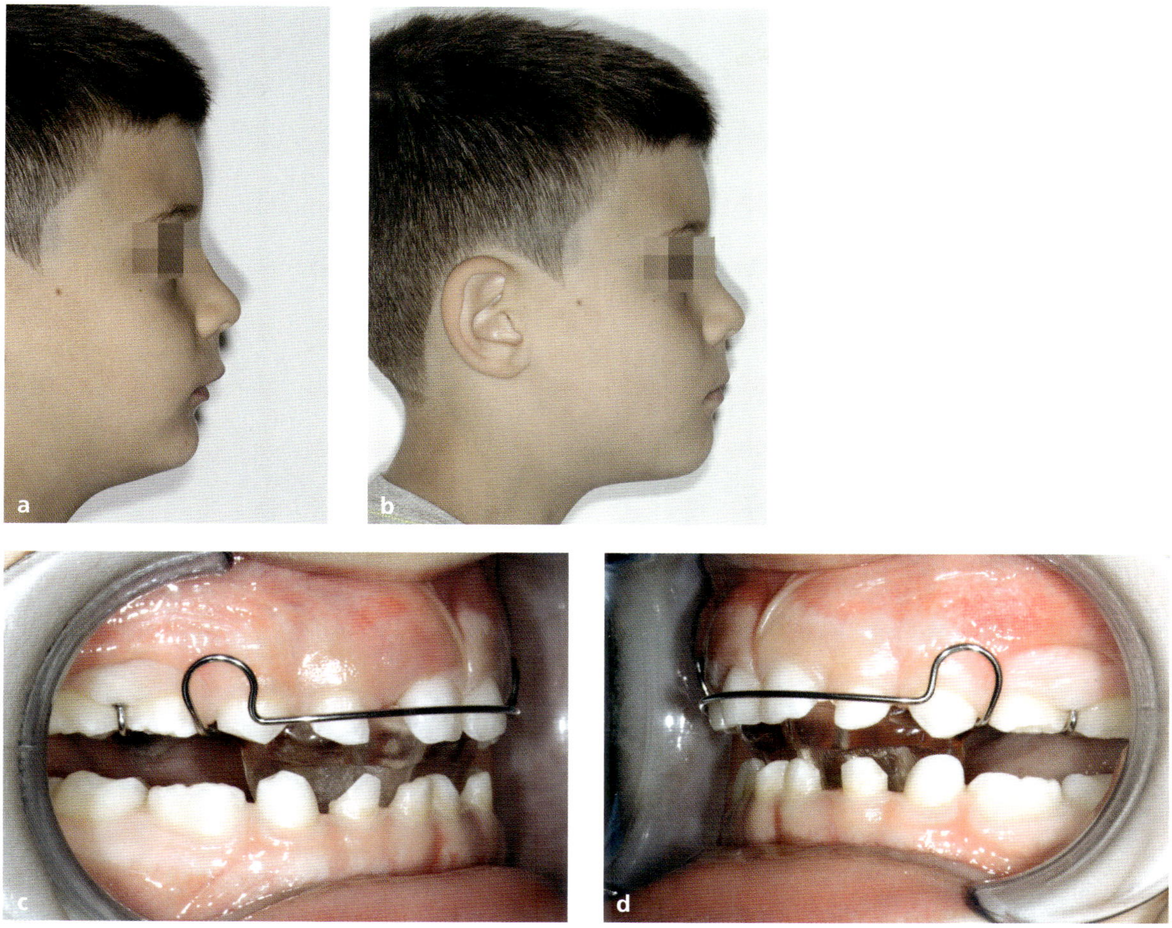

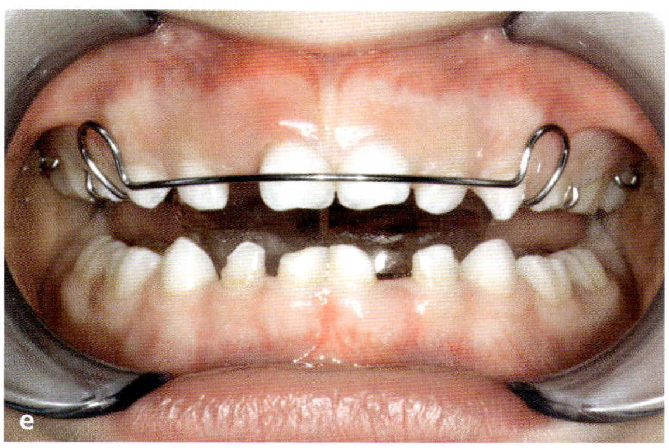

Figure 17.10 Clinical application and intraoral view of the functional device for mandibular advancement; lateral photograph of the face with (**a**) and without (**b**) the advancement device and dental arches (**c–e**).

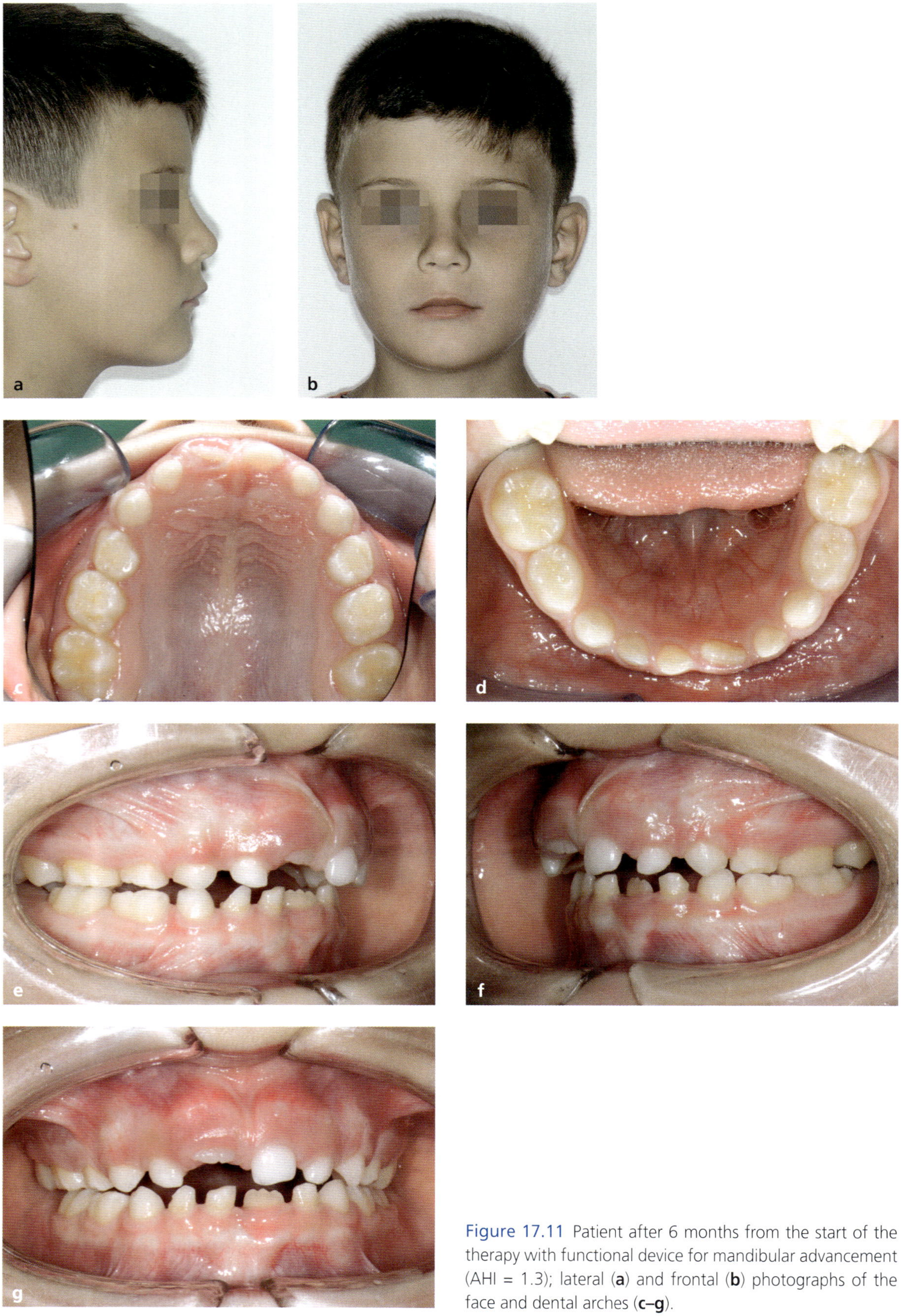

Figure 17.11 Patient after 6 months from the start of the therapy with functional device for mandibular advancement (AHI = 1.3); lateral (**a**) and frontal (**b**) photographs of the face and dental arches (**c–g**).

References

Cozza P, Polimeni A, Ballanti F. A modified monobloc for the treatment of obstructive sleep apnoea in paediatric patients. Eur J Orthod 2004;26:523-30.

De Luca Canto G, Singh V, Major MP, Witmans M, El-Hakim H, Major PW, Flores-Mir C. Diagnostic capability of questionnaires and clinical examinations to assess sleep-disordered breathing in children: a systematic review and meta-analysis. J Am Dent Assoc 2014;145:165-78.

Haviv Y, Benoliel R, Bachar G, Michaeli E. On the edge between medicine and dentistry: review of the dentist's role in the diagnosis and treatment of snoring and sleep apnea. Quintessence Int 2014;45:345-53.

Hultcrantz E, Larson M, Hellquist R, Ahlquist-Rastad J, Svanholm H, Jakobsson OP. The influence of tonsillar obstruction and tonsillectomy on facial growth and dental arch morphology. Int. J. Pediatr Otorhinolaryngol 1991;22:125-34.

Iwasaki T, Saitoh I, Takemoto Y, Inada E, Kanomi R, Hayasaki H, Yamasaki Y. Improvement of nasal airway ventilation after rapid maxillary expansion evaluated with computational fluid dynamics. Am J Orthod Dentofacial Orthop 2012;141:269-78.

Jennum P, Ibsen R, Kjellberg J. Morbidity and mortality in children with obstructive sleep apnoea: a controlled national study. Thorax 2013;68:949-954.

Katyal V, Pamula Y, Daynes CN, Martin J, Dreyer CW, Kennedy D, Sampson WJ. Craniofacial and upper airway morphology in pediatric sleep-disordered breathing and changes in quality of life with rapid maxillary expansion. Am J Orthod Dentofacial Orthop 2013;144:860-71.

Linder-Aronson S, Woodside DG, Lundström A. Mandibular growth direction following adenoidectomy. Am J Orthod 1986;89:273-84.

Marcus CL, Moore RH, Rosen CL et al. A randomized trial of adenotonsillectomy for childhood sleep apnea. N Engl J Med 2013;368:2366-76.

Ministero della Salute. Linee guida nazionali per la prevenzione e il trattamento odontoiatrico della sindrome delle apnee ostruttive nel sonno (osas). 2014.

Nazarali N, Altalibi M, Nazarali S, Major MP, Flores-Mir C, Major PW. Mandibular advancement appliances for the treatment of paediatric obstructive sleep apnea: a systematic review. Eur J Orthod 2015;37:618-26.

Ong KC, Clerk AA. Comparison of the severity of sleep- disordered breathing in Asian and Caucasian patients seen at a sleep disorders center. Respir Med 1998;92:843-8.

Pavoni C, Cretella Lombardo E, Franchi L, Lione R, Cozza P. Treatment and post-treatment effects of functional therapy on the sagittal pharyngeal dimensions in Class II subjects. Int J Pediatr Otorhinolaryngol 2017;101:47-50.

Pavoni C, Cretella Lombardo E, Lione R, Bollero P, Ottaviani F, Cozza P. Orthopaedic treatment effects of functional therapy on the sagittal pharyngeal dimensions in subjects with sleep-disordered breathing and Class II malocclusion. Acta Otorhinolaryngol Ital 2017;37:479-485.

Villa MP, Miano S, Rizzoli A. Mandibular advancement devices are an alternative and valid treatment for pediatric obstructive sleep apnea syndrome. Sleep Breath 2012;16:971-6.

Chapter 18

Preformed orthodontic appliances in pediatric dentistry

G. Ierardo, G. Farronato, A. Polimeni

For the past several years, preformed appliances, which are important aids in the treatment of patients in the developmental age, have been widely used in interceptive orthodontics along with conventional appliances. These appliances, via the correct diagnosis and case selection, allow interceptive orthodontic treatment to be managed by combining therapeutic effectiveness, comfort, and ease of use, leading to a reduction in the treatment duration. One of the primary advantages of these devices is their versatility, which allows the timing and treatment goals to be diversified; in addition, the technology associated with these devices allows patients with special needs, in whom the use of conventional appliances may be contraindicated, to be treated.

The *positioner* is among the most used resilient appliances in orthodontics. It is a removable appliance constructed using the patient's model *set-up* with bite reconstruction on a terminal hinge axis composed of resilient material, which acts through muscle strength and deforms and comes into contact with the entire tooth surface, thereby acting in a constant, intense, continuous, and controllable manner. When there is residual growth, apart from actively restricting the residual growth, the positioner allows improved and consolidated results.

The positioner was developed in 1945 as a result of the brilliant intuition of H.D. Kesling, a young student of Charles H. Tweed, with the aim of perfecting dental inclinations and relationships. After the fixed appliance stage, it has remained unchanged in terms of construction principles and usage to the present day.

Previously, rubber was the material of choice because its resilience allowed its deformation following muscle contraction; this allowed the whole tooth surface to come into contact with the appliance, which then acted in a constant and controllable manner.

Currently, in compliance with the EC regulations, the material of choice is a biocompatible vinyl resin called Elvax® (ethylene and vinyl acetate copolymer), which can be either transparent, semitransparent, or composed of various colors and flavors.

It is used in the correction of minor anteroposterior and transversal discrepancies; it enables the closure of small diastemas, correction of mild overbite and slightly increased overjet, and minor rotations of the incisors and molars. In addition, because of the application of *socket liners* (steel grids corresponding to the central and lateral elements of both arches), it can modify the buccolingual inclination, thereby achieving movement on three levels.

Orthodontic elastodontic therapy

The *positioner* is the forerunner of all resilient appliances that are currently available and widely used in clinical practice; it is therefore the forerunner of the field of *elastodontics*.

The term elastodontics refers to the branch of orthodontics dealing with preformed and non-shaped appliances composed of resilient material suitable for both orthopedic and dental work.

The orthopedic action of elastodontic appliances is somewhat inconvenient compared with standard equipments that are currently the gold standard in orthopedic functional therapies, but they are currently used in clinical practice because of the combination of the *set-up* of the dental elements on an articulator and a constructed preformed bite that may help resolve various cases of malocclusion.

Therefore, elastodontics enters the context of orthodontic treatment at a retainer stage, but given the multifaceted nature of the construction of appliances, it plays an important role at all other treatment stages.

It is important to note the use of elastodontic appliances in the preventive treatment phase because in pediatric orthodontics, the orientation toward prevention is linked to the hypothesis of the functional theory, which states that *by modifying the function, we can modify the form*. In other words, early intervention for an altered function can modify bone plasticity. Eliminating bad habits early allows the recovery of orthological development.

The phrase "*bad habit*" is often generic and imprecise. Parafunctions that can cause dysmorphisms, such as prolonged sucking of pacifiers, fingers, or other objects, atypical swallowing, and mouth breathing, are usually considered bad habits. They belong to the group of extrinsic etiological factors that must be eliminated as early as possible to promote correct recovery of the growth of the stomatognathic apparatus consistent with the multiple functions that it performs.

Psychoanalytic theory considers parafunctions as symptoms of an underlying mental disorder that may be more or less enduring and more or less severe. Psychoanalytic theory recommends the treatment of such conditions with two types of therapies.

The first type is entrusted to specialized psychologists; therefore, it is considered a *behavioral* therapy; the second is the *orthodontic* type and it makes use of functional appliances.

Elastodontic appliances are helpful in the elimination of bad habits and guiding the eruption of dental elements in pediatric patients because they are constructed by considering the ideal position of the tongue and other perioral muscles.

Various parts of elastodontic appliances are modeled using the ideal mouth as a reference and are indicated in malocclusion cases in which, at other instances, rigid appliances would have sufficed. For instance, they are used in cases of lower anterior crowding caused by mentalis muscle hyperactivity, in which a *lip bumper* is commonly used; in cases of open anterior bite caused by an exaggerated tongue thrust or prolonged thumb sucking, in which a lingual grid is usually selected; in cases of deep bite with lesions on the palatal mucosa; in cases of exaggerated overjet due to the interpositioning of the lower lip; or in cases of loss of space in the arch, in which, owing to the presence of an ideal arch shape, it allows the arrangement of the elements according to the new arch shape.

Orthodontic elastodontic appliances

Some of the interceptive elastodontic appliances available are described below.
This field is constantly being updated both at the industrial and research level, which is an indication of the strong interest in such appliances and the need to develop simpler therapies where possible, particularly for younger patients.
All the appliances listed below are characterized by a preformed bite taken in mandibular advancement in a head-to-head ratio between the incisors, channels for the creation of a muscle corridor, spaces for the guidance of the eruption of the first dental elements, and more protruding fins or labial arches for the so-called *lip bumper effect*, i.e., the ability to counteract the hypertonic mentalis muscle.
With regard to the orthopedic phase, elastodontic appliances are necessary to guide the growth of maxillary bones, combining specific spaces for each individual tooth with the preformed bite.
In some cases, the spaces are present for all dental elements, including the second molars; in others, they descend distally to the premolars to facilitate the opening of the bite, acting as inclined planes to allow the extrusion of posterior sectors.

Trainer® T4K appliances

These appliances are characterized by a buccal and lingual screen; they facilitate lingual repositioning and control the abnormal interpositioning of muscles (tongue and lips) using an element called "tongue-climbing appliance" and lower ribs having a *lip bumper* effect. They allow mandibular repositioning from class II to class I malocclusions.
They are primarily used to correct bad habits (Fig. 18.1). They are available in two versions: one for deciduous teeth (infant Trainer®) (Fig. 18.2) and one for mixed teeth, and are used in patients aged 4–8 years for approximately 1 hour every day and night.

Myobrace®

The Myobrace® is primarily composed of two materials: a soft and flexible external area and a rigid internal center (DynamiCore®). The prefabricated shape of the arch in DynamiCore® allows it to extend, thereby correcting the shape of the front arch (Fig. 18.3).
Additionally, the appliance has all the well-known features of myofunctional training according to the myofunctional effect. It can be used in mixed or permanent dentition, but the optimal treatment time is the eruptive phase of growth in the late mixed dentition.

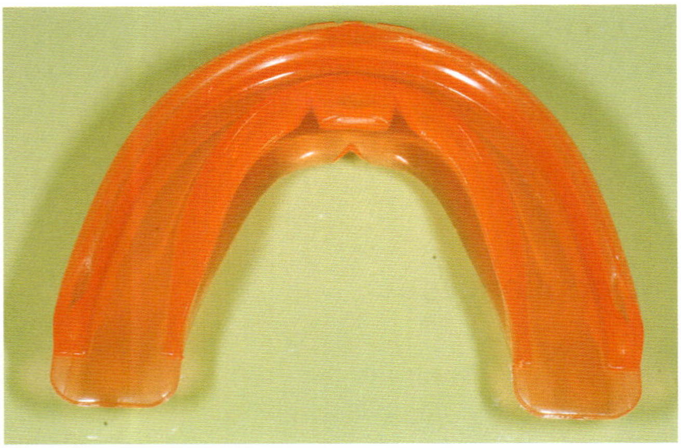

Figure 18.1 Trainer® T4K appliance.

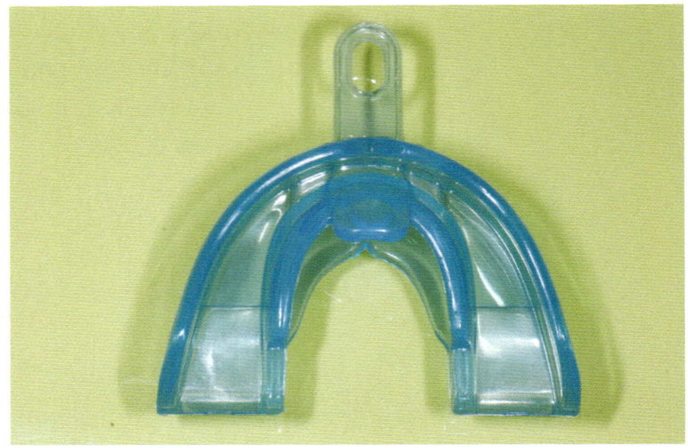

Figure 18.2 Infant Trainer® appliance.

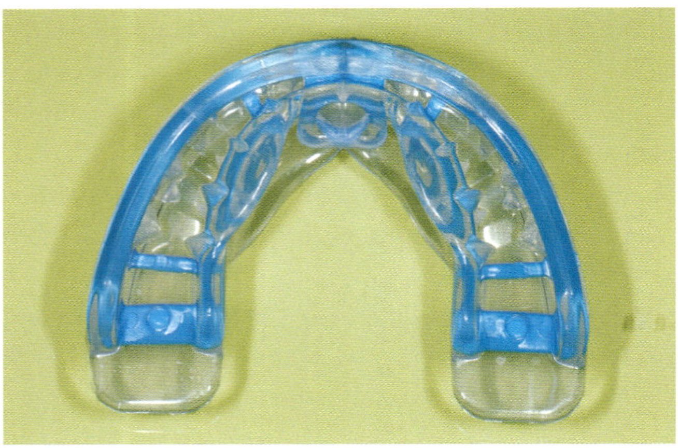

Figure 18.3 Myobrace® appliance.

The effectiveness of Myobrace® decreases with time, particularly when the permanent dentition has stabilized. Patient cooperation, degree of myofunctional correction, and malocclusion are influential factors. However, similar to other orthodontic treatments, individualized programs are necessary.
Regarding the choice of appliance, a specific ruler must be used to measure the width of the four upper incisors.
The appliance is available in six sizes, which is sufficient to deal with most cases encountered on a daily basis. The application must take place for a minimum of 2 hours each day and throughout the night to obtain the appropriate arch expansion and the alignment of the anterior group.

Multi-P®

The Multi-P® is another similar appliance currently in the market; compared with the abovementioned appliances, it is composed of holes for the flow of air through the appliance in the buccolingual direction.

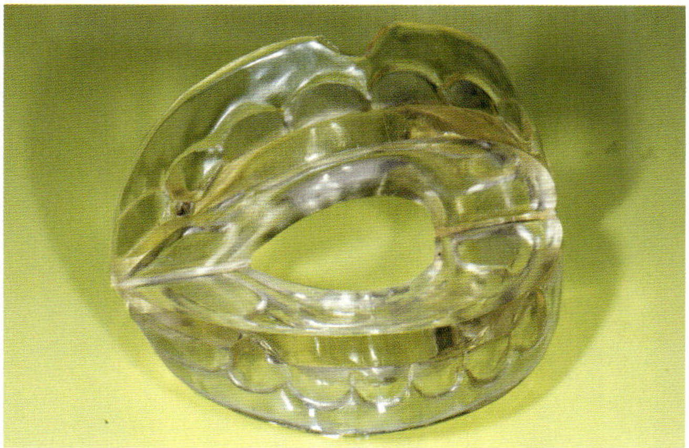

Figure 18.4 Nite-Guide® appliance.

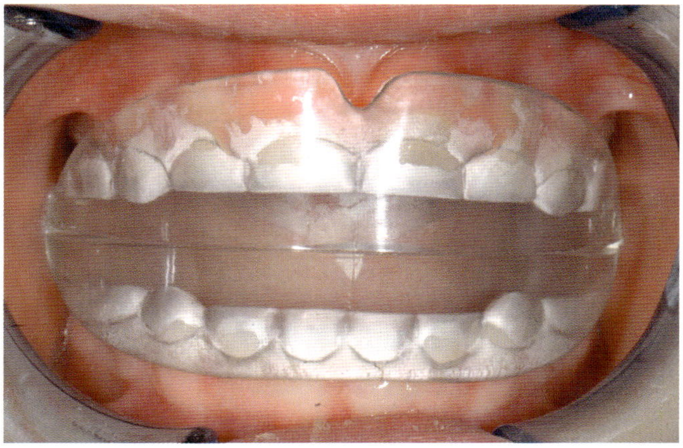

Figure 18.5 Application of Nite-Guide® appliance.

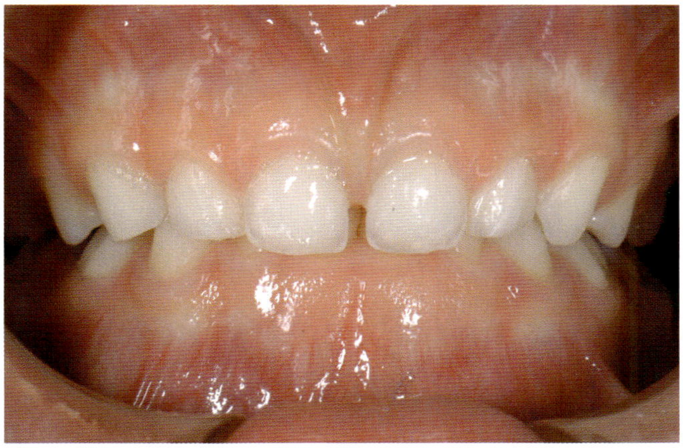

Figure 18.6 Deep bite in the deciduous dentition.

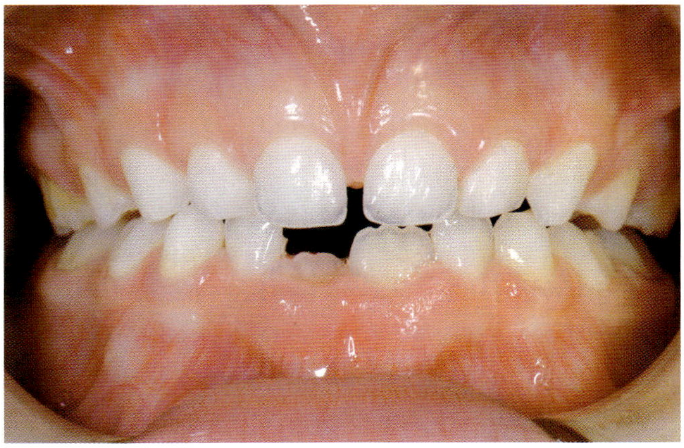

Figure 18.7 Resolution of deep bite using Nite-Guide®.

Nite-Guide®

The Nite-Guide® is indicated in patients aged 5–7 years. It guides the lower permanent incisors during eruption to achieve an optimal class I occlusion and can correct overbite and overjet of various extents (Fig. 18.4 and 18.5).

This appliance is recommended to be applied only at night. Nite-Guide® is a functional appliance for deciduous dentition because with very simple management it allows intervention in complications such as deep bite, class II with increased mandibular retrusion, and increased overjet (Fig. 18.6 and 18.7).

It can be useful in the elimination of bad habits, bruxism, and sleep apnea (obstructive sleep apnea syndrome, OSAS) characterized by mandibular retrusion.

The choice of appliance size is made using a special ruler to measure the distance between the mesial surfaces of the deciduous canines. Nite-Guide® is available in 13 sizes; therefore, it is suitable for most situations. The main, absolute contraindication is the third skeletal class.

It is generally replaced at the age of 7 years with the Occlus-o-Guide® G-series.

Occlus-o-Guide®

Among the appliances available in the market, the Occlus-o-Guide® is the most well known and widely used because of its specific features and extreme versatility of use. It is available in various series, the G-series being the main one used for the orthopedic phase, particularly for mixed dentition (Fig. 18.8 and 18.9).

Occlus-o-Guide® is a preformed *positioner*-like appliance designed in an attempt to shorten the treatment period with multiband.

As a result of its use, in certain clinical cases, it has helped achieve results comparable to those of standard orthodontic treatment, thereby considerably simplifying the treatment process.

As with the principle of the *set-up* of dental elements in the *positioner*, it is possible to observe specific spaces for each individual dental element within the Occlus-o-Guide® to ensure alignment.

Thus, it can also be used to guide the eruption of canines and premolars toward a perfect occlusal relationship, aligning them simultaneously.

It also acts as an activator, and because it is constructed for maintaining the jaw in an advanced position with the upper and lower incisors in a head-to-head ratio, it stimulates mandibular growth, inhibits maxillary growth, and creates a permanent change in the skeleton in horizontal overjet.

It provides depressive forces to the anterior teeth and encourages the posterior elements to erupt in their ideal vertical position (Fig. 18.10).

Furthermore, it is a myofunctional regulator that correctly balances the muscular forces: it rehabilitates the posture of the tongue, re-educates atypical swallowing, and stimulates correct breathing.

The Occlus-o-Guide® can be used to treat certain dysgnathic forms and malocclusions at any age, including adults. At early ages, it is indicated in the treatment of various degrees of overbite, overjet up to 10 mm, early crowding of the lower incisors, lingual eruption or rotations of permanent incisors of the upper and lower arch, interincisive diastemas, interception of class II malocclusions, interception of bad habits, and certain cases of dental crossbite (Figs. 18.11-18.16).

In adults, the Occlus-o-Guide® allows the resolution of slight dental misalignments and resolves cases of mild overjet and overbite as well as slight incoordination of the median lines.

The size selection is made using a ruler. The scale for the upper and lower arch is shown on this ruler.

Using the scale for the upper arch, the ruler's tab is placed on the distal wall of the left lateral incisor and folded along the incised edges, and the measurement is recorded at the level of the distal surface of the right lateral incisor. The same steps are followed for the lower arch (Fig. 18.17).

The correct size of the appliance must be used for perfect adaptation to the dental elements in case there is spacing or crowding. In the case of diastemas, a half-measure less than that detected is recommended; in contrast, in case of crowding, a greater measurement is necessary. Each half-measure varies by 1.5 mm for the upper arch.

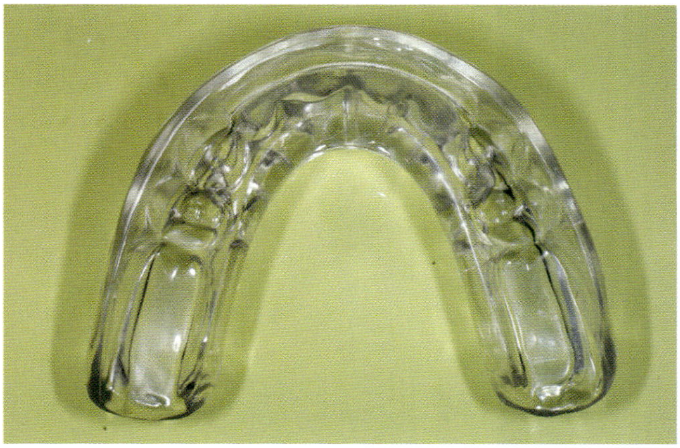

Figure 18.8 Occlus-o-Guide® G-series appliance.

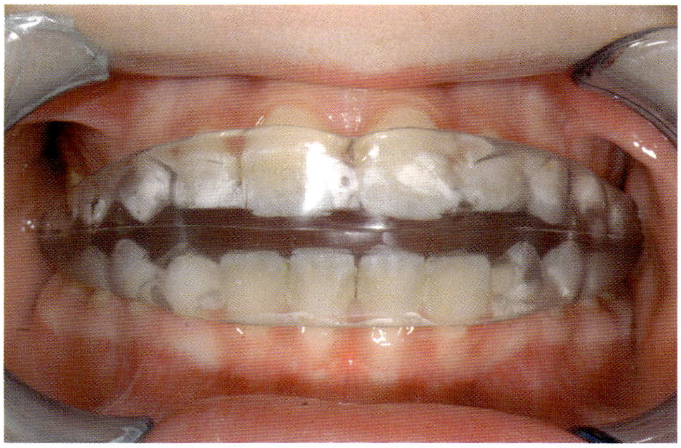

Figure 18.9 Application of Occlus-o-Guide®.

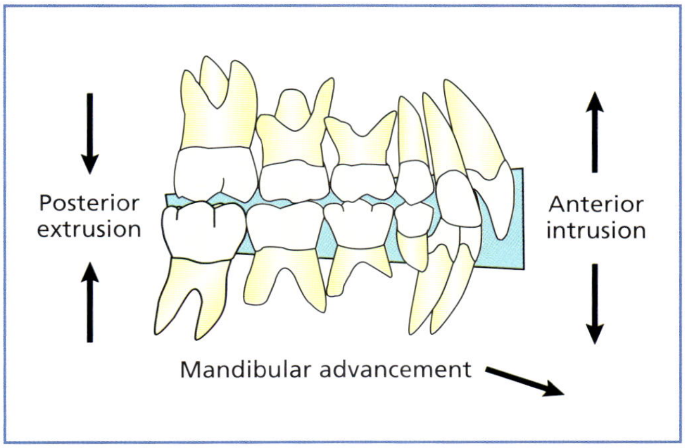

Figure 18.10 Effects of Occlus-o-Guide®.

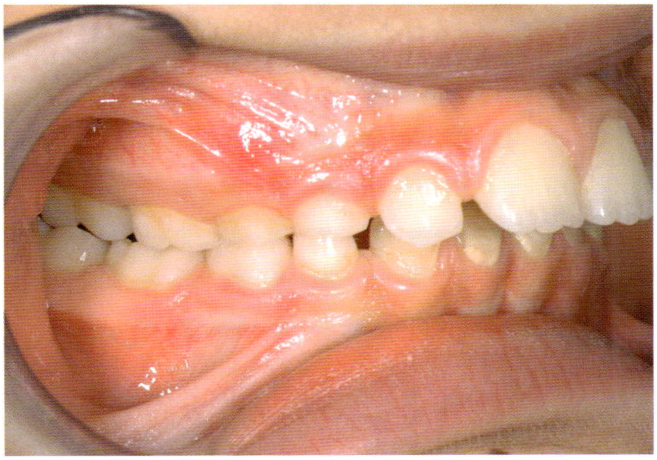

Figure 18.11 Class II in mixed dentition.

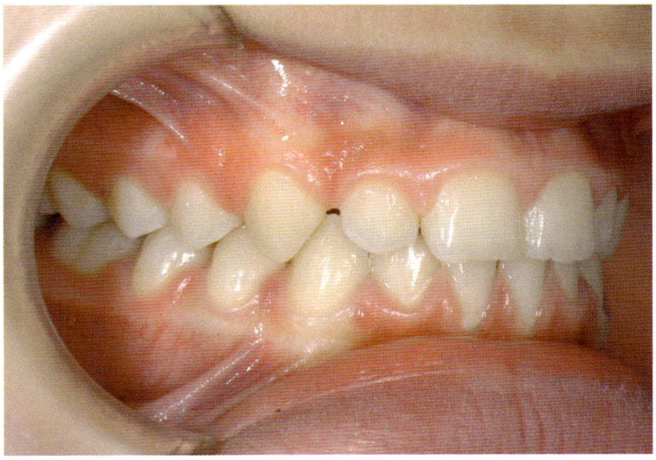

Figure 18.12 Resolution of Class II using Occlus-o-Guide®.

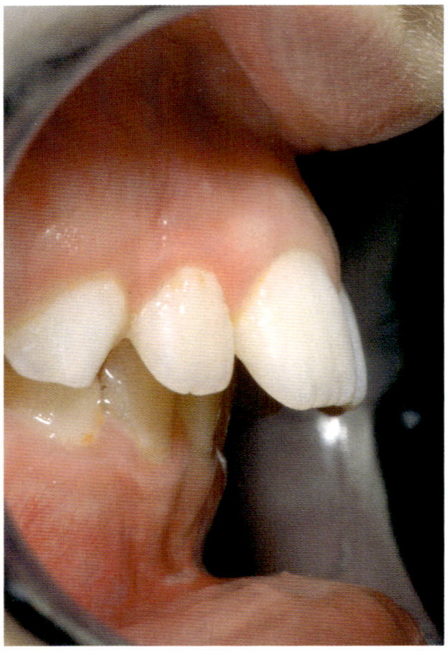

Figure 18.13 Increased overjet.

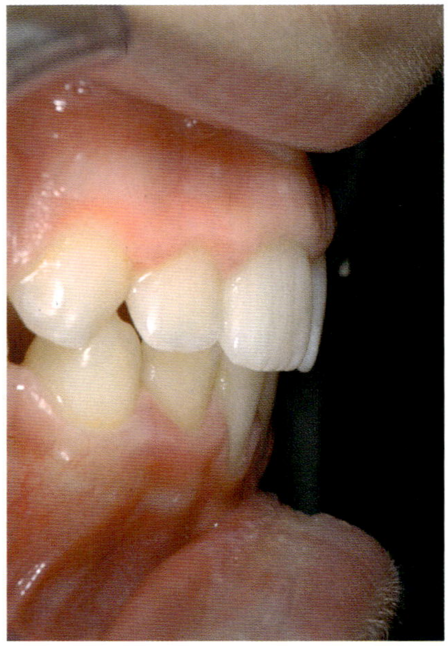

Figure 18.14 Correction of increased overjet using Occlus-o-Guide®.

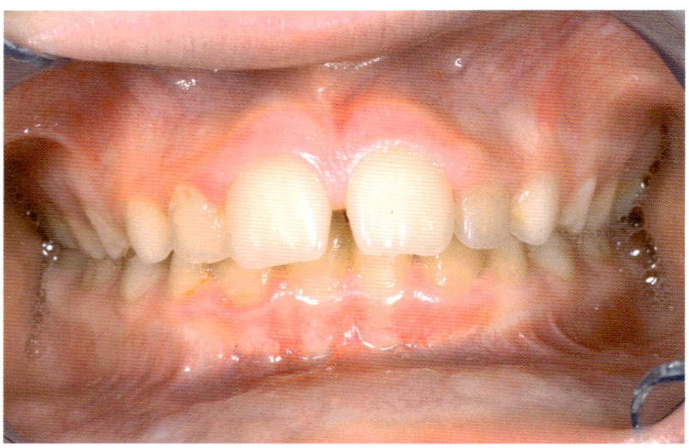

Figure 18.15 Deep bite in the mixed dentition.

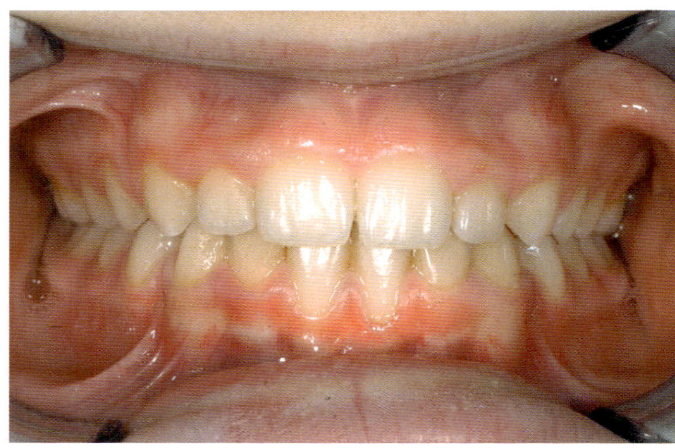

Figure 18.16 Resolution of deep bite using Occlus-o-Guide®.

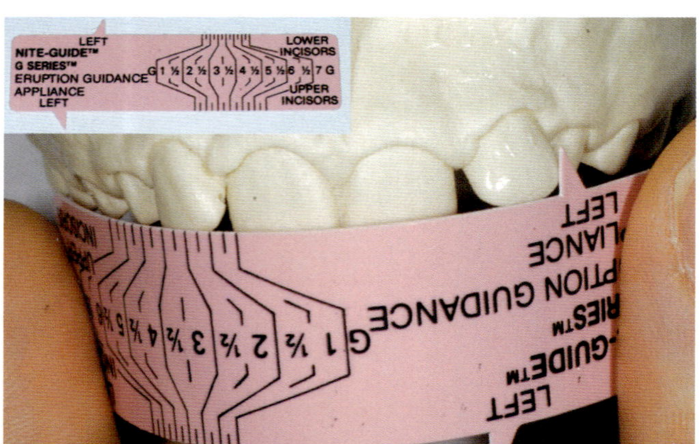

Figure 18.17 Measurement for selection of the appliance.

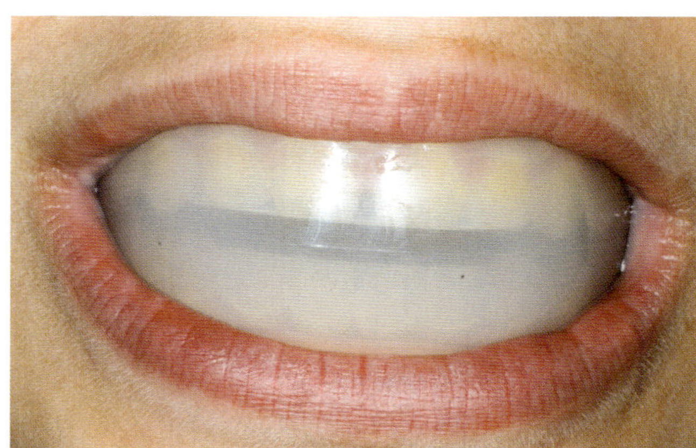

Figure 18.18 Change of color of the appliance.

The appliance should be cold sterilized because it is made of resilient material that undergoes deformation in the autoclave.
All Occlus-o-Guide® appliances contain a material called *cooperation detector*, which, in contact with oral fluids, gradually opacifies the appliance, and assumes a milky color when transparent (Fig. 18.18).
Therefore, if the patient cooperates, there is opacification of the appliance during various follow-up examinations.
If, for any reason, the appliance is not consistently used a further color change toward the initial one is observed.
The patient is instructed to gradually increase the use of the appliance up to 2–4 hours per day, including all night; thus, after 2–6 months of regular application, a remarkable improvement can be observed.
This appliance is available in the market and is commercially grouped in specific *series* depending on the dentition phase of the patient and the type of clinical condition to be treated.

G-series. These appliances are specifically used for patients with mixed dentition until the eruption of the second permanent premolars.
They are highly effective in correcting any type of vertical overbite, horizontal overjet, rotations, slight crowding, diastemas, labiolingual positions of anterior elements, and crossbite in the premolar region.
This appliance has specific spaces for each dental element up to the premolars of both arches to guide the eruption. It descends posteriorly to facilitate the eruption of posterior sectors, correct deep bite, and flatten the curve of Spee.
The recommended period for starting the correction is when the upper incisors begin to erupt permanently, but it is possible to apply this appliance even after this stage.
To achieve an optimal result, we recommend using it for 4 hours a day and throughout the night.

N-series. This is specifically used for patients with permanent dentition after eruption of the second permanent molars (Fig. 18.19). It can also be used in adult patients.
It can help correct overbite of various degrees, horizontal overjets, rotations, slight crowding, diastemas, labiolingual positions of the front elements, and crossbite in the area of the premolars.
The appliance was developed as a *positioner* to be applied after the multibanding of class II cases.
It has specific spaces for each dental element up to the second permanent molars and does not descend posteriorly as the previous one; therefore, in the authors' clinical practice, it has allowed the resolution of less serious overjet conditions compared with the G-series, and because the patient's growth phase was at a more advanced stage.
Additionally, this series of Occlus-o-Guide® appliances is to be worn from 1 to 4 hours a day, plus all night, and can be applied for fine-tuning after the G-series.

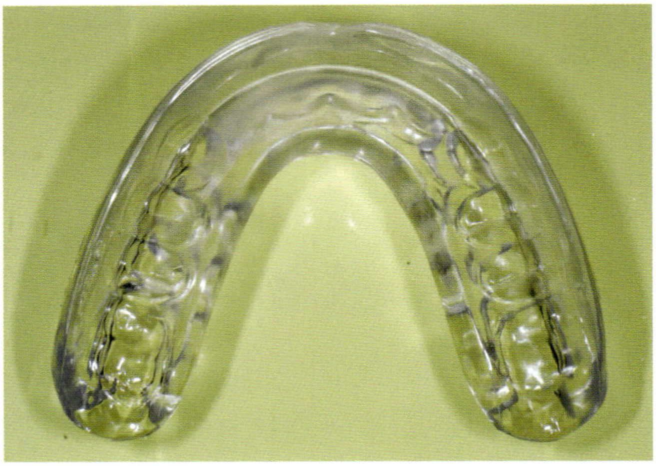

Figure 18.19 Occlus-o-Guide® N-series appliance.

X-series. This appliance is specifically used for patients with significant dental crowding where it is necessary to extract the first four deciduous molars and the first four permanent premolars and where the unerupted permanent canines are distally located between the lateral incisor and the first deciduous molar in a high position.
The canines, if not already erupted, are guided into the position of the first premolars; if instead the permanent canines have erupted and an extraction needs to be performed, the application of multiband is necessary, although it is possible to remove it early enough to allow the Occlus-o-Guide® of the X-series to refine the case.
It should be applied for 2–4 hours a day until the teeth have attained the correct position, after which it should be applied for only 1 hour per day and night until all the permanent elements are erupted.

U-series. This series is specifically used for cases in which only the first two upper premolars are extracted. It is rarely used in our clinical practice and is mostly employed as a positioner following a fixed orthodontic treatment in which two upper premolars have been extracted.

H-Series. This appliance is specifically used in cases of mixed dentition with a severe overjet. The appliance causes a displacement of the lower jaw 5 mm beyond the upper jaw. Once the overjet has been corrected, the appliance has to be replaced with the G/N-series or multiband to finalize the case.
We have used this appliance as an orthopedic appliance and have noted its effectiveness. However, it is advisable to take advantage of the corrective capacity of the G-series before using the H-series because the extreme protrusion causes considerable discomfort to the patient and, in cases of severe mandibular retrusion, it often causes pain in the temporomandibular joint.

Interim-G-series®. To complete the Occlus-o-Guide® system, the interim-G is also available; comprises colored plastic materials of softer consistency and allows the

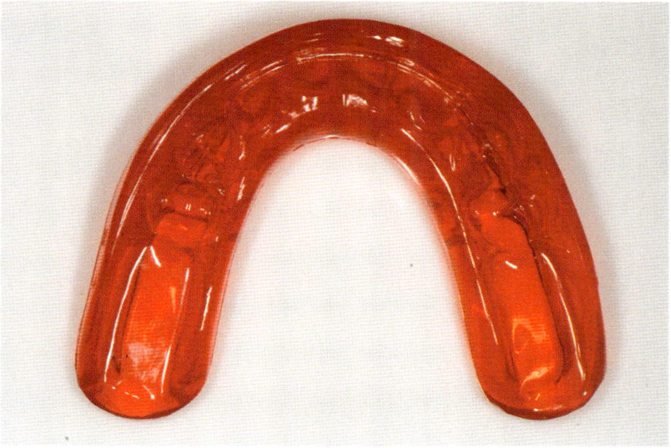

Figure 18.20 Interim-G® appliance.

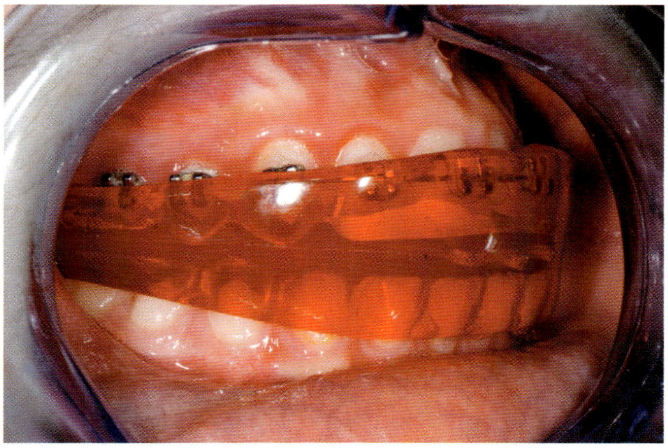

Figure 18.21 Application of interim-G® with fixed appliance.

same corrections as those of the Occlus-o-Guide® of the G-series. In addition, owing to its consistency, it can be used as a support during multiband phases instead of class II elastic bands (Fig. 18.20 and 18.21).

Once the class I relationship between the maxilla and the mandible is restored, dental misalignment and the subsequent maintenance of stability of the results are the only remaining problems.

In this regard, elastodontic appliances are of great value because they combine the ideal *set-up* of dental elements with all the features already described, and therefore, it is possible to observe a progressive alignment of the dental elements until the ideal positions are attained.

The *positioner* described above is the most commonly used elastodontic appliance in the orthodontic corrective phase for mild dental misalignment and is subsequently used as a retainer. Nevertheless, because it is designed following the same principle, the Occlus-o-Guide® in the specific N-series for permanent dentition also provides valuable assistance to clinicians.

The wide versatility of the Occlus-o-Guide® appliances should be appreciated because it is possible to use them in combination with many clinical supports to further improve their effectiveness.

Rotating *cleats* can be inserted to accelerate the correction of rotations. Australian wire can be a valuable aid in recovering ectopic elements, for closing diastemas, or for correcting dental crossbite.

It is possible to use the Occlus-o-Guide® in combination with other appliances such as the *lip bumper* to achieve further recovery of space, thereby allowing a slight distalization of the posterior region or extraoral tractions, for instance, with high separated arched traction to correct a gummy smile and to allow a better orientation of the bispinal plane or in combination with appliances for upper arch expansion such as the rapid palate expander or the Quad Helix, obviously by deactivating the appliance at the points of interference with the other.

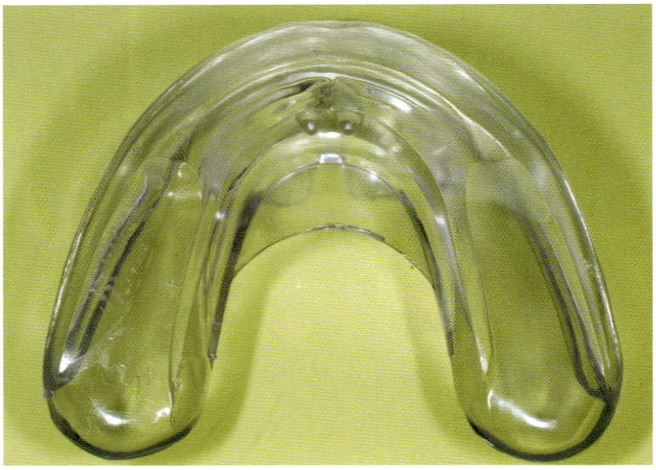

Figure 18.22 Habit-Corrector® appliance.

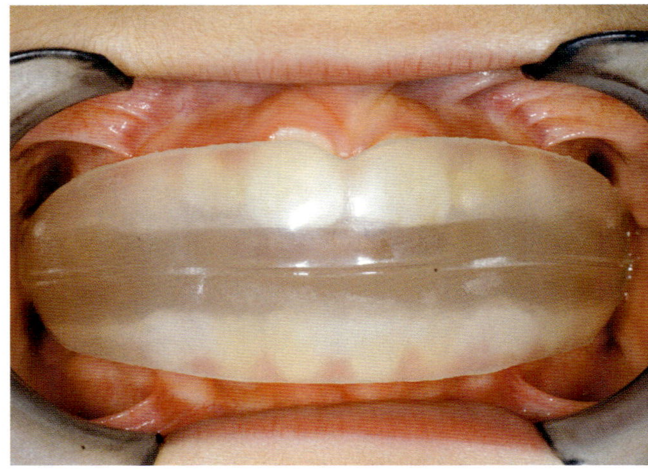

Figure 18.23 Application of Habit-Corrector®.

Habit-Corrector®

This appliance is indicated in pediatric patients for the correction of open bite due to bad habits. The design is characterized by a vestibular shield, smooth and thick posterior surfaces, a groove for positioning the upper and lower dental elements, and two elements for lingual re-education: a tongue-climbing plane and two projections for the tip of the tongue.

It does not have individual spaces for the teeth; therefore, no measurement is needed for size selection because it can be adapted to all patients with the correct indication (Fig. 18.22 and 18.23).

It needs to be applied for 2–3 hours a day, during which tongue re-education is performed, and during the night.

The child places the tongue on the plane and moves the projections with the tip of the tongue, practicing to find a high position and avoid an abnormal interposition. This appliance can be used in combination with classic muscle exercises or speech exercises.

It is indicated in cases of atypical swallowing, finger or pacifier sucking, and habitual mouth breathing. The action of the Habit-Corrector® consists of lingual control and re-education, posterior extrusion blockage, and anterior extrusive action for open bite closure.

The appliance is available in two versions: closed and open Habit-Corrector®; the second type is used in cases of mouth breathing. In addition, it can be used as a substitute for eliminating the bad habit and facilitate treatment in children who still suck their fingers or pacifiers. It is contraindicated in cases of class III skeletal dysgnathia and skeletal deep bite.

It is usually prescribed in the early and late deciduous or mixed dentition period as a retainer; it may be helpful in patients in whom treatment has been performed using other appliances but there is still a need to evaluate the lingual interposition to avoid recurrence (Figs. 18.24–18.28).

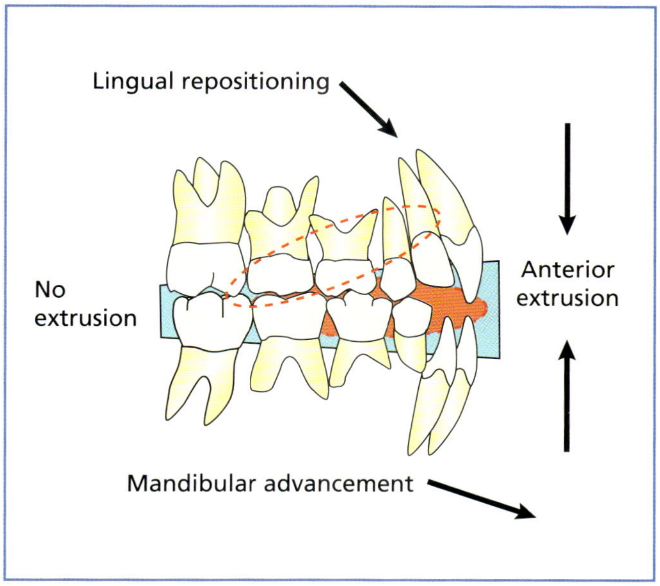

Figure 18.24 Effects of Habit-Corrector®.

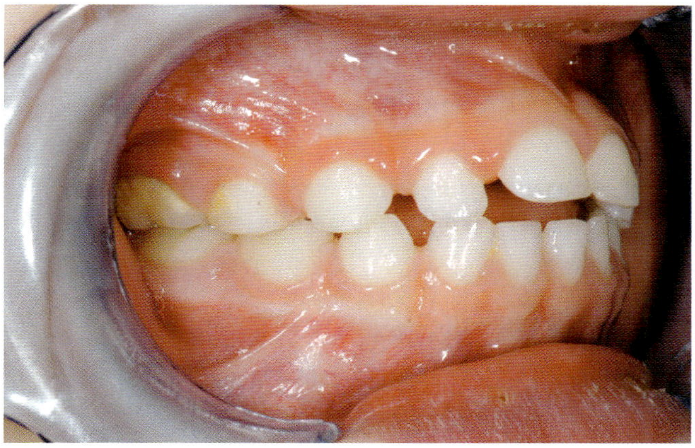

Figure 18.25 Open bite and increased overjet in the deciduous dentition.

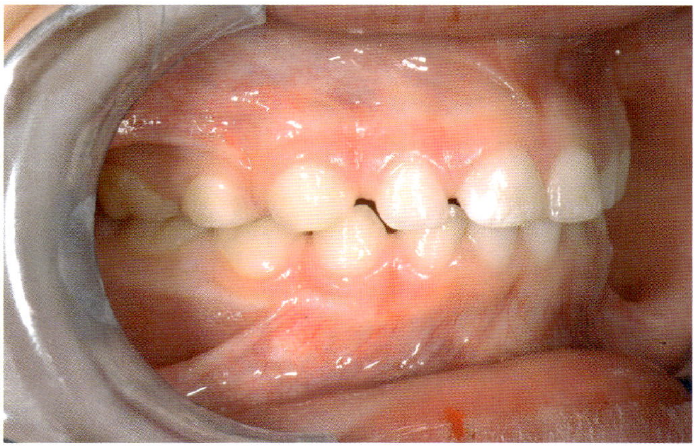

Figure 18.26 Resolution of malocclusion using Habit-Corrector®.

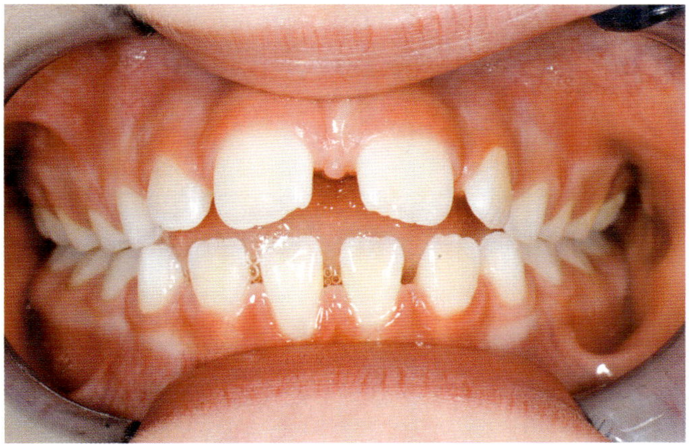

Figure 18.27 Open bite and atypical swallowing in the mixed dentition.

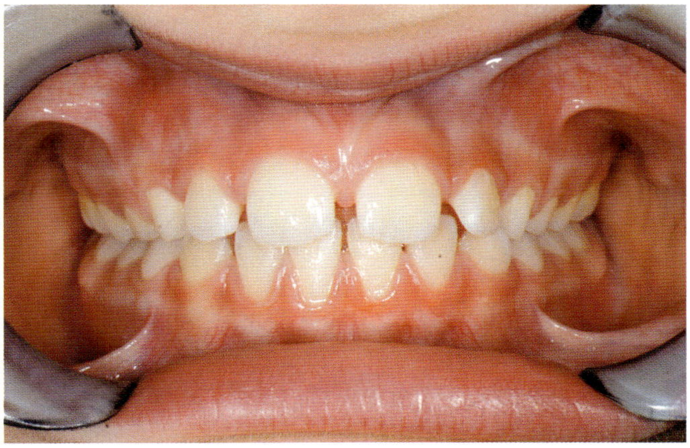

Figure 18.28 Resolution of malocclusion using Habit-Corrector®.

Conclusions

One of the major advantages of the above-described appliances is their versatility; they can be used in the prevention, correction, and retention phases, alone or in combination with other appliances.

With the objective to *minimize intervention*, these appliances enable patients with *special needs* to be treated, making it possible to simplify and optimize the treatment. In our experience, these appliances can be used for patients with general complications, such as heart disease, hemophilia, immune deficiency, and disability, as well as for patients with odontostomatological complications, such as amelogenesis imperfecta and dentinogenesis imperfecta, who have not experienced complications related to the application of fixed and rigid appliances.

In Table 18.1, indications and contraindications for using the various types of elastodontic equipment are summarized, emphasizing that appropriate case selection and precise diagnosis matter the most.

Table 18.1 Use of elastic orthodontic devices

• Skeletal Class I and skeletal deep bite • Skeletal Class II normal overbite and skeletal deep bite • Overbite of various degrees • Overjet up to 10 mm • Interception of bad habits • Early crowding of lower incisors • Lingual eruption or rotation of upper and lower permanent incisors • Interincisive diastema • Dental crossbite • Resolution of temporomandibular joint problems	• Skeletal Class III • Skeletal hyperdivergence • Overjet greater than 10 mm • Dental open bite after 11 years of age • Severe lower dentition crowding • Basal crossbite • Severe problems related to the temporomandibular joint

References

Bergersen EO. A longitudinal study of anterior vertical overbite from eight to twenty years of age. Angle Ortho 1988;58 237-56.

Bergersen EO. Preventive and interceptive orthodontics in the mixed dentition with the myofunctional eruption guidance appliance: correction of crowding, spacing, rotations, crossbites and TMJ. J Pedodont 1988;12:386-414.

Bergersen EO. Preventative eruption guidance in the 5 to 7-year-old. J Clin Ortho 1995;29: 382-95.

Bergersen EO. The preformed orthodontic positioner and eruption guidance appliance. Chicago: Northwestern University; 1981.

Bergersen EO, Manzini P. L'utilizzo dei dispositivi Nite-Guide e Occlus-o-guide in terapia ortodontica preventiva e intercettava. Torino: Utet; 2005.

Farronato GP, Bruno E, Calderini A, Giovannoni R. Posizionatore: nota I. Tecnica di costruzione e suo significato clinico. Odontoiatria Oggi 1988;5(1).

Farronato GP, Bruno E, Calderini A, Giovannoni R. Posizionatore: nota II. Casistica clinica. Odontoiatria Oggi 1988;5(2).

Frassanito P, Paini L, Alicino C, Farronato D. Proposta di una nuova classificazione diagnostica delle disgnazie. Mondo Ortodontico 2003;2:115-21

Farronato GP, Paini L, Alicino C et al. Attuali orientamenti in ortognatodonzia. Il Dentista Moderno 2003;23-42.

Giannì E. La nuova ortognatodonzia, vol. 1-2. Padova: Piccin; 1980-1986. Problemi e soluzioni. Mondo Ortodontico 2002;2.

Ierardo G, Luzzi V, Manes Gravina G et al. Eruzione ectopica degli incisivi inferiori: intercettamento precoce con dispositivi preformati Nite-Guide e Occlus-o-Guide. Doctor Os 2004;1.

Ierardo G, Luzzi V, Trapani D et al. Intercettamento delle abitudini di suzione con dispositivi preformati. Doctor Os 2007;2.

Ierardo G, Luzzi V, Vassallo D et al. Nuovi concetti di management in ortodonzia preventiva. Efficacia ed efficienza. Dental Cadmos 2000;15:98-103.

Janson G, de Souza JE, de Freitas MR et al. Occlusal changes of Class II malocclusion treatment between Fränkel and the eruption guidance appliances. Angle Orthod 2004;74(4):521-5.

Janson G, Nakamura A, Chiqueto K, Castro R, de Freitas MR, Henriques JF. Treatment stability with the eruption guidance appliance. Am J Orthod Dentofacial Orthop 2007;131(6):717-28.

Keski-Nisula K, Hernesniemi R, Heiskanen M et al. Orthodontic intervention in the early mixed dentition: a prospective, controlled study on the effects of the eruption guidance appliance. Am J Orthod Dentofacial Orthop 2008;133(2):254-60.

Keski-Nisula K, Keski-Nisula L, Salo H et al. Dentofacial changes after orthodontic intervention with eruption guidance appliance in the early mixed dentition. Angle Orthod 2008;78(2):324-31.

Levrini A. Terapia miofunzionale. Rieducazione neuromuscolare integrata. Milano: Masson; 1997.

Lorentz H. Treatment with preformed positioner. Trans Eur Orthod Soc 1973;207.

Luzzi V, Ierardo G, Ladniak B et al. L'intercettamento precoce delle deviazioni mandibolari funzionali in dentatura decidua mediante l'utilizzo del dispositivo Nite Guide: Case Report. Mondo Ortodontico 2003;3.

Manzini P, Collini M. Trattamento ortodontico preventivo con dispositivi rimovibili. Il Dentista Moderno 1999.

Chapter 19

Pharmacological therapy in pediatric dentistry

G. Giuliana, N. D'Alessandro

The administration of drugs during the developmental age involves considerable responsibility as it may affect the safety and health of the child undergoing treatment.
Children should not be considered as "young adults" when prescribing drugs. The route of administration, absorption, metabolism, and excretion of drugs in children are different from those in adults for anatomical and physiological reasons. However, the use of drugs that do not have a pediatric indication, known as *off-label* use, i.e., outside the indications given in the license, is still widespread. The majority of drug-related incidents affecting children are caused by the considerable lack of specific clinical trials conducted on children.
In many cases, dentists must resort to pharmacological therapies that, depending on the case, are purposed toward the control of pain and inflammation, treatment or prevention of infectious processes, and treatment of emergencies. In general professional practice, pediatric orthodontists frequently deal with patients undergoing treatment for systemic diseases. Intervention by pediatric orthodontists involving prescription or direct administration of drugs may interfere with pharmacological treatment implemented in pediatric patients; therefore, it is important to have appropriate interdisciplinary liaison.
Prescription or administration of drugs in pediatric patients is therefore a complex occupational activity that requires the pooling of scientific knowledge, practical skills, respect for ethical principles, and educational skills. The educational role is particularly relevant where the patient's parents are concerned, who must be guaranteed comprehensive, correct, and adequate information on why, how, when, and where the drug is to be administered, and involves adequate training on administration.

Prescription of drugs for pediatric use

It is of paramount importance to verify the indications of the drug and to know whether it is authorized for pediatric use and, if so, in which pharmaceutical form. Different formulations of the same drug containing the same amount of active ingredient and administered via the same route may produce different pharmacological responses.
Additionally, via careful collection of family and personal medical history, it is important to ascertain whether adverse reactions have occurred following drug administration. The prescription should clearly indicate the generic name of the drug next to the brand name. Once the drug to be administered has been selected, a treatment sched-

ule should be established to determine the route of administration, dose, dose range, and duration of treatment following instructions on the package leaflet. Precautions regarding use and possible interactions should be clearly stated (Randall, 2005). It is preferable to state the patient's weight on the prescription and reduce the duration of the prescription to the minimum. As mentioned parents should be informed about the type of drug and the route of administration. They should also be made aware of the risks associated with the interruption of dosage, possible adverse effects, or interactions with other drugs.

Dosage

The pediatric population includes several heterogeneous groups ranging from infants to adolescents; consequently, doses of the same drug can vary by up to ten times. No rules guarantee the efficacy and safety of drugs in children. The most rational approach is offered by pharmacokinetic data according to age group. If the dosage is calculated per unit of body weight, there is a high risk of a simple mathematical error. This error in dosage calculation affects children up to 4.94 times more than it affects adults and results in overdose in 56% of cases (Conroy et al, 2008).

Routes of administration

Various routes of administration are available and they should be assessed for clinical needs at the time of drug prescription. The most common is the *enteral* route, through which, in descending order of bioavailability, solutions, suspensions, capsules, tablets, and coated tablets can be administered. The effect of the pharmaceutical form is predominantly in terms of absorption and varies depending on the route of administration. Tablets are not indicated in children aged up to 5 years for whom liquid administration is preferred. In prolonged treatments, it is advisable to prescribe sugar-free, non-cariogenic drugs. Generally, rectal medications are prescribed in very young children who are unable to consciously swallow drops and syrups or in cases in which the child is experiencing gastrointestinal complications.

Administration via *inhalation* is mainly used for the treatment of respiratory diseases. Its use in dentistry consists of the administration of nitrous oxide (N_2O) for analgesic purposes.

Administration via injection (intramuscular, subcutaneous, or intravenous) allows a rapid systemic effect. It is recommended for children with vomiting, diarrhea, or other gastrointestinal complications. Local anesthetics are examples of injectable solutions.

Topical administration of drugs is preferred when the active ingredient must have a localized effect in a particular area of the body. In dentistry, preparations for local use are frequently used.

Pharmacological interactions

Concomitant administration of two or more drugs is a common clinical practice aimed at achieving one or more desired therapeutic results. However, the effects of a drug may be altered by the concomitant administration of other compounds, which include herbal remedies, foods (Table 19.1), ethanol, and tobacco. Pharmacological interactions may be *pharmacokinetic* (absorption, distribution, metabolism, and elimination) or *pharmacodynamic*, such as antagonism and receptor enhancement.

For example, drugs commonly used in the treatment of epilepsy, such as carbamazepine, phenobarbital, phenytoin, and primidone, are metabolized in the liver and induce cytochrome P450 (CYP). Treatment along with other drugs that are metabolized through the same route, e.g., oral contraceptives, oral anticoagulants, calcium channel blockers, statins, and some antibacterials, may reduce the efficacy of antiepileptic and associated drugs or may reduce tolerability by requiring an adjustment of the daily doses administered. These possible limitations in handling and tolerability should always be considered when selecting a treatment option, especially in patients particularly at risk, such as children. Every adverse event should be reported via the pharmacovigilance system regulated by the Italian Medicines Agency.

Table 19.1 Influence of food on major antibiotics

Influence	No influence
• Ampicillin (oral)	• Amoxicillin
• Rifampicin	• Amoxicillin + clavulanate
• Macrolides	• Cephalexin
• Tetracyclines	• Doxycycline
• Lincosamides	• Minocycline
• Erythromycin ethylsuccinate	
• Metronidazole	

Commonly used drugs

Antimicrobials

Antibiotics

In pediatric dentistry, antibiotics are used for the treatment of oral cavity infections for which supporting or prophylactic antibiotic therapy is required in patients with cardiovascular disease, those at risk of bacterial endocarditis, or immunocompromized patients (American Academy of Pediatric Dentistry, 2010-2011a; Fisher et al, 2005). According to the antimicrobial spectrum, antibiotics can be classified into *broad-spectrum* (the molecule is active against multiple microorganisms, both gram-positive and gram-negative bacteria), *medium spectrum* (for example, the molecule is active against gram-positive and certain gram-negative bacteria), and *narrow-spectrum* compounds (the molecule is only active against gram-positive or gram-negative bacteria or has exclusive antitubercular action).
The type of action, whether *bactericidal* (the antibiotic causes death of the bacteria) or *bacteriostatic* (the antibiotic blocks bacterial reproduction), depends on the mechanism of action. Bactericidal antibiotics act on fundamental structures on or within the bacterial cell, such as the cell wall and nucleic acids. Bacteriostatic antibiotics, many of which act by reversibly inhibiting ribosomal protein synthesis, leave the task of eliminating microorganisms to the immune system (Table 19.2); therefore, their use in immunocompromized patients should be avoided.
Antimicrobial agents commonly used in pediatric dentistry include *penicillins*, *macrolides*, and *cephalosporins*, while the use of *clindamycin* has decreased because of the fear of complication of pseudomembranous colitis from *Clostridium difficile*. *Tetracyclines* are not used in pediatric patients as they cause dental dyschromia.

Broad-spectrum penicillins

Broad-spectrum penicillins such as ampicillin, amoxicillin, and amoxicillin + clavulanate are authorized for pediatric use.

Table19.2 Bactericidal and bacteriostatic antibiotics

Bactericidal	Bacteriostatic
• Penicillins	• Macrolides
• Cephalosporins	• Tetracyclines
• Glycopeptides	• Chloramphenicol
• Carbapenems	• Sulfonamides
• Monobactams	• Lincosamides
• Aminoglycosides	• Oxazolidinones
• Quinolones	• Streptogramins

Ampicillin. Ampicillin is a semisynthetic broad-spectrum aminopenicillin with bactericidal action (similar to all β-lactams, it inhibits bacterial cell wall synthesis) against gram-positive and gram-negative cocci including strains of *Escherichia coli*, *Haemophilus influenzae*, *Salmonella* sp., and *Proteus mirabilis*. It frequently causes gastrointestinal disorders and diarrhea as well as urticarial or maculopapular skin rashes. Its use is contraindicated in cases of known hypersensitivity to β-lactams; patients with infectious mononucleosis frequently develop rash owing to the administration of this antibiotic.

Amoxicillin. This is also a semisynthetic penicillin that is similar to ampicillin; it has the same spectrum as ampicillin, although it is less active against *Shigella*. It is indicated for the prophylaxis of infective endocarditis. Absorption after oral administration is more complete and rapid than that after amoxicillin administration, with gastrointestinal disorders occurring less frequently. It is contraindicated in cases of known hypersensitivity to β-lactams. The increase in resistance to both ampicillin and amoxicillin suggests that both antibiotics should be used judiciously.

Amoxicillin + clavulanate. The combination of these drugs forms a powerful inhibitor of β-lactamases; it allows the "protection" of the antibiotic by extending its spectrum of activity to the β-lactamase-producing strains of staphylococci, *Haemophilus*, *Escherichia*, *Proteus*, *Enterobacter*, *Aeromonas*, and *Bacteroides*. The use of this combination is contraindicated in cases of hypersensitivity to penicillins and cephalosporins.

Macrolides

Macrolides such as erythromycin, azithromycin, clarithromycin, and roxithromycin are antibiotics with a complex chemical structure. They have the same features as streptogramins and lincosamides.

Erythromycin. Erythromycin is the first member of this class to be isolated. The antibiotic has a bacteriostatic effect; it can be bactericidal depending on the dosage and the bacterial species targeted. Elective indications of erythromycin include streptococcal infections in case of penicillin allergy, staphylococcal infections resistant to β-lactams, and respiratory, skin, and urogenital tract infections. Erythromycin is the drug of choice in the treatment of legionellosis, brucellosis, diphtheria, and whooping cough. It is contraindicated in patients with severe liver impairment or biliary obstruction. It increases the blood levels of terfenadine and astemizole, resulting in severe arrhythmias. It also increases the blood levels of carbamazepine, cyclosporine, digoxin, and ergotamine and reduces the clearance of theophylline and methylprednisolone. Coadministration of warfarin may prolong prothrombin time and promote bleeding. Oral administration may lead to gastrointestinal complications. It is authorized for pediatric use.

Clarithromycin and azithromycin. They have a broad therapeutic spectrum. *Clarithromycin* is well absorbed orally with increased tolerability, especially in gastrointestinal disorders. Its use in pediatric patients is authorized, but not intravenously. *Azithromycin* (an azalide) is characterized by its long elimination half-life, which allows administration in a single daily dose, and by its good bioavailability in saliva and especially in the gum and alveolar bone. Both clarithromycin and azithromycin inhibit CYP to a lesser extent than erythromycin, with less significant interactions.

Roxithromycin. This antibiotic is active against some microorganisms that are normally resistant to other macrolides.

Cephalosporins

Cephalosporins are a group of β-lactam antibiotics with bactericidal action. They have a broad spectrum of action and are classified into four generations. The generations after the first generation tend to have increased activity against gram-negative bacteria and increased resistance to β-lactamases, usually at the expense of coverage against gram-positive bacteria. Only first-generation variants are active against anaerobic bacteria. Cephalosporins should be used with caution in patients with hypersensitivity to penicillins. Cephalosporins for oral use include cefaclor, cefadroxil, and cephalexin. Administration of cephalosporins is not considered advantageous in dental therapy. Such drugs should be used only for serious infections, such as hospital infections and post-surgical complications.

Antibiotic prophylaxis in cardiopathic patients

In 2007, the American Heart Association published updated guidelines for the management of antibiotic prophylaxis in cardiopathic patients (Wilson et al, 2007). These guidelines restrict the use of prophylactic antibiotics to smaller categories than those provided in the previous (1997) version. In particular, prophylaxis is indicated for patients at high risk of bacterial endocarditis, which includes patients with prosthetic heart valves, history of bacterial endocarditis, congenital heart defects, particularly cyanotic heart disease, and valvular pathologies developed after cardiac transplantation (Table 19.3). Other indications for antibiotic prophylaxis concern the type of dental intervention at the highest risk: tartar ablation, periodontal interventions, biopsies, dental extractions, endodontic surgery, the placement of orthodontic bands, and all procedures performed on gum tissues, in the periapical region of the teeth, and interventions involving perforation of the oral mucosa. However, tooth brushing, chewing, and other daily activities also cause episodes of bacteremia (Forner et al, 2006). Thus, maintaining oral health and an optimal incidence of oral hygiene may reduce the incidence of bacteremia to a greater degree than that achieved using antibiotic prophylaxis to prevent endocarditis during certain dental treatments (Wilson et al, 2007).
With regard to the route of administration of antibiotics, the objective of prophylaxis is to achieve high concentrations of the prophylactic agent during bacteremia. It follows that administration should be performed immediately prior to surgery, over a period of time (depending on the type of antibiotic and route of administration) sufficient to achieve and maintain high concentrations during the most probable period of bacteremia. The therapeutic protocol recommended by the American Heart Association in 2007 for prophylaxis of bacterial endocarditis in children is shown in Table 19.4.

Table 19.3 Heart conditions associated with a high risk of bacterial endocarditis for which antibiotic prophylaxis is recommended in patients undergoing dental treatment*

Valvular cardiac prostheses	
Previous bacterial endocarditis	
Congenital heart disease	• Untreated congenital cyanotic heart disease • Recent surgical correction (within 6 months) of congenital cardiovascular defects • Surgical correction of congenital cardiovascular defects with residual defects in the prosthesis that inhibit endothelialization of the prosthetic material
Valvular disease following cardiac transplantation	

(Source: Wilson W et al. Prevention of bacterial endocarditis. JADA 2007;138:739-60; adapted.)

* Dental procedures on gum tissues or periapical region of the teeth and interventions on the oral mucosa.

Table 19.4 Recommended prophylactic antibiotic regime for pediatric dental procedures

Patient's conditions	Medication	Dosage
No contraindication	Amoxicillin	50 mg/kg orally (1 hour earlier)
Impossibility of oral intake	Ampicillin	50 mg/kg IM or IV (<30 minutes earlier)
	Cefazolin or Ceftriaxone	50 mg/kg IM or IV (up to 30 minutes earlier)
Allergy to penicillins	Cephalexin*	50 mg/kg orally (1 hour earlier)
	Clindamycin	20 mg/kg orally (1 hour earlier)
	Azithromycin or Clarithromycin	15 mg/kg orally (1 hour earlier)
Impossibility of oral intake	Clindamycin	20 mg/kg IM or IV (<30 min)
Allergy to penicillins	Cefazolin* or Ceftriaxone*	50 mg/kg IM or IV (<30 min)

(Source: Wilson W et al. Prevention of bacterial endocarditis. JADA 2007;138:739-60; adapted.)

* Cephalosporins should not be used in subjects with immediate hypersensitivity reaction (angioedema, urticaria or anaphylaxis) to penicillins.

Antibiotic resistance

Drug resistance is the reduction or absence of the efficacy of a drug in the treatment of a disease or its symptoms. In the case of antibiotics, it refers to the ability of bacteria to be resistant to these drugs from the beginning or to gain resistance to them. Misuse of antibiotics outside indications and their inappropriate use in terms of dosage and duration of treatment, as well as the use of broad-spectrum drugs or those that are slowly eliminated from the tissues and body, have contributed to the development of antibiotic-resistant bacteria. The problem is further aggravated by the self-prescription of antibiotics by individuals taking them without the prescription of a qualified doctor. Resistance can be innate or acquired. *Innate resistance*, is genetically determined; for example, it is typical of mycoplasmas that are free of cell walls to be resistant to β-lactams, antibiotics specifically targeting this structure; it is also characteristic of enterococci, which, by absorbing preformed folic acid from the external environment, are resistant to sulfamidics. *Acquired resistance* is generally developed by prior exposure of the pathogen to the antibiotic, and it acts through various mechanisms, such as modification of the bacterial target and formation of specific enzymes, such as β-lactamases, which block antibiotic activity. An example of antibiotic resistance is methicillin-resistant staphylococci. Methicillin-resistant staphylococci are a major cause of nosocomial infections. An emerging phenomenon, particularly important in pediatric patients, concerns the dual resistance (to penicillin and macrolides) or multiple resistance of the most important airway pathogen, *Streptococcus pneumoniae*.

In this case, the antibiotic resistance is particularly stimulated by the use of long-acting antibiotics, which persist in low concentrations for long periods in tissues and act on the microbial flora by selecting resistant strains (Dagan et al, 2006). Airway disorders are among the primary reasons for prescribing antibiotics in pediatric patients, and aggressive infections caused by resistant strains of pneumococci are often associated with high mortality levels because of the lack of response to treatment. Multidirectional interventions addressed to both physicians and patients may reduce the inappropriate prescription of antibiotics and the phenomenon of antibiotic resistance.

Antifungal drugs

Mycetes, belonging to the genus *Candida*, particularly *C. albicans*, are components of the normal flora colonizing the oral mucosa and gastrointestinal tract. The invasion of colonized tissues, which causes the onset of lesions, occurs primarily in immunocompromized patients. The most common form of infection during childhood is pseudomembranous candidiasis (thrush). The predisposing conditions are associated with the use of broad-spectrum antibiotics, inhaled or systemic corticosteroid therapy, antiblastic therapy (especially during severe immunosuppression and neutropenia, Alberth et al, 2006), the condition of patients with HIV infection (Gaitan-Cepeda et al, 2010), and those with diabetes or undergoing organ transplantation. Oral candidiasis

in pediatric patients unassociated with immune deficiency is generally treated using topical antifungals such as *nystatin* (oral suspension), which is the first drug of choice, and *amphotericin B* (oral suspension).
In the event of failure or in patients at risk of systemic infection, a systemic active antifungal is used. With regard to systemic therapy, it is important to note that there are substantial differences in the pharmacokinetics of antifungal drugs in adults compared with that in children and data on the efficacy and safety of systemic antifungals in children are limited (Zaoutis et al, 2005).

Nystatin (oral suspension). Nystatin is virtually nontoxic and nonallergenic and is well tolerated by patients of all ages, including frail infants. It should not be used in the treatment of systemic mycosis because its activity is essentially local. If administered in combination with an oral antibacterial agent, it is advisable to continue its use for the same duration as that of the antibacterial agent. Half of the drug dose should be kept as long as possible in each side of the mouth before swallowing. For prophylaxis in infants, the product is introduced directly into the mouth using a dropper.

Amphotericin B (oral suspension). The oral suspension should not be used for systemic fungal infections because the drug is not absorbed by the gastrointestinal tract. Local treatment should be associated with oral treatment by administering the suspension directly into the mouth using a swab. Amphotericin B is tolerated well and rarely induces gastrointestinal disorders. The drug contains parahydroxybenzoate, which may cause delayed allergic reactions such as contact dermatitis. More rarely, it may cause immediate reactions with urticaria and bronchospasm.

Antiviral drugs

Primary HSV-1 infection is the most frequent cause of serious ulcerative lesions of the oral mucosa in children (Shulman, 2005). HSV-2 infection has also been described; they are caused via orogenital contact. Symptoms include irritability, loss of appetite, fever, gum inflammation, and painful mouth ulcers. The infection is self-limiting, typically lasts 10–14 days, and requires symptomatic treatment, including systemic analgesics (paracetamol) and topical anesthetics (2% lidocaine). Younger children have difficulty feeding and face dehydration. In such cases, the volume of parenteral fluids should be restored. In severe conditions, such as disseminated neonatal disease, encephalitis, or immunocompromized patients, antiviral drugs such as *acyclovir*, *valacyclovir*, and *famciclovir*, administered either orally or intravenously, should be used according to the severity of infection (James and Whitley, 2010). There is evidence that early oral administration of acyclovir (within 36 hours of onset) may significantly reduce the clinical course and symptomatology of primary herpetic stomatitis.

Pain control

Over the past 20 years, *research on pain experiences in children* has considerably developed, and various tools are currently available for pediatric pain assessment that in children with communication impairments or neuromotor disabilities. It has been determined that from the 23rd week of gestation, the nociceptive system is, from an anatomical and functional perspective, ready for the perception of pain; however, children aged less than 4 years do not have a sufficiently defined body map to allow them to specify the type, location, and intensity of pain and are not always able to identify the condition that caused it. The memory of pain already exists in the first years of life, and the psycho-behavioral consequences of untreated pain are confirmed. In pediatric dentistry, when possible, treatment should be etiological, oriented toward eliminating the cause of pain; however, it is sometimes necessary, at least until control of causal factors is achieved, to use analgesic drugs to relieve painful symptoms.

Non-narcotic analgesics

Non-narcotic analgesics are the drugs most frequently used to control painful symptoms in children.

Paracetamol. This is the first-choice drug when seeking an antipyretic and analgesic effect; it is indicated for the treatment of mild and moderate pain. Paracetamol should not be considered a genuine nonsteroidal anti-inflammatory drug (NSAID). It has no anti-aggregating activity, and its anti-inflammatory activity is very weak. It is rapidly absorbed at the gastrointestinal level and acts within 30–60 minutes of oral administration. The duration of action is approximately 4–6 hours. Paracetamol can be administered via several routes and has a high bioavailability; it is predominantly excreted in the form of conjugated metabolites. In the case of overdose, paracetamol is potentially toxic to the liver and kidney. In patients receiving oral anticoagulant drugs such as warfarin, administration of paracetamol doses equal to or greater than 2 g/day for several days requires more frequent international normalized ratio (INR) testing than scheduled (due to pharmacological interaction, INR could increase, thereby increasing the risk of bleeding). In pediatric dentistry, the use of paracetamol is indicated to counteract pain or fever due to the eruption of teeth. It is important to avoid overdosage; moreover, children can inadvertently mistake paracetamol tablets for treats and take them. NSAIDs may be used if an anti-inflammatory drug is actually needed. Acetylsalicylic acid can cause Reye's syndrome and bleeding and, therefore, rarely used in pediatric patients. A significant limitation of NSAIDs is the restricted use related to the patient's age and unavailability of pharmaceutical products with a formulation suitable for use in children.

Ibuprofen. Among pediatric NSAIDs, ibuprofen (for children aged >6 months) is the most studied drug with regard to the safety profile. Similar to all NSAIDs, ibuprofen has an anti-inflammatory, analgesic, and antifebrile action. Side effects of NSAIDs include gastrointestinal disorders, gastric mucosa lesions, allergies, and changes in liver and renal functions. Although these are considered to be rare, they are possible in cases of dehydration. Therefore, it is appropriate to assess the hydration status or the risk of dehydration of the child before prescribing the drug. The most important limitation to the use of NSAIDs is complications of blood coagulation, which constitute a risk to be assessed in clinical conditions related to the presence of hematological diseases or the postoperative period, as well as trauma. "Nonopoid" drugs are drugs that have a *ceiling* effect, i.e., the effect cannot be increased by increasing the dosage and changing the route of administration, but the occurrence of side effects is increased; therefore, if the analgesic response is insufficient, the most appropriate approach is to switch to medium-intensity opioids.

Narcotic analgesics

Codeine, *tramadol*, *morphine*, *fentanyl*, and *methadone* are the most commonly used opioid drugs in children.

Codeine. Codeine is a weak opioid and is the most commonly used drug in pediatric pain control, usually in combination with paracetamol. For codeine and tramadol, once the dose limit is exceeded, the analgesic efficacy remains unchanged, while the adverse effects increase (*ceiling* effect); this effect does not occur for major opioids (morphine, methadone, fentanyl, hydromorphone, and oxycodone) for which, increased dosage increases the analgesic effect, although the adverse effects still pose a limitation to dose increases. The multiple adverse effects of opioids, such as addiction, respiratory depression, gastrointestinal effects, urinary retention, hallucinations, and seizures, require close monitoring of the patient.

Pharmacological control of operating pain, anxiety, and behavior

The prevention of *pain* during dental procedures is essential for establishing a favorable relationship between the patient and dentist and promoting an appropriate approach to dental care. Generally, the elimination of pain in the dental field is achieved at a peripheral level using local anesthetic drugs or at a central level using general anesthesia. In case the management of *anxiety* and *behavior* is needed, sedation may be appropriate, which may involve nonpharmacological, pharmacological, or both techniques (Damia et al, 1988; American Academy of Pediatric Dentistry, 2010-2011b). Nonpharmacological techniques are essentially divided into physical, cognitive, and behavioral methods. The effectiveness of nonpharmacological treatments is primarily determined by the greater plasticity characterizing the circuits involved in children's physiological and cognitive learning than that in adults. Various pharmacological techniques are available, which should be selected on an individual basis.

Local anesthetic drugs

Local anesthesia in dentistry is generally indicated in response to the requirement of the healthcare professional to operate instrumentally on various tissues of the mouth while exceeding the pain threshold. Local anesthetics are of two main types: *amino esters*, such as procaine, benzocaine, and tetracaine, and *amides*, such as lidocaine, mepivacaine, bupivacaine, and articaine. Both types have the ability to block sodium channels in excitable cells with the possible occurrence of toxicity in the central nervous system (with manifestations of excitation because of the blocking of inhibitory pathways and even convulsions, after which a phase of depression may occur with respiratory arrest) and cardiovascular system (cardiac depression and vasodilation) when present in high systemic concentrations.
Amides differ among themselves in several features; for example, bupivacaine is more powerful and has a longer duration of action but also results in greater cardiac toxicity than lidocaine; single-enantiomer derivatives that have less cardiotoxicity, such as ropivacaine and levobupivacaine, have been developed from bupivacaine. Amino esters are affected by a high frequency of allergic reactions, and only some are still used, which are limited to surface anesthesia.
The addition of a vasoconstrictor, such as adrenaline, to the injected local anesthetic solution slows down its passage into the bloodstream, thereby reducing the risk of systemic toxicity and prolonging local action. However, the addition of a vasoconstrictor should be avoided or considered with great caution in patients with significant cardiovascular disease, thyroid dysfunction, diabetes, and sulfite allergy or in those undergoing treatment with certain types of medication, such as nonselective β-blockers (due to the danger of significant hypertension) or halothane, which sensitizes the heart to catecholamines.

Articaine. Articaine is a local anesthetic that is widely used in pediatric dentistry. It differs from other amides in that it contains a thiophene aromatic ring instead of a benzene ring and an additional ester allowing rapid hydrolysis by plasma esterases. These features reduce possible cross-reactivity with other amides and the risk of overdose. Articaine has a rapid onset time and a short duration of action and is used in 4% solution with adrenaline 1:100,000 or 1:200,000. Allergy and methemoglobinemia associated with articaine are rare, but it is important to adhere to the recommended doses: for example, in a child weighing 15 kg, the maximum recommended dose is one vial (72 mg). Due to weight adjustments, there are no age-related pharmacokinetic differences that justify the need to set a dose (mg/kg) that is lower in children than in adults. Alternatively, 2% lidocaine with adrenaline may be used. A randomized trial meta-analysis comparing articaine with lidocaine in local anesthesia for routine dental treatments indicated a certain superiority of articaine in terms of anesthetic efficacy in the region of the first molar, with a safety comparable to that of lidocaine. However, the study did not recommend the use of articaine in children aged <4 years because of the lack of supporting data (Katyal, 2010).

Lidocaine. The topical application of an anesthetic such as lidocaine in the form of an ointment may be useful to minimize the pain caused by needle puncture performed for local anesthesia. Topical administration of lidocaine is associated with an extremely low incidence of allergic reactions but is systemically absorbed and can be added to another amide compound used for actual anesthesia, with an increased risk of overdose. Its use is not authorized in children aged <1 year.

Sedatives

Conscious sedation by inhalation

N_2O is an inhaled analgesic–anxiolytic drug with rapid onset and elimination of effects. Noncompetitive N-methyl-D-aspartate antagonism for glutamate contributes to its mechanism of action. It is almost completely eliminated in an unchanged form by the pulmonary route. Conscious sedation with N_2O and oxygen is a suitable technique in pediatric dentistry. The child, inhaling the mixture from a nasal mask, enters a state of mild sedation and analgesia without the loss of consciousness; therefore, he/she can cooperate without fear. Sedation is initiated using 50% N_2O, and depending on the response, can be reduced to 40% or 35% or increased in 5% increments. In any case, devices administering N_2O for dental use should not dispense <30% oxygen. At the end of the session, the patient is asked to inhale pure oxygen for 5 minutes to avoid diffusion hypoxia.

A precaution is to recommend consuming only a light meal at most 2 hours before the procedure to avoid nausea and vomiting. The dosage of the local anesthetic should not be changed when N_2O is administered. A careful medical history should be made to evaluate the general state of the patient and intake of other medications.

N_2O in this form is authorized in all pediatric age groups provided the child can breathe through the nose. It is contraindicated in patients with an obstruction of the upper respiratory tract, sinusitis, infections of the middle ear or respiratory tract, chronic obstructive pulmonary diseases, psychic disorders, myasthenia gravis, multiple sclerosis, dependence on abuse compounds, and in the first trimester of pregnancy and may interfere with vitamin B12 and cause megaloblastic anemia and neurological toxicity, especially in predisposed patients. If N_2O is used with other sedatives, such as hydrochloride hydrate, midazolam, and opioids, or if it is administered in concentrations >50%, it increases the possibility of switching to a moderate or deep degree of sedation (Tab. 19.5).

Table 19.5 Sedation

Degree of sedation	Level of sedation	Patient's state
1	Minimum sedation	• Relaxed • He/she autonomously maintains the patency of the airways • He/she answers verbal commands in an appropriate manner
2	Moderate sedation	• Sleepy • He/she autonomously maintains the patency of the airways • He/she answers verbal commands and responds to mild physical stimulus in an appropriate manner
3	Deep sedation	• Can be woken only with intense stimuli • Partial or total loss of protective reflexes
4	Anesthesia	• Temporary total loss of consciousness and protective reflexes • Cannot be woken by surgical stimuli

Enteral and parenteral conscious sedation

In children who are unable to breathe voluntarily through their nose, are reluctant, or in whom N_2O is less effective, oral, rectal, sublingual, intranasal, intramuscular, or intravenous sedation may be considered, with the possibility of choosing among various drugs belonging to sedative-hypnotic barbiturates (*pentobarbital*) and non-barbiturates (*hydrochloric hydrate*), anxiolytics (*benzodiazepines*), and narcotic-analgesic (*opioids*). Intranasal administration and injection can be performed only in hospital dental departments, and it is always advisable to use a pulse oximeter for every sedation procedure.

The international literature has numerous controlled and randomized studies of small groups of pediatric patients who have been evaluated at different degrees of sedation; however, the inadequate quality of reporting, variety of treatment regimens and performance indicators adopted, as well as other difficulties, have prevented systematic reviews in determining which drugs and methods are the most effective for sedation (Matharu and Ashley, 2006).

The most commonly used agents are *benzodiazepines*, primarily because of their anxiolytic effects, such as sedation, amnesia, and anticonvulsant activity. Benzodiazepines bind to the gamma-aminobutyric acid (GABA)A receptor site (Cl^- ion-permeable ionotropic receptor) of the inhibitory neurotransmitter GABA and allosterically facilitate the interaction of GABA with its receptor site. The wide safety margin of benzodiazepines is derived from the fact that they enhance the physiological inhibitory mechanism and that they cannot lead to depression of the generalized central nervous system such as that induced by other agents (alcohol or barbiturates) capable of increasing the frequency of opening of Cl^- channels, regardless of the presence of GABA. In addition, in the case of benzodiazepine overdose, *flumazenil*, a competitive receptor antagonist, is available as a specific antidote. The pharmacokinetics are crucial for the choice of benzodiazepine. At present, the most suitable drugs for short- or medium-duration sedation in pediatric dentistry are *diazepam* (indicated for hyperactive children with psychomotor agitation), available in drops; *midazolam* (in Italy, authorized only by injection; however, enteral or intranasal routes conform to a number of internationally accredited studies); and, to a lesser extent, *triazolam* (in Italy, available orally but not recommended for children). Diazepam is characterized by its long duration of action, primarily because of the prolonged presence of its active metabolites in the organism. Midazolam and triazolam are both powerful and have short latency; elimination is rapid for both parent drugs and their active metabolites. However, there is a variability in the pharmacokinetics of these two agents, also in terms of bioavailability after administration by various routes; therefore, titration is important depending on the desired effects. Used alone, these drugs have minor but defined influences on cardiovascular and respiratory functions; triazolam appears to be associated with an increased frequency of residual effects on psychomotor functions.

It should be noted that the activity of these benzodiazepines can be enhanced via association with other substances that depress the central nervous system and by the simultaneous intake of compounds, such as erythromycin, diltiazem, verapamil, azole antifungals, HIV protease inhibitors, and grapefruit juice, which inhibit the metabolic enzyme cytochrome P450 (particularly the CYP3A4 isoform). As a general rule, an oral dose of 0.25–0.75 mg/kg midazolam is adequate to induce effective sedation in children, while the intravenous dose is lower, whereas patients aged <5 years may require substantially higher doses than older children and adolescents.

Some antihistamines such as hydroxyzine and diphenhydramine, although not indicated for sedation, possess sedative-hypnotic and antiemetic properties that can be advantageous in dentistry; these compounds show enhanced effects when used concomitantly with other sedative-hypnotic agents.

A regimen known as analgosedation has been described in international literature. It involves the addition of compounds such as *opioids* or *ketamines* to sedative-hypnotics, usually benzodiazepines such as midazolam. The purpose of these combinations is to improve the quality of sedation with an analgesic component or to prolong its duration; they can also precede general anesthesia when required. In general, both local anesthetics and sedatives depress the central nervous system, and there is evidence of increased toxic reactions to local anesthetics when they are combined with opioids. The use of sedative drugs to achieve conscious sedation requires caution, especially by those who are unfamiliar with their dosage and possible adverse effects. Except for the use of N_2O by inhalation, the use of these drugs is reserved for medical staff specialized in anesthesia and resuscitation.

Specific pathological conditions and emergency drugs

Allergic reactions

Acute allergic reactions are disconcerting events, and the main drugs involved are β-lactams, and to a lesser extent, local anesthetics. The most frequent reactions according to increasing severity are urticaria, asthma, Quincke's edema, and anaphylactic shock. In case the only symptom is urticaria, it may be sufficient to administer intramuscular antihistamine anti-H1, such as *chlorphenamine* (0.3 mg/kg with a maximum dose of 10 mg; it should be noted that according to the technical data sheet, the safety of chlorphenamine for injection has not been established in children aged <12 years, for whom use is not recommended) or, if the situation is more severe, a rapid-acting corticosteroid (such as *hydrocortisone sodium succinate* 100 mg). Bronchial asthma usually resolves with the inhalation of a 2-stimulant bronchodilator with rapid onset and short duration of action, such as *salbutamol* (dosed aerosol, 100 µg per dispensed dose using a VHC spacer and a mask in younger children; or as aerosol solution, one drop, 0.05 ml = 0.25 mg per 2 kg, with the dose diluted in 3 ml of saline solution and not exceeding 20 drops). Such treatments are repeatable, e.g., up to four deliveries in children aged between 6 months and 5 years, and low-flow oxygen helps normalize the condition. If bronchospasm does not subside promptly after salbutamol administration, hospitalization is necessary. In severe cases, adrenaline (0.1 mg/10 kg) is administered subcutaneously or intramuscularly for faster absorption; if necessary, the 1:1000 vial is further diluted to ensure accurate dosing in younger children. Intravenous administration is indicated only in severe conditions and should be performed under myocardial monitoring. It should be noted that adrenaline is light- and heat-sensitive, and unless the self-injectable formulation is used, adrenaline must be kept in a refrigerator. Adrenaline is capable of fully stimulating all types of adrenergic receptors (with vasoconstriction, β1 with reactivation of cardiac function, and β2 with bronchodilator effects) and is the primary emergency pharmacological agent for the treatment of Quincke's edema and anaphylactic shock. The action of the adrenaline is rapid but short-lived, and its timely administration, which may be repeated every 10–20 minutes, is useful to antagonize the most threatening immediate symptoms. Oxygen administration is also of primary importance. Concomitant administration of chlorphenamine and intravenous hydrocortisone succinate is primarily intended to counteract the later stages or recurrence of the aforementioned allergic events. There is an urgent need to transfer the patient to a hospital setting, where treatment should be implemented to restore blood volume, correct metabolic acidosis, and prevent relapses. Conversely, adrenaline is not used in *cardiogenic shock*; in such cases, it is preferable to use a selective β1-receptor agonist, *dobutamine*, combined with low doses of dopamine to preserve renal function.

Seizures

Without considering febrile convulsions, at the time of a dental procedure, most young patients with epilepsy normally have their condition kept under control by specific treatment. However, it is possible that a generalized seizure may occur with tonic–clonic convulsions and loss of consciousness. A possible trigger is respiratory alkalosis from hypercapnia secondary to stimuli such as emotional tension and pain. As mentioned above, local anesthetics can cause convulsions even in healthy children, usually after accidental intravascular injection. The possible association between pediatric administration of N_2O and seizures has also been described in the literature (Zier and Doescher, 2010).

These events have rarely been documented, and the responsibility of N_2O has not been definitively proven; however, for dentists, this is a further recall to their pharmacovigilance duties so that all possible adverse reactions are reported, particularly those that are serious or unexpected.

Usually, the seizure is short-lived and resolves spontaneously, so the procedure consists of preventing injury to the patient and controlling the airway. Care should be taken to not insert any object in the patient's mouth or between the teeth with the mistaken belief that this can protect the patient from biting their tongue. This is rare, and a forced tetanic contraction can cause a fracture of the teeth or jaw. Drug administration (benzodiazepines) should only be performed when seizures are prolonged (movements last 5 minutes or longer) or recur rapidly. In these cases, the patient must visit a hospital.

Hypoglycemia

In children with diabetes, it is advisable to establish procedures to prevent accidents and intra- and postoperative complications associated with metabolic disorders, microangiopathy, and immunological deficit. Treatment should be restricted to well-controlled cases. Stress should be limited because it promotes the secretion of adrenaline, which has hyperglycemic effects. Moreover, dentists should be prepared to recognize the early symptoms of hypoglycemia, including sweating, hunger, paresthesia, palpitations, tremors, and anxiety. However, younger children and 10% of older children do not show warning reactions and directly exhibit neuroglycopenic symptoms such as drowsiness, confusion, and apathy. Hypoglycemia is usually effectively controlled by consumption of a sugar-containing drink. In cases when the patient is unable to swallow, for example, because of loss of consciousness, a 50% glucose solution for intravenous infusion should be available. If intravenous administration is not possible, intramuscular administration of glucagon (vials stored in the refrigerator) may be a solution.

References

Alberth M, Majoros L, Kovalecz G et al. Significance of oral candida infections in children with cancer. Pathol Oncol Res 2006;12:237-41.

American Academy of Pediatric Dentistry. Guideline on use of antibiotic therapy for pediatric dental patients, special issue: reference manual. Pediatr Dent 2010-2011a;32:246-8.

American Academy of Pediatric Dentistry. Guideline on use of nitrous oxide for pediatric dental patients, special issue: reference manual. Pediatr Dent 2010-2011b;32:163-6.

Conroy S, North C, Fox T et al. Educational interventions to reduce prescribing errors. Arch Dis Child 2008;93:313-5.

Dagan R, Barkai G, Leinovitz E et al. Will reduction of antibiotic use reduce antibiotic resistance? Pediatr Infect Dis J 2006;25:981-6.

Damia G, Caprioglio D, Vernole B. La sedazione cosciente in pedodonzia. Quaderni di odontoiatria infantile. Milano: S.p.a. Alberto Matarelli; 1988.

Fisher RG, Boyce TG, Moffet HL. Pediatric infectious diseases a problem-oriented approach. Philadelphia: Lippincott Williams & Wilkins; 2005.

Forner L, Larsen T, Kilian M et al. Incidence of bacteremia after chewing, tooth brushing and scaling in individual with inflammation. J Clin Periodontol 2006;33:401-7.

Gaitan-Cepeda LA, Dominguez-Sanchez A, Pavia-Ruz N et al. Oral lesions in HIV+/AIDS adolescents perinatally infected undergoing HAART. Med Oral Pathol Oral Cir Bucal 2010;15:e545-50.

James SH, Whitley RG. Treatment of herpes simplex virus infections in pediatric patients: current status and future needs. Clin Pharmacol Ther 2010;88:720-4.

Katyal V. The efficacy and safety of articaine versus lignocaine in dental treatments: a meta-analysis. J Dent 2010;38:307-17.

Matharu L, Ashley PF. Sedation of anxious children undergoing dental treatment. Cochrane Database Syst Rev 2006;(1):CD003877.

Randall C. Pharmaceutical prescribing for children. Part 1. Introduction and general principles of prescribing for children. Prim Dent Care 2005;12:123-6.

Shulman JD. Prevalence of oral mucosal lesions in children and youths in the USA. Int J Paediatr Dent 2005;15:89-97.

Wilson W, Taubert KA, Gewitz M et al. American Heart Association Rheumatic Fever, Endocarditis, and Kawasaki Disease Committee. Research Interdisciplinary Working Group 116: 1736-1754, 2007.

Zaoutis TE, Benjamin DK, Steinbach WJ. Antifungal treatment in pediatric patients. Drug Resistance Updates 2005;8:235-45.

Zier JL, Doescher JS. Seizures temporally associated with nitrous oxide administration for pediatric procedural sedation. J Child Neurol 2010;25:1517-20.

Chapter 20

Laser therapy in pediatric dentistry

U. Romeo, A. Galanakis, R. Kornblit

Physical characteristics of lasers

A laser is a device that emits electromagnetic radiation through a process of optic amplification based on the stimulated emission of photons. The term "*laser*" is an acronym for Light Amplification by Stimulated Emission of Radiation. The light beam emitted by laser has peculiar characteristics that can be summed up as follows:

- *monochromaticity*: the emitted radiation always has the same wavelength, which in spectroscopic terms corresponds to a limited spectral line width
- *directionality*: unlike standard electromagnetic sources, a laser emits radiation in a single direction
- *brilliance*: the quantity of energy emitted by lasers per unit surface is much higher than that emitted by standard sources. This characteristic is a direct consequence of the above two characteristics
- *coherence*: each photon in the stimulated emission has the same phase as the one that has induced the emission. The phase is maintained over time and space; consequently, the electromagnetic radiation in a particular moment has the same phase on the whole wavefront.

Generally, a laser comprises three basic components (Fig. 20.1)

- *active medium*: a series of physical processes take place inside an active medium that lead to the emission of the laser radiation. The active medium can be in a solid, liquid, or gaseous state or can comprise a semiconductor. The active medium determines the specific wavelength of the light at which the laser operates
- *energy* or *pumping source*: in many devices, a flash lamp is used to stimulate the atoms of the active medium
- *optical resonator* or *resonant optical cavity*: the optical resonator has two flat and parallel mirrors with which photons, which bounce on them, manage to cross the active material several times and contribute to the stimulation of the emissions before leaving the semireflective mirror.

The produced laser radiation can be funneled and transmitted to a specific target via various optic systems. The components used in the transport of laser light include the following:

- articulated arm (Fig. 20.2)
- hollow fiber (Fig. 20.3)
- optical fiber (Fig. 20.4).

The light beam emission can be

- *continuous*, if the emission is uninterrupted and constant
- *semicontinuous*, if there is emission interruption that lasts within a range of 10 msec–1 sec
- *pulsed*, when emission peaks last for around 1 msec
- *superpulsed*, when emission peaks are of 10 nsec, interrupted by a 10-psec interval.

The light emitted by a laser is contained within the electromagnetic spectrum that lies in the infrared, visible, and ultraviolet regions; in other words, its wavelength is between 10^{-7} and 10^{-3} m (Fig. 20.5).

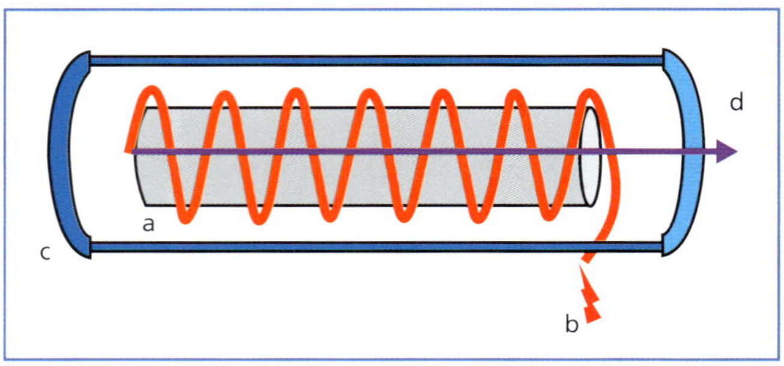

Figure 20.1 A diagram showing the basic laser components: a) active medium; b) energy or pumping source; c) optical resonator comprising mirrors; d) outgoing laser beam.

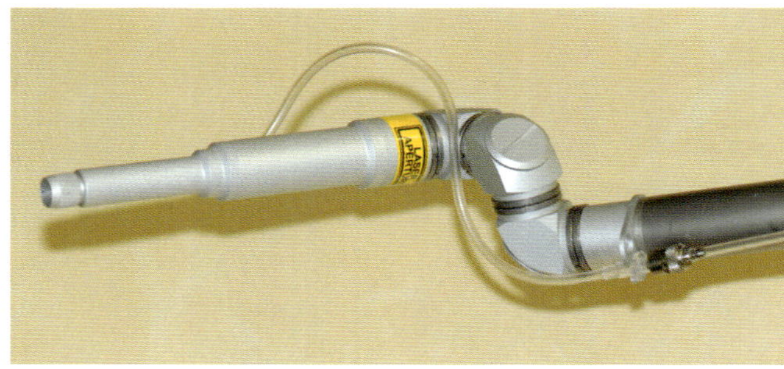

Figure 20.2 Articulated arm.

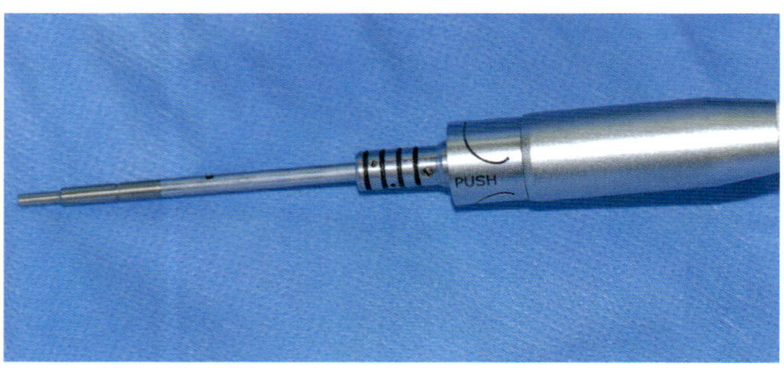

Figure 20.3 Hollow fiber.

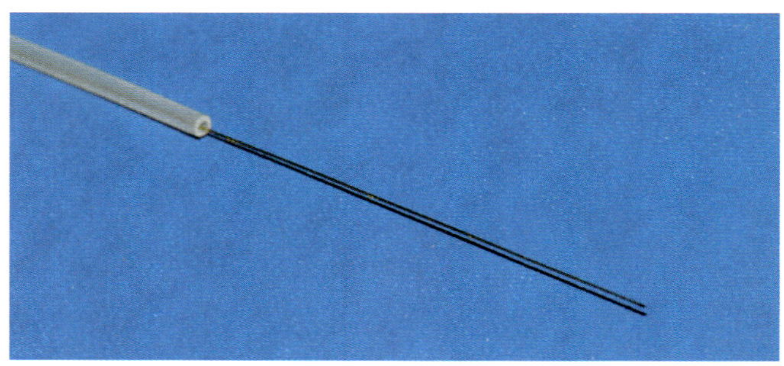

Figure 20.4 Optical fiber.

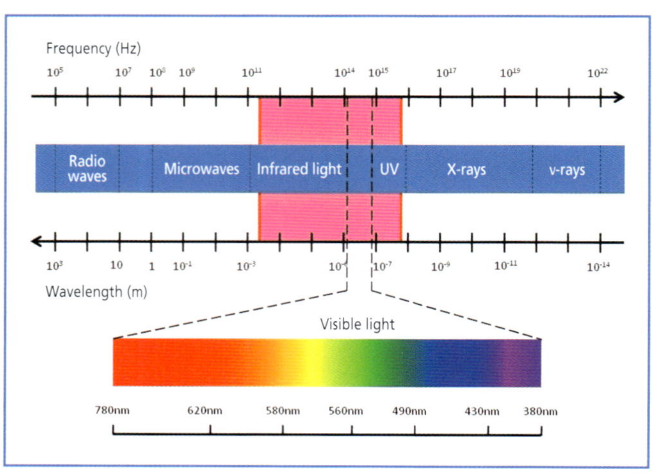

Figure 20.5 Electromagnetic spectrum. The red band indicates the band of wavelengths used by lasers.

Physical interaction between laser light and biological tissues

In general, the interaction between light radiation and biological tissues depends on both the wavelength of the emitted radiation and the optical properties of the tissue concerned. From an optical point of view, biological tissues can be defined as homogeneous and isotropic media in which the propagation of light radiation is described on the basis of fundamental optical properties such as reflection, absorption, transmission, and diffusion (Anderson and Parrish, 1981).

The different modalities of propagation include three types of interactions: photochemical, photothermal, and photomechanical; these exhibit low, intermediate–high, and high intensities, respectively. The possible interaction combinations are well summarized by the map of interactions shown in Figure 20.6. The x-axis shows exposure time (in seconds), and the y-axis shows the power density of the laser beam used. Photochemical interactions (in other words, chemical reactions stimulated by light radiation) take place for low power densities and long exposure times; photothermal and photomechanical interactions take place for high power densities and much shorter exposure times (10^{-3}–10^{-9} sec) and are based on the transformation of light radiation into thermal or mechanical energy (Vogel and Venugopalan, 2003; Boulnois, 1986).

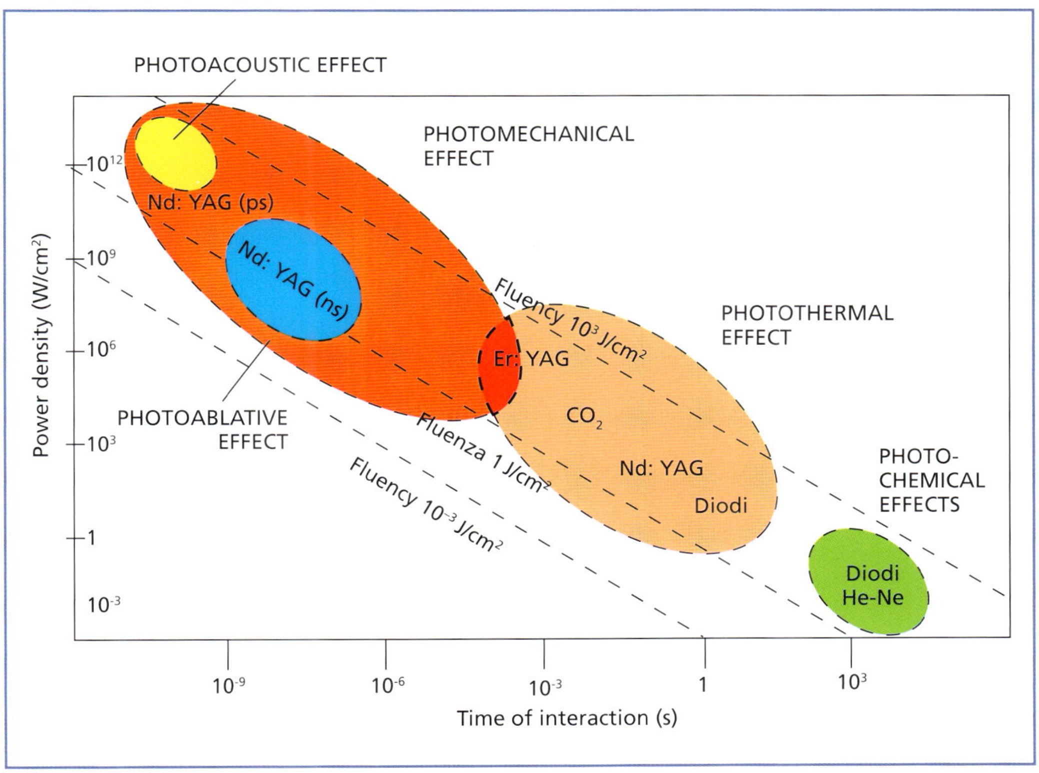

Figure 20.6 Map of interactions between laser radiations and tissues. For each interaction, at least one type of laser is indicated that can achieve the required effect. (From: Boulnois, 1986; modified.)

Dental hard tissues

In dentistry, most recently, lasers have been applied for hard biological tissues; in July 1997, the Food and Drug Administration approved the use of the Er:YAG laser for cavity preparation and caries removal. The laser energy is converted into kinetic energy, and little heat remains in the tissue concerned; this renders the mechanical and thermal damage to surrounding tissues minimal, if not negligible (Tokonabe, 1999). For fluence values between 6 and 10 J/cm^2, the photoablation effect is obtained with impulses that last from 150 to 250 µsec (Apel et al, 2002). Practically speaking, all the interactions between Er:YAG laser radiations and dental tissues depend on the parameters with which the equipment is used (for example, fluence, pulse repetition frequency, pulse energy, and duration) in addition to the water content of the target tissue and the use of air/water cooling sprays (Apel et al, 2002; Kim et al, 2003).

Soft tissues of the oral cavity

For the treatment of soft tissues inside the oral cavity, several wavelengths can be used. This is possible because various wavelengths have an affinity for the chromophores inside the target tissues, specifically hemoglobin and melanin. Together with the use of appropriate parameters, this allows obtaining photometric effects (coagulation, vaporization with cutting effect) that are functional to the intended procedure.
On a macroscopic level, depending on the heating generated, the thermal damage can be gradual and selective:

- 42–45°C: initial hyperthermia, structural modifications, and collagen breakdown
- 50°C: enzymatic activity reduction
- 60°C: protein denaturation, collagen coagulation, membrane permeabilization
- 100°C: tissue dehydration and vacuole formation
- >100°C: initiation of tissue vaporization and carbonization
- 300–1000°C: tissue thermoablation, photoablation, and destruction.

These effects are typically detected with continuous emission lasers for power densities > 10 W/cm^2 or with irradiation through pulsed lasers lasting longer than microseconds. In general, different thermal effects are produced in biological tissues depending on the laser parameters used.
The diagram presented in Figure 20.7 shows the stratification of effects that can be detected in soft tissues depending on the temperature reached in the volume of the tissue concerned. In general, it is possible to observe an area of vaporization within the target tissue at the point where energy is mostly absorbed and the greatest thermal rise is detected, with the ensuing transformation of the water contained in the target tissue into vapors. Below this area, there is an area of carbonization surrounded by a wide area of coagulation. The sizes of these areas can vary depending on the parameters and wavelengths used.

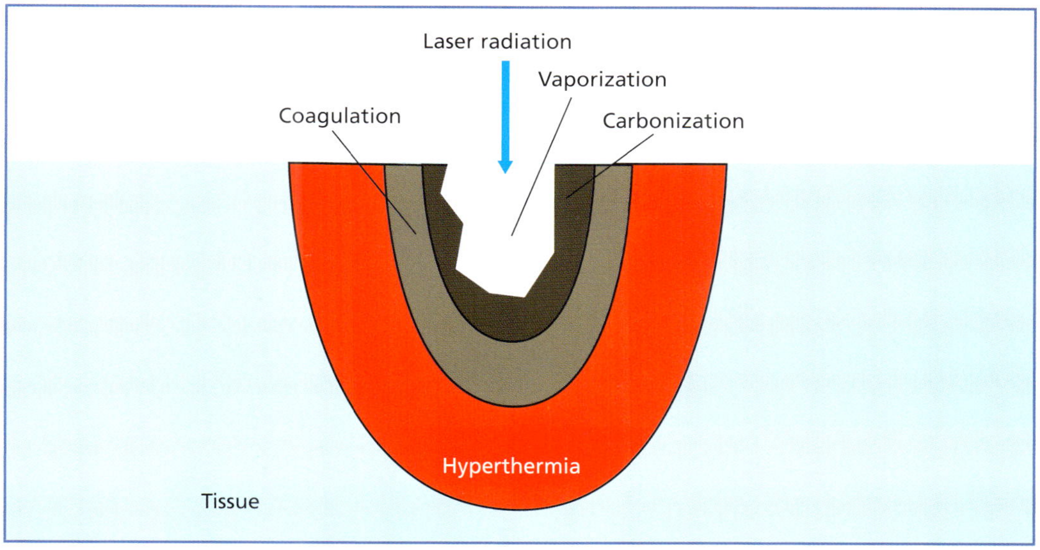

Figure 20.7 Photothermal effects of laser radiations on target tissues. There is an area of carbonized tissue under the vaporized tissue. If thermal effects are conspicuous, but not enough for carbonization, it is possible to detect a portion of tissue where proteins are coagulated and denatured. A large area of hyperthermia can be observed at the margins of the healthy tissue.

Treatment of carious lesions in deciduous and permanent teeth using erbium laser

At present, erbium lasers, whose electromagnetic radiation is absorbed by water, are the only ones that can be used for the removal of dental hard tissues. Two types of erbium lasers are used in dentistry:

- erbium chromium: yttrium, scandium, gallium, garnet (Er, Cr:YSGG) laser (2780 nm)
- erbium: yttrium, aluminum, garnet (Er:YAG) laser (2940 nm).

The efficacy of the erbium laser in the ablation of enamel, dentin, and carious tissues is well documented in the literature (Mir et al, 2008; Liu et al, 2006). It has been shown that during the ablation of dental hard tissues, the intrapulpal temperature increase induced by the laser with air/water cooling sprays is identical to the one generated by rotary devices. So far, no study has detected a temperature increase > 5.5°C, a critical limit for pulp vitality, and this aspect guarantees the preservation of dental pulp healing potential after laser irradiation (Krmek et al, 2009; Kilinc et al, 2009; Contente et al, 2010).

Using an erbium laser in a focused manner, it is possible to vaporize surfaces with a diameter of around 0.8–1 mm. Ablation occurs layer by layer. If an erbium laser is used with a handpiece without a tip (remote handpiece), ablation visibility and control are optimal (Fig. 20.8).

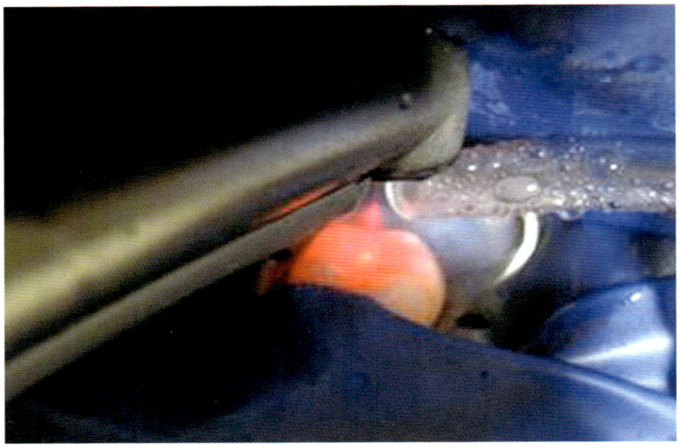

Figure 20.8 Ablation using the erbium laser (remote handpiece), with which it is possible to outline an ablative area around 1 mm in diameter by focusing the tip.

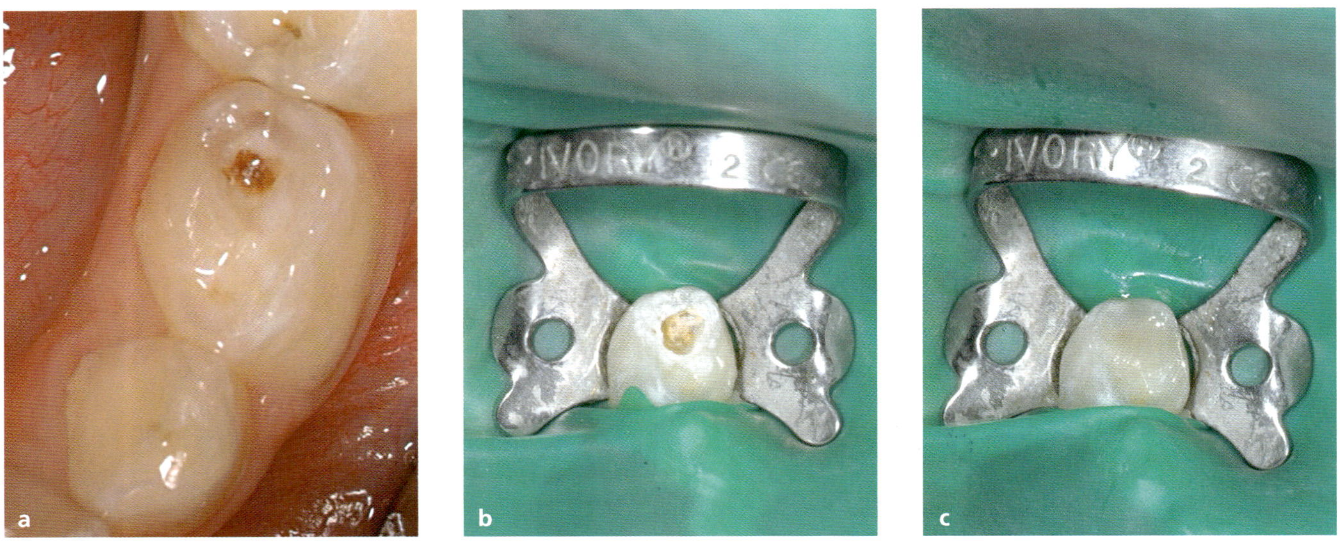

Figure 20.9 (**a**) Occlusal caries in the first lower deciduous molar treated using Er:YAG laser. (**b**) Cavity preparation performed using Er:YAG laser. (**c**) Direct filling using composite material.

The laser technology used for the vaporization of carious dental tissue enables meeting one of the most important requisites of minimally invasive dentistry, i.e., preservation of the healthy dental tissue, which is particularly important when it comes to the deciduous dentition because enamel and dentin thicknesses are lower in the deciduous teeth than in the permanent teeth (Kornblit et al, 2008).

The bactericidal effect produced by the erbium laser (Schoop et al, 2004) allows decontamination of the layer of the affected dentin after the removal of the amorphous layer of the infected dentin, thus permitting the possible remineralization of the former, in which collagen fibers are intact.

After reviewing the literature (Gentil et al, 2010) regarding the treatment of cavity margins using erbium lasers instead of tooth etching with 37% phosphoric acid solution, it is possible to understand the importance of enamel etching at cavity margins to obtain an adequate marginal seal with composite restorations.

Some studies based on the use of a scanning electron microscope have shown non-selective destruction of the enamel prisms of the permanent teeth after laser irradiation (Kornblit et al, 2009). Furthermore, it has been found that the strength of the bond between the intertubular dentin and the related composite material is very poor in a cavity prepared using the erbium laser compared with that in a cavity prepared using the standard equipment (Firat et al, 2010; Moretto et al, 2010); this is due to the damage caused by the laser to the collagen fibers inside the intertubular dentin, preventing the penetration of the adhesive system into the interfibrillar spaces and as well as formation of a hybrid layer. Therefore, it is advisable to treat the irradiated dentin with a 5% sodium hypochlorite (NaOCl) solution for 30 sec to remove the organic components damaged by laser irradiation, exposing new layers of intact collagen fibers for the formation of an adequate hybrid layer.
Figure 20.9 shows the treatment of a carious deciduous tooth using an Er:YAG laser.

Endodontic treatment with laser for deciduous and permanent teeth

The use of laser in endodontics dates back to 1971, albeit with very poor initial results; since then, an increase has been observed in the experimental and clinical research regarding the use of different types of lasers in various endodontic applications.
In pediatric dentistry, the most sought-after applications of laser are, undoubtedly, pulp capping and root canal decontamination.

Pulp capping

The laser devices indicated for pulp capping procedures include diode, Nd:YAG, potassium titanyl phosphate (KTP), and erbium lasers. Capping procedures are performed using a double layer of calcium hydroxide (cementing paste). Specifically, calcium hydroxide placed in direct contact with the pulp tissue forms a mummification area of around 0.2–0.5 mm that is induced by chemical cauterization achieved with high pH levels. Subsequently, a dentin bridge forms that will act as a protective barrier against the attack by bacteria and their by-products on the exposed pulp. However, the problem that ensues involves bacterial infiltration, as the dentin bridge newly formed by calcium hydroxide does not constitute a continuous barrier. Therefore, in the last decade, a material called mineral trioxide aggregate (MTA) has been introduced in the market, which seems to get around this problem. However, the difficult handling and management of this material, together with the many problems associated with high cost and lack of decontamination activity, suggest that the introduction of new materials is necessary. Meanwhile, according to some authors, lasers can provide very satisfactory outcomes thanks to their capacity to offer "bloodless" operating fields and to "decontaminate" the exposed pulp if used with non-excessively high parameters.

Melcer et al in 1987 first highlighted the usefulness of lasers in these endodontic procedures in animals, whereas Moritz et al in 1998 highlighted the importance of these procedures for direct pulp capping in humans. However, in 2000, Kimura et al stated that "to use lasers for pulp capping and pulpotomy, appropriate usage parameters should be selected. In fact, if energy levels are too high, the treatment might be unsuccessful." An important study in this regard was conducted by Santucci et al (1999); these authors assessed the efficacy of Nd:YAG lasers in direct capping in association with a glass ionomer cement (3M Vitrebond).
The results of this study showed a higher radiographic and clinical success at 54 months in the laser group (90.3%) than in the control group (43.6%).
The operating protocol for pulp capping using laser equipment is simple and repeatable. After isolating the operating area using a rubber dam and cleaning the cavity, it is possible to proceed with laser irradiation using different parameters depending on the wavelength used. In all cases, the end of the optical fiber should be placed as close as possible to the pulp but not in direct contact with it (*no contact mode*). After laser irradiation, it is possible to proceed with the application of a double layer of calcium hydroxide and MTA and, lastly, with the final restoration.
A case of capping, which also requires the clinical use of lasers, is shown in Figures 20.10 and 20.11.

Root canal disinfection

Root canal disinfection can be achieved with correct cleaning and shaping of the root canals. This method enables the removal of infected pulp residue and of a 1–2-μm-thick layer of organic and inorganic materials adhering to the canal walls, which constitutes the so-called *smear layer*. To achieve the bactericidal effect and sterilize the canal, the irrigating agents must penetrate inside the canal system, including the lateral canals and dentinal tubules. Many experimental studies have shown that several bacterial

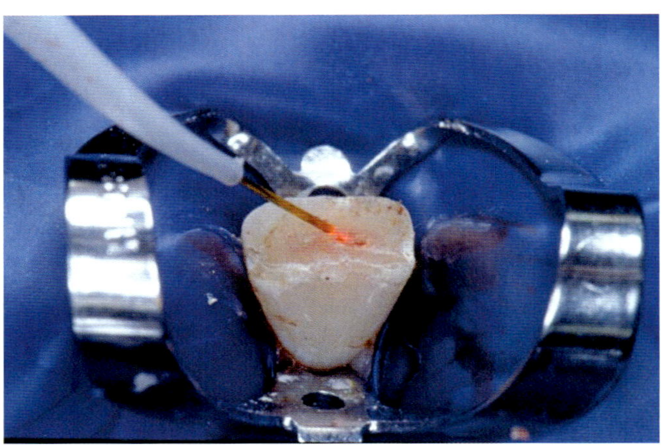

Figure 20.10 Pulp exposure in dental element 1.1, following complex enamel–dentin coronal fracture.

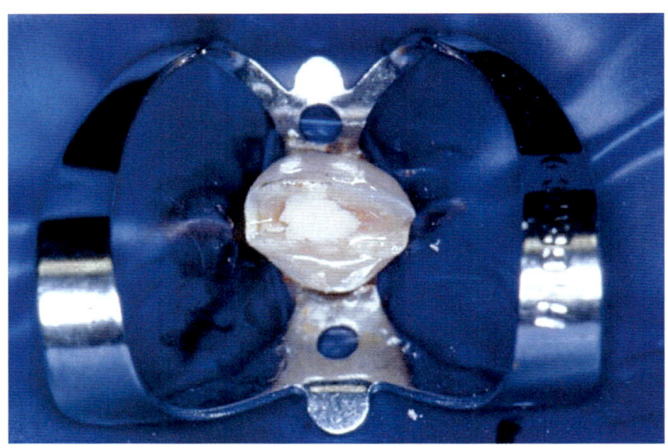

Figure 20.11 Application of calcium hydroxide as a paste and cement over the decontaminated pulp.

species are able to invade and penetrate dentinal tubules up to a considerable extent. Perez et al (1993) showed that *Streptococcus sanguinis* manages to penetrate dentinal tubules to an average depth of 458.8 µm, with peaks up to 792 µm. On the other hand, according to Gutierrez et al (1990), the bacterial penetration depth is around 250 µm. Berutti et al (1997) showed that NaOCl can penetrate along dentinal tubules to a maximum depth of up to 130 µm. The discrepancy between the penetration depths of microorganisms and irrigating solutions is frequently responsible for the cases of long-term failure, which can be seen in standard endodontic treatments.

It has been commonly believed by an increasing number of experts (Kreisler et al, 2003; Romeo et al, 2003; Moritz et al, 1997) that the bactericidal effect of laser irradiation, used together with an adequate cleansing action and the necessary mechanical equipment, can increase the rates of long-term success of endodontic treatments. For example, Klinke et al (1997) showed significant bacterial reduction obtained using Nd:YAG lasers within the first 300 µm of the dentinal tubule length and a bactericidal effect, although slightly weak, up to a depth of 1000 µm; the bactericidal effect of lasers is superior to that of irrigating solutions, which manage to penetrate only up to a depth of 100 µm, thus reducing the potential discrepancy between the penetration depth of bacteria in the dentinal tubules and the bactericidal agent in question. Finally, it has been shown (Levy et al, 1996) that laser irradiation can provide, if performed in a liquid medium such as NaOCl, the cavitation effect generally sought with ultrasounds, thus enhancing the germicidal effect of irrigating solutions.

The antibacterial properties of laser can help resolve persistent canal infections that would require repeated antimicrobial dressings. These properties are useful in cases of chronic apical periodontitis (fistulized or granulomatous) that may be successfully treated in a single session using laser endodontic treatment (Fig. 20.12–20.14), with all the operational and managerial advantages that can be derived from laser (Romeo et al, 2005; 2010) (Tab. 20.1).

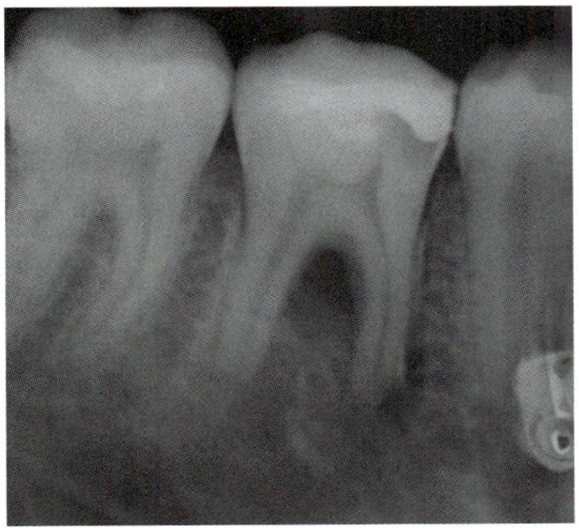

Figure 20.12 *Single-visit* laser-assisted endodontic treatment. A preoperative radiograph of dental element 4.6 with a large carious lesion on the mesial side and a chronic granulomatous apical periodontitis located on the tip of the mesial root.

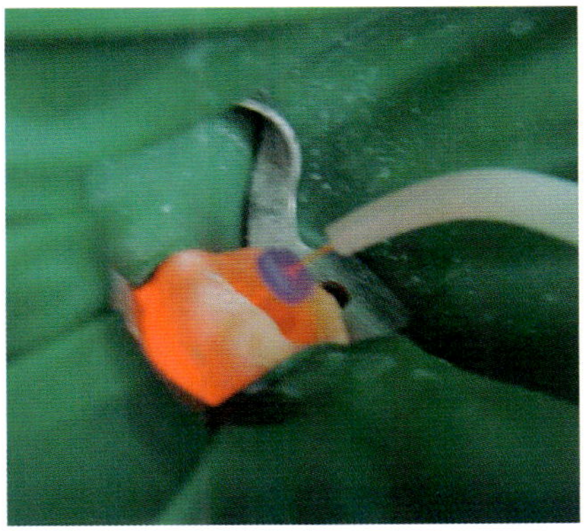

Figure 20.13 Irradiation using Nd:YAG laser (200 µm fiber) in sodium hypochlorite solution.

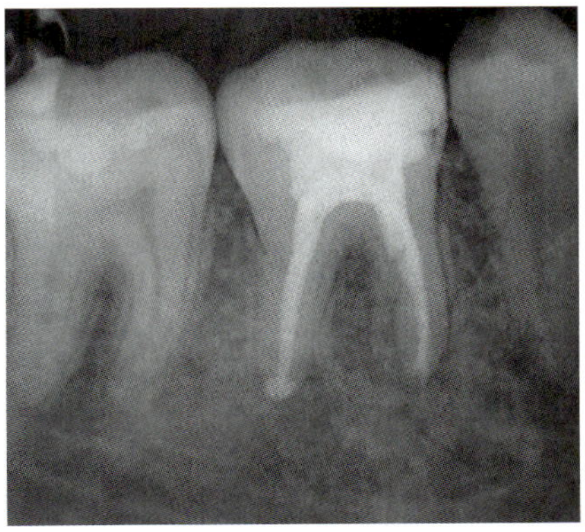

Figure 20.14 Radiographic follow-up performed 1 year after root canal closure, with the healing of periradicular radiographic lesion.

Table 20.1 Advantages and disadvantages of *single-visit* endodontic treatment

Advantages	Disadvantages
• Saves patient's and dentist's time • Reduced discomfort (related to the need to repeat the operating procedures of endodontic therapy) • Continuity with the canal instrumentation phase • No need for repeated fillings	• Inability to adequately dry the endodontic canals • Lack of sufficient time to complete therapy • Patient discomfort related to the long temporary duration of the appointment (temporomandibular joint pain, psychological discomfort)

The steps of laser endodontic treatment involve initial and complete cleaning and shaping of the root canals using mechanical Ni-Ti instrumentation, together with the use of chemical agents such as NaOCl and ethylenediaminetetraacetic acid, and three laser irradiations in NaOCl solution, with parameters that vary depending on the wavelength used. Afterward, the canal is dried using paper points and subsequently filled using the most appropriate filling method.

Endodontic treatment of soft tissues inside the oral cavity using laser

Soft tissue surgery undoubtedly figures prominently among the fields of dentistry most influenced by laser development. The most commonly used lasers are the ones that show the greatest affinity to hemoglobin and, consequently, allow the greatest level of intraoperative hemostasis, which in turn helps perform the surgical intervention in a short time without being too traumatic for pediatric patients.

For this reason, several authors (Walinski, 2004; Jinbu et al, 2003; Epstein, 1991; Gontijo et al, 2005; Stübinger et al, 2006; Romeo et al, 2008; Marangoni et al, 2005; Lee, 2006) have proposed gingivectomy–gingivoplasty, frenectomy, and operculectomy, as well as bioptic procedures for soft tissues using CO_2, diode, Nd:YAG, KTP, Er:YAG, and Er,Cr:YSGG lasers.

The surgical treatment of oral frenula is indicated when these are considered pathological or in the presence of orthodontic, prosthetic, and periodontal abnormalities; breastfeeding difficulties; language articulation disorders; or incorrect postures as in the case of a short lingual frenulum (Tenore et al, 2009; Lalakea and Messner, 2003; Segal and Stephenson, 2007; Kotlow, 2004).

Frenulotomy involves a simple interruption of frenular fibers to therapeutically reduce tension forces; on the other hand, frenulectomy involves the excision of the frenulum itself. Considering the poor predictability of the outcomes of frenulotomy, most au-

Table 20.2 Advantages of lasers in oral surgery

• Good patient compliance
• Hemostasis in the operating field
• Anesthesia and suturing are sometimes not required
• Optimal healing for the second intervention

thors reserve this intervention exclusively for the treatment of small lower vestibular frenula, scarring fibers, and short lingual frenula at an early age (Lalakea and Messner, 2003; Segal and Stephenson, 2007; Kotlow, 2004).
The surgical treatment of frenula can be performed using laser, which offers important advantages (Kotlow, 2004) (Tab. 20.2).
The operative steps do not differ from those of the standard cold knife surgery, apart from the cases in which it is possible to perform the treatment only by applying an anesthetic gel and achieve healing of the surgical wound by secondary intention.
In cases of lingual frenulectomy, to restore labial and/or lingual function as soon as possible and further reduce relapses, it is advisable to perform certain functional exercises several times a day for about a month.
Figures 20.15 and 20.16 show two clinical cases of frenulectomy both performed using diode lasers: a case of upper labial frenulectomy and a case of lingual frenulectomy.

Biopsy

Biopsy can be incisional or excisional. In incisional biopsy, one or more fragments of a lesion are resected to proceed with the subsequent treatment based on the histological diagnosis. On the other hand, excisional biopsy requires complete resection of the lesion concerned; therefore, it serves both diagnostic and therapeutic purposes. The use of lasers in the study of soft tissue lesions has brought undeniable advantages to the management of particularly problematic pathological cases; however, it has also generated considerable perplexities in the study of lesions with suspected dysplastic or clearly neoplastic potential. The harmful effect is naturally related to the photothermal effect of the laser and is strictly related to its mode of action within the tissues concerned.
However, several *in vitro* studies (Romeo et al, 2007; 2010; 2011; 2009) have shown that, with controlled parameters, it is always possible to perform laser biopsies of oral soft tissues without the formation of thermal artifacts that interfere with the correct "reading" of the histological sample.
Based on these experiences, it is considered appropriate to subdivide soft tissue lesions within the oral cavity on the basis of their dysplastic potential into nonsuspicious and suspicious lesions. In nonsuspicious lesions (for example fibromas), the use of

Clinical cases

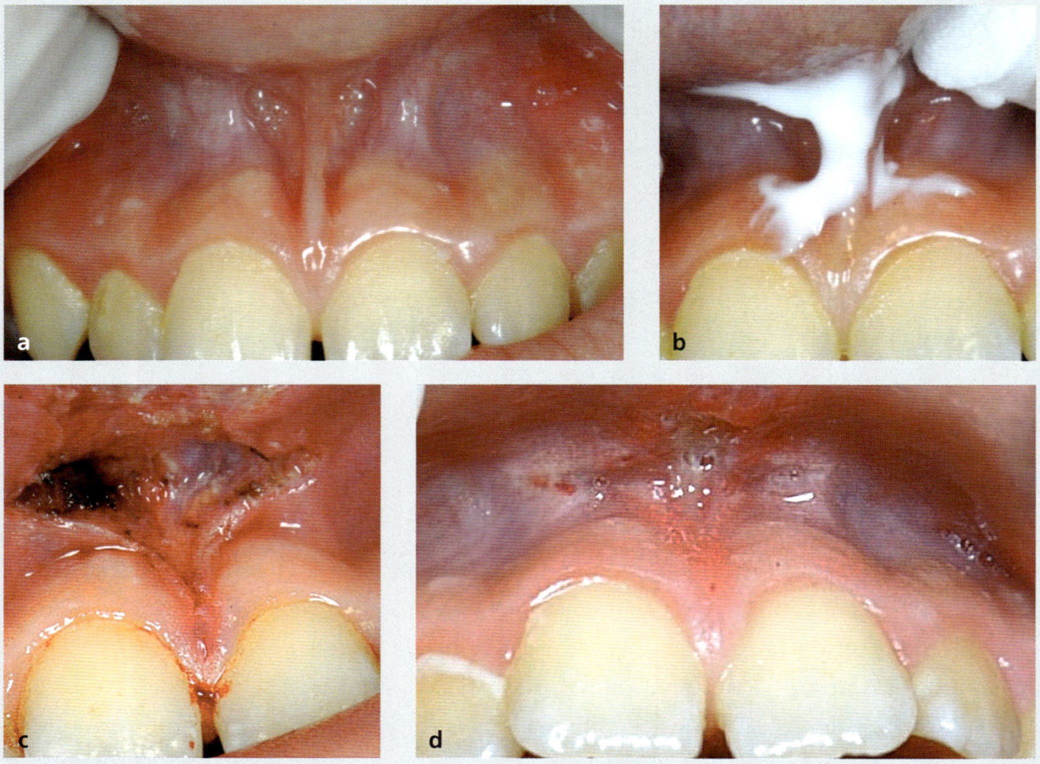

Figure 20.15 (**a**) Pathologic upper median labial frenulum. (**b**) Topic application of anesthetic gel at the level of the labial frenulum and over the gingival and labial mucosa. (**c**) Intraoperative phase of frenulectomy using diode laser. (**d**) Follow-up after 20 days showing almost complete healing of the surrounding mucosal tissues.

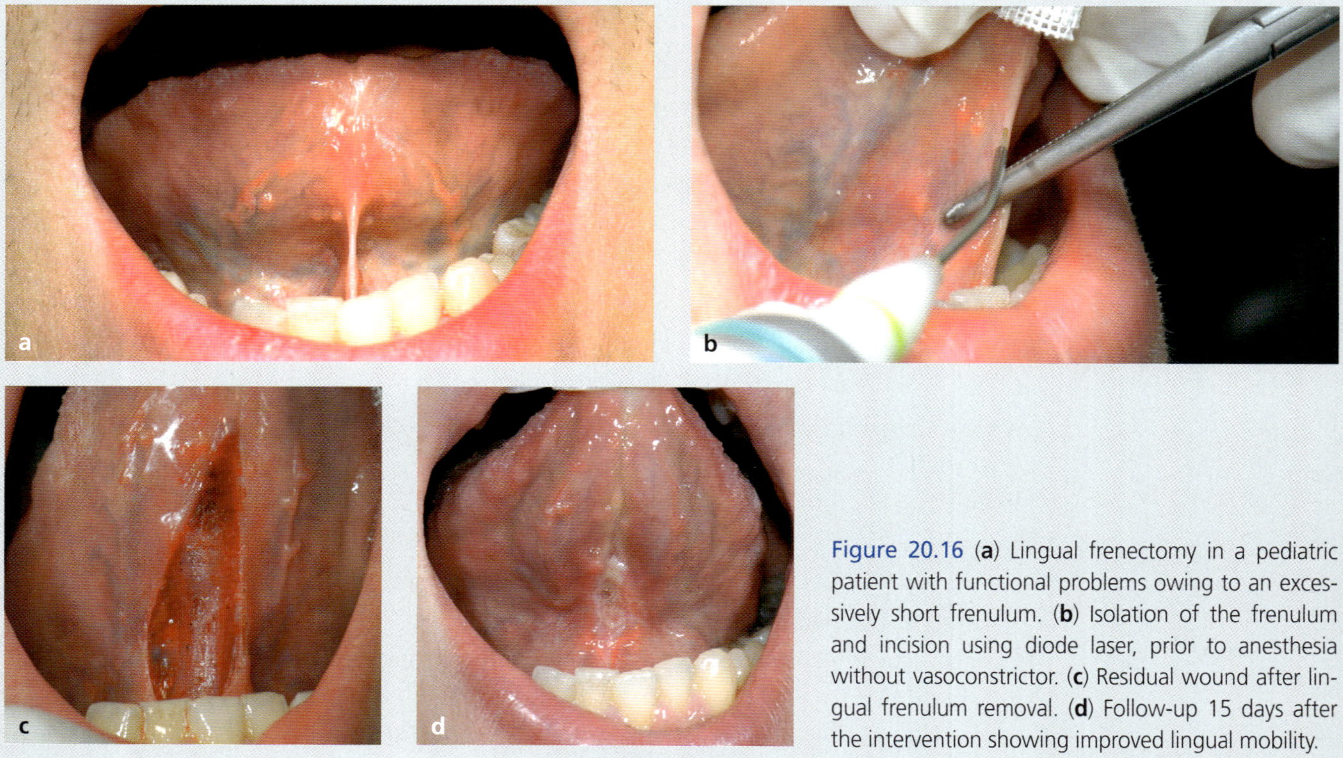

Figure 20.16 (**a**) Lingual frenectomy in a pediatric patient with functional problems owing to an excessively short frenulum. (**b**) Isolation of the frenulum and incision using diode laser, prior to anesthesia without vasoconstrictor. (**c**) Residual wound after lingual frenulum removal. (**d**) Follow-up 15 days after the intervention showing improved lingual mobility.

lasers proves to be decisive, as it helps resolve different clinical cases. In dysplastic or suspicious lesions (for example, precancerous lesions and conditions), the presence of peri-incisional damage does not make the use of lasers entirely risk-free. This does not mean that laser devices should not be used but means that operating margins should be enlarged (Catone and Alling, 1997) by at least 0.5 mm compared with the hypothesized margins for cold knife biopsy. After making this due premise, it can be said that the most commonly used lasers for oral soft tissue biopsy are diode, KTP, CO_2, and Nd:YAG lasers (Tab. 20.3).

These devices can guarantee the following to varying degrees:

- the handling of a bleeding area, which turns out to be fundamental for the treatment of vascular pathologies (for example, hemangiomas)
- the possibility of performing the procedure using only topical anesthesia in some cases
- no requirement of sutures, which is particularly useful in areas such as the soft and hard palate, where suture placement would be very difficult
- limited postoperative symptoms
- the relative ease and speed of performing the surgical procedure, even though it is always important to remember that the laser requires a learning curve and, if not correctly used, can cause unintended damage.

The steps of laser biopsy are very similar to those of the standard cold knife biopsy and include the following:

- topical anesthesia application for 20 min using an anesthetic gel based on a 2.5% lidocaine solution
- perilesional infiltration anesthesia, to avoid altering the surgical sample, using an anesthetic without a vasoconstrictor to keep the surgical area vascularized to better exploit the physical characteristics of the laser
- lesion immobilization without causing any trauma
- lesion excision with variable parameters depending on the wavelength used
- hemostasis, if necessary, using the laser in a defocused and continuous manner

Table 20.3 Lasers mainly used in oral biopsies

Laser	Wavelength (nm)	Target chromophore
Diodes	808–980	Oxyhemoglobin and melanin
KTP	532	Oxyhemoglobin and melanin
CO_2	10,600	Water
Nd:YAG	1064	Oxyhemoglobin and melanin

- application of a sterile gauze swab to achieve complete hemostasis
- storage of the removed sample in a dark-colored test tube that contains a 10% buffered formalin solution and its delivery to the pathologist. The test tube that contains the histological sample is accompanied by a sheet with the related clinical information
- prescription of a nebulizer based on a 0.2% chlorhexidine solution as well as a gel based on hyaluronic acid and amino acids, which should be applied twice daily for a week on the surgical wound.

Subsequent follow-up shows excellent healing by secondary intention, with the absence of complications such as hemorrhage and pain. Initially, there is fibrin layer formation, which is very clear on the seventh day; this layer is subsequently and gradually replaced by newly formed healthy tissue. In general, the complete healing of a laser wound occurs in the third week after the intervention.
An example of laser excisional biopsy performed in a pediatric patient is shown in Figure 20.17.

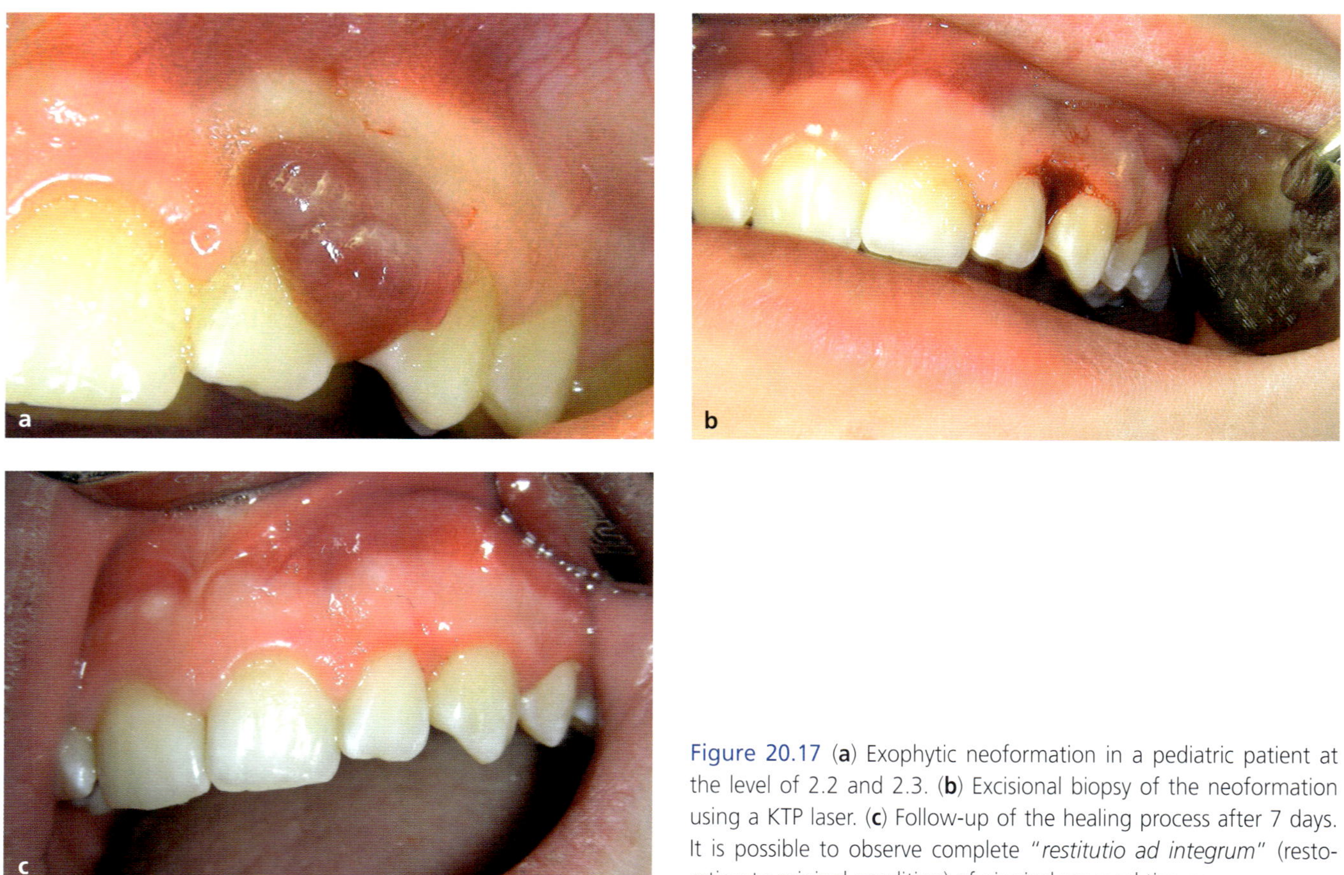

Figure 20.17 (**a**) Exophytic neoformation in a pediatric patient at the level of 2.2 and 2.3. (**b**) Excisional biopsy of the neoformation using a KTP laser. (**c**) Follow-up of the healing process after 7 days. It is possible to observe complete "*restitutio ad integrum*" (restoration to original condition) of gingival mucosal tissues.

References

Anderson RR, Parrish JA. The optics of human skin. J Invest Dermatol 1981;77(1):13-9.

Apel C, Franzen R, Meister J et al. Influence of the pulse duration of an Er: YAG laser system on the ablation threshold of dental enamel. Lasers Med Sci 2002;17(4):253-7.

Berutti E, Marini R, Angeretti A. Penetration ability of different irrigants into dentinal tubules. J Endodontics 1997;23(12):725-7.

Boulnois JL. Photophysical processes in recent medical laser developments: a review. Lasers Med Sci 1986;1:47-66.

Catone GA, Alling CC. Laser application in oral and maxillofacial surgery. 1st ed. Philadelphia: W.B. Saunders Company; 1997.

Contente MM, de Lima FA, Galo R, Pécora JD et al. Temperature rise during Er:YAG cavity preparation of primary enamel. Lasers Med Sci 2012;27(1):1-5.

Epstein SR. The frenectomy: a comparison of classic versus laser technique. Pract Periodontics Aesthet Dent 1991 Aug;3(5):27-30.

Firat E, Gurgan S, Gutknecht N. Microtensile bond strength of an etch-and-rinse adhesive to enamel and dentin after Er:YAG laser pretreatment with different pulse durations. Lasers Med Sci 2010 Aug 31; [Epub ahead of print].

Gentil De Moor RJ, Delme KI. Laser-assisted cavity preparation and adhesion to erbium-lased tooth structure: part 2. present-day adhesion to erbium-lased tooth structure in permanent teeth. J Adhes Dent 2010 Apr;12(2):91-102.

Gontijo I, Navarro RS, Haypek P et al. The applications of diode and Er:YAG lasers in labial frenectomy in infant patients. J Dent Child (Chic) 2005 Jan-Apr;72(1):10-5.

Gutierrez JH, Jofre A, Villena F. Scanning electron microscope study on the action of endodontic-irrigants on bacteria invading the dentinal tubules. Oral Surg Oral Med Oral Pathol 1990;69(4): 491-501.

Jinbu Y, Tsukinoki K, Kusama M, Watanabe Y. Recurrent multiple superficial mucocele on the palate: histopathology and laser vaporization. Oral Surg Oral Med Oral Pathol Oral Radiol Endod 2003 Feb;95(2):193-7.

Kilinc E, Roshkind DM, Antonson SA et al. Thermal safety of Er:YAG and Er,Cr:YSGG lasers in hard tissue removal. Photomed Laser Surg 2009 Aug;27(4):565-70.

Kim ME, Jeoung DJ, Kim KS. Effects of water flow on dental hard tissue ablation using Er:YAG laser. J Clin Laser Med Surg 2003;21(3):139-44.

Kimura Y, Wilder-Smith P, Matsumoto K. Laser in endodontics: a review. Int Endod J 2000;33(3): 173-85.

Klinke T, Klimm W, Gutknecht N. Antibacterial effect of Nd:YAG laser irradiation within root canal dentin. J Clin Laser Med Surg 1997 Feb;15(1):29-31.

Kornblit R, Bossù M, Mari D et al. Enamel and dentine of deciduous teeth Er:YAG laser prepared. A SEM study. Eur J Paediatr Dent 2009 Jun;10(2):75-82.

Kornblit R, Trapani D, Bossù M et al. The use of Erbium:YAG laser for caries removal in paediatric patients following Minimally Invasive Dentistry concepts. Eur J Paediatr Dent 2008 Jun;9(2):81-7.

Kotlow LA. Lasers in pediatric dentistry. Dent Clin N Am 2004;48(4):889-922.

Kreisler M, Kohnen W, Beck M et al. Efficacy of NaOCl\H202 irrigation and GaAlAs laser in decontamination of root canals in vitro. Lasers Surg Med 2003;32(3):189-96.

Krmek SJ, Miletic I, Simeon P et al. The temperature changes in the pulp chamber during cavity preparation with the Er:YAG laser using a very short pulse. Photomed Laser Surg 2009 Apr;27(2):351-5.

Lalakea ML, Messner AH. Ankyloglossia: does it matter? Pediatr Clin N Am 2003;(50):381-97.

Lee EA. Laser-assisted gingival tissue procedures in esthetic dentistry. Pract Proced Aesthet Dent 2006 Oct;18(9):suppl 2-6.

Levy G, Rizoiu I, Friedman S, Lam H. Pressure waves in root canals induced by Nd: YAG laser. J Endod 1996 Feb;22(2):81-4.

Liu JF, Lai YL, Shu WY, Lee SY. Acceptance and efficiency of Er:YAG laser for cavity preparation in children. Photomed Laser Surg 2006 Aug;24(4):489-93.

Marangoni O, Melato M, Longo L. 808-nm laser with exogenous chromophores for the treatment of benign oral lesions. Photomed Laser Surg 2005 Jun;23(3):324-7.

Melcer J, Channette MT, Melcer F. Dental pulp exposed to the CO_2 laser beam. Laser Surg Med 1987;7(4):347-52.

Mir M, Meister J, Franzen R et al. Influence of water-layer thickness on Er:YAG laser ablation of enamel of bovine anterior teeth. Lasers Med Sci 2008 Oct;23(4):451-7.

Moretto SG, Azambuja N Jr, Arana-Chavez VE et al. Effects of ultramorphological changes on adhesion to lased dentin-Scanning electron microscopy and transmission electron microscopy analysis. Microsc Res Tech 2011 Aug;74(8):720-6.

Moritz A, Gutknecht N, Goharkhay K et al. In vitro irradiation of infected root canals with a diode laser: results of microbiologic, infrared spectrometric, and stain penetration examinations. Quintessence Int 1997 Mar;28(3):205-9.

Moritz A, Schoop U, Goharkhay K, Sperr W. The CO2 laser as an aid in direct pulp capping. J Endod 1998;24(4):248-51.

Perez F, Rochd T, Lodter JP et al. In vitro study of the penetration of three bacterial strains into root dentine. Oral Surg Oral Med Oral Pathos 1993;76(1):97-103.

Romeo U, Del Vecchio A, Palaia G et al. Evaluation of bone damage induced by different cutting instruments: an "in vitro study". Braz Dent J 2009;20(2):162-8.

Romeo U, Del Vecchio A, Ripari F et al. Effects of different laser devices on oral soft tissues: an "in vitro" experience. J Oral Laser Appl 2007;7(3):155-9.

Romeo U, Libotte F, Palaia G et al. Histological "in vitro" evaluation of the effects of Er:YAG laser on oral soft tissues. Laser Med Sci 2011. DOI:10.1007/s10103-011-0969-z.

Romeo U, Palaia G, Del Vecchio A et al. Effects of KTP laser on oral soft tissues. In vitro study. Lasers Med Sci 2010 Jul;25(4):539-43.

Romeo U, Palaia G, Kornblit R et al. Endodontic treatment of periapical chronic periodontitis. A laser assisted technique. Laser magazine 2010;2(1):26-9.

Romeo U, Palaia G, Pacifici L et al. Antimicrobial activity of Nd:YAG laser in endodontics. J Dent Res 2003;82 (Spec. Iss.B):184.

Romeo U, Palaia G, Tenore G et al. Impiego del laser a diodi 808 nm nella biopsia escissionale delle patologie della mucosa orale. Doctor Laser 2008 Mag-Ago;2(2):50-6.

Romeo U, Ripari F, Palaia G, Tenore G. Trattamento di fistola cutanea in unica seduta con terapia endodontica laser-assistita. Caso clinico. Giornale italiano di endodonzia 2005;19(2):127-9. ISSN: 1121-4171.

Santucci PJ. Dycal Versus Nd:YAG laser and Vitrebond for direct pulp capping in permanent teeth. J Clin Laser Med Surg 1999;17(2):69-75.

Schoop U, Kluger W, Moritz A et al. Bactericidal effect of different laser systems in the deep layers of dentin. Laser Surg Med 2004;35(2):111-6.

Segal LM, Stephenson R et al. Prevalence, diagnosis, and treatment of ankyloglossia. Can Fam Physician 2007;53(6):1027-9.

Stübinger S, Saldamli B, Jürgens P et al. Soft tissue surgery with the diode laser-theoretical and clinical aspects. Schweiz Monatsschr Zahnmed 2006;116(8):812-20.

Tenore G, Zicari S, Palaia G et al. Il trattamento dei frenuli orali patologici mediante laser KTP 532 nm. Atti del Congresso Nazionale dei Docenti in discipline Odontostomatologiche e Chirurgia Maxillo Facciale; Roma, April 2009.

Tokonabe H. Morphological changes of human teeth with Er:YAG laser Irradiation. J Clin Laser Med Surg 1999;17(1):7-12.

Vogel A, Venugopalan V. Mechanisms of pulsed laser ablation of biological tissues. Chem Rev 2003;103(2):577-644.

Walinski CJ. Irritation fibroma removal: a comparison of two laser wavelengths. Gen Dent 2004 May-Jun;52(3):236-8.

Chapter 21

Sedation and anesthesia in pediatric dentistry

R. Favaro, P. Tordiglione

The main objective of sedation in pediatric dentistry should be the alleviation of fear and/or pain of the dentist and the specific causes that determine their occurrence. There can be many causes for pain and fear, including the negative view of dentists by children's parents, friends, and the society, which can intentionally or unintentionally give rise to fear in children. Sometimes, the causes are identifiable in previous painful or otherwise traumatic experiences with dentists or other healthcare professionals or in the instinct of self-preservation, which causes the person to defend themselves against any form of pain.

The inability to treat children who have fear and anxiety poses a barrier to treatment and simultaneously causes anxiety and frustration to the dentist, thereby establishing a vicious circle that makes the patient's visit and the dental treatment more and more annoying and unwelcome to the child, with the possibility that an unconscious transfer of anxiety occurs from the dentist to the child.

Social causes and negative experiences are the root causes of anxiety in children, which can manifest via physiological modifications associated with the release of catecholamines. Table 21.1 lists the actions that can modify the heart rate to a greater extent during dental examination.

Table 21.1 Changes in the child's heart rate (HR) at different times during the dental examination

Actions	Variation HR/min
The dentist puts on the gown	10 beats
He gets ready	15 beats
He positions the chair	12 beats
He adjusts the lamp	10 beats
Intraoral examination	–1 beat
End of the examination	–3 beats

Methods of evaluating anxiety in children

The decision to use a sedation technique cannot be made without proper diagnosis and quantification of anxiety, for which dentists use tests that are particularly important for children. The most commonly used tests are based on questionnaires, which are preferably used in children aged less than 7-8 years, together with tests for the self-evaluation of anxiety by means of figures or colors and tests that focus on the observation of children when they relate to dental procedures, instruments, and the appearance of the dentist.

Questionnaires. Questionnaires are generally addressed to the mother and child. One such questionnaire aims at identifying the nondental and dental variables of anxiety (Holst et al, 1988).

Tests for self-evaluation. Among self-evaluation the ones, the best known test is certainly the Venham picture test (Venham, 1979), which involves displaying eight numbered cartoons to the child. The final score quantifies the child's anxiety.

Tests on observation. These tests include tests used to evaluate the child's behavior (North Carolina Behavior Rating Scale) as well as treatment acceptability by assessing the relationship between the type of treatment and its acceptability.
Cooperation tests provide useful elements in the study of the evolution of the child's overall behavior in relation to the iterative nature of dental care (five-point test: one point indicates full cooperation; five points indicate resorting to physical constraints).

The use of these tests has enabled the identification of the various ways of classifying the child's behavior in relation to the success of dental care. In particular, using the Frankl Behavior Rating Scale, the observer can classify the child's behavior into four categories according to their attitude:

- decidedly positive attitude
- positive attitude
- negative attitude
- decidedly negative attitude.

A further classification identifies three major groups of children:

- cooperative children: this group includes the majority of the patients, who can be approached using the *tell–show–do* technique
- uncooperative children
- potentially uncooperative children. This group is further classified into subgroups.

Psychosedation

Treatment success in pediatric patients who show little or no cooperation is closely linked to the use of psychosedation techniques, which include iatrosedation techniques and/or nonpharmacological psychosedative techniques and pharmacological sedation techniques.
Iatrosedation is a technique that involves communication between the dentist and patient, leading to the establishment of a relationship of absolute trust between them. Iatrosedation and other pharmacological sedation techniques such as hypnosis, acupuncture, audio-analgesia, *biofeedback*, and transcutaneous electronic nerve stimulation are often not very effective in children, who should therefore be treated with pharmacological sedation.

Sedation

Until 2002, the American Dental Association (ADA) classified sedation in dentistry into four levels:
- anxiolysis
- vigilant sedation
- deep sedation
- general anesthesia.

Anxiolysis. Decrease/elimination of anxiety by pharmacological or nonpharmacological methods without any depression of the state of consciousness

Vigilant sedation. Minimum depression of the state of consciousness, produced by pharmacological or nonpharmacological methods, without affecting the patient's ability to communicate with the dentist and without compromising airway patency

Deep sedation. Depression of the state of consciousness such that verbal contact may fail and airway control may be compromised (absence of protective reflexes)

General anesthesia. A state of pharmacologically induced unconsciousness associated with the loss of protective reflexes and the ability to keep the airways accessible. Subsequently, the ADA proposed a different definition of the sedation levels (ADA, 2002):
- minimum sedation (already anxiolytic)
- moderate sedation (already vigilant sedation)
- deep sedation
- general anesthesia.

In addition to this new definition, the "*rescue*" concept was introduced, according to which, as there is no solution of continuity between the different levels of sedation, the dentist, who is considered responsible for the treatment of anxiety, must be able to manage a level of sedation deeper than that planned (Table 21.2).

Table 21.2 Evolution from minimal sedation to general anesthesia without continuous solution

Minimum sedation		Moderate sedation	Deep sedation	General anesthesia
Type of response	Normal to verbal stimuli	Purposeful to verbal and tactile stimuli	Purposeful to repeated and/or painful stimuli	Absent
Airways	Not altered	Does not require any intervention	Possible intervention	Required intervention
Spontaneous ventilation	Not altered	Adequate	May be adequate	Often inadequate

Objectives

The main objectives of sedation in pediatric dentistry are listed below:

- ensure the patient's cooperation by achieving a state of comfort
- decrease the patient's anxiety
- reduce the stress on the dental staff
- minimize the need for hospitalization, with all the related drawbacks.

The concept of the ideal level of sedation varies widely. For some dentists, the ideal level of sedation occurs when the patient does not move and cry during treatment (deep sedation). Others prefer to work in a relaxed atmosphere, both for the team and for the patient, even if the patient moves and speaks (moderate sedation). A minimum level of sedation may be more suitable in older, moderately apprehensive children.

Pathology of the pediatric patient

Pediatric dentists who select sedation should keep in mind some important differences that exist at the anatomical and physiological level between children and adults. Indeed, the sedation procedures cannot completely disregard the knowledge of the possible interferences of sedation drugs in the main functions of the body. In many situations involving inexperienced personnel, the risks associated with the pharmacological treatment could prevail over the benefits, thereby determining the impairment of the respiratory and/or cardiovascular systems in case of incorrect drug titration.

If differences in height, weight, and age as indicators of the development of the different body systems are fairly obvious, the differences in basal metabolism between adults and children are less obvious but equally important. In this case, baseline metabolic activity is increased, thereby interfering not only with the drug response but also

Table 21.3 Vital parameters at different ages

Age (years)	HR (beats/min)	BP (mmHg)	RR (breaths/min)
1–3	70–110	90–105/55–70	20–30
3–6	65–110	95–110/60–75	20–25
6–12	60–95	100–120/60–75	14–22
12	55–85	110–135/65–85	12–18

HR: heart rate; RR: respiratory rate; BP: blood pressure.
Source: Behrman RE. Nelson textbook of pediatrics. 17th ed. Philadelphia: Elsevier Science; 2004.

with vital parameters. Because the oxygen demand in children is greater but the alveolocapillary apparatus is less developed, the respiratory frequency is noticeably higher (Table 21.3). This should be carefully considered when administering drugs that can cause respiratory depression.

The static functional residual capacity (FRC), which represents the lung volume remaining in the lungs during normal ventilation, is lower in children (10% of the total lung capacity) than in adults (40%–50% of the total lung capacity). Such an FRC would cause the appearance of atelectasis, which the child prevents through a dynamic functional attitude, namely tachypnea and an increase in intercostal muscle tone. Tachypnea reduces the respiratory time and contributes to increasing the FRC, while the increase in intercostal muscle tone prevents pulmonary atelectasis via an increase in pulmonary volume. These compensatory mechanisms can be attenuated during deep sedation, representing a limit to their application in children because of the resulting breathing complications.

In the airway management of children, some important anatomical features should be considered. In fact, lower caliber of the upper airways, together with adenotonsillar hypertrophy, greater relative volume of the tongue, and an increase in secretions lead to a greater risk of airway obstruction. Therefore, these should be carefully evaluated before sedation by performing a careful examination of the oropharyngeal cavity (Fig. 21.1). From these considerations, it can be deduced that the child presents a reduced tolerance to respiratory obstruction together with an increased incidence of sleep apnea, which constitute an absolute contraindication to sedation.

The fact that the heart rate (HR) is higher and the arterial pressure (AP) is lower means that children are more susceptible to bradycardia, decreased cardiac output, and hypotension. Unlike in adults, in children, HR is the main factor in the regulation of AP. Compensatory mechanisms for adjusting the AP in the event of a decreased HR are not well developed in children. Therefore, a decrease in HR leads to a corresponding decrease in AP and tissue oxygenation. This should be considered during the administration of potentially bradycardic substances.

The effectiveness and duration of drug action are much more variable in children. The action of lipophilic agents can be prolonged, particularly in children who are overweight. In addition, improved peripheral perfusion accelerates the action of intramuscularly administered drugs.
The anatomical and physiological differences between children and adults lead to the conclusion that anesthesia dosing is not a simple application of a percentage-derived formula for the drug dose and that this dosage should be carefully adjusted according to established guidelines.

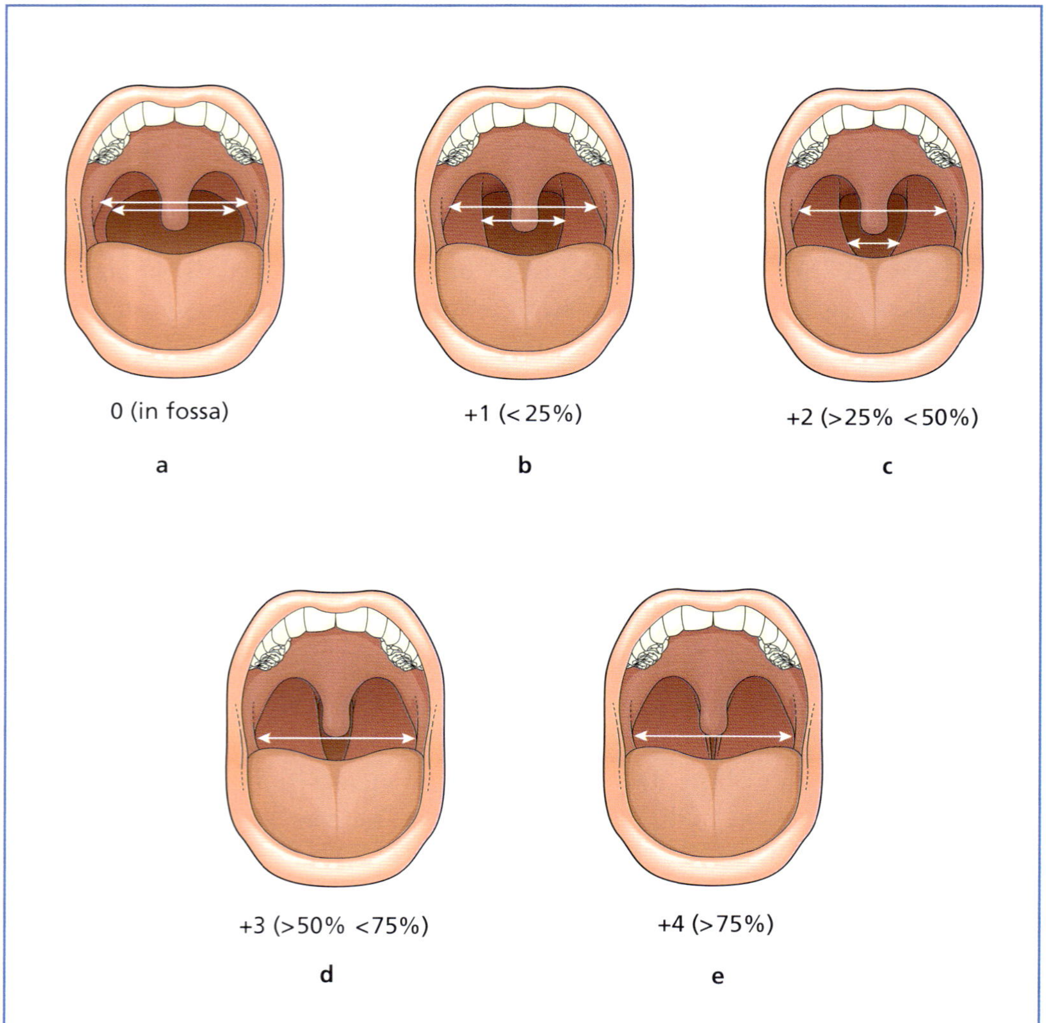

Figure 21.1 Evaluation of free pharyngeal space based on tonsil volume. In patients classified as ≥3, there is an increased risk of airway obstruction.

Indications

Sedation can only be used after having properly evaluated the following factors:

- assessment of the required treatment
- cooperation of the patient
- cooperation of the patient's relatives
- selection of the most suitable technique
- assessment of the preoperative health status
- preoperative assessment of behavior
- preparation and experience of the dentist and his/her collaborators.

Assessment of the required treatment. In the case of minimal dental treatment, e.g., caries, the use of sedation is generally superfluous.

Cooperation of the patient. Most pediatric dentists believe that at least two attempts, including iatrosedation, should be made before using pharmacological sedation or general anesthesia. Crying in the absence of very agitated behavior may not be a valid indication for sedation.

Cooperation of the patient's relatives. The dentist should take into consideration the advice and suggestions of the relatives without being influenced by them as the final decision is only left to the dentist.

Selection of the most suitable technique. There is no single effective method for all patients. The failure rate of sedation in children is considerably higher than that in adults. Recent studies report a failure rate of 40%–50% in case of oral sedation compared with a failure rate of 5% with intramuscular/intravenous sedation techniques. The younger the patient, the greater is the likelihood of failure, the incidence of which is linked to the number of sedation techniques that the dentist is familiar with.

Assessment of the preoperative health status. The collection of accurate medical history and a scrupulously conducted clinical examination can help determine whether the pediatric patient can be sedated. In this regard, the classification of the American Society of Anaesthesiologists (ASA) may be helpful (Table 21.4).

Patients in ASA class I can definitely be sedated. Some patients in ASA classes II and III may benefit from this method after consultation with the pediatrician. The American Academy of Pediatric Dentistry (AAPD) guidelines require ASA class III and IV patients with special needs showing airway abnormalities or significant tonsil hypertrophy to be hospitalized.

Using the medical history and the clinical examination findings, it is possible to collect information regarding the following aspects:

- allergies
- ongoing medical therapy (drugs, dosage, timing, and route of administration);
- comorbidities (OSAS, etc.)
- previous hospitalizations

Table 21.4 ASA classification

Class I	Normal, healthy patient
Class II	Patient with mild systemic disease
Class III	Patient with severe systemic disease, e.g., a child with active bronchospasm
Class IV	Patient with severe life-threatening systemic disease, e.g., a child with asthmatic disease
Class V	Moribund patient unable to survive without surgery

- previous general sedation/anesthesia and any associated complications of the pediatric patient and close family members
- clinical evaluation of the various equipment
- age, body weight, vital parameters (HR, blood pressure, respiratory rate, and body temperature), presence of anatomical abnormalities, e.g., mandibular hypoplasia, that may increase the risk of airway obstruction, ASA classification, and name and telephone number of the family doctor.

Informed consent. As sedation is not an integral part of dental treatment, consent to it should be separate and distinct from consent to dental care.

Instructions to relatives. Detailed information should be given, especially regarding the diet:
- clear liquids (water, pulpless fruit juice, soft drinks, and light tea) may be taken up to 2 hours before the intervention
- breast milk up to 4 hours before the intervention
- freeze-dried milk up to 6 hours before the intervention
- light meal (toast, biscuits, and light liquids) up to 6 hours before the intervention.

Fried or fatty foods should be avoided, including any food that delays gastric emptying. The reason for these recommendations is twofold. Initially, vomiting that may occur during or immediately after sedation may lead to serious complications (laryngospasm or obstruction of airways by inhalation of foreign matter) or mild complications (interference in the management of scheduled activities). It is also widely established that drugs taken orally are more effective on an empty stomach. The relatives should also be informed that the pediatric patient may sleep for several hours and be sleepy and irritable for 24 hours following sedation.
It is recommended to provide all the above written instructions in view that complete knowledge by the relatives of any possible event contributes to making the postsedation period peaceful, comfortable, and uncomplicated.

Techniques of sedation

The common routes of administration of drugs are oral, rectal, sublingual, intramuscular, intravenous, intranasal, and inhalation; these routes can be used alone or in combination with each other.
Oral and inhalation techniques of sedation, both alone and combined, are preferred by dentists. These methods are undoubtedly safe and easy to learn; for this reason, this chapter will focus on these two administration routes more extensively than the others, which will only be briefly mentioned.

Oral sedation

Oral sedation is a valid technique although not always effective. The failure rate varies from 40% to 50%, especially if the goal is to achieve moderate sedation in pediatric patients.
The drugs that are used for this purpose have been and still are benzodiazepines. In 1965, gastrointestinal diazepam was the first drug to have been used with good results. More recently, lorazepam, temazepam, oral prazepam, triazolam via sublingual administration, and midazolam have been used. The use of neuroleptics and barbiturates should be completely avoided in children. The former, in fact, have a prevalent and prolonged sedative activity with little amnesic action and with a possible state of psychomotor agitation, while the latter have hypnotic effects that are difficult to handle in the dental setting.
In accordance with the AAPD guidelines, it is absolutely not advised to have the drug administered at home.

Diazepam. This drug is indicated in hyperactive, highly anxious children aged more than 4 years. The effectiveness is greater in children with cerebral palsy and in children with mental retardation.

Midazolam. Midazolam is currently the most commonly used drug for oral sedation. It is particularly indicated in the management of children who have behavioral problems and are in need of minor interventions.
The latency period is approximately30–40 minutes. As midazolam is not commercially available in the form of drops or syrup, oral administration of the injectable preparation may be used. However, in Italy, this procedure is limited to hospital facilities as the injectable pack is not for sale to the public.

Promethazine. It is typically used in combination with other drugs. As a single agent, it is indicated only in the sedation of children with moderate anxiety.
Other drugs for gastrointestinal sedation have been proposed, either to be used alone (chloral hydrate, hydroxyzine, and meperidine) or in combination. Because of their

Table 21.5 Doses of benzodiazepines commonly used in paediatric dental patients

	Gastrointestinal Dose	Rectal	Intramuscular	Intravenous
Promethazine	2.2 mg/kg	12–25 mg	1 mg/kg	
Diazepam	0.3–0.5 mg/kg	0.7 mg/kg		0.2 mg/kg
Midazolam	0.5 mg/kg	0.3–0.5 mg/kg	0.1–0.2 mg/kg	0.05–0.1 mg/kg
Flurazepam	15–30 mg			
Lorazepam	2–4 mg			

scarce availability and unsatisfactory outcomes, the authors do not consider it appropriate to focus on these drugs.

The optimal doses of the mentioned drugs are summarized in Table 21.5.

Rectal sedation

This is an alternative technique to oral administration if the latter is rejected by the child. In the opinion of the authors, this method may acquire a particular relevance in presedation for the administration of associated analgesics such as codeine and paracetamol, which, in addition to ensuring a state of periprocedural analgesia, contribute to sedation.

Inhalation sedation

At present, inhalation is the closest sedation technique to the ideal one in the field of pediatric dentistry. It is used by 85% of American pediatric dentists and by approximately 1,500 Italian dentists.
According to AAPD guidelines, the objectives of inhalation sedation are as follows:

- reduction or elimination of anxiety
- reduction of reactive movements
- improvement of communication and cooperation
- increase of pain threshold
- increased willingness to accept prolonged treatment
- facilitation of treatment in patients with physical and/or mental disabilities
- reduction of retching
- enhancement of the sedative effects of other drugs.

Furthermore, according to the AAPD guidelines, the limitations of this technique are as follows:

- variation in sedation level
- the results are greatly influenced by the relationship of trust that the dentist can establish with the patient
- interference of the nasal mask with local anesthetic injection at the premaxilla level
- ability of the patient to engage in nasal respiration
- issues regarding environmental pollution.

Concept of pharmacokinetics and pharmacodynamics. The low solubility of nitrous oxide (N_2O) in plasma gives it a short latency and rapid reemergence. Its saturation in blood is completed within 3–5 minutes, there is no biotransformation, and it is rapidly eliminated from the lungs once the delivery is stopped. N_2O is easily titratable owing to these features. The absence of airway irritability allows it to be used in asthmatic patients without bronchospasm. In addition, N_2O is completely cardiostable. These features make N_2O safe for use in the sedation of children with severe heart disease.

Technique. The success of the proposed technique is largely linked to the relationship of empathy established between the dentist and patient. For this purpose, the first approach between the two parties is very important (along with the decisive contribution of relatives and assistant staff), during which a positive emotional and behavioral relationship between the child and the dentist should be sought. Feelings of danger and fear should be alleviated by involving the child via simple explanations, such as asking the child to choose the color and perfume of the mask and performing tests of nasal respiration (Fig. 21.2). In this regard, it may be useful to show a video of a peer who successfully received the inhalation sedation. Furthermore, during the first approach, in which the child is reassured that no action will be taken inside the mouth, the so-called demonstrative administration should be performed, delivering an equal mixture of $N_2O/O2$. A few minutes are sufficient to achieve a good level of sedation, ascertained from a clear symptomatology (eyes that look into the void, absence of reactivity). It is important not to perform any type of dental treatment during demonstrative sedation; this could cause a reaction of rejection in the child, which could be difficult to reverse over time. In the course of the next session, the dentist should start practical application, during which he/she will communicate every single procedure to the child, suggesting them through sounds and noises that characterize his/her recreational activity and his/her fantasies, resorting to positive reinforcements (Fig. 21.3).

The vast majority of children are adequately sedated with 30%–45% N_2O. If the nasal mask is not accepted by the child (especially children aged less than 3 years or those who are very apprehensive), two options can be pursued. In the first case, oral, nasal, or rectal pre-sedation is used, followed by inhalation of the anesthetic gas supplied with a nasal mask placed on the mouth; once the patient has been calmed, the same mask should be positioned in the usual way (Fig. 21.4a). The second option involves positioning of the nasal mask near the face, with delivery of N_2O at maximum concentration (70%) and high flow rate (10–15 L/min) (Fig. 21.4b). Subsequently, the concentration may be reduced by titrating the gas to the level best suited to the patient.

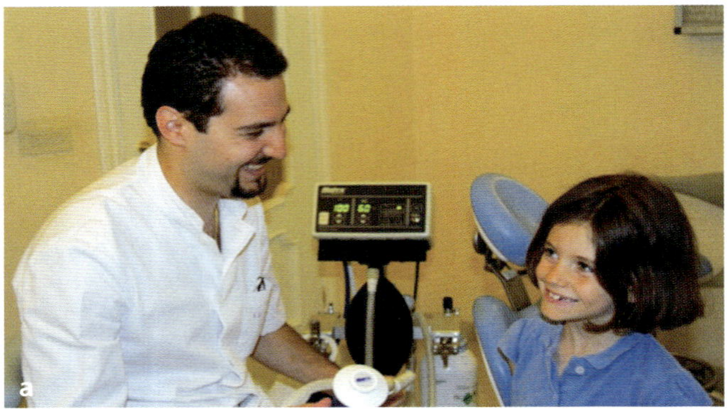

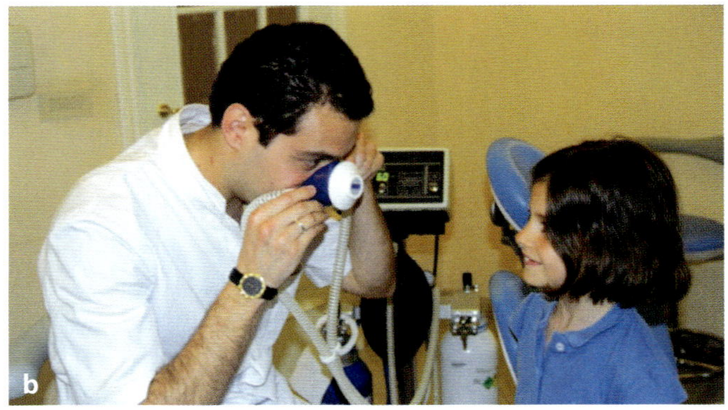

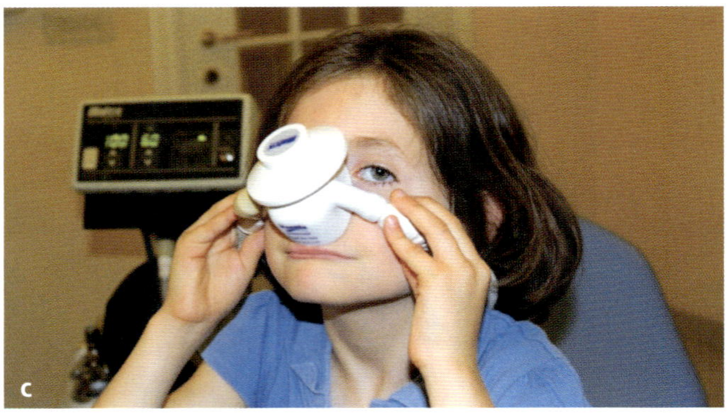

Figure 21.2 Demonstration phase.

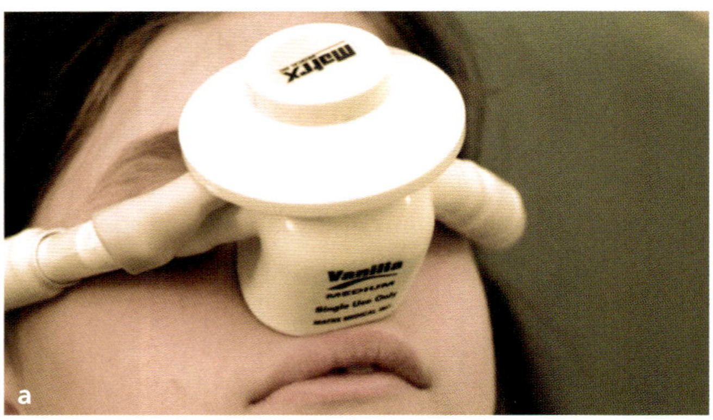

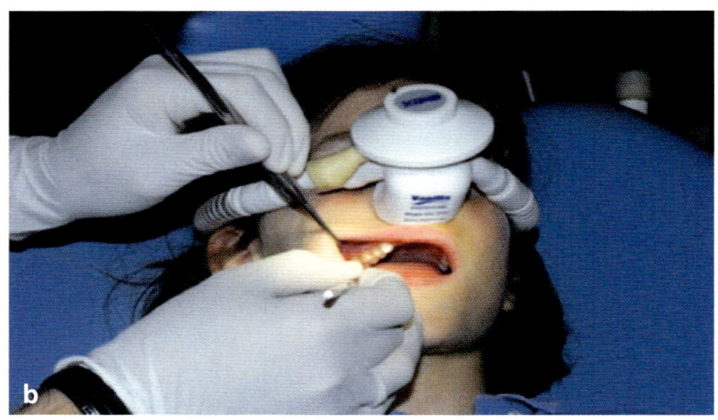

Figure 21.3 Operating phase.

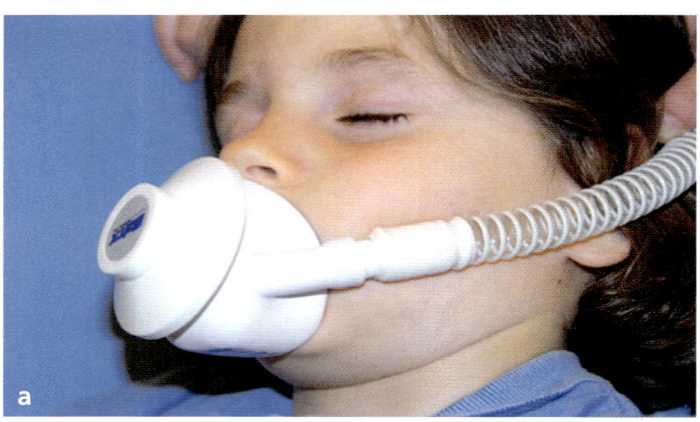

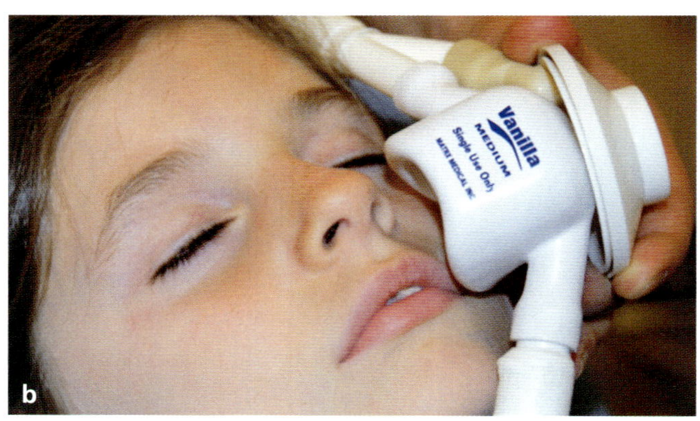

Figure 21.4 Phases of N2O inhalation.

Discharge should occur after interrupting the administration of N_2O, followed by administration of 100% O2 for a few minutes to avoid diffusion hypoxia (see *Complications*). The child should then be placed in a sitting position and may often report having had pleasant dreams. After approximately 30 minutes in the waiting room, the patient can be discharged with the accompanying relative.

The use of this technique allows the maximum possible performance to be achieved in conditions of absolute safety even if in relation to the pathology to be treated and the capacity of the dentist. In this regard, it should be noted that, within the framework of the ADA Council on Dental Materials, Instruments, and Equipment programme to prevent hypo-anoxia hazards, the minimum permissible O2 concentration should be 20% (ADA, 2002) (incidentally, in almost all commercially available appliances, the lower limit has been increased to 30%). No instrumental monitoring is required, and careful clinical observation is sufficient.

Complications and toxicity. Nausea and vomiting are the most common side effects; their incidence is variable (1%–10%) and is associated with the concentration of anesthetic gas dispensed (>50%), duration of the procedure, too frequent changes in concentrations, and the excessive speed at which the patient is induced and resurfaced. However, pretreatment fasting is not required, although it is a good idea to avoid the intake of liquids at least 2 hours prior to surgery.

To overcome diffusion hypoxia, a phenomenon of little clinical importance that can occur at the end of sedation, it is sufficient to administer 100% O2 for approximately 2 minutes once the supply of anesthetic gas ceases.

Toxicity, which is clinically negligible to patients, is certainly a more important problem for the staff owing to chronic exposure. Research in this field is very extensive and generally agrees that inhalation of N_2O at concentrations higher than the safe levels can cause abortions in the first trimester of pregnancy, malformations, and, in case of exposure to very high and continuous concentrations, myeloneuropathy. To prevent complications associated with chronic toxicity, dental surgeries should minimize environmental pollution by using laminar air flows and adequate exhaust and ventilation systems, which alone can reduce the environmental concentration of the gas by up to 90%. The antipollution efficacy also depends on the tightness of the nasal masks, the proper functioning of the other components of the dispensing system (tubes, flasks, fittings, etc.), and the patient's behavior (Table 21.6).

Sedation by parenteral route

The parenteral routes of administration include the intranasal, intramuscular, and intravenous routes. The first two are certainly more important in pediatric patients than in adults, as cooperation is not required. One limitation, however, is the nonretitration of the two methods, which increases the risk of overdose. The latency of the two techniques is superimposable (30–40 minutes).

Intranasal route. Midazolam is the drug of choice, which, at a dose of 0.3–0.5 mg/kg, is 79%–90% effective in children aged 4 years. Administration can proceed via drop-by-drop instillation or via atomizer spray. A disadvantage of the first procedure is the irritant power of the drug and its unpleasant taste when in contact with the oropharynx. These drawbacks can be overcome with the use of the atomizer.

Intramuscular route. This is a technique that is not appreciated by the child and the dentist because it is painful and not titratable. Midazolam is the drug of choice as it is less irritant than diazepam (see Table 21.5).

Intravenous route. This technique has seen success because of it titrability and fast implementation. However, the intravenous route must be reserved for professionals who have undergone specific training courses. This method should be used for moderate sedation as the requirements of deep sedation are indeed the same as those for general anesthesia. The anesthesiologist must be a person other than the clinician.
There are two techniques: mono- and poly-pharmacological. The latter is reserved for very experienced clinicians (in Italy, specialists in anesthesia and resuscitation are preferable according to the authors, who are experts in dental complications). The mono-pharmacological technique can be practiced by experienced dentists (sedationist) and involves the use of midazolam or diazepam (see Table 21.5). This technique causes more marked anterograde amnesic effects and can more easily cause "liberation" phenomena (disinhibition and arousal).

Combined techniques

The most common techniques used in combination are inhalation as preparation for moderate/deep sedation by the intravenous route and oral or rectal sedation as preparation for inhalation or parenteral techniques.

Table 21.6 Main causes of N_2O environmental pollution

Causes	Incidence
Speaking	48%
Moving	48%
Poor grip of the mask	36%
Technical problems	9.5%

Monitoring

The type of monitoring is obviously linked to the level of sedation achieved and allows the control of vital parameters. Monitoring can only be clinical (observation) in case of oral and/or inhalation sedation; it should be instrumental in case of intramuscular and/or intravenous sedation. In this respect, instruments that allow accurate and precise monitoring of vital parameters, such as pulse oximeter and capnometer, are currently available. In the opinion of the authors, a pulse oximeter (Fig. 21.5) is absolutely indispensable in any dental surgery in which sedation is practiced. It is an inexpensive instrument that continuously displays the state of arterial oxygenation and HR. Hypoxemia occurs when saturation decreases to less than 95% (PaO2 = 80 mmHg). With saturation values of <90% (PaO2 = 60 mmHg), the patient quickly desaturates. The pulse oximeter is even more useful in association with the capnometer (Fig. 21.6), with which the quality of ventilation is monitored.

Patient discharge

The following are the criteria for the discharge of pediatric patients:

- ability to answer questions, stand up, and walk
- stable vital signs
- the responsibility for discharge rests with the dental sedationist.

At the time of discharge, precise instructions regarding the diet to be taken, the activity that the child will be able to perform, any analgesics to be administered, and the telephone number to be used in case of need should be provided by the assistant staff and signed by the accompanying relative.

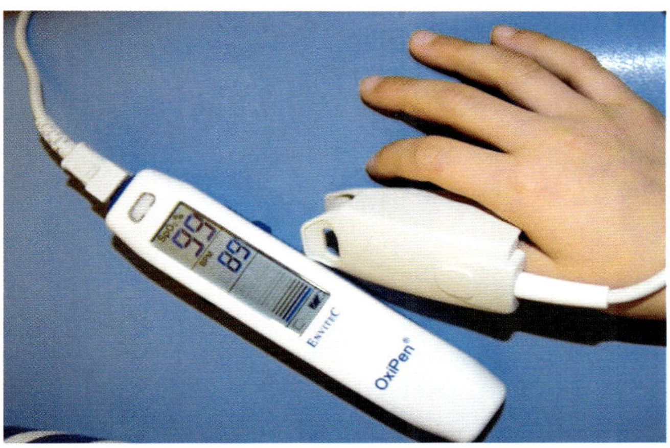

Figure 21.5 Pulse oximeter.

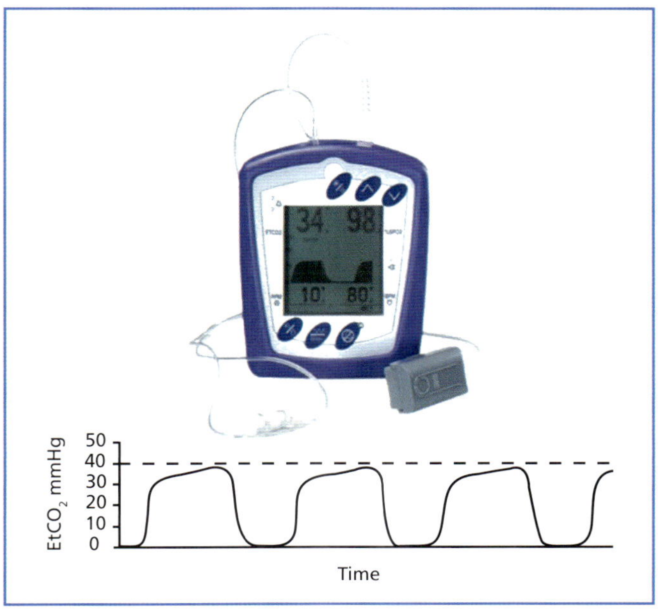

Figure 21.6 Capnometer and normal capnometry curve.

General anesthesia

It is important that every dentist knows that the indication for general anesthesia will be his/her exclusive task, while the task of the anesthesia specialist will be to evaluate the associated risks. In the opinion of the authors, this is a very important point because, if complications should occur following general anesthesia, the dentist will have to demonstrate (also in the context of a medical and legal evaluation) that general anesthesia was the only possible option. In fact, every other alternative must be considered before giving the indication and proceeding to general anesthesia. It is widely believed that at least two attempts should be made using conventional behavioral management or sedation techniques before using general anesthesia.

In recent years, the prevalence of general anesthesia in dentistry has decreased significantly in accordance with the recommendations of the General Dental Council, which suggests that neither general anesthesia nor deep sedation should be used without adequate equipment necessary for their implementation and without suitable equipment readily available for resurfacing (GDC, 1999).

The indications for general anesthesia in pediatric dentistry can be summarized as follows:

- extended dental treatment in uncooperative patients who resist any conventional procedure, including sedation and acceptable restraint methods
- extended dental treatment in immature adolescents and uncooperative children whose behavior hinders dental care
- multiple pulp lesions in children suffering from heart diseases, in which there is an indication for urgent treatment
- extended dental treatment in patients with severe sensory or physical disabilities, such as blindness and deafness, with whom communication is not possible
- relevant dental treatments in children with severe blood disorders that may require blood transfusion
- extended dental treatment in children with mental retardation whose behavior hinders treatment and makes communication with the dentist difficult or impossible.

General anesthesia can be administered for outpatients and inpatients. The recent availability of short-term anesthetic drugs has made it possible to use the first option with perfectly acceptable safety margins considering that this solution should be reserved for patients in ASA class I and II, whereas hospital care should be provided for patients in ASA classes III and IV.

Conclusions

To minimize the risk of complications in sedated patients undergoing dental treatment, professionals should remember the following ADA recommendations:

- use drugs and techniques that are well known by the clinician
- limit the use of such techniques only when necessary (extensive treatment, psychological problems, or medical conditions)
- perform a detailed preoperative assessment, with a complete medical history
- perform visual and/or instrumental monitoring from the start of treatment to discharge
- ensure the availability of medicines and equipment needed to deal with emergencies
- take note of the drugs used and their dosage, the monitored vital parameters, and any complications and related treatments
- ensure the availability of personnel with adequate and specific training for the assigned tasks
- appropriately manage high-risk patients (ASA class III and IV) in hospitals or similar facilities.

Finally, remember that *any single or combined sedation technique is never a pain control method*. Therefore, whatever the level of sedation achieved (minimum, moderate, or deep), local anesthesia, where necessary, should be administered correctly without assuming that the sedation can justify less accuracy in its implementation.

References

ADA Council on Dental Materials, Instruments and Equipment. ADA Guide to Dental Therapeutics. Chicago: 2nd American Dental Association; 2002.

American Dental Association. Guidelines for the use of conscious sedation, deep sedation and general anaesthesia for dentists. Oct 2002, ADA House of Delegates, American Dental Association.

GDC. New guidelines for sedation. SAAD 1999;16,17.

Holst A, Schroder U, Hallonstein AL et al. Prediction of behavior management problems in children. Scan J Dent Res 1988;96:457.

Venham LI. The effect of mother's presence on child's response to dental treatment. J Dent Child 1979;46:221.

Further reading

Malamed SF. Sedation. A guide to patient management. 5th ed. Saint Louis: Mosby Elsevier; 2010.

Manani G, Facco E, Zanette G. Anestesia odontoiatrica ed emergenze. 3a ed. Napoli: Idelson Gnocchi;2011.

McDonald RE, Avery DR, Dean J. Dentistry for the child and adolescent. 9a ed. Maryland: Mosby Elsevier; 2011.

Chapter 22

Therapeutic procedures in patients with systemic disorders or syndromes

G.L. Sfasciotti, G. Ierardo, M. Bossù

Introduction

G.L. Sfasciotti

The term disability refers to one or more impairments that reduce an individual's ability with interact with the social environment compared with what is considered as the norm.

The World Health Organization presented a classification that indisputably clarifies the meaning of impairment, disability, and handicap. Impairment refers to the loss of physical or mental functions and represents the extension of a pathological state; disability is the inability to perform a task or activity due to an impairment; the term handicap defines the disadvantage or limitation of an individual, caused by impairment or disability, compared with another person of equal age, sex, and education. Currently, no clear definition of the term is used internationally, although the concept of disability was discussed at the UN Convention on the Rights of Persons with Disabilities, and a final document was adopted by the UN General Assembly on August 25, 2006.

A standing ovation of all the delegations of the member countries of civil society welcomed the final verdict of the *ad hoc* committee with the words "*So it is decided*" pronounced by the Extraordinary President of the Committee, Don MacKay. The first International Convention on the Rights of Persons with Disabilities was adopted on August 25, 2006 at the UN Glass Palace.

The health of the oral cavity is of the utmost importance in some patients and represents a real challenge for dental staff; above all, it is essential to establish simple and repeatable guidelines to be able to better approach and treat oral ailments. Imagination, ingenuity, and flexibility are needed for those involved in the treatment of patients with disabilities; modification of routine procedures to include patience, calmness, and kindness are the keys to approach these patients.

Dentists and their staff can make important contributions to the well-being and personal value of patients with disabilities, beginning with precise objectives: motivate the patient and the caregiver; develop practices for the personal care of the oral cavity, aiming for the maintenance of healthy oral tissues; and contribute to the patient's overall health, of which oral health is an integral part.

Preventing the loss of dental elements primarily helps in mastication, which in turn is essential to prevent malnutrition and increase resistance to infections. It is also useful in preventing the need for major interventions that the patient would not be

able to bear due to a reduction in physical resistance or lack of cooperation. Last but not least, it aims at improving esthetics and thus contributing to social acceptance of these patients.
Many patients with disabilities or at least those with an acceptable degree of cooperation can be treated in an outpatient setting in a completely safe manner, both for themselves and for the professional who provides the treatment. The levels of cooperation are variable, and sometimes, even the help of parents, additional staff, or special aids (such as sedative drugs) are needed to increase the level of cooperation; in most cases, the results are very satisfactory. Among the auxiliary staff, it is also possible to take advantage of the socio-sanitary staff, who have the task of minimizing dental practices and negative emotions, using the clown therapy, thereby favoring positivity and cooperation (Fig. 22.1).
Patients who show a lower degree of cooperation or are uncooperative may be treated under general anesthesia in hospitals (Fig. 22.2). This possibility, however, must always be considered as a last option; the real challenge is to cure them in the dentist's chair by attempting to implement simple protocols that are effective and safe not only for the dentist but also for the patient.

First visit

G.L. Sfasciotti

The first visit and clinical examination represent one of the main instances for approaching such patients, being their first instance of contact with the outpatient dental environment.
The medical record serves the main purpose of reconstructing the medical history of the patient; it is composed of the three classic bases of medical history:
1. family history, which aims to identify the presence of hereditary diseases

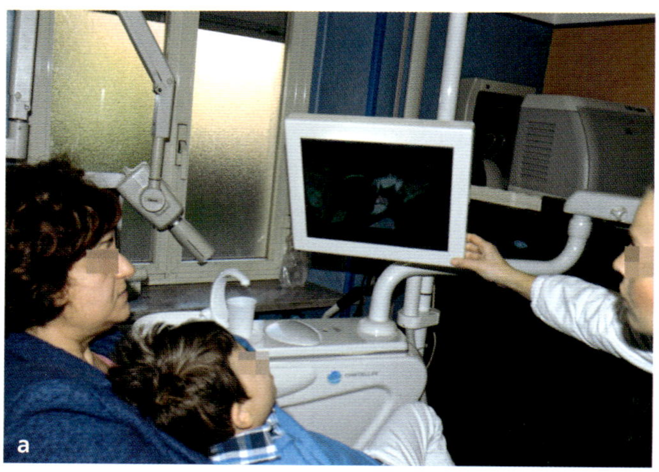

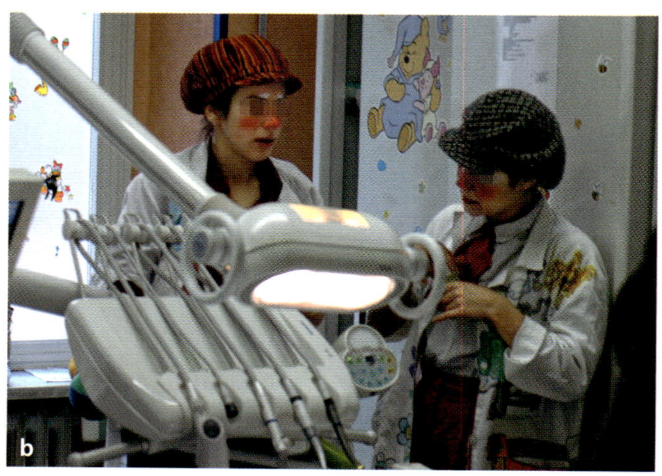

Figure 22.1 Collaboration: parents' help and clown therapy.

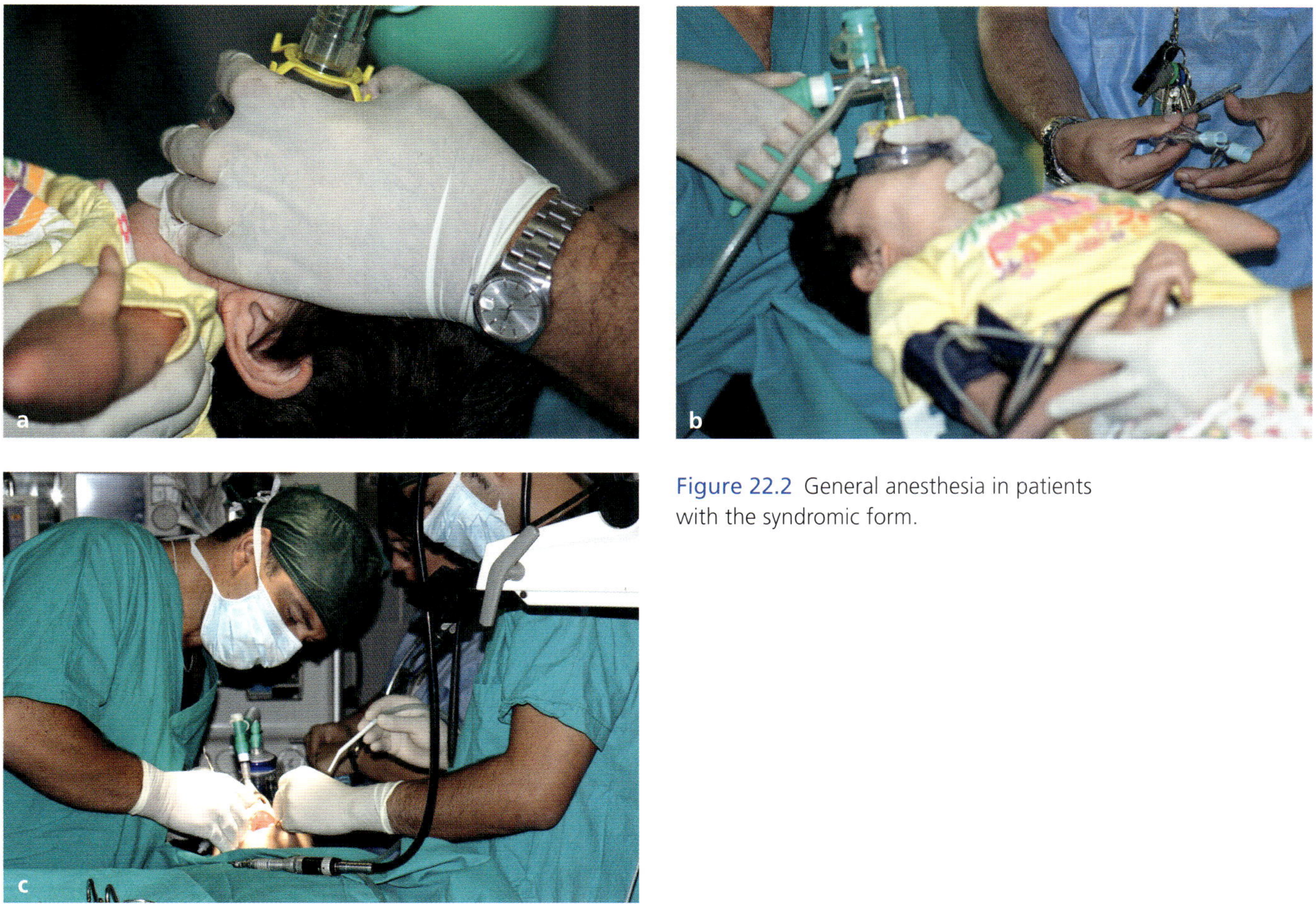

Figure 22.2 General anesthesia in patients with the syndromic form.

2. physiological history, which collects information about the various stages of development of a patient
3. pathological history, which is classified as long-term (information about the various pathologies of the patient from birth to the current observation) and short-term (which takes into account the reason for the specialist visit).

Thus, the pathology that affects the patient, with its possible causes, and primarily the applicable drug therapy, can be identified. Additionally, it is important to know whether the patient has ever had any experience in the field of dentistry as this information is necessary for the professional to decide which approach to take and how to customize it. Finally, the consent form for the treatment of the patient is filled and signed by the parent or caregiver/guardian, who should be over the age of 18 years.

Another important aspect is the assessment of the parent's personality profile, which could influence the child's behavior, such as in the following cases:

- reasonable, quiet, and relaxed = cooperative child
- anxious, indecisive, and doubtful = anxious child and difficult cooperation
- aware of the problems of the child, but provides contradictory education = cooperative child only to resolve urgencies
- superb, aggressive, pretentious, and uncooperative = fearful and uncooperative child.

The parent's figure is of great help to dentists because it can help identify the degree of cooperation and the most effective methods to obtain cooperation. In order to increase the compliance of overindulgent or overprotective parents, it is necessary to describe to them the cooperation and assistance that is needed during the session and provide instructions to them about home oral hygiene maneuvers, if these are incorrect or insufficient. Reading and filling in the folder will allow the dentist to speak with the parents and thus better understand the problems related to the child, not only from the point of view of dental care but also from that of everyday life. Knowing the physical and mental limitations of the patient, the clinician can better implement the treatment plan.

During the clinical examination, classic semiological maneuvers are performed, and rubber mouth openers (Fig. 22.3) and steel fingers (Fig. 22.4) can be used as aids for the examination. Parents or guardians participate in the examination itself; they cooperate directly by helping the professional during the armchair maneuvers. It is

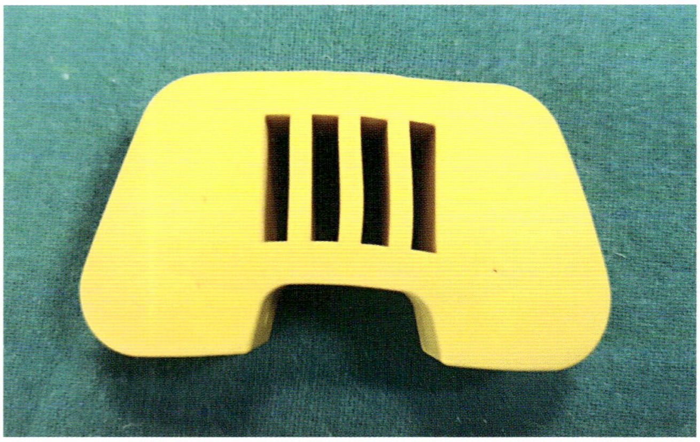

Figure 22.3 Rubber mouth opener.

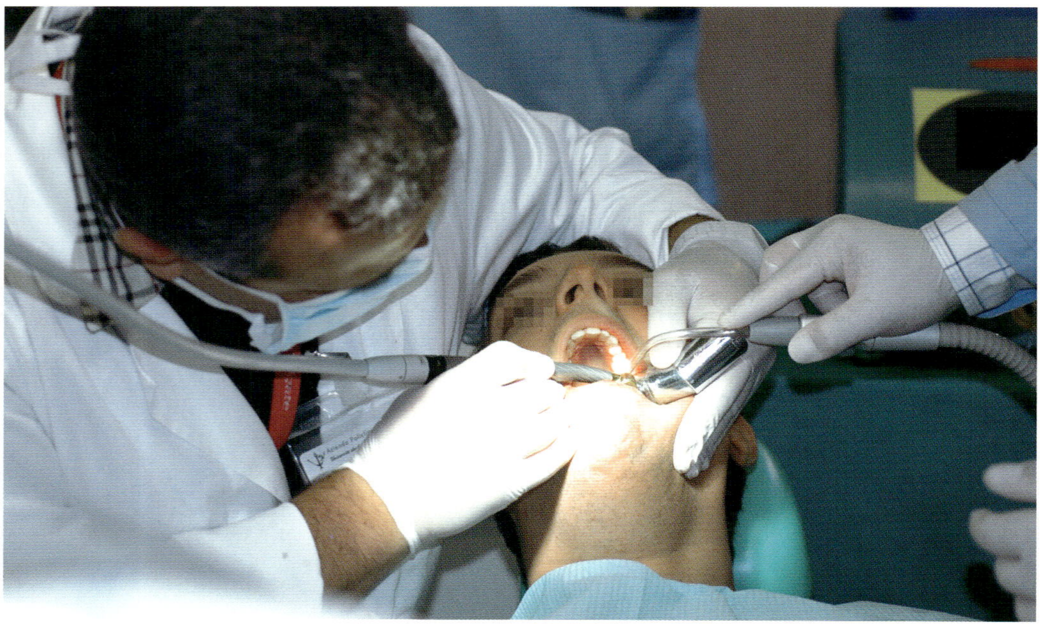

Figure 22.4 Use of the steel finger.

very important to try to gradually bring the child to cooperate between maneuvers; after the first time the patient opens the mouth, he is allowed to rest, is told to close it, and is rewarded with positive verbal reinforcements. After a short interval, the dentist can start again, trying to always be faster in visually grasping the alterations of the oral cavity.
In addition to the dental elements, soft tissues are also examined as the patient may have changes in them.

Oral health management in patients with disabilities

The management of oral health of patients with disabilities is intricately linked to the physical and mental deficiencies and poses a challenge for the dental staff. The main problem to be addressed is the maintenance of oral health; therefore, the role of parents or caregivers is crucial.
Already during the first visit, the dentist has the opportunity to ask them how they face daily what for them, unlike for others, is a fundamental problem. To confirm this, based on findings in the international literature, the main oral manifestations in such patients are oral hygiene sessions, conservative care, and extractions.
The first fundamental step in maintaining good oral hygiene is the removal of calculus, which can also be useful as an approach toward the patient. Once seated in the armchair, the dentist can illustrate and describe each instrument, so that, knowing well every tool that is going to be used, the patient can be less fearful and more motivated.
This is the so-called "*tell–show–do*" technique: it consists of a preliminary explanation of the functioning of the instrumentation and the sensations that might be felt, with practical–clinical demonstration. Understandable and psychologically acceptable terms should be used. In patients who are less cooperative, pharmacological sedation using diazepam or midazolam is very useful, which, in addition to having a calming effect on the patient, leads to a reduction in muscle tone and postsurgery amnesia.
The necessary tools are as follows:
- probe
- small mirror
- ultrasound
- abrasive paste similar to toothpaste
- curettes.

The following aids may help:
- pharmacological sedation
- sedation with nitrous oxide
- rubber mouth opener
- giant model of mouth and toothbrush.

The dentist has to proceed for short periods with the scaler, then stop and ask the patient if everything is alright; in this way, the patient understands that there is nothing to fear. Then, the dentist starts again and continues working in short periods, occasionally interrupting the work and using verbal positive reinforcements.
The dentist can ask the parents what methods of oral hygiene are used for the child at home; in most cases, they reply that there is no method at all because the child's disability compromises home hygiene; in other cases, they indicate that mainly sodium carbonate, gauzes soaked with mouthwash, or electric toothbrush are used; these methods are very useful in case of almost complete noncooperation. The electric toothbrush is one of the main indications for patients with disabilities, but such toothbrushes with soft bristles should be carefully used and should be replaced after 2 months. In most cases, the parents take care of the child, but they should let him/her do as much as possible in a completely autonomous manner. Feelings of self-esteem and achievement of the goal are the most important things. This is also central from the professional's perspective because a patient who has achieved a good level of self-esteem is even more motivated to perform any dental treatment. Various alternatives can be used at home depending on the manual skills.

- Patients who permanently hold their fingers fixed in a fist position: insert the handle of the toothbrush into the grip. In such cases, the parent can help the patient during the maneuvers, but if the patient is able to perform the maneuver autonomously, it is better to let him/her do them without interfering.
- Patients who cannot grasp or hold anything in their hands: in such cases, a Velcro band tied around their hand can be used, with a slit at the level of the palm into which the handle of the toothbrush is inserted. Alternatively, the operator can attach the handle of a nail brush to the toothbrush using a waterproof adhesive tape.
- Patients unable to handle the toothbrush because of a limited closing of the hand: it is necessary to increase the diameter of the handle; then, the operator can use the knob of a bicycle handlebar to insert the handle of the toothbrush or a tennis ball to insert the handle through a hole; otherwise, the operator can insert both in a tin can.
- Patients unable to lift an arm or hand: the toothbrush handle should be extended. A wooden cylinder with the cemented toothbrush handle inside or two toothbrushes in which the handles are joined (using a tape for instance) can be useful to increase the length.
- Patients able to hold and position the toothbrush but not handle it: in such cases, a toothbrush that wraps around all the faces of the tooth (vestibular, oral, and occlusal) and requires only a single back and forth movement is very useful. Research has shown a reduction in residues and bacterial plates similar to that achieved using a conventional toothbrush.
- The electric toothbrush remains one of two major indications for patients with disabilities.

Another important instrument is dental floss; in this case, the help of the parent is necessary because the wrong use of this instrument can result in damage at the level of the interpapillary zone.
During the same session, the dentist can suggest positions that facilitate oral hygiene at home so that the parent can independently take care of the child. In this case, there are three options:

- Standing parent: standing behind the patient, the parent places the arm around the head of the child and the chin rests on the cupped hand, while the thumb and forefinger of the same hand are used to pull the lips and cheeks back. The other hand uses a toothbrush, the floss, or other instruments. This technique can be used when the patient is of a short stature, when he is sitting on the wheelchair and can therefore recline his head, ensuring that the wheelchair brakes are applied.
- Sitting parent: the patient sits on the ground with the parent behind him and the back resting on his knees. The parent in turn holds the patient's arms firmly with his legs to prevent any sudden gestures; he can use both hands for oral hygiene maneuvers. If the patient is forced to stay in bed, the parent can sit next to him with the patient's head resting on the parent's legs.
- In the third case, the patient may need help from another parent to keep his arms or hands still. If the child is very young, the two parents can sit one in front of the other, with the patient lying between them; one blocks the head, wipes the teeth, and passes the dental floss; the other holds the arms, hands, or legs still.

If there is a need for conservative care or dental extractions, these must be conducted following normal procedures, but the patient's condition still obliges the dentist to use special procedures. First, if the patient is uncooperative, the presence of one of the parents is of fundamental importance because, on one hand, it reassures him, and on the other, it can be useful to hold the arms and legs. The dentist's assistant must also be ready to address any sudden gesture by the patient and, using the aspirator, must try to not allow the operating field from getting contaminated with saliva. If necessary, sedation using benzodiazepines may be useful due to their hypno-inducing, myo-relaxing, and amnesic effect as already mentioned. The "*all-in-one*" system is very useful (Fig. 22.5) as it contains mordant, primer, and agents bonding together in a single product, thereby allowing reduction in the number of passages and reduction in dental sessions. This is important: reduced intervention time allows the patient to get less tired and reduces stress so that he can face the sessions with greater confidence.
The rubber mouth opener and steel finger lead to excellent results and can be used in case of dental extractions, all associated with the good will of the dentist, a minimum level of flexibility with regard to normal procedures, and a great deal of patience.

In the case of extractions, the role of the assistant and of those who, like the parent, assist the professional assumes greater importance because the instruments used for extractions can be more damaging than the previous ones. The maneuvers for the

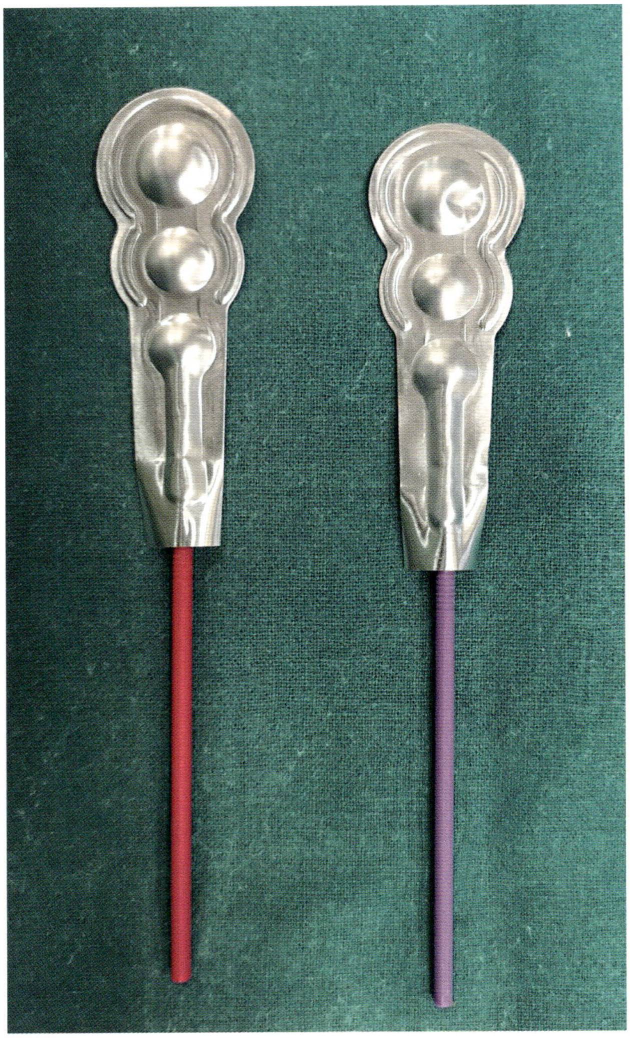

Figure 22.5 *All-in-one* system.

extractions of dental elements follow the classic phases that are at the base of the extractions in patients not affected by any systemic pathology. One person will have to hold the patient's head, one the hands, and the other the legs, in addition to the assistant at the chair.
It is necessary to illustrate and describe some of the main systemic alterations in addition to the normal alterations of odontostomatological interest and the systemic features attributable to particular conditions.
The pathologies are subdivided into groups: syndromic, genetic, neuropsychiatric, and hematological.

Three diseases will be described: autism, ectodermal dysplasia, and osteogenesis imperfecta.

Autism spectrum disorder: an update on oral health management in children

M. Bossù, D. Corridore

Definition, diagnosis, and prevalence

Autism is a behavioral syndrome caused by a developmental disorder that is biologically determined, with onset in the first 3 years of life. Children with autism are physically healthy with a normal physical appearance and undergo the same development as their healthy peers, but their cognitive performance profile is rather uneven and involves various brain functions; autism manifests itself through a wide range of symptoms of different modes and degrees of severity for each child, and this leads to the phrase "autistic spectral disorders" (ASD) being used in place of "autism." The disorders of the autism spectrum are described and classified using internationally recognized diagnostic tools: the *Diagnostic and Statistical Manual of Mental Disorders, 5th Edition* (DSM-5) by the American Psychiatric Association and the *International Classification of Diseases*, 11th edition (ICD-11), by the World Health Organization, which include ASDs in neurodevelopment disorders.

The diagnosis of ASDs has become unique, and all subtypes that were previously present in DSM-4 (Asperger syndrome, childhood disintegrative disorder, and pervasive developmental disorder not otherwise specified) have been eliminated.

With regards to the diagnosis, there are two domains of interest considered by the pathology:

- **Criterion A.** Persistent lack of social communication and social interaction in multiple contexts, as manifested by the following factors, which are present currently occurring or have occurred in the past:
  - *Deficit of socio-emotional reciprocity*, which ranges from abnormal social approach and failure to normally reciprocate in conversation to a reduced sharing of interests, emotions, or feelings, as well as the inability to initiate or respond to social interactions.
  - *Deficit of nonverbal communication behavior for social interaction*, which includes poorly integrated verbal and nonverbal communication, abnormalities in eye contact and body language, lack of understanding and use of gestures, and total lack of facial expression and nonverbal communication.
  - *Deficit in the development, management, and understanding of relationships*, which includes difficulties in adapting the behavior to various social contexts, difficulty in sharing imagination or making friends, and the absence of interest in peers.

- **Criterion B.** Restricted and repetitive patterns of behavior, interests, or activities that are manifested by at least two of the following factors, which are present currently occurring or have occurred in the past:
  - Movements, use of objects, or stereotyped or repetitive speech, e.g., simple motor stereotypes, lining up toys or flipping objects, echolalia, and idiosyncratic phrases.
  - Insistence in similarity, adherence to routine without flexibility or rituals of verbal or nonverbal behavior, e.g., extreme discomfort in facing small changes, difficulties in the transition stages, rigid thought patterns, ritual greetings, and the need to walk the same path or eat the same food every day).
  - Very limited, fixed interests that are abnormal in intensity or depth, e.g., strong attachment or concern for unusual patients and excessively circumscribed or persevering interests.
  - Hyper- or hypo-reactivity in response to sensory stimuli or unusual interests toward sensory aspects of the environment, e.g., apparent indifference to pain/temperature, aversion to specific sounds or tactile textures, sniffing or touching objects in an excessive manner, and being fascinated by lights or movements.

The first aspect comprises three criteria that must all be met to obtain the diagnosis, while the second aspect requires at least two out of four criteria to be met. In particular, the presence of narrow and stereotyped behaviors (criterion B) becomes crucial to establish the diagnosis of ASDs, making differential diagnosis with other types of disorders such as social communicative disorder introduced in the manual. Furthermore, the manual also specifies that the disorder is present early but can fully manifest itself in different ages depending on social demands (criterion C). Finally, the diagnosis of ASDs is accompanied by an indication of the severity of symptoms (criterion D), according to which the patient can be classified as in need of very significant, significant, or modest help (Santocchi andMuratori, 2012) (Table 22.1).
DSM-5 presents an additional novelty: if a child with ASD also presents symptoms of another disorder, it is possible to diagnose the child with two or more disorders without having to identify and diagnose only the prevalent one.

ICD-10 is currently being revised, and the new version will come into force from January 2022. In its new interpretation, ICD-11 differs from DSM-5 in several key points. Among the features of DSM-5, there is the preeminent treatment of sensory anomalies, such as over- or under-sensitivity to sound and touch. The definition of autism in ICD-11, on the contrary, makes no mention of sensory anomalies. In addition, ICD-11 does not require a fixed number or a combination of features for a diagnosis but lists identifying features and allows clinicians to decide whether a person's traits coincide with those of autism. ICD-11 also makes a distinction between autism with and without intellectual disabilities and highlights the fact that older individuals and women sometimes mask their traits of autism.
Recent studies do not detect any geographical, ethnic, or socio-cultural prevalence for ASDs; however, it has been widely established that the incidence rate is 4-5 times higher in males than in females, with an average ratio of 4:1. Several hypotheses have

Table 22.1 Severity level of symptoms according to DSM-5

Severity level	Social communication	Restricted, repetitive behaviors
LEVEL 3 There is a need for very significant support	Severe deficits in social, verbal, and nonverbal communication skills cause severe impairment of functioning, very limited initiation of social interactions, and minimal reactions to social interactions initiated by others.	Inflexibility of behavior, extreme difficulty in dealing with change, or other restricted/ repetitive behaviors interfere markedly with all areas of operation. Considerable discomfort/difficulty in changing the object of attention or action.
LEVEL 2 There is a need for significant support	Marked deficiencies in verbal and nonverbal social communication skills, social impairments visible even in the presence of support, limited initiation of social interaction, and reduced or abnormal reactions to social interactions initiated by others.	Inflexibility of behavior, difficulties in coping with change or other restrictive/repetitive behaviors are sufficiently frequent as to be apparent to the casual observer and interfere with functioning in various contexts. Discomfort/unease in modifying the object of attention or action.
LEVEL 1 There is a need for support	In the absence of support, deficits in social communication cause significant compromises. Difficulty in initiating social interactions and clear examples of atypical or unsuccessful responses to social openings by others. The individual may show little interest in social interaction.	The inflexibility of behavior causes significant interference with functioning in one or more contexts. Difficulty in switching from one activity to another. Problems in organization and planning hinder independence.

been put forward: a greater vulnerability related to the male sex or, on the contrary, the presence of protective factors in the female sex that determine the need for a more severe organic lesion and a greater genetic influence; in fact, it has been observed that females are affected by a more severe cognitive deterioration in which the pathology manifests. In the United States, a prevalence of approximately 1:750 children affected by AS is reported, which increases to 1:150 when referring to ASDs (these data are related to studies conducted in the 1990s). More recently, epidemiological studies conducted in the United States, Europe, and Asia show a general increase in ASD diagnoses, with a significant increase in the last decade (equivalent to double). This increase is linked to a better capacity of diagnosis by specialists, leading to the ability to establish diagnoses at an increasingly early age (currently, the threshold is 18 months) and to the widening of the diagnostic criteria. In Italy, the growing perception and attention to the problem of children affected by ASDs has led the National Institute of Statistics to consider the disease in its specificity. According to the data, in

2016-2017, the disability affected 25.6% of the 90,000 *special-needs* pupils in primary schools and 21.7% of the 69,000 *special-needs* pupils in first-grade secondary schools, for a total of 38,000, with a prevalence of 0.84% in total; this was slightly higher than the data for the previous year, 2015-2016, but in line with international data. A recent research on cases of pediatric autism in children aged 7–9 years conducted in the Province of Pisa within the framework of the European project Autism Spectrum Disorders in the European Union concluded that this figure can be expected to reach 1% of the total number of pupils. The figure of 1% is however much higher than the one derived from the registry of the information system of the Italian Society of Neuropsychiatry in Childhood and Adolescence of Emilia-Romagna (SINPIA-ER), which reported a prevalence of 0.44% in children aged 6–10 years in the year 2016. In Emilia-Romagna, too, the absolute value of the prevalence of autism recorded by child neuropsychiatry services doubled from 2011 to 2017, and an increase is expected in all age groups.

Etiology

ASD cannot be considered as a single disorder but as a multifactorial disorder resulting from genetic and nongenetic risk factors and their interactions.

Genetic causes, including chromosomal defects and abnormalities, were found in the literature in 10%–20% of patients with ASD. Siblings born in families with a patient with ASD have a 50-fold greater risk of presenting the disorder. The concordance rate reaches up to 82%–92% in monozygotic twins compared with 1%–10% in dizygotic twins. Genetic studies have suggested that individual mutations alter the developmental pathways of neuronal and axonal structures involved in synaptogenesis. Genome-wide association studies have identified chromosomes 2q, 7q, 15q, and 16p as the sites of susceptibility genes, although the mechanism has not been fully determined. These chromosomal anomalies are involved in the breakdown of neural connections, brain growth, and synaptic/dendritic morphology. Recently, the correlation between the gene responsible for cerebellar development (Engrailed2) and autism has been reported. It is the first identified genetic allele that contributes to susceptibility in at least 40% of ASD cases. Other genes were considered as predisposing genetic factors.

Several environmental causal factors, including prenatal, perinatal, and postnatal factors, also contribute to the occurrence of ASD. Prenatal factors associated with ASD include exposure to teratogenic drugs such as thalidomide (withdrawn from the market in Italy in 1963, which was also prescribed in pregnant women), some viral infections (congenital rubella syndrome), and maternal anticonvulsants such as valproic acid. The weight at birth, the gestation period, and asphyxiation at birth comprise the perinatal factors. Postnatal factors associated with ASD include autoimmune disease, viral infection, hypoxia, mercury toxicity, and others.

In recent years, researchers have suggested that ASD is the result of complex interactions between genetic and environmental risk factors. Understanding the interaction between these components will lead to an optimal treatment strategy.

Prognosis

In the case of autism, prognosis is complex due to the uncertainties of the related etiopathogenesis. However, autism is a lifelong disorder for which there is currently no possibility of definitive treatment; only the recourse to specific psycho-educational programs can partially adapt social interactions. These programs represent an effective intervention in many directions, such as in personal autonomy, socialization, cognitive activity, motor activity, and communication, and minimize undesired behaviors.

Oral risk and health factors

Potential risk factors in patients with ASD, as well as for the rest of the population, mainly include diet, oral hygiene, and age. The predilection for soft and sticky foods and the use of sweet foods/drinks as rewards in psycho-pedagogical therapies make diet a significant risk factor for caries. The prevalence level of deciduous and permanent tooth decay in children with ASD was analyzed in a series of studies, and the results were inconsistent. Some report a lower prevalence of caries in deciduous, mixed, and permanent teeth and no significant association between this prevalence and severity of ASD; others, on the contrary, report a higher prevalence.

However, oral hygiene is the most influential risk indicator in children with autism, and special attention should be given to the presence of visible plaques and gingivitis in individual patients.

Most studies have found poor oral hygiene in the affected children and adults, and the level of oral hygiene was associated with increased experience of caries and the presence of generalized gingivitis and increased severity of ASD symptoms. Concern about periodontal disease as a consequence of poor oral hygiene in patients with ASD was supported by the evidence of significantly worse periodontal status in children with autism compared with children not affected by it. Indeed, the degree of severity is also accompanied by the level of cooperation in carrying out home oral hygiene maneuvers and by the same ability to perform them more or less effectively. In most cases, the executors are not the patients but their parents or guardians, for whom the success of the maneuvers is subject to numerous variables. The lack of attention is another risk factor that parents/guardians of patients have toward the prevention of caries, considering the state of oral health as a secondary issue in the management of ASD. This behavior is defined as the *halo effect* and leads to a worsening of the oral conditions, which are only considered when a painful symptomatology is presented by the patient. The xerostomic side effects of psychoactive drugs in many studies were not considered as a risk factor for caries; however, no hypotheses for these findings have been provided.

Another risk factor is orthodontic malocclusion, which in patients with ASD compared with healthy individuals include a greater tendency toward open anterior bite and dental crowding. Other studies reported increased interdental spaces, reverse overjet, and a class II molar relationship. Furthermore, the presence of malocclusion is also associated with an increased risk of dental trauma in patients with ASD, particularly in those with tendencies to self-harm.

Therapeutic approach

Providing oral care to individuals with intellectual disabilities requires modification of ordinary skills. In fact, many individuals with mild or moderate intellectual disabilities can be successfully treated in daily practice using an effective overall approach that does not pose significant behavioral problems and complicate dental treatments. In contrast, anxiety regarding the treatment of patients with ASD often occurs and involves the patient, the parent/guardian, and often the operator too. Individuals with ASD slowly and often with difficulty learn ordinary daily life activities such as brushing their teeth or dressing up and have problems in understanding the behavior of others as well as their own. This can pose as a real challenge for themselves and especially for their relatives. Those who do not know about dental surgery and its equipment and instruments could show fear. Some react to fear with uncooperative behavior, such as crying, aggressive language, or anything that helps them avoid the treatment. In children with autism, it is more difficult to interpret the signs of fear and identify them before losing cooperation. It is possible to perform oral care in a more reassuring context for patients if the clinician can recognize their anxiety.
The hypersensitivity of these patients to sensory inputs is of particular importance for dentistry, although hyposensitivity and indifference to pain or extreme temperature may also occur. The consequent sensory overload can quickly lead to overstimulation and subsequent avoidance reactions. Therefore, considerable attention must be paid to the modalities and times with which certain treatments are intended to be conducted.

Basic behavioral techniques

Traditional approaches

The basic guide techniques currently used include positive reinforcement, "*tell–show–do*" (TSD), distraction methods, nonverbal communication, and voice control. These techniques are effective in treating patients of development age; however, they may not always be successful in patients with ASD in whom speech deficits and receptive language can have a negative impact on their use. Limitations in social interactions, such as the inability to participate in imitation games, may represent a significant obstacle to the effective use of TSD methods because they require the child to project the simulation actions of the dentist for a given procedure in his mouth. Prior consultation with parents/guardians is needed to assess the behavior and symptoms of the patient in order to customize the use of behavioral guidance technique (BGT).

Visual pedagogy

Visual pedagogy is a nontraditional approach to behavioral guidance that takes advantage of the ability of children with autism to respond better to images than to words. It involves the use of books with colored photographs, social stories, or videos and can be combined with traditional BGT as positive reinforcement and TSD to adapt to neurocognitive deficits in patients with ASD. Bäckman et al demonstrated the effectiveness of visual pedagogy, which involves the use of a book with a series of colored photographs that describe the different stages of a dental examination for children with autism. The authors reported improved cooperation by patients exposed to this behavioral approach compared with children with ASD who have not undergone visual pedagogy techniques.

Social stories

Visual pedagogy has also been used for the development of "social stories," which is a widely used strategy for children with ASD. Initially developed by a special education teacher, Carol Gray, the technique of social histories attempts to promote an accurate understanding by the child of the social information given to him from the explanation of an activity and the related behavioral expectations. Social stories are generally short and are based on a relationship of descriptive, perspective, and/or affirmative phrases, as well as visual signals. They are easy to construct and are adaptable to the specific needs of each specialist.
In children with ASD, social stories can improve social behaviors, such as washing hands, greeting people appropriately, and sharing toys. There is evidence that a disruptive behavior can also be reduced by the repetitive use of a social story. In addition to visual signals, social stories are based on reading and hearing processing skills.

Video modeling

For patients with limited reading and hearing abilities, video modeling can be an alternative method based on visual pedagogy, which is in turn based on the increasing propensity for children with autism to use electronic media. Although there is limited evidence regarding the use of video modeling in dentistry, the viewing of videos studied specifically and agreed in advance with the specialist to make the visit to the dentist less anxiety-inducing can be very effective. In addition, the projection of themed cartoons or of cartoon that are of particular interest to the patient can be helpful.

Desensitization

Desensitization sessions are designed to repeatedly expose a child to the dental environment and to promote trust and adaptation. The use of desensitization can lead to greater cooperation for performing dental examinations and debridement in children with ASD and other intellectual disabilities. The process begins with a cognitive interview with the parents for acquiring the preferences of the patient to establish the type of positive reinforcement for their child, e.g., stickers and stamps. Thus, steps associated with a procedure such as a dental examination are performed in a simulated environment, e.g., their home, combining the use of positive reinforcement with praise. Ideally, practice sessions should be followed up by visits to the dentist, where the actual clinical examination occurs. However, professional desensitization requires time and availability of dental facilities and staff. Thus, consultation/collaboration with the child's therapist is desirable to practice simulations of dental examinations before the actual dental examination, even in the facilities where the child undergoes his or her own therapy.

Nitrous oxide

There are contradictory reports about the success of nitrous oxide (N_2O) as BGT for dental patients with autism. Some authors have claimed that N_2O is not effective because it only works well when combined with BGT based on communications such as distraction, TSD, and positive reinforcement, to which patients with autism may not be susceptible. Others, however, recommended the use of N_2O for patients with mild behavioral problems. In a recent prospective study, patients with autism showed a success rate between 50% and 87.5% with the use of N_2O.
Faced with limited evidence, parents/guardians may be further confused by fears of systemic adverse effects due to the interaction of N_2O with potential mutations of the methylene tetrahydrofolate reductase gene or abnormalities in folate metabolism. Dentists should discuss the use of N_2O with interested parents and help them make informed decisions by explaining the risks and benefits and exploring other treatment modalities. Consultation with the patient's doctor on possible genetic mutations or abnormalities in folate metabolism will contribute to the decision-making process, especially in cases of longer and higher concentrations and exposure to N_2O.

Advanced Behavioral Techniques

Protective restraint

Patients with autism may require active or passive protective restraint for urgent diagnosis or treatment as part of a scheduled sedation or because they show uncontrolled movements that can jeopardize their own safety and that of the dental staff and families. The protective restraint can actually calm children with autism because of the deep pressure produced by its positioning. However, it should be considered with due care as lesions may occur in patients who do not always respond positively. In such cases, minor scratches and bruises may occur, but more serious injuries are possible. The doctor should be very careful on how tightly the casing is placed on the patient as it may limit breathing or may lead to overheating. It has been shown that fewer injuries occur with the passive method compared with the active method and in situations in which passive stabilization has been used in a planned manner rather than for emergencies.
Parents of children with autism may be reluctant to use this technique, but acceptance can be improved by positive explanations and detailed informed consent that takes into account their concerns and preferences. The presence of parents during the use of protective restraints should be encouraged.

Sedation

The use of sedation is a feasible option that can be considered for patients with autism when basic and advanced BGTs have failed. Benzodiazepines such as diazepam and midazolam are recommended, in combination with nitrous oxide administration, with reported success rates of 77%–100%. Midazolam is more successful in regulating the patient's behavior than diazepam but has a shorter working time, and this should be considered when choosing between the two agents. The doctor should rule out other comorbidities that contravene the use of sedation and medications that may negatively affect the success of a sedation regimen or compromise it.

General anesthesia

For patients that show uncertainties related to the safety of a sedation regimen, general anesthesia (GA) serves as an advanced approach to providing complete dental care, but the severity of the lesions and their resolution should be proportional to the inherent risks for such a procedure.

Among dental patients with special needs, autism is one of the most frequently indicated syndromes to provide dental care under GA due to factors such as high caries activity requiring extensive/extractive treatment and uncooperative behavior. However, this option should be considered when other therapeutic alternatives have been ruled out or when the patient is planned for treatment under GA because of other medical services that can be combined with the dental treatment.

Parents of children with autism are likely to have a positive attitude toward GA. The hospital environment, however, can produce defensive responses in the minor, increasing the stress of the family. While GA is generally considered a safe procedure, adverse events related to its use in patients with autism include destructive behaviors (12%) and postoperative vomiting that delays disposal (6%),whereas lethality is very rare. Other less frequent adverse events include postoperative bleeding extended by patient handling of surgical sites and postoperative seizures requiring hospitalization.

The risk of perioperative complications and the general hypersensitivity of patients with autism require appropriate preoperative planning. The use of visual pedagogy may also be useful in this regard and may include books or videos describing the processes involved in the GA procedure.

The dentist should provide relevant information on the specific ASD diagnosis to the anesthesiologist, as well as the presence of related comorbidities, and any potentially challenging preoperative behavior, as these will determine the choice of pre drug and the need for additional staff or restrictions. In the case of related comorbidities, such as uncontrolled epilepsy, a pre surgical examination can predict the risk of postoperative complications. In any case, the resolution of the case in GA should not restrict the treatment of these patients even with the above-mentioned techniques to prevent further use of surgery.

Treatment of the autistic patient in developmental age with pedagogical intervention

There are multiple aspects in the manifestation of the pathology in the diagnosis of autism. This step is essential because the dentist must adopt a diversified, flexible, and adaptable approach to each case.
The need for a specifically trained team to improve conditions on the chair of autistic patients becomes apparent, in order to improve their quality of life. This approach has seen in theory the possibility of perfecting dental treatment, both to limit traumatic experiences in the autistic patient allowing continuity in his care and to improve the level of cooperation in the operating room, with consequent use of GA for small interventions (minimal carious lesions, seals, and debridement, *follow-up*). The team works in a synergistic and continuous way to identify which needs have priority for both the dentist and the individual patient, trying to exercise a certain amount of control on some variables, if not all, especially on the environmental ones.

Sequence (with possibility of modification)

The first and perhaps the most important phase is the fact-finding one and that of the interview with the patient's parents, in which all the useful information to optimize and personalize the therapy of ASD patient and the expectations of the parents regarding the therapy are collected. This cognitive phase is performed in the dental surgery in a free and unconstrained way for the patient, so that the dentist can observe him in the medical environment, be able to detect positive or negative behaviors, and provide the young patient with the opportunity to interact with the dental environment and the doctor in a very natural way.
Naturally, the environment must be prepared in advance and made safe for the patient and for the team; it should be possible to have a monitor with pictures or cartoons or relaxing music (Fig. 22.6).
The time devoted to the treatment of the patient must be adapted to his possibility of endurance, increased in a slow but constant way in the meetings, and agreed with the parents, who will perform simple simulation maneuvers at home, in an environment that is favorable and known.
Once on the chair, all four senses are stimulated in the patient, in particular the touch, through which he recognizes the instrumentation (gloves, cotton, water, air, mirror,probe, excavator, and turbine) and the parts of his mouth. The autistic patient learns what is the state of his teeth and gums, as well as the treatment methods and tools that are used. He can also know the intentions of doctors by building relationships of trust. Naturally, in order to create a link with the patient by inserting the dental examination/treatment experience into an accepted and known routine, the medical team must necessarily plan the use of the same operators for each patient in order to ensure continuity that becomes tranquillity (Fig. 22.7).

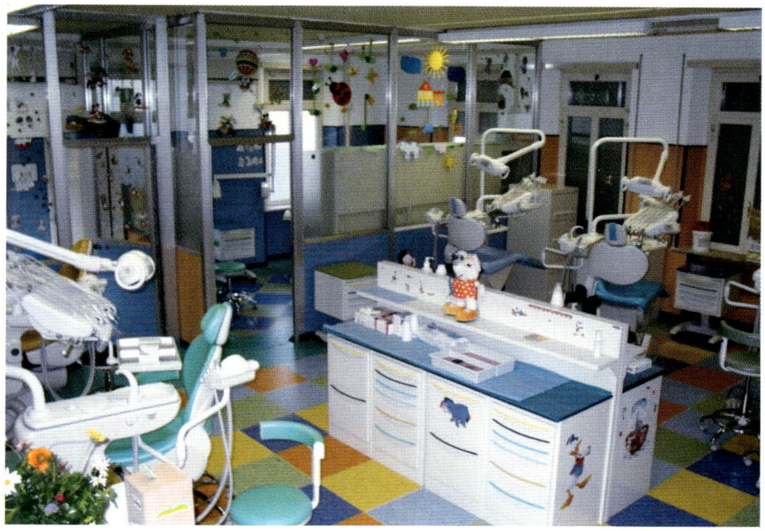

Figure 22.6 Environment designed for the necessities of pediatric patients with *special needs*.

Phases of the educational-sensory approach

- The child will play, along with the dentist, with a big plastic mouth and a toothbrush, will count the teeth by touching them, and will stop on those to be treated. The dentist teaches him how to use the toothbrush on the plastic mouth with particular attention to the sick teeth.
- The child will look at his mouth in the mirror where he will see the sick tooth (it is important to indicate it so that the child sees it, even by carrying his finger in his mouth). If the mirror creates a state of tension, avoid it and use only the child's finger to touch the tooth that hurts him.

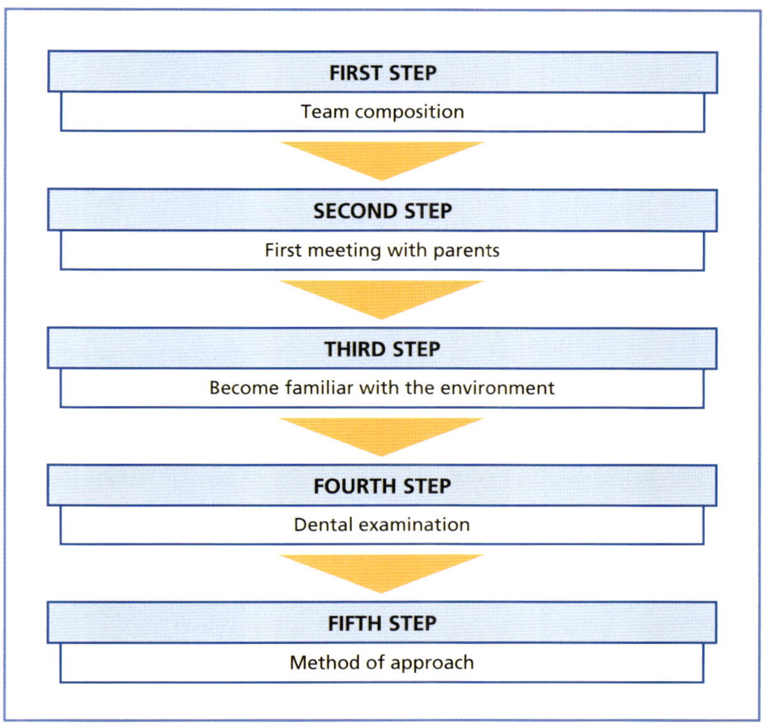

Figure 22.7 Operating sequences.

- The dentist, on the instructions of the educator, will start touching the patient's face with his fingers first, to subsequently get to the teeth and massage them slowly; finally, wrapping the finger with a gauze, the dentist will begin to massage the gums. At this stage, the educator interacts with the patient through gestural communication or alternative and augmentative communication (AAC, a whiteboard on which are placed images related to the dentist and instruments and which provides as final image a prize; fig. 22.8-22.9), favoring the dentist–patient relationship.
- Sensory knowledge of instruments is also a decisive stage in educational intervention. The autistic child will touch all the tools, including water and air that will then be gradually brought to the mouth even by the child himself, following the behavioral approach method called "*tell–show–do*."
- The execution times will be established by the doctor in order to give the child the possibility to perceive them and relax.

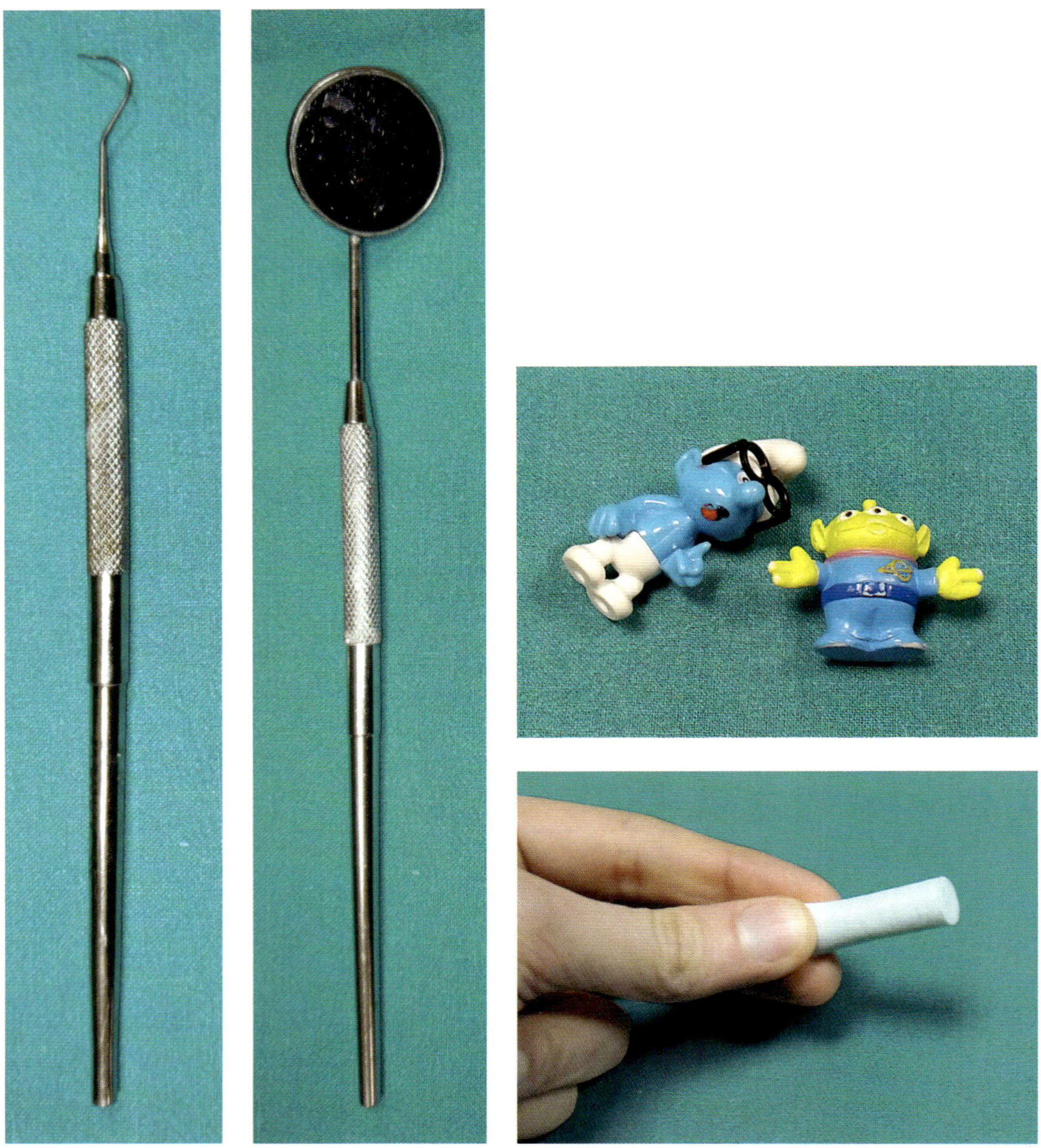

Figure 22.8 Example of a sequence of images in AAC.

During the sensory approach, the educator is constantly observing the child to identify his needs or particular reactions that may require new strategies. The sensory approach can last even for several sessions, as many as it takes for the autistic patient to gain confidence with the dentist and all the instrumentation.
Once confidence has been established, dental therapy is initiated.
A dental department or surgery can become not only a place of care but also an opportunity of growth for children and, therefore, of learning to acquire skills and competences.

Prevention

The evidence that poor oral hygiene frequently occurs in individuals with autism, associated with an increased risk of gingivitis, periodontitis, and caries guides prevention strategies aimed at improving the oral hygiene of these patients. Having a deficiency in their motor skills, some should be guided in the oral hygiene maneuvers so as to avoid too aggressive brushing damage. The parent/guardian should be instructed in the best oral hygiene techniques and the most effective type of instrument that can be adapted to the child's needs. Prevention strategies must account for the patient's profile and the difficulties of acceptance and hypersensitivity of children with autism who may not like too strong smells and flavors and above all may not be able to rinse or expectorate. These individual features should guide the dentist in choosing the best preventive strategy and, particularly, in choosing the primary and secondary prevention therapies (fluorine, casein, etc.). Visual pedagogy, with the insertion, for example, of colored photographs of oral hygiene steps in the patient's bathroom, is useful when combined with close references for the evaluation of therapy success.

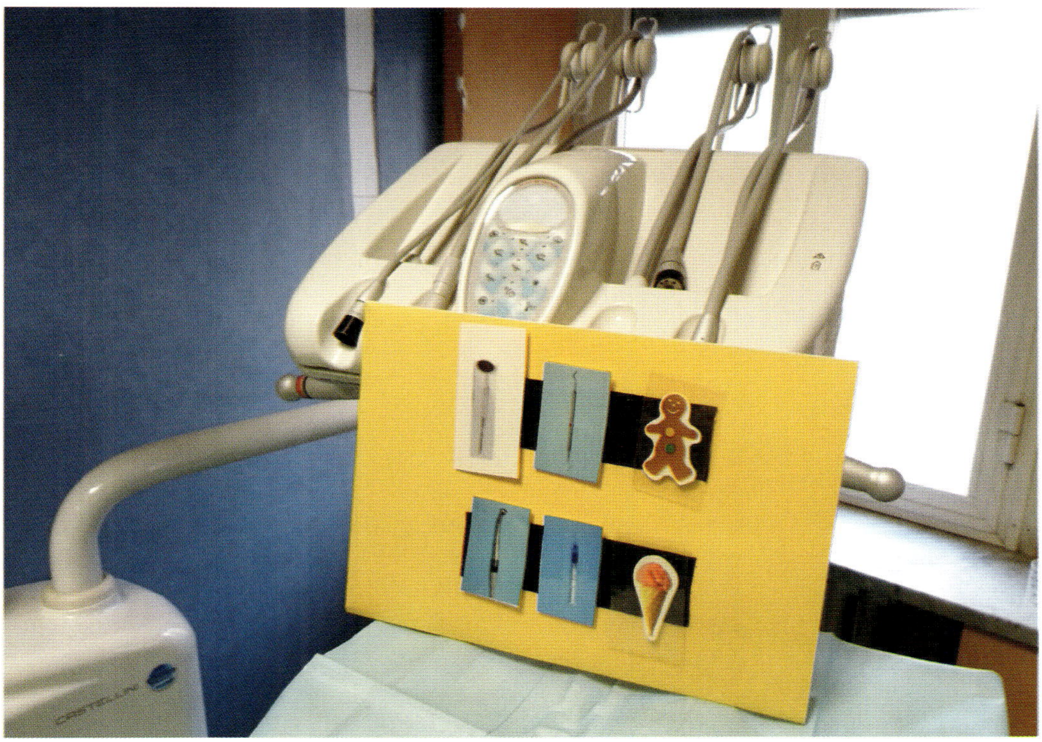

Figure 22.9 Example of AAC.

Preventive, restorative, and extractive treatments

In literature, the materials used for ASD patient restorations include amalgam, resin-based composites, glass-ionomer cements (GIC), and metal crowns according to the ART technique.

The use of amalgam is increasingly declining in accordance with the new EU regulation, which aims to eliminate the current gaps in EU legislation in order to ensure the perfect alignment of EU law with Minamata Convention on Mercury, enabling its ratification and implementation by the EU and its Member States.

In Italy, its use in children under the age of 6 years is not recommended in the dental recommendations of the Italian Ministry of Health issued in 2014 (*Raccomandazioni Cliniche in Odontostomatologia* del Ministero della Salute, 2014). The same document recommends the use of resinous GIC as effective means for restoring deciduous elements or as a temporary treatment in patients with socio-sanitary fragility.

These considerations lead us to consider GICs as the material of choice in the restorative treatment and caries prevention in uncooperative patients with special needs in whom a dam cannot be mounted. In these individuals, indeed, the use of composite resins is hindered by the inability to adequately isolate the operating area due to compliance, which is a factor that limits the use of the composite and does not guarantee an optimal adhesion to the dental tissues, facilitating its detachment and the possible recurrence of carious lesions. In many cases, the only effective way of treating carious lesions with composite resins in *special-need* patients could be to use GA. This step can be avoided with the use of GICs, which have hydrophilic properties that predispose them to be used as restoration materials and sealing agents, both in normal and in humid conditions; furthermore, their easy application reduces the number of steps necessary to perform restoration/sealing.

In the case of stainless steel preformed crowns, parents can be reassured that the levels of nickel, chromium, and iron released into the oral cavity are low and have no impact on systemic health. However, their application may involve the presence of pre contacts, which can create even more discomfort for the patient and exacerbate existing tics. Even the execution of low or medium difficulty extractive interventions can be performed on patients with ASD with the help of the right approach technique and the aid of tools aimed at performing nontraumatic anesthesia.

References

American Academy of Pediatric Dentistry Reference Manual. Protective stabilization for pediatric dental patients, 2012-2013;34(6).

American Psychiatric Association. Diagnostic and Statistical Manual of Mental Disorders. 5th ed. Arlington, VA: American Psychiatric Association, 2013. [Trad. it. Manuale Diagnostico e Statistico dei Disturbi Mentali, DSM-5®. 5 ed., Milano: Raffaello Cortina Editore, 2014].

Amira A, El Khatib AA, Magda M et al. Oral health status and behaviours of children with Autism Spectrum Disorder: a case-control study. Int J Paediatr Dent 2014;24:314-23.

Bäckman B, Pilebro C. Visual pedagogy in dentistry for children with autism. ASDC J Dent Child 1999;66(5):325-31.

Bartolomé-Villar B, Mourelle-Martínez MR, Diéguez-Pérez M et al. Incidence of oral health in paediatric patients with disabilities: Sensory disorders and autism spectrum disorder. Systematic review II. J Clin Exp Dent 2016;8(3):e344-51.

Bhat S, Acharya UR, Adeli H et al. Autism: cause factors, early diagnosis and therapies. Rev Neurosci 2014;25(6):841-50.

Bossù M, Corridore D, D'Errico A et al. Education and dentistry: advanced synergy in the dental treatment of children with autism; a pilot clinical trial. Senses Sci 2014;1(3).

Cagetti MG, Mastroberardino S, Campus G et al. Dental care protocol based on visual supports for children with autism spectrum disorders. Med Oral Pathol Oral Cir Buccal 2015;20(5):e598-604.

Capozza LE, Bimstein E. Preferences of parents of children with autism spectrum disorders concerning oral health and treatment. Pediatr Dent 2012;34(7):480-4.

Crozier S, Tincani M. Effects of social stories on prosocial behavior of preschool children with autism spectrum disorders. J Autism Dev Disord 2007;37(9):1803-14.

Faulks D, Hennequin M, Albecker-Grappe S et al. Sedation with 50% nitrous oxide/oxygen for outpatient dental treatment in individuals with intellectual disability. Dev Med Child Neurol 2007;49(8):621-5.

Gandhi RP, Klein U. Autism spectrum disorders: An update on oral health management. J Evid Base Dent Pract 2014;14S:115-126.

Hurlbutt M, Young DA. A best practices approach to caries management. J Evid Base Dent Pract 2014;14S:77-86. ISTAT, L'integrazione degli alunni con disabilità nelle scuole primarie e secondarie di primo grado. Anno scolastico 2016-2017 (www.istat.it/it/archivio/60454).

Kupietzky A, Ram D. Effects of a positive verbal presentation on parental acceptance of passive medical stabilization for the dental treatment of young children. Pediatr Dent 2005;27(5):380-4.

Loo CY, Graham RM, Hughes CV. The caries experience and behavior of dental patients with autism spectrum disorder. J Am Dent Assoc 2008;139(11):1518-24.

Marshall J, Sheller B, Mancl L. Caries-risk assessment and caries status of children with autism. Pediatr Dent 2010;32(1):69-75.

Maskey M, Warnell F, Parr J et al. Emotional and behavioral problems in children with autism spectrum disorder. J Autism Dev Disord 2013;43(4):851-9.

Messieha Z. Risks of general anesthesia for the special needs dental patient. Special Care Dent 2009;29(1):21-5.

Mineo B, Ziegler W, Gill S, Salkin D. Engagement with electronic screen media among students with autism spectrum disorders. J Autism Dev Disord 2009;39(1):172-87.

Ozdemir S. The effectiveness of social stories on decreasing disruptive behaviors of children with autism: three case studies. J Autism Dev Disord 2008;38(9):1689-96.

Pilebro C, Backman B. Teaching oral hygiene to children with autism. Int J Paediatr Dent 2005;15(1):1-9.

Rada RE. Treatment needs and adverse events related to dental treatment under general anesthesia for individuals with autism. Intellect Dev Disabil 2013;51(4):246-52.

Rayner CS. Video-modelling to improve task completion in a child with autism. Dev Neurorehabil 2010;13(3):225-30.

Selzer RR, Rosenblatt DS, Laxova R et al. Adverse effect of nitrous oxide in a child with 5,10-methylenetetrahydrofolate reductase deficiency. N Engl J Med 2003;349(1):45-50.

Nunes Da Silva S, Gimenez T, Souza RC et al. Oral health status of children and young adults with autism spectrum disorders: systematic review and meta-analysis. Int J Paediatr Dent 2016.

Vozza I, Cavallè E, Corridore D et al. Preventive strategies in oral health for special needs patients. Annali di Stomatologia 2015;VI(3-4):96-9.

Wilson K. Teaching social-communication skills to preschoolers with autism: efficacy of video versus in vivo modeling in the classroom. J Autism Dev Disord 2013;43(8):1819-31.

Ectodermal dysplasia

G. Ierardo, V. Luzzi

Definition and classification

The term ectodermal dysplasia (ED) includes a vast and complex group of pathologies characterized by an abnormal development of tissues and organs with ectodermal origin and their appendices, in particular teeth, hair, nails, and sweat glands. EDs are congenital, diffuse, and nonprogressive forms.

Ectoderm is one of the three germinative layers formed during the gastrulation during the third week of intrauterine life together with endoderm and mesoderm. They give rise to all the primordial tissues and organs: skin, nails, hair, dental enamel, sweat glands, sebaceous glands, central nervous system, peripheral and autonomous, sensory epithelium of eye, ear, and nose, mammary gland, epiphysis, pituitary, and medullary gland of the adrenal gland.

Changes do not always involve ectoderm only: mesodermal structures may also be affected and more rarely endodermal structures too. This is because the physiological maturation of the ectodermic structures of the tegument is fundamental for the determination and development of the underlying mesenchymal structures.

Among the almost 200 forms of ED, with extremely variable manifestations and with wide overlap in the clinical presentation, only for 30 of them the gene responsible for the pathology has been precisely identified. The most common forms are X-linked recessive hypohydrotic ED (Christ–Simens–Touraine syndrome) and hydrotic ED (Clouston syndrome).

There are currently four different classifications:

- Clinic classification
- Molecular–biochemical classification
- Molecular–genetic classification
- Biological classification.

The first classification of ED dates back to the scientific activity of Freire-Maia and Pinheiro in 1984 and 1994; they used as classification criteria the clinical aspects of the pathology, thus obtaining cases of the group A and cases of the group B. The first includes all the EDs in which defects in at least two of the classical ectodermic structures (hair, teeth, nails, and sweat glands) are present; the second includes all the cases where there are defects in a single classical structure, plus another ectodermal defect (abnormality of ears and lips, dermatoglyphics on the palm of the hand or the sole of the foot). Clinically, there may be two large families of ED: the hypohidrotic (anhidrotic) and the hydrotic type, related to the degree of impairment of the glandular system (sweat glands and salivary glands). EDs generally have an incidence of 7:10000 internationally; instead, hypohydrous or anhydrous ectodermal dysplasia, the most frequent type of ED, has an incidence of 1:100000.

According to a study of Freire-Maia and Pinheiro published in 1994, among 154 types of ED, three possible forms of inheritance were identified: dominant autosomal (41 cases), recessive autosomal (52 cases), and X-linked (8 cases) inheritance; the related cause for the remaining 53 cases was unknown. As to anhydrous ectodermal dysplasia (EDA), it was observed that the most frequent form is that linked to alterations of the gene EDA1 localized on the X chromosome (Xq12- q13), which codes for ectodysplasin A, a membrane protein expressed in keratinocytes, hair follicles, and sweat glands, involved in the cell–cell or cell–matrix interactions.

Clinical manifestations

The following clinical manifestations are found in the Clouston syndrome form:

- alopecia
- nail dystrophy
- palmar and plantar hyperkeratosis
- mental deficit (occasionally)
- atrophic rhinitis
- atopic dermatitis
- noncharacteristic facies.

The following clinical manifestations are found in the hypo-anhydrous form:

- hypo-anhidrosis
- hypotrichosis
- thin, wrinkled, pale skin (ichthyosiform appearance) (Fig. 22.10)
- flattening of epidermal ridges at palm-plantar level
- blonde and hypopigmented hair as viewed using optical microscopy,
- nail alterations
- typical facies.

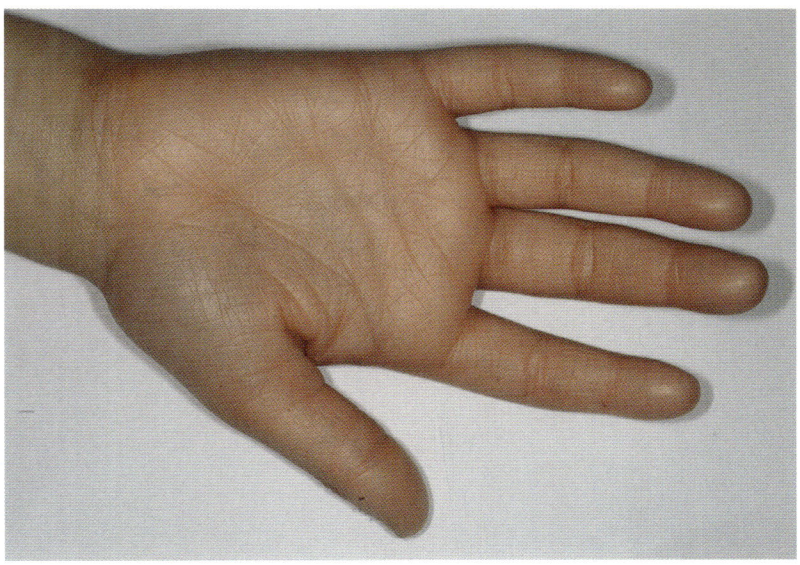

Figure 22.10
Apperance of skin.

The absence or deficiency of the eccrine sweat glands causes frequent hyperthermia with a strong intolerance to heat. Hyperpyrexia, typical of the summer season, can occur in childhood.

These patients exhibit the following characteristic *facies*:
- Old look
- Crowned, prominent, and squared forehead
- Protruding eyebrow arches
- Wrinkles and pigmentations in the periocular zone
- Small nose with hypoplastic wings and enlarged root (saddle nose)
- Small chin
- Acute nose-labial angle.

Protruding lips.
1/3 middle facial retraction (caused by hypoplasia of the jaw). Large ears with low structure.

As for the odontostomatological aspects, patients with ED show anomalies of the dental elements in terms of number, shape, and structure, which can already be found in the deciduous dentition (Fig. 22.11).
The number abnormalities involve rounded down teeth numbers and include cases of hypodontia (congenital absence of one or more dental elements) or anodontia (total absence of teeth). Due to the lack of numerous dental elements, especially the deciduous teeth, alveolar processes may show growth abnormalities in the edentulous sites due to the loss of functional matrixes caused by tooth eruption mechanisms.
Hypodontia and anodontia not only cause crestal atrophy but also hypoplasia of both jaws (Fig. 22.12).

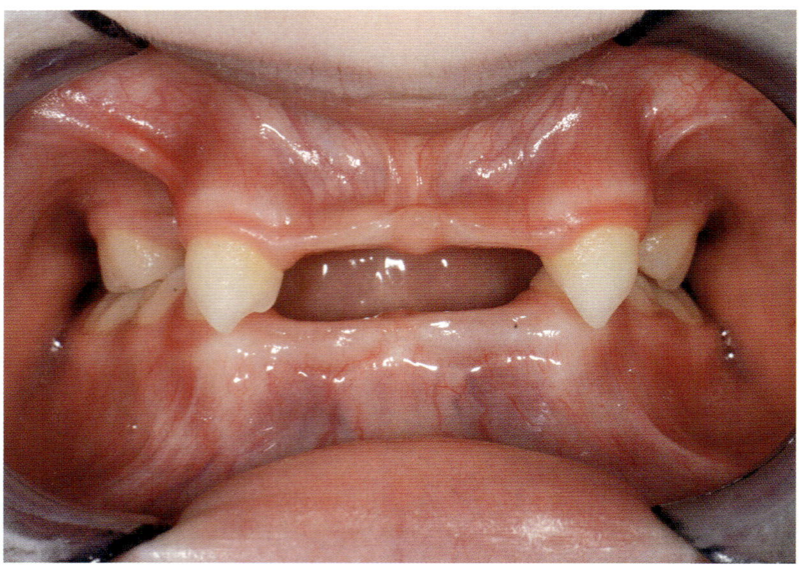

Figure 22.11 Typical arch with multiple agenesis.

This alveolar and maxillary growth deficit, combined with the reduction in occlusal vertical height, causes a reduction in the patient's facial height. Among the anomalies of shape, the presence of conical teeth is typical. More frequently, the upper central incisors and the upper and lower canines have a conoid shape. Some teeth may have taurodontism (tooth with pulpar chamber wider than normal, short roots, and elongated root canals).

Diagnosis and therapy

The diagnosis of ED involves a multidisciplinary approach that involves many professionals such as pediatricians, dermatologists, otorhinolaryngologists, ophthalmologists, and dentists, and generally occurs during childhood.
The diagnosis of ED is achieved from an accurate medical history combined with clinical examination and specific instrumental tests.
The aid tests that can lead to the diagnosis are as follows:

- Hypohidrosis test
- Saliva test
- Hair test
- Radiographic test
- Molecular test

The therapeutic approach should be early and multidisciplinary with relevance given to the pediatric dentist.
Therapies should be planned according to the severity of the case and age group of the patient.
They can range from preventive interventions to the implant prosthetic rehabilitative ones (Fig. 22.13).

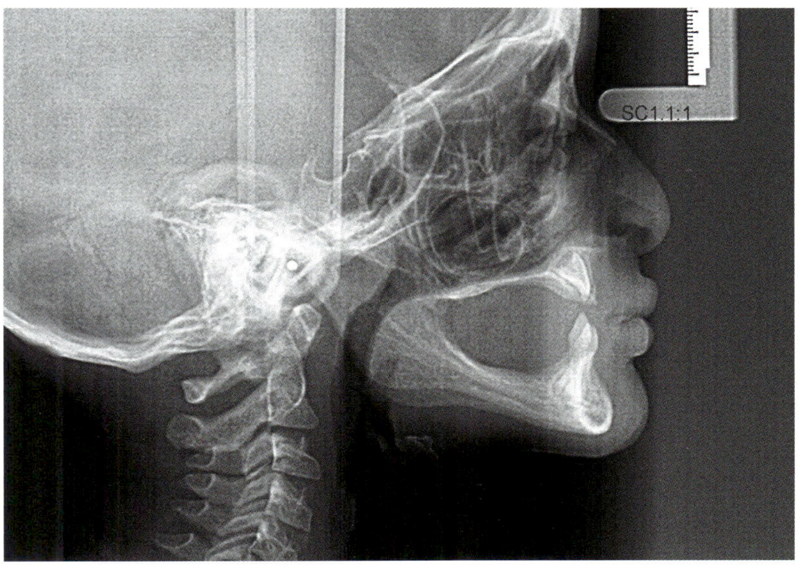

Figure 22.12 Teleradiograph in a patient with severe ED.

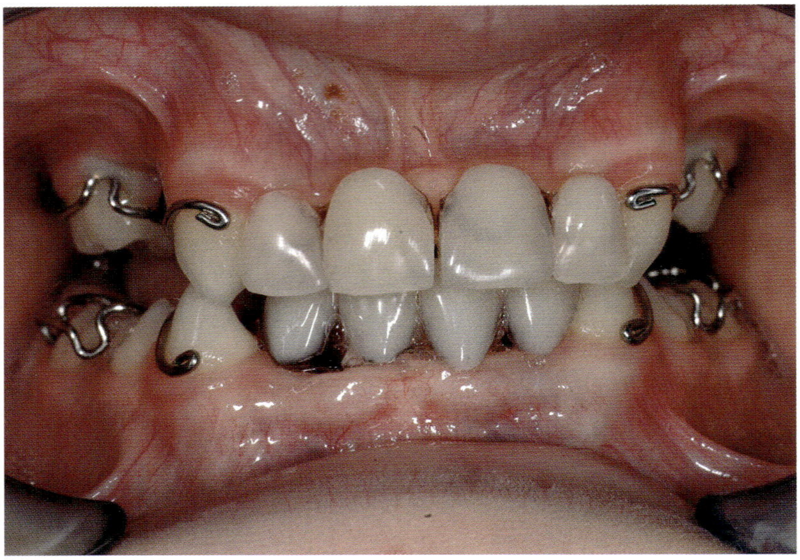

Figure 22.13 Upper plate with dental elements.

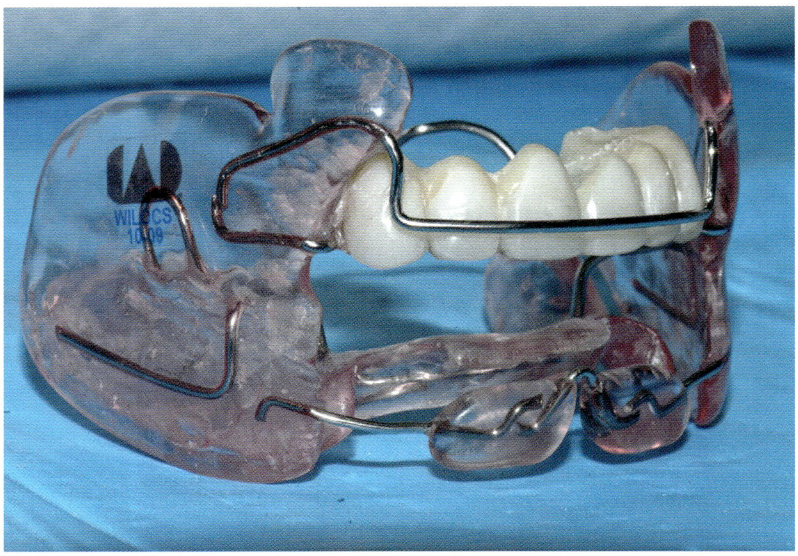

Figure 22.14 Frankl device with dental elements.

First of all, it is necessary to prevent the loss of dental elements due to carious processes, with preventive interventions such as fluoride prophylaxis with fluorine gel for topical use, careful oral hygiene, and proper nutrition.

Children with ED are very sensitive to carious lesions for both the xerostomy present in most cases and for structural abnormalities, which are typical of tooth enamel, such as hypoplasia, hypocalcification, or immaturity.

Already in the first years of life, removable prostheses can be created to allow the phonatory, chewing, and esthetic function of the stomatognathic apparatus and to begin to lead the facial growth (Fig. 22.14).

These devices should be managed by providing replacements every 2-3 years to adapt to the patient's growth.
With growth, the following orthodontic problems should be managed:
1. Reduced vertical growth of the lower facial height
2. Reduced sagittal and transverse development of the upper jaw
3. Superior anterior rotation of the jaw
4. Labial protrusion
5. Vertical hypodevelopment of cellular processes.

The aim of orthodontic treatment are as follows:
- Optimum space management
- *Up-righting* and alignment of some teeth
- Correction and control of *overbite*
- Control of maxillomandibular relationships on the sagittal plane
- Occlusal stability.

The choice of orthodontic equipment should consider dental and skeletal diagnosis, the presence of anchor teeth, and the age of the patient.
Therapies may include orthopedic phases such as the use of rapid expanders and facial masks, functional phases such as the use of elastodontic or Frankel appliance and orthodontic appliances during pre prosthetic correction.
In some cases of anchorage deficiency, the use of orthodontic mini-implants could be evaluated (Fig. 22.15).
The appliances can often be accompanied by dental elements, in order to obtain a good esthetics during the orthodontic phases.

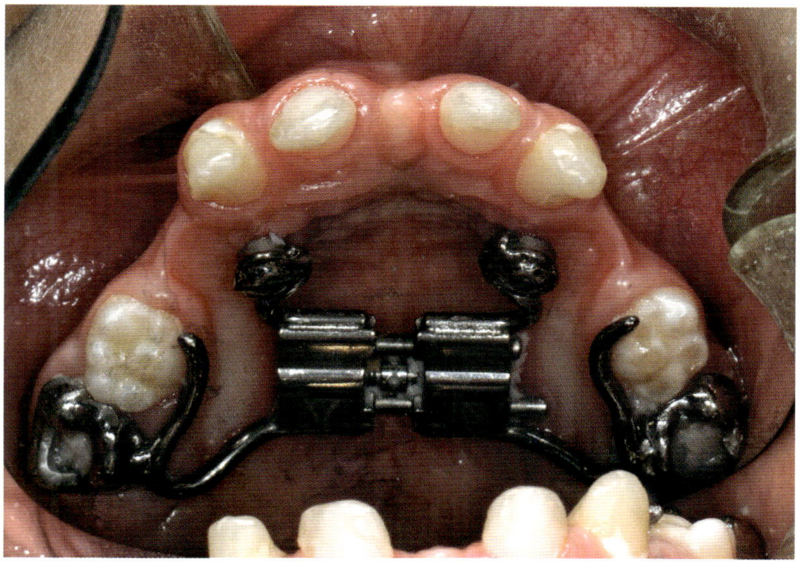

Figure 22.15 REP on orthodontic mini-implants.

References

Bondarets N, Jones RM, McDonald F. Analysis of facial growth in subjects with syndromic ectodermal dysplasia: a longitudinal analysis. Orthod Craniofac Res 2002;5(2):71-84.

Boujtat K, Rouf S, Boutahar I, Skiker I, Tajir M et al. Ellis-Van Creveld syndrome and Dandy-Walker malformation: an uncommon association. Pediatr Endocrinol Rev 2018;16(2):275-83.

Celli D, Manente A, Grippaudo C, Cordaro M. Interceptive treatment in ectodermal dysplasia using an innovative orthodontic/prosthetic modular appliance. A case report with 10-year follow-up. Eur J Paediatr Dent 2018;19(4):307-12.

De Santis D, Sinigaglia S, Faccioni P, Pancera P, Luciano U et al. Syndromes associated with dental agenesis. Minerva Stomatol 2019;68(1):42-56.

Freire-Maia N, Lisboa-Costa T, Pagnan NA. Ectodermal dysplasias: how many? Am J Med Genet 2001;104(1):84.

Guckes AD, Roberts MW, McCarthy GR. Pattern of permanent teeth present in individuals with ectodermal dysplasia and severe hypodontia suggests treatment with dental implants. Pediatr Dent 1998; 20:278-80

Hsieh YL, Razzoog M, Garcia Hammaker S. Oral care program for successful long-term full mouth habilitation of patients with hypohidrotic ectodermal dysplasia. Case Rep Dent 2018;2018:4736495.

Ioannidou-Marathiotou I, Kotsiomiti E, Gioka C. The contribution of orthodontics to the prosthodontic treatment of ectodermal dysplasia: a long-term clinical report. J Am Dent Assoc 2010;141(11):1340-5.

Itin PH, Fistarol SK. Ectodermal dysplasias. Am J Med Genet C Semin Med Genet 2004;131C(1):45-51.

Itin PH. Etiology and pathogenesis of ectodermal dysplasias. Am J Med Genet A 2014;164A(10):2472-7.

Kearns G, Sharma A, Perrott D, Schmidt B, Kaban L et al. Placement of endosseous implants in children and adolescents with hereditary ectodermal dysplasia. Oral Surg Oral Med Oral Pathol Oral Radiol Endod. 1999;88(1):5-10.

Mehrtens SH, Shankar S. A case of focal facial dermal dysplasia type 4. Pediatr Dermatol 2019;36(1):e58-e59.

Nordgarden H, Storhaug K, Lyngstadaas SP, Jensen JL. Salivary gland function in persons with ectodermal dyslasias. Eur J Oral Sci 2003;111(5):371-6.

Omondi BI, Chepkwony F, Ariemba RM, Miyogo JO, Opinya GN. Prosthodontic rehabilitation of a child with ectodermal dysplasia: a preliminary report. Int J Prosthodont 2019;32(1):107-9.

Polimeni A, Perfetti G, Ghirlanda Pippi R. Displasia ectodermica. Considerazioni su di un raro caso. Annali di stomatologia 1989;38(4).

Priolo M. Ectodermal dysplasias: an overview and update of clinical and molecular-functional mechanisms. Am J Med Genet A 2009;149A(9):2003-13.

Suri S, Carmichael RP, Tompson BD. Simultaneous functional and fixed therapy for growth modification and dental alignment prior to prosthetic habilitation in hypohidrotic ectodermal dysplasia: a clinical report. J Prosthet Dent 2004; 92: 428-33.

Wright JT, Fete M, Schneider H, Zinser M, Koster MI et al. Ectodermal dysplasias: classification and organization by phenotype, genotype and molecular pathway. Am J Med Genet A 2019;179(3):442-7.

Yenisey M, Guler A, Unal U. Orthodontic and prosthodontic treatment of ectodermal dysplasia: a case report. Br Dent J 2004;196(11):677-9.

Zhang XJ, Chen JJ, Yang S, Cui Y, Xiong XY et al. A mutation in the connexin 30 gene in Chinese Han patients with hidrotic ectodermal dysplasia. J Dermatol Sci 2003;32:11-7.

Osteogenesis imperfecta

G. Ierardo, M. Celli

Definition, epidemiology, and classification

Osteogenesis imperfecta (OI), also called "glass bone disease," is a heterogeneous group of connective tissue disorders involved in the appearance of numerous fractures, which, in the most serious cases, can also compromise the survival of the affected individual.

The pathology has an estimated incidence of about one case in 20,000–50,000 births; this number is often underestimated because less serious cases are often misdiagnosed and/or diagnosed later. The male:female ratio is 1:1, with both dominant and recessive transmission. Numerous studies have highlighted a correlation between OI and *COLIA1* and *COLIA2* (located on chromosomes 7 and 17) related to the production of type 1 collagen.

The OI classification still in use today is that drawn up by Sillence in 1979, which is based on the clinical features and severity of the disease, but in recent years the advancements of medical genetics have widened this classification: at present, 15 types are distinguished, although this number is estimated to increase as not all the genes responsible for the disease have been identified.

Type I OI is the mildest and the easiest to detect; it has a dominant autosomal transmission and the diagnosis is difficult in mild cases, even if other cases are present in the family.

Because this protein is one of the major components not only of bones but also of other noncalcified tissues, this disease can involve different body structures and need, therefore, a multidisciplinary approach.

Clinical manifestations

The extra-skeletal manifestations of OI are represented by the presence of blue sclera and dentinogenesis imperfecta, hearing loss, and ligamentous laxity. The dentist plays an important role in the diagnosis of the disease: as collagen is the major component of the tissues of the dental elements, a genetic anomaly in the production of this protein will lead to an altered production and mineralization of dentin.

Dentinogenesis imperfecta is the most common dental alteration and is manifested in 5%–15% of cases, more frequently in type III and IV and rarely in type I OI.

The involved teeth have a bulbar crown and an increased coronal angle and can also able to be without pulp cavities (Fig. 22.16-22.17). Permanent teeth are less affected than deciduous ones. The electronic microscopy of the dentin shows a disorganization of the tubules that prevents the adhesion of the enamel to the dentin and leads to the rapid abrasion of the teeth (Fig. 22.18).

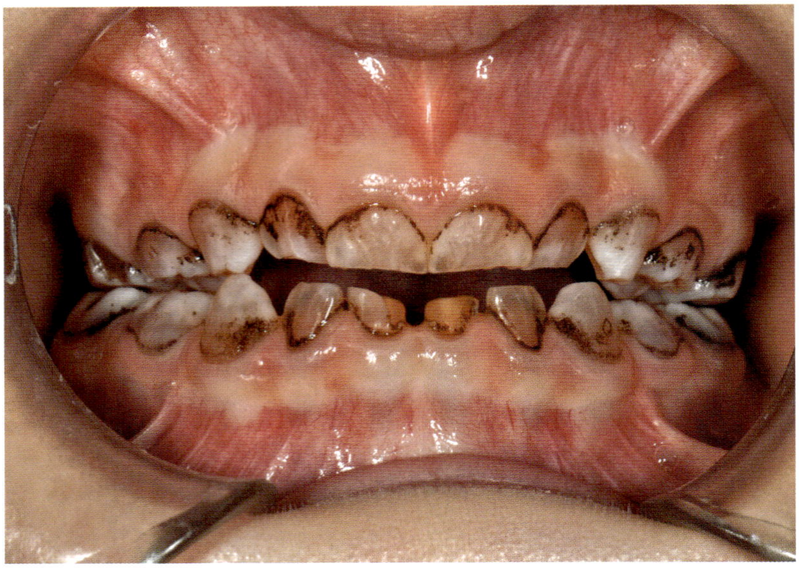

Figure 22.16 Dentinogenesis imperfecta in a patient with OI.

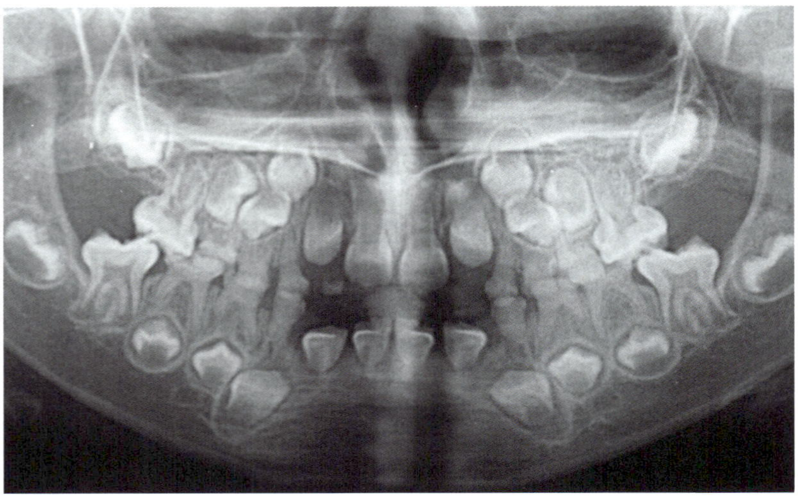

Figure 22.17 Radicular abnormalities in patients with dentinogenesis imperfecta.

Dental eruption may be delayed or early and does not appear to be related to the type of OI.

In addition to dentinogenesis imperfecta, further dental implications include high incidence of skeletal class III malocclusion with anterior and/or posterior crossbite and posterior open-bite, as well as craniofacial deformities (in many cases, there is evidence of a triangle-shaped face, protrusion of both temporal bones, and prominence of frontal bone) (Fig. 22.19).

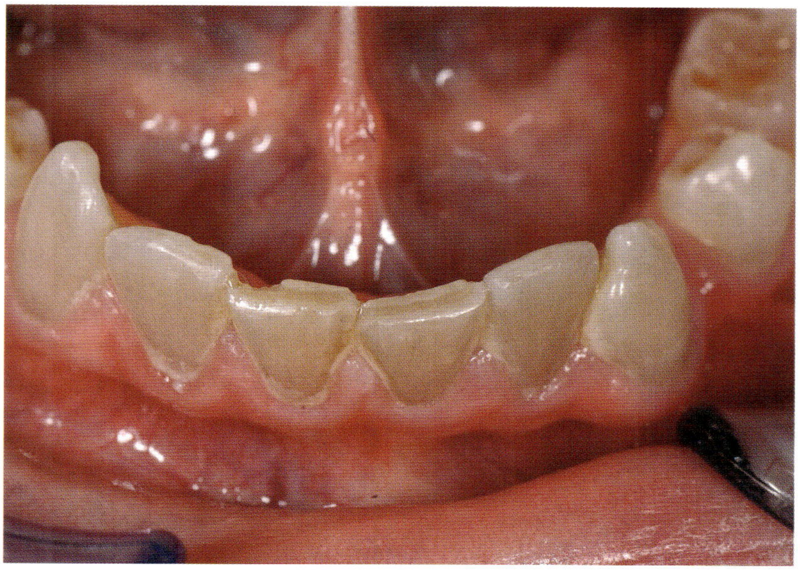

Figure 22.18 Typical wear in dentinogenesis imperfecta.

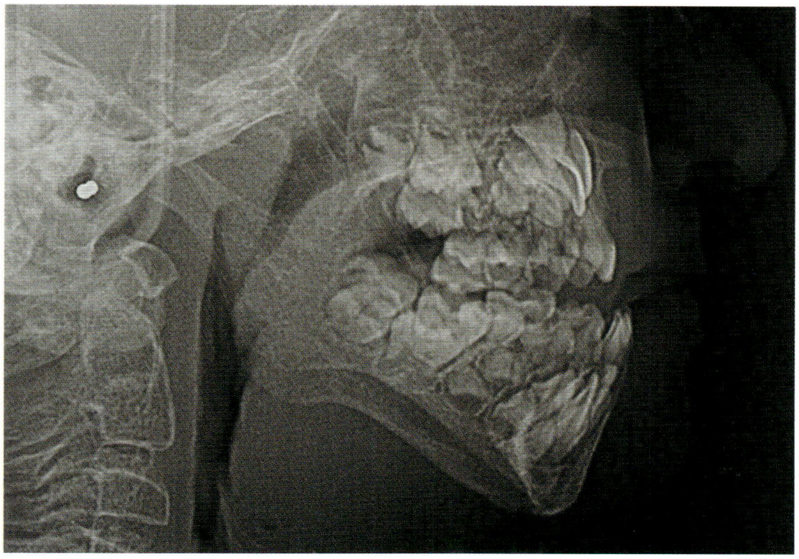

Figure 22.19 Class III skeletal growth in a patient with OI.

Diagnosis and therapy

The diagnosis of OI is sometimes difficult, both for the wide phenotypic variability and for the increasing number of recessive forms discovered, with clinical aspects less characteristic than the first four forms. The diagnosis can be made in the presence of positive genetic or biochemical tests or, if they are not possible or negative, through clinical and radiological examinations. Some of the most common manifestations are bone fragility with fractures for even trivial traumas or traumatic fractures of unexplained nature, marked and progressive deformity of bones, radiological evidence of

osteoporosis, evidence of bone mineral density reduced by age, blue discoloration of sclera, and dentition changes. Genetic tests make it possible to diagnose the specific form of OI and direct prenatal diagnosis in cases of mutation in one of the first degree family members, although in some cases these mutations are *new*.
Genetic analysis can be used to diagnose all forms of OI for which the molecular defect is known.
These patients generally follow therapies that are customized and differentiated on the basis of age and severity:

1. Medical therapy, by the use of drugs that increase bone resistance and reduce the number of fractures (bisphosphonates)
2. Orthopedic surgical treatment
3. Nonsurgical treatment (physical therapy, rehabilitation, and use of corsets and supports).

To date, there is no cure for this disease, and the use of bisphosphonates (BFs) is the only symptomatic treatment for patients with OI, especially in pediatric age.
These drugs are able to significantly increase bone mineral density, halve the number of fractures, and reduce pain.
BFs are also inhibitors of osteoclast-mediated bone resorption and cause bone remodeling, which is necessary for dental movement, to occur more slowly in patients taking these medicines.
BFs have been studied extensively in recent years, due to the presence in literature of numerous cases of osteonecrosis affecting the jaws in adult patients. To date, however, there is no documented case of this problem in pediatric age.
In pediatric dentistry, the orthodontic approach of patients with OI is not a routine approach, as demonstrated by the limited availability of reports in this field.
The studies conducted so far review a treatment that is both surgical and orthodontic, showing in the majority of patients a malocclusion that requires the repositioning of the skeletal bases, preceded and followed by a supportive orthodontic treatment (Fig. 22.20).
An interceptive orthodontic approach can certainly be a valid example for orthodontists who have to intervene in a growing patient with skeletal and/or dental–skeletal problems, without having to procrastinate the resolution of the case to a future orthodontic treatment, which, as amply demonstrated, is however extremely difficult to perform.
Orthopedic therapies (rapid expander and facial mask) and functional therapies (activators and elastodontic appliances) are very important in such patients to reduce the severity of malocclusion and eliminate or limit the use of fixed *multibracket* appliances.
Orthopedic therapy may require temporary withdrawal of the drug, but this decision must always be agreed with the referring pediatrician.
Most of the cases in which fixed orthodontic *multibrackets* treatment has been implemented have not shown positive results, being certainly conditioned to a therapy, such as that with bisphosphonate, which, because of the same underlying mechanism, is in itself a limiting factor. Therefore, treating a skeletal malocclusion, even if of a mild

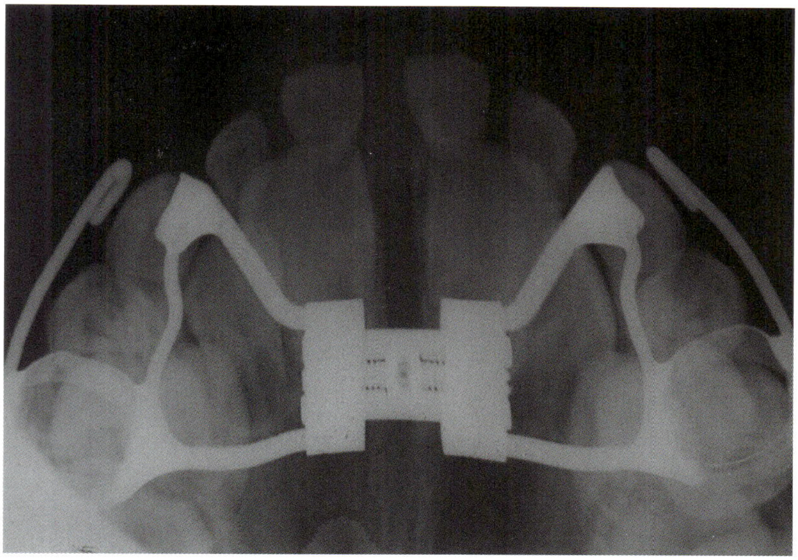

Figure 22.20 REP applied to a patient with OI: opening of the median palatine suture.

type, with a dental camouflage cannot be considered the key to success in a patient who takes bisphosphonates.

The prevention of caries and their infectious and orthodontic complications is very important. All specific preventive measures must be implemented from the early years of life.

Surgical therapies in children, from the simplest to the most invasive ones such as germectomy, can be planned in such patients.

It is always important to implement adequate antibiotic measures and to agree with the pediatrician the best time for such interventions based on the radiological and laboratory analysis.

Moreover, the main problem that the clinician must take into consideration is often not the type of treatment but rather the need to know when intervention is required. Thus, the collaboration with pediatricians and other specialists is essential.

References

Burgeson R, Nimni M. Collagen types. Molecular structure and tissue distribution. Clin Orthop1992;282:250-72.

Engelbert RH, Pruijs HE, Beemer FA, Helders PJ. Osteogenesis imperfect in childhood: treatment strategies. Arch Phy Med Rehab 1998;79:1590-94.

Flanagan AM, Chambers TJ. Inhibition of bone resorption by bisphosphonates: interaction between bisphosphonates, osteoclasts, and bone. Calcif Tissue Int 1991;49:407-15.

Freedus MS, Schaaf NG, Ziter WD. Orthognatic surgery in osteogenesis imperfect. J oral Surg 1976;34:830-4.

Ierardo G, Bossù M, D'Angeli G, Celli M, Sfasciotti GL. Bisphosphonates therapy in children with osteogenesis imperfecta: clinical experience in oral surgery. Oral Implantol 2017;10(3):311-6.

Ierardo G, Calcagnile F, Luzzi V, Ladniak B, Bossu M, Polimeni A. Osteogenesis imperfecta and rapid maxillary expansion: Report of 3 patients. Am J Orthod Dentofacial Orthop 2015;148(1):130-7.

Ierardo G, Luzzi V, Vestri A, Sfasciotti GL, Polimeni A. Evaluation of custom satisfaction at the department of Paediatric dentistry of Sapienza University of Rome. Eur J Paediatr Dent 2008;1.

Igarashi K, Mitani H, Adachi H, Shinoda H. Anchorage and retentive effects of a bisphosphonate (AHBuBP) on tooth movements in rats. Am J Orthod 1994; 106:279-289.

Kuivaniemi H, Tromp G, Prockop DJ. Mutations in fibrillar collagens (types I, II, III, and XI), fibril-associated collagen (type IX), and network-forming collagen (type X) cause a spectrum of diseases of bone, cartilage, and blood vessels. Hum Mutat. 1997;9(4):300-15.

Libman RH. Anesthetic considerations for the patients with osteogenesis imperfecta. Clin Orthop Related Res 1981;159:123-5.

Ma MS, Najirad M, Taqi D, Retrouvey JM, Tamimi F et al. Caries prevalence and experience in individuals with osteogenesis imperfecta: A cross-sectional multicenter study. Spec Care Dentist. 2019. doi: 10.1111/scd.12368.

McKusich V, Scott CI, A nomenclature for constitutional disorders of bone, J Bone Joint Surg Am 1971;53:978-86.

McKusich V. Hereditary disorders of connective tissue. Bull NY Acad Med 1959;35(5):143-56.

O'connell AC, Marini JC. Evaluation of oral problems in an osteogenesis imperfecta population. Oral Pathol Oral Radiol Endod 1999;87:189-96.

Petersen K, Wetzel WE.Recent findings in classification of osteogenesis imperfecta by means of existing dental symptoms. ASDC J Dent Child 1998;65:305-9.

Prockop D, Osteogenesis imperfecta: phenotypic heterogeneity, protein suicide, short and long collagen, Am J Hum Genet 1984;36:499-505.

Prockop DJ, Kivirikko KI. Collagens: molecular biology, diseases, and potentials for therapy. Annu Rev Biochem 1995;64:403-34.

Rinchuse DJ, Sosovicka MF, Robison JM, Pendleton R. Orthodontic treatment of patients using bisphosphonates: a report of 2 cases. Am J Orthod Dentofacial Orthop 2007;131:321-6.

Rogers MJ, Frith JC, Luckman SP, Coxon FP, Benford HL, et al. Molecular mechanism of action of bisphosphonates. Bone 1999;24:S73-S79.

Chapter 23

Emergencies and urgencies in pediatric dentistry

G. Piana, S. Pizzi, R. Botto

Access to the dental emergency department or urgent dental examination is required when a child needs immediate intervention because of an accident or signs and symptoms affecting the oral cavity.

Medical history

Pain is the reason that most often leads a child to seek emergency dental treatment. Everything concerning childcare must be aimed at preventing, avoiding, and alleviating pain and must consider the concomitant emotional and psychological aspects of illness and trauma. The elimination of pain, therefore, must be a priority for all health professionals (Pinto et al, 2008).

Pain usually indicates the presence of tissue damage, and its intensity is not necessarily proportional to the extent of the damage; occasionally, pain may occur in the absence of organic damage. In the presence of tissue damage, the pain, originating at the level of the peripheral nervous system caused by the stimulation of receptors, is processed at the level of the central nervous system (CNS). For this reason, the perception of pain is influenced by emotional, cultural, and cognitive factors (for example, attention and distraction) and past painful experiences. Pain is a subjective symptom; therefore, it cannot be visually assessed and must be investigated through medical history. To accurately frame the clinical picture of a cooperating patient with good language skills, it is necessary to ask the following questions: "what adjectives would you use to explain your pain (sharp, dull, or pulsating)?"; "where is it stronger?"; "where does it start?"; "how strong is it?"; "does it allow you to sleep or does it wake you up?"; "when did it start?"; "is it continuous or intermittent?"; "if it is intermittent, how long does it last each time?"; "is there a trigger that makes it start?"; "is there something that makes it better?"; "is there something that makes it worse?"; "are there any other problems?".

Medical history provides numerous indications that help develop a correct diagnosis, which is a prerequisite for implementing the most appropriate treatment plan. The collection of information can be extremely difficult during the initial years of a child's life because of the incomplete level of maturity and the scarcity of linguistic background; the interlocutors (parents and guardians) can answer questions only partially.

Features. Pain described as *acute* is often associated with exposed dentin (due to caries, traumatic fracture, or fractured filling), reversible pulpitis, irreversible pulpitis, or trigeminal neuralgia (rare in the developmental age). Pain described as *dull-pulsating* is often associated with endodontic apical abscess, periodontal abscess (rare in the developmental age), necrotizing ulcerative gingivitis, postextraction alveolitis, herpes zoster, sinusitis, and temporomandibular joint pathologies.

Intensity. Regarding medical history data, pain is described as *not intense* if the patient has not used analgesics and as *intense* if it prevents the child from sleeping and/or eating. The intensity of pain can be assessed using Scott, Ansell, and Huskisson's visual analog scale. The scale of facial expressions can also be used in the most known variants such as Wong and Baker's scale and Bieri's scale.

Location. Pain localization is often difficult; pulpal pain may be irradiated (dento-dental, dento-mucosal, and dento-cutaneous synalgia) but is always within the same hemisoma; sinusitis can cause pain in multiple teeth in the upper arch.

Duration. Short-term pain that recedes after the removal of the triggering stimulus (cold, sugars, etc.) is a symptom of reversible pulpitis; a lasting spontaneous pain is a symptom of irreversible pulpitis or abscess.

Exacerbating factors. Pain triggered by thermal (cold and hot) or osmotic (sugar and acids) stimuli is usually of pulp origin, whereas that felt during chewing or percussion is of periodontal origin.

Physical examination and diagnosis

After obtaining the medical history, it is necessary to proceed with the physical examination to identify the tooth responsible for the symptoms. Physicians should focus on carious lesions; previous extensive fillings and/or fillings with marginal infiltration, changes in tooth color, and swelling and/or fistulae.

In children, thermal and electrical pulp sensitivity tests are not very reliable, particularly for deciduous teeth with reabsorbed apex and permanent teeth with incompletely formed apex. The cold thermal test can be used for differential diagnosis between reversible (pain recedes as soon as stimulus is removed) and irreversible (pain lasts even after stimulus removal) pulpitis (Gopikrishna et al, 2009). Intraoral radiographic examinations show carious lesions and periapical pathologies with extensive bone resorption and also evaluate the level of resorption of the deciduous teeth, determining the treatment plan.

Most frequently, pain in the oral cavity is of dental origin (Tab. 23.1) (Milsom et al, 2002; Lewis and Stout, 2010). A study on 1166 children (age range: 0–14 years) reported the causes that most frequently bring a child to the dentist for an emergency visit: 62% for pain caused by carious lesions, 18% for dental trauma, and 14% for eruption problems (Sakai et al, 2005).

Pain of pulpal origin

Pulpitis

In a carious tooth, which is initially asymptomatic, pain occurs when an inflammatory process develops in the pulp. In the initial phase of *reversible pulpitis*, pain is caused by certain stimuli (cold, hot, sweet, etc.) and resolves spontaneously after a few seconds. The treatment involves removal of the decayed tissue and restoration of the tooth.

If the carious lesion causing reversible pulpitis is not treated, the pulpitis becomes *irreversible*. Pain becomes intense, spontaneous, and long-lasting, and is not resolved

Table 23.1 Pulpar emergencies

Diagnosis	Definition	Symptoms	Complications	Therapy
Reversible pulpitis	Reversible pulp inflammation	Pain as a result of thermal (cold and warm) and osmotic (sugars and acids) stimuli	Irreversible pulpitis Periapical abscess, phlegmon	Conservative
Irreversible pulpitis	Irreversible pulp inflammation	Intense, spontaneous, persistent, vaguely localized pain	Acute apical periodontitis, periapical abscess, phlegmon	Endodontic or extraction
Apical acute periodontitis	Bacterial infection limited to the periapical area	Severe, spontaneous, persistent, localized pain	Acute apical periodontitis, periapical abscess, phlegmon	Pharmacological pain therapy, endodontic therapy, or extraction
Abscess	Bacterial infection limited to periapical tissues	Localized pain and swelling	Phlegmon	Antibiotic treatment, drainage, and incision, followed by endodontic therapy or extraction
Phlegmon	Widespread soft tissue bacterial infection	Widespread pain, erythema, and swelling	Systemic complications	Antibiotic treatment, followed by endodontic therapy or extraction

in a few seconds if triggered by a stimulus and can radiate to other regions. Urgent treatment comprises pulpotomy or tooth extraction (when endodontic therapy is contraindicated during the transition period from deciduous to permanent dentition). The urgency of dental treatment is determined by the patient's pain; in case of deferred treatment, pharmacological therapy according to pain intensity is indicated:

- **mild pain**: paracetamol 10–15 mg/kg oral administration (rectal 20 mg) per dose, repeatable every 4–6 hours (maximum dosage 80 mg/kg/day); 1–5 years, 120–250 mg; 6–12 years, 250–500 mg
- **medium pain**: ibuprofen 5–10 mg/kg every 8 hours (maximum dosage 40 mg/kg/day) or 1–2 years, 50 mg; 3–7 years, 100 mg; 8–12 years, 200 mg 3–4 times/day; max, 2.4 g/day
- **intense pain**: codeine or codeine and paracetamol.

Periodontitis

The passage of bacteria and toxins from the pulp and the site of irreversible inflammation and/or necrosis causes *acute apical periodontitis*. The pain is intense, spontaneous, and persistent, but unlike that of irreversible pulpitis, it is localized in the concerned tooth. The tooth is sensitive to percussion. Regional lymphadenopathy may be present. Pharmacological pain therapy with paracetamol or ibuprofen is indicated as emergency treatment. The ultimate treatment is endodontic therapy or extraction.

Apical abscess

Apical abscess is a localized and purulent form of apical periodontitis. Clinically, it manifests as a fluctuating buccal or palatal swelling with or without fistula. Often regional lymphadenopathy is present. If the pus is draining, pain is usually not intense. The urgent treatment to facilitate drainage of the abscess—when the patient's level of cooperation permits—is the opening of the pulp chamber and instrumentation beyond the apex of approximately 1 mm with respect to the working length assessed on preoperative radiography. If drainage is achieved, this should be facilitated using high suction speed and possibly a gentle compression of the mucosa at the site of swelling. After the completion of exudate leakage, the opening created in the tooth is plugged after positioning cotton pellets at the pulp chamber level with temporary filling. A mucosal incision using a scalpel is reserved for cases of swelling with a declivous floating zone. Antibiotic therapy with penicillin or macrolides (in case of penicillin allergy) is always recommended and is indispensable when drainage is not possible. In case of pain, paracetamol or ibuprofen therapy is indicated. The final treatment is endodontic therapy or extraction.

Phlegmon

Phlegmon represents an abscess complication and is caused by the spread of septic inflammation in the surrounding tissues of a site of diffuse, tense, and painful swelling (Fig. 23.1). Regional lymphadenopathy is frequent and fever may be present.

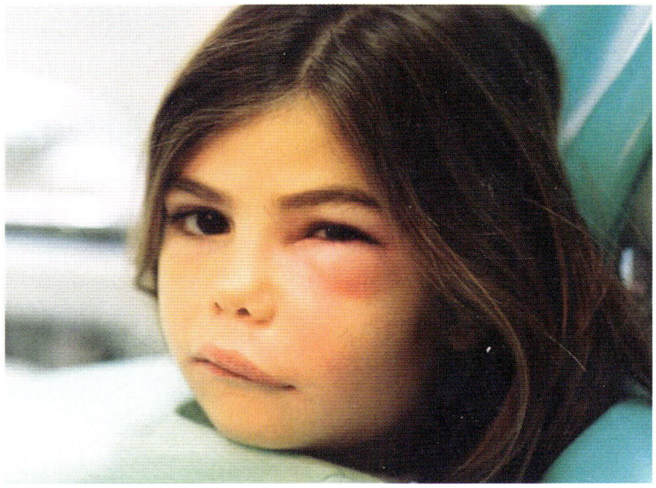

Figure 23.1 Phlegmon.

Antibiotic therapy must be initiated, and the patient must be monitored every 1–2 days; if the clinical picture does not improve, it is necessary to consult a maxillofacial surgeon. Systemic effects of infection are most pronounced in young children, such as a rapid rise in temperature, increased risk of dehydration, and rapid spread of infection. Infection can spread into the fascial head and neck spaces with the consequent risk of impaired airways; in the maxilla, infection can also spread in the periorbital area, leading to the risk of serious complications such as loss of vision, cavernous sinus thrombosis, and involvement of CNS. Phlegmon cases of dental origin in which the patient has direct access to a pediatric emergency department and in which hospitalization for intravenous antibiotic therapy is necessary are frequent (Thikkurissy et al, 2010). The ultimate therapy is endodontic therapy or extraction. It should be noted that in all cases with swelling, the extraction should be deferred until resolution of the swelling, both due to the reduced effectiveness of local anesthetic for pain control and increased risk of bacteremia. In this regard, in all patients at risk of bacterial endocarditis (for example, patients with congenital heart disease) with swelling, antibiotic therapy should be initiated immediately as a prophylaxis of endocarditis.

Dental injuries of traumatic origin

When urgency is the consequence of a dentofacial trauma, a careful and scrupulous examination of the child is necessary to develop a correct and complete diagnosis of soft and hard tissue injuries, followed by intervention with the most appropriate therapy (Andreasen and Andreasen, 1985; Bakland and Andreasen, 1996; Andreasen et al, 2007) (see Chapter 9). Therefore, it is necessary to perform the following:

- *cleanse the face and oral cavity with water or a physiological solution*. If soft tissue wounds are present, a mild detergent may be used. This cleaning will provide comfort to the patient and will facilitate extra- and intraoral examination

- *collect a short medical and dental history*. Medical history may reveal allergies, blood disorders, and other information that may influence therapy (for example, a congenital heart disease requiring antibiotic prophylaxis for bacterial endocarditis). Dental history may reveal past traumas that explain radiological findings such as pulp canal obliteration and apical pathologies.

During the first examination of an injured child, answers to some questions related to the trauma can be very useful:
- *Where did the trauma occur?* This information may have legal implications for the patient and may sometimes indicate the possibility of contamination, and therefore, the need for prophylactic measures (tetanus).
- *How did the trauma occur?* This can lead to the identification of affected parts; for example, a chin lesion is often accompanied by coronal or corono–radicular fractures of the premolars or molars and, especially in young patients, fractures of condyles of the jaw.
- *When did the trauma occur?* This information can be crucial for many injuries. In case of tooth avulsion, the time elapsed and the conditions of extraoral storage are decisive for subsequent treatment.
- *Was there a period of loss of consciousness? If so, how long?* Amnesia, nausea, and vomiting are all signs of brain damage and require urgent medical attention.
- *Are there any changes in occlusion?* An affirmative response may indicate dental dislocation or an alveolar, maxillary, or condylar fracture.
- *Do teeth react to exposure to cold or hot temperature?* A positive response indicates the exposure of dentin or pulp.

During clinical examination, it is important to perform the following:
- *examine* the face, lips, and oral muscles to check for soft tissue lesions
- *palpate* the facial skeleton to detect signs of fractures
- *inspect* the mouth for fractures, dental dislocations, tooth mobility, and abnormal responses to percussion. It is necessary to observe the direction of the tooth in case of a dislocation and to observe the relationship with the gingival sulcus in case of fractures to exclude pulpal involvement
- *pulp tests* (usually electrical) complete the clinical examination, although the responses from children may not be reliable.

Once a clinical examination of the affected area has been performed, a radiographic examination is required to further inspect the area. The objective is to identify both the dislocation of the tooth in the alveolus—also crucial in cases of avulsion where the tooth cannot be seen to make a differential diagnosis with the intrusive dislocation with complete ascent of the tooth into the alveolus—and the presence of root fractures (Andreasen and Andreasen, 1985). Intraoral radiographs are the most suitable radiographic examination modality; orthopantomographs may be required when skeletal base lesions are suspected.
In case of penetrating wounds of the lips, obtaining radiographs of the soft parts may be necessary for identifying foreign objects.

Alveolar hemorrhages

Dental emergencies include immediate and late alveolar hemorrhages, which are complications of tooth extraction.

Immediate alveolar hemorrhages are more frequent in surgical extractions; they are primarily related to the involvement of an intraosseous artery during the extraction, and the hemostasis is controlled immediately after the hemorrhage occurs.

The situation is slightly more complex when a *late postextraction hemorrhage* occurs. In such cases, it is necessary to investigate any blood coagulation disorders that are not known to be present in the patient. These problems can be both congenital and acquired and can affect both primary (platelet defects) and secondary (coagulation factor defects) coagulations.

From a therapeutic point of view, if immediate hemorrhage is complex enough, requiring the application of all local hemostasis measures, systemic intervention is also necessary in cases of coagulation factor defects.

Local hemostasis can be performed by compression, using local hemostats such as oxidized cellulose or collagen sponges, suturing with alveolar mucosal flaps (Della Valle et al, 2003), and in critical cases, using bipolar clamps, quantum molecular resonance scalpels, or laser.

Systemic therapy should also be administered in cases of coagulation defects. If platelet defects are involved, platelet concentrate infusion may be required; if a congenital coagulation factor defect such as hemophilia is present, it is often necessary to infuse substitution factors or drugs that amplify the residual factors. Therefore, it is necessary for the child to visit a pediatric department or a hemostasis center (Brewer and Correa, 2006). In any case, a local tamponade with a fibrinolytic drug such as tranexamic acid is always advisable.

Pediatric emergencies in dentistry

A dentist must bear in mind that while providing care to young patients during his or her professional practice in a public or private facility, he or she may face emergencies because of certain maneuvers, child's pathological history, or random events (Vanelli, 2006).

Among the emergencies in dentistry, breathing difficulties have been reported, which may exacerbate to acute respiratory arrest, following an episode of bronchospasm in a an asthmatic patient or bronchospasm after an allergic reaction caused by exposure to an allergen (drugs: anesthetic, antibiotic, etc.; latex: gloves, rubber dam, etc.; or insect bites). Bronchospasm may also be caused by acute obstruction of the upper airways by a foreign body (a tooth, a tool or part of it, etc.).

Many clinical pictures may be encountered in dental surgery prior to the initiation of a treatment, such as during or after a pharmacological treatment (for example, treatment with anesthetics and/or adrenaline, antibiotics, etc.), an extraction maneuver, suture placement, and during or at the end of a dental session.

Pain, in particular, can be the sign of a vagal response, which can cause a lipothymic–syncopal episode or a seizure, which in turn can cause the patient to fall to the ground, leading to head trauma.

Lipotimia and syncope

Lipotimia means the sensation of imminent loss of consciousness (presyncope) following the onset of premonitory symptoms such as loss of strength, dizziness, sweating, shivering, blurred vision, polypnea, and nausea.
Syncope means transient and acute loss of consciousness caused by cerebral hypoxia or hypoglycemia; it lasts from a few seconds to a few minutes and usually does not accompany abnormal movements and urinary incontinence (unlike a seizure). After regaining consciousness, the patient appears normal or slightly confused.
The following may be the causes:

- *metabolic*: hypoglycemia
- *psychological*: hysteria and/or anxiety
- *vasomotor*: closed and warm environments, painful stimuli
- *cardiovascular*: tachycardia or orthostatic hypotension.

Fainting episodes that are not correlated to obvious reasons require immediate assessment by a pediatrician.

What to do

If a change in consciousness is noted, blood supply to the brain should be facilitated by laying the subject in the Trendelenburg position and keeping the airways patent. If fainting due to hypoglycemia is experienced, for example, following prolonged fasting or after taking medicines (such as insulin or oral antidiabetic drugs), the patient should drink water and consume sugar after awakening. However, it is necessary to contact the emergency service at 118 in case of the following:

- a second fainting occurs shortly after the first
- in the event of fainting that does not resolve rapidly
- if chest pain, shortness of breath, headache, dizziness, and sharp increase in heart rate occur
- if back or abdominal pain occurs
- if pain associated with paresthesia or burning sensation in the arms or legs occurs
- if convulsions occur
- if blood loss occurs (hematemesis or enterorrhagia).

Epilepsy

Epilepsy is a disease of the nervous system causing a sudden discharge of electrical signals into the brain, triggering seizures. A single episode of convulsions is not considered epilepsy as it is not the only cause of seizures in children and individuals with epilepsy experience several seizures over time.

The severity, frequency, and duration of seizures varies widely depending on the involved areas of the brain. Seizures can last from a few seconds to several minutes. Two main types of epileptic seizures are known: *generalized* (which involve the whole brain) and *partial seizures*, also called focal seizures (which involve only some areas of the brain).
The most striking clinical signs are represented by tonic–clonic convulsive movements with the turning of the eyeballs, associated with prolonged unconsciousness; urinary incontinence, and release of the anal sphincter may also occur along with these signs. Mild convulsive syncope leaves children confused or unaware of their surroundings with disorientation that can last from approximately 10 minutes to a few hours (post-critical phase).

Little epileptic disease. It often affects children and is characterized by a sudden loss of consciousness (approximately 5–10 seconds) with sudden stopping of activity, fixed gaze, and often upward rotation of the eyes. These absences can be simple (only the loss of consciousness) or complex (accompanied by clonic contractions, muscle hypotonia, and hypertonia of axial muscles). After recovery from the absence, the child realizes what has happened from the astonished and questioning gazes of those present.

Great epileptic disease. It is a more severe type of epilepsy and is characterized by an initial maximum spasm of all skeletal muscles (tonic phase), followed by a few tens of seconds of rapid muscle contractions, which are more or less regular with wide and fast movements (clonic phase), loss of consciousness for 5–10 minutes, possible urinary incontinence, and release of the anal sphincter.

What to do

In case of seizures, it is necessary to perform the following:

- insert a rubber mouth opener or a Mayo or Guedel airway in the patient's mouth
- transfer the patient to the floor in a supine position while protecting the head from possible traumas and removing surrounding furniture and objects without countering convulsions
- ensure airway patency by extending the neck and freeing it from constraints caused by clothing
- aspirate saliva from the oral cavity to prevent its accidental inhalation
- monitor heart rate and blood pressure for differential diagnosis with cardiovascular accidents
- after the convulsions stop, put the patient in a comfortable position and calm him or her down; in case the patient falls asleep, do not force him or her to wake up; and ensure that the patient has fully recovered before accompanying him or her to the waiting room
- if the crisis does not resolve spontaneously in a few minutes, benzodiazepines (diazepam or midazolam) should be administered either intravenously or rectally, and an ambulance should be requested for immediate transfer to a hospital.

Hypoglycemia

Hypoglycemia in children means the detection of whole-blood glucose levels < 70 mg/dl. Hypoglycemia is a common occurrence that can happen occasionally in a healthy child because of a prolonged fasting. When it occurs in a diabetic child, it is often possible to identify the causes:

- failure to take a meal or a snack
- incorrect use of insulin; insulin overdose and/or administration of the wrong type of insulin (for instance, rapid insulin instead of Lantus insulin)
- injection at the lipodystrophy site
- injection too deep into a muscle
- injection into a blood vessel
- increased blood flow at the injection site because of overheating: hot shower or bath after injection
- excessive rubbing before or after injection
- injection in a region subjected to muscle strain
- recent hypoglycemia
- intense physical exercise.

Symptoms

The symptoms and effects of hypoglycemia caused by hormone regulation systems (adrenaline and glucagon) that trigger a decrease in blood glucose can be distinguished from those of neuroglycopenia caused by insufficient glucose supply to the brain.
The clinical picture of a hypoglycemic episode is related to the duration and severity of the event; it may vary from the occurrence of faint symptoms to hypoglycemic coma. The activation of the autonomic nervous system with catecholamine release is responsible for cold sweating, tremors, tachycardia, paleness, and anxiety; neuroglycopenia is responsible for confusion, headache, fatigue, convulsions, and coma.

Treatment

Blood glucose dosing is important. It is necessary to stop the activity underway and immediately consume simple sugars (sugar powder, sweetened drinks, juice, fruit, sweets, etc.), which are rapidly absorbed and can rapidly increase blood glucose levels. The treatment takes approximately 10 minutes to be effective and is repeatable after 15 minutes if the condition does not improve. Considering that 10 g of glucose increases the blood glucose levels of an adult by 35 mg/dl in 15 minutes, children will need approximately 1.5 g/10 kg body weight of glucose to achieve the same glycemic effect. For example, in a baby weighing 10 kg, 1.5 g of glucose increases blood glucose levels by 35 mg/dl, whereas 3 g of glucose increases blood glucose levels by 70 mg/dl. The following are equivalent to 10 g of glucose: 1 and a half sachets of sugar, 1 tablespoon of honey, half a glass of orange juice.
In case of severe hypoglycemia, if the child is partially conscious, sugar should be put in his or her mouth, under the tongue if possible, to allow regaining of consciousness. If the situation does not improve or if the seizure is more severe, glucagon (1 mg vial)

is injected intramuscularly and *not* subcutaneously, and is effective within 10–15 minutes. However, if the situation still does not improve, the injection is repeated after 30 minutes. If no results are obtained, it is necessary to contact the emergency room (ER) to inject 30% glucose solution into a vein as soon as possible and then 10% glucose solution in a continuous infusion until glycemia stabilizes. It should be kept in mind that both hypoglycemia and glucagon may have an emetic effect, so the patient should not be placed in a supine position to avoid *inhalation*.

Head trauma

Head injuries are among the most important causes of morbidity and mortality in children. Dentists must be able to recognize and manage a head trauma if during the first surgery for a dental trauma, a child shows signs that may indicate CNS involvement. There are characteristic features of anatomical–physiological and developmental origin that differentiate head trauma in a child from that in the adult population.
In children, the brain is better protected by the flexibility of the cranial vault with independent bones, large fontanelles, and a highly developed subarachnoid space.
The high vascularization of the cranial bones and dura mater explains the considerable frequency of subcutaneous and epidural hematomas in children, even in the absence of skull fractures. Extracranial hematomas can be observed very frequently.
The clinical symptoms of head trauma in a child are related to the cause and age. It is necessary to distinguish head trauma into the following:

- mild
- moderate
- severe.

Mild head trauma is usually the result of accidental falls or direct shocks to the cranial case. There are no immediate signs other than crying and, in some cases, vomiting; the state of consciousness is never compromised. Headache and vomiting may occur, which may last for several hours. Confusional headache may be observed in adolescents.
Moderate head trauma is characterized by short and immediate loss of consciousness, often followed by posttraumatic amnesia. Signs and symptoms are loss of consciousness, vomiting, headache, paleness and irritability, and retrograde and anterograde amnesia.
In both situations, no special maneuvers are necessary. It is recommended to hospitalize the child for an observation period and to avoid administering food via the mouth within the first 4 hours of the trauma or after the most recent vomiting episode.
Severe head trauma is characterized by prolonged loss of consciousness, which may not be immediate; in some situations there may be an interval between the occurrence of trauma and appearance of neurological signs. In most cases, a child with head trauma visits the ER in a conscious state; the initial loss of consciousness is observed in 25% of cases. In 30% of traumatized children, drowsiness, confusion, and irritability are observed. Vomiting is the most common symptom in young children (aged <3 years), whereas it is present in 15%–30% of older children. Consciousness should be

assessed on the basis of the Glasgow Coma Scale (GCS) for children aged 2 years and above and the Children Coma Scale for children aged <2 years.
The immediate treatment comprises neuroanesthesiologic assessment, airway management, and cerebral oxygenation parameter stabilization. Immediate transfer to a pediatric intensive care unit is necessary after complete monitoring of all ventilator-derived pressure parameters.

Complications of local anesthetics

Paresthesia

Paresthesia is persistent anesthesia beyond the expected duration. One cause may be a nerve lesion resulting from surgery. Another cause may be the trauma caused by the needle during injection, when the patient feels an "electric shock-like sensation" during anesthetic inoculation in the region of the involved nerve. Paresthesia can also be caused by bleeding around the concerned nerve. Paresthesia unrelated to surgery more often involves the tongue, followed by the lip, and it is more common if 4% articaine or prilocaine solutions are used. Most cases are resolved in approximately 8 weeks.

Postoperative soft tissue injuries

Self-induced soft tissue trauma is an unpleasant clinical complication of local anesthesia in the oral cavity. Most of the lesions caused by the biting of the lips and cheeks are self-limiting and heal without complications; however, bleeding and infection may occur.
Tongue bites causing heavy bleeding require the application of sutures. The use of a bilateral mandibular block does not increase the risk of soft tissue trauma compared with that of unilateral mandibular block or ipsilateral maxillary infiltration; the frequency of soft tissue trauma is in fact higher when only one side is anesthetized (Fig. 23.2). Maxillary infiltration does not reduce the risk of injury compared with mandibular block.

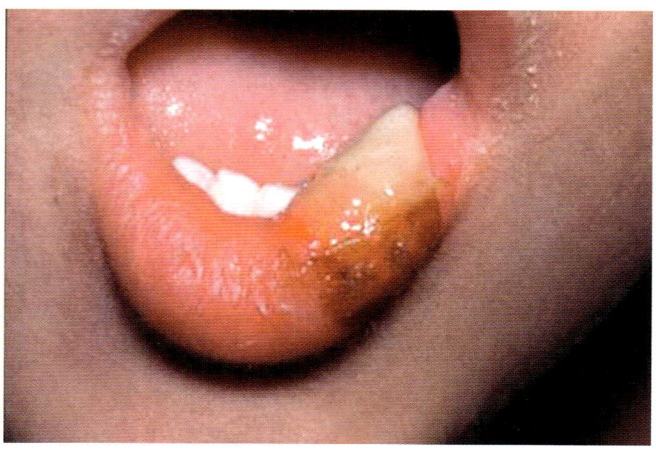

Figure 23.2 Lower lip lesion caused by biting after truncal anesthesia.

Toxicity (overdose)

Most adverse reactions to anesthetics occur during injection or within the first 5–10 minutes of their administration. Overdose of a local anesthetic may result in its high blood levels caused by a single inadvertent intravascular injection or repeated injections. Local anesthetics cause a biphasic reaction (for example, excitation followed by depression) in CNS. Early subjective signs of toxicity involve CNS and include dizziness, anxiety, and confusion; these may be followed by diplopia, tinnitus, somnolence, numbness, and perioral tingling. Objective signs of toxicity may include convulsive contractions, tremors, loquacity, slow speech, and chills.

The response of the cardiovascular system (CVS) to local anesthetic toxicity is also biphasic. CVS is more resistant to anesthetics than CNS. Initially, during CVS stimulation, the patient's heart rate and blood pressure may increase. As soon as the plasma levels of the anesthetic increase, vasodilation occurs, followed by myocardial depression with a subsequent drop in blood pressure; bradycardia and cardiac arrest may follow. Cardiodepressive effects of local anesthetics do not manifest until considerably high blood levels of a local anesthetic are reached.

The local toxicity of these anesthetics may be prevented by a cautious injection technique, careful observation of the patient, and knowledge of the maximum dosage in relation to weight. Before each injection, it is necessary to aspirate and inject slowly. After the injection, the dentist, hygienist, or assistant should stay with the patient while waiting for anesthetic effects to appear. Early recognition of a toxic reaction is crucial for effective management. When signs and symptoms of toxicity appear, local anesthetic administration should be suspended. The management of the emergency depends on the severity of the reaction.

Allergies

Allergic reactions are not dose-dependent but are caused by a patient's increased ability to react even to a small dose. Allergies may manifest in various ways: dermatitis, urticaria, angioedema, fever, photosensitivity, or anaphylaxis. The management of the emergency depends on the speed and severity of the reaction.

Hypersensitivity events triggered by contact with an allergen may occur during a dental session. The most common allergens are drugs (antibiotics and anesthetics) and dental materials. Latex allergy is clinically important and should be taken into account as many materials and supplies used in dental environments contain latex (Tab. 23.2). The *prevalence* increases according to the *frequency of exposure*; early exposure (for example, in children undergoing surgery during the initial years of life) conditions the appearance of allergy. Moreover, cross-allergy may occur with numerous foods, especially fruits and vegetables (pineapple, avocado, banana, orange, egg whites, apple, grapes, etc.). Therefore, latex may be responsible for *allergic skin reactions* (contact dermatitis, urticaria, and angioedema) (Fig. 23.3), *respiratory reactions* (oculorhinitis and asthma), and *generalized reactions* (anaphylaxis) (Tab. 23.3).

It is the duty of the dentist to identify through the medical history those at risk of allergic manifestations to latex, focusing in particular on those who have undergone surgery and frequent hospitalizations during the initial years of life (Tab. 23.4). In case

Table 23.2 Primary medical devices containing latex

• Gloves • Patches • Dropper • Components of syringes • Lacci emostatici • Armbands for sphygmomanometer • Catheters • Ambu balloons	• Anesthetic masks • Anesthesia circuits • Intratracheal and dental drainage tubes • Needle cannulas • Elastic laces for metallic orthodontic appliances and rubber handles • Rubber braces • Rubber dam • Mouth opener	• Saliva aspirator • Equipment protection • Dental instruments • Chair components • Emergency kits

Table 23.3 Primary clinical manifestations of latex allergy

• Contact dermatitis • Common urticaria • Conjunctivitis • Bronchial asthma • Rhinitis	• Periorbital edema • Angioedema • Oedema of the lips • Anaphylaxis

Table 23.4 Major diseases that risk the development of latex allergy in children

- Spina bifida
- Urogenital malformations
- Nonperforated anus
- Tracheoesophageal fistula
- Esophageal atresia
- Vater's syndrome

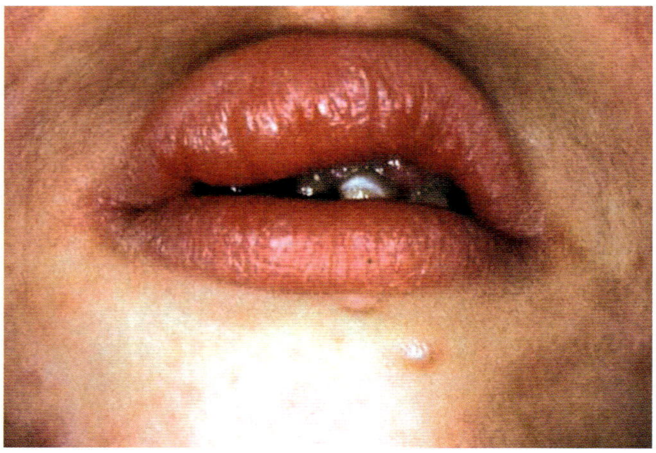

Figure 23.3 Latex allergy.

of a suspected or documented allergy, a *latex-free* environment should be provided, and alternative materials (vinyl, polyurethane, silicone, nylon, styrene–butadiene, and plastic) should be used for all materials and devices that come into contact with the patient (gloves, rubber dam, orthodontic elastics, etc.). The setting up of a latex-free clinic does not present any particular difficulties at present as companies produce a large number of latex-free materials. However, because latex particles can disperse in

the environment, in anticipation of a session with an allergic patient, it is necessary to aerate the operating area and schedule the session at the beginning of the day.
Allergic reactions may occur in unidentified latex-allergic patients during or after surgery. In case of contact manifestations, remove the latex-containing device and wash the affected surface thoroughly. However, it is recommended to consult the allergist, providing him or her with the devices considered as responsible for the allergic reaction, to document the allergy condition with diagnostic tests. The most serious cases—from asthmatic crisis to anaphylactic shock—should be pharmacologically treated in time, as the survival of the patient is at risk (Cocchi and Piana, 2000; Piana, 2005; Clark and Ewan, 2002; Hashim Nainar, 2001).
Relatively frequent contact allergies to nickel–chromium and cobalt should be taken into account when the treatment plan includes the application of orthodontic and/or prosthetic devices, both fixed and mobile.
Acrylic resins used in the fabrication of prosthetic and orthodontic appliances can also be responsible for allergic skin and respiratory reactions. The responsible agent is considered to be the free fraction of methyl methacrylate monomer. At present, resins are produced in a way such that the quantity of free monomer is reduced as much as possible. In patients with allergic reactions to acrylic resins, the use of micro- or macrofilled composite resins is recommended.

Treatment

The optimal strategy for the prevention of allergic reactions is to identify the subjects at risk and eliminate substances and materials that cause allergic reactions. In cases of allergic reactions, the treatment depends on the type of event.
Medicines used for the treatment of *allergic contact reactions*, *angioedema*, and *bronchial asthma* are presented in Table 23.5 with the relevant doses and routes of administration. *Anaphylactic shock*, an emergency condition that endangers the patient's life, must be promptly recognized and requires immediate treatment of laryngeal edema, bronchospasm, and hypotension.
In the event of an anaphylactic reaction, the following measures should be taken:

- contact ER
- check the airways and maintain their patency
- lay the patient down and lift his or her legs to facilitate blood pressure recovery
- intramuscular administration of the following: in children, a dose of 0.01 mg/kg of adrenaline 1:1000; in adults, a dose of 0.3–0.5 mg/kg of adrenaline 1:1000 (according to USA guidelines) or 0.5–1 mg/kg of adrenaline 1:1000 (according to European guidelines); alternatively, subcutaneous or sublingual administration is possible. If the patient's weight cannot be determined, dosing is decided according to age (Tab. 23.6)
- avoid hydrocortisone administration in the initial treatment of anaphylactic shock, as its pharmacological action begins only after a few hours
- administer oxygen
- support circulation with an infusion of liquids, to which an antihistamine such as chlorpheniramine hydrochloride may be added to prevent recurrence

Table 23.5 Drugs for the treatment of allergic contact reactions, angioedema, and bronchial asthma

Drug	Formula	Dosage	Route of administration
Antihistamines (e.g., chlorphenamine maleate)	1 mL (10 mg) vial	• <1 year: 250 mcg/kg • >1 year: 2–5 mg • 2–5 years: 2.5–5 mg • 6–12 years: 5–10 mg • >12 years: 10–20 mg	sc, im If iv: diluted in 5–10 mL of saline solution
Corticosteroids (e.g., hydrocortisone)	100 mg vial in 1 mL (1 and 5 mL vials)	• 0-1 month: 2.5 mg/kg • 1 month to 12 years: 4 mg/kg (up to 100 mg) • >12 years: 100–500 mg	iv, im
Bronchodilators topical use (e.g., salbutamol)	vial or inhaler	• 1-2 puffs every 5–10 min up to three administrations • or five drops in 3 mL of saline solution (repeatable after 15 min)	Aerosol

Table 23.6 Dose of adrenaline 1:1000 depending on age

Age	Dose
2–6 months	0.07 mL
12 months	0.10 mL
18 months to 4 years	0.15 mL
5 years	0.20 mL
6–9 years	0.30 mL
10–13 years	0.40 mL
≥14 years	0.50 mL

Table 23.7 Main allergic and non-allergic symptoms

Non-allergic symptoms	Allergic symptoms
• Agitation • Disorientation • Nausea • Apprehension • Tremors and convulsions • Hypotension • Myocardial depression • Respiratory depression	• Hypotension • Bronchospasm • Warm feeling • Edema • Erythematous maculae • Papules • Dyspnea • Nausea • Laryngeal/pharyngeal edema

- in case of worsening of symptoms, administer β2-agonists (salbutamol in bottles or puffs: up to 3 doses or 5 drops in 3 ml of physiological solution repeatable after 15 minutes or 1–2 puffs every 5–10 minutes) and prepare for assisted breathing and possible emergency tracheotomy.

The correct diagnosis of anaphylactic shock must be made through the recognition of basic symptoms (Tab. 23.7).

Vital parameters

For each intervention, the dentist must ensure his or her and the pediatric patient's safety; following this, the patient must be evaluated to understand the health problem, quantifying the degree of severity of the condition.

Vital parameters provide immediate and objective information on the severity of a child's clinical situation and are essential to determine the type of care that should be provided; via the initial evaluation of signs and symptoms, problems threatening the patient's survival can be identified and addressed promptly with immediate intensive care, without the assistance of resuscitators or emergency professionals.

The accuracy of measurement of vital parameters is fundamental; a wrong value or its misinterpretation can have crucial consequences for life.

Evaluation is a dynamic process that, in addition to a series of procedures to be performed according to a specific sequence, allows for accurate and constant monitoring of the child, showing sudden changes in condition in a timely manner. Through comparison with previous assessments, the deterioration, improvement, or stability of the condition can be observed and the intervention can be appropriately managed by requesting the emergency service to send the most suitable resources to the site of event.

The primary vital parameters include the following:

- state of consciousness
- breathing
- circulation
- skin
- body temperature.

State of consciousness

The state of consciousness is generally defined by the degree of awareness that the child has of himself/herself and of the surrounding environment. The alterations are always related to events that suggest a traumatic or pathological alteration of brain function; evaluation is performed through sensory examination using the AVPU scale (Tab. 23.8) or the GCS modified for children and infants.

Table 23.8 AVPU Scale

Alert	The child is awake, alert, and well-oriented
Verbal (clouded)	The child is not alert but can respond to verbal stimuli more or less consistently
Painful (reactive to pain)	The child reacts to a pain stimulus through coordinated movements to ward off the stimulus or with uncoordinated or inefficient movements if the pain is severe
Unresponsive	The child does NOT respond to any stimulus, whether verbal or painful

Breathing

Cardiorespiratory arrest (CRA) in children commonly originates from respiratory arrest. The following may be the most frequent causes:

- foreign body obstruction
- trauma
- sudden infant death syndrome
- drowning
- respiratory diseases (diphtheria, laryngitis, and asthma)
- anaphylactic shock
- neurological diseases.

It is therefore essential to ensure in rapid succession (1) airway patency; (2) artificial respiratory activity; and at the same time, (3) artificial blood circulation through a procedure called ABC (airway, breathing, circulation).

Obstruction of the airways

Airway obstruction is a common cause of CRA in pediatric patients during the early years of life. Inhalation of foreign matter causes approximately 27% of all accidental deaths of children aged <4 years every year. Usually, airway obstruction occurs when the child is eating or playing due to the aspiration of food (grapes, peanuts, sweets, ham), rubber balloons, and small objects. During a dental session, bronchospasm may occur following acute obstruction of the upper airway by a foreign body, for example, a tooth during extraction, an instrument or part of it following accidental breakage, or an infiltrated restoration.
The child has persistent cough and/or stridor and/or wheezing in the expiratory phase, while being in an otherwise healthy condition, associated with breathing difficulties of varying severity, depending on the anatomical location and degree of obstruction.

Partial obstruction. The child is alert, coughing, making sounds, and breathing, even if with difficulty. He or she must be calmed, encouraged to cough, and kept in the position he or she prefers, avoiding intervening with maneuvers that could turn partial obstruction into complete obstruction. The effective cough (noisy) is a sign of a certain

degree of spontaneous ventilation, which, if maintained, can allow rapid hospitalization through the emergency service, transporting the patient in a semisitting position. If the child continues to cough, oxygen may be administered (5–8 L/min). He or she must be placed bent on the forearm or prone on the thighs of the rescuer, with the head in a more tilted position than the trunk. Four interscapular blows are given with the palm of the hand with a lateral escape route followed by four blows to the middle of the sternum, inducing an artificial cough that can favor the expectoration of the foreign body. Care should be taken to *never* hold the child upside down holding the ankles: this position, because of the disproportion between the large size of the head and the weak spine, muscles, and ligaments, may cause vertebral lesions.
In case of emergency, if the child is older than 1 year, it is possible to perform the Heimlich maneuver (strong and abrupt epigastric compression from the bottom to the top with the superimposed fists, standing behind the patient).

Total obstruction. The child does not cough, stops breathing, and does not make any sound. Only when the cough is no longer effective, and there is a simultaneous rapid change in the state of consciousness (up to the level of nonconsciousness), resuscitation measures for freeing the airways must be undertaken. For children, the cardiopulmonary resuscitation sequence is started with 30 chest compressions and 2 ventilations, while ensuring to check the possible presence of surfacing foreign bodies in the oral cavity; 3 complete cycles; and patient revaluation after 1 minute (30/2 ratio) (ILCOR; AHA, 2010; ERC, 2010) (Tab. 23.9).

Table 23.9 Cardiopulmonary resuscitation

Part A	Part B	Part C
Evaluation of consciousness Call the child's name out loud Apply a painful tactile stimulus	**Evaluation of respiratory activity** Perform LLF within 10 seconds	**Evaluation of circulatory activity and presence of vital signs** Search for the central pulse and vital signs for no more than 10 seconds
If the child moves or responds Quickly evaluate if the child has any obvious traumatic injury and if he/she needs medical assistance	**If the child is breathing** Put him/her in the safe side position (in the absence of trauma) and perform periodic revaluations	**If vital signs are present** Support respiratory activity (20 acts/minute)
If the child does not move or does not answer Quickly call for help (118) Place the child in the appropriate position and establish the patency of the airway	**If the child is not breathing** Perform five rescue breaths	**If vital signs are not present** Begin cardiopulmonary resuscitation maneuvers

30 compressions and two breaths for a total of three cycles (approximately 1 minute). After 1 minute: revaluation of the patient (C-B-A). At the first negative evaluation: activation of the advanced first aid. LLF, look–listen–feel.

References

American Heart Association. Guidelines for cardiopulmonary resuscitation and emergency cardiovascular care science. Circulation 2010 November 2;122(18 suppl. B).

Andreasen FM, Andreasen JO, Tsukiboshi M. Examination and diagnosis of dental injuries. In: Andreasen JO, Andreasen FM, Andersson L (eds). Textbook and color atlas of traumatic injuries to the teeth. 4th ed. Oxford: Blackwell; 2007. P. 255-79.

Andreasen FM, Andreasen JO. Diagnosis of luxation injuries: the importance of standardized clinical, radiographic and photographic techniques in clinical investigations. Endod Dent Traumatol 1985;5:160-9.

Bakland LK, Andreasen JO. Examination of the dentally traumatized patient. Calif Dent Ass J 1996;24:35-44.

Brewer A, Correa ME. Guidelines for dental treatment of patients with inherited bleeding disorders. Treatment of Hemophilia 2006 n. 40 © World Federation of Hemophilia, 2006.

Clark AT, Ewan PW. The prevention and management of anaphylaxis in children. Current Paediatrics 2002;12:370-5.

Cocchi S, Piana G. L'allergia al lattice in ambito odontoiatrico. Dental Cadmos 2000;2:11-6.

Della Valle A, Sammartino G, Marenzi G et al. Prevention of postoperative bleeding in anticoagulated patients undergoing oral surgery: use of platelet-rich plasma. Gel J Oral Maxillofac Surg 2003;61:1275-8.

European Resuscitation Council. Guidelines for Resuscitation 2010, www.CPRguidelines.eu.

Gopikrishna V, Pradeep G, Venkateshbabu N. Assessment of pulp vitality: a review. Int J Paediatr Dent 2009 Jan;19(1):3-15.

Hashim Nainar SM. Dental management of children with latex allergy. Int J Paed Dent 2001;11:322-7.

ILCOR Pediatric Life Support worksheet, www.americanheart.org

Lewis C, Stout J. Toothache in US children. Arch Pediatr Adolesc Med 2010 Nov;164(11):1059-63.

Manuale di rianimazione cardiopolmonare pediatrica di base, defibrillazione precoce e manovre di disostruzione da corpo estraneo per la popolazione secondo nuove linee guida internazionali ILCOR 2010.

Milsom KM, Tickle M, Blinkhorn AS. Dental pain and dental treatment of young children attending the general dental service. Br Dent J 2002 Mar 9;192(5):280-4.

Piana G. Patologie sistemiche e patologie del cavo orale in età evolutiva. Linee guida di prevenzione e di terapia. Cap.15, Bononia: University Press; 2005. P. 187-90.

Pinto A, Balasubramaniam R, Arava-Parastatidis M. Neuropathic orofacial pain in children and adolescents. Pediatr Dent 2008 Nov-Dec;30(6):510-5.

Sakai VT, Magalhães AC, Pessan JP et al. Urgency treatment profile of 0 to 15 year-old children assisted at urgency dental service from Bauru Dental School, University of São Paulo. J Appl Oral Sci 2005 Dec;13(4):340-4.

Thikkurissy S, Rawlins JT, Kumar A et al. Rapid treatment reduces hospitalization for pediatric patients with odontogenic-based cellulitis. Am J Emerg Med 2010 Jul;28(6):668-72.

Vanelli M. (ed). Emergenze in pediatria. Linee-guida della Scuola di Specializzazione in Pediatria dell'Università degli Studi di Parma. 3rd ed. Mattioli 1885; 2006.

Subject Index

Page numbers followed by "f," "t," or "d" indicate figures, tables, or diagrams, respectively.

B

C

D

E

F

M

N

O

P